Noninvasive Cardiac Imaging

NONINVASIVE CARDIAC IMAGING

Edited by

JOEL MORGANROTH, M.D.

Professor of Medicine and Pharmacology, Hahnemann University
Director, Sudden Death Prevention Program,
Likoff Cardiovascular Institute, Philadelphia, Pennsylvania

ALFRED F. PARISI, M.D.

Associate Professor of Medicine, Harvard Medical School,
Chief of Cardiology, West Roxbury VA Medical Center
West Roxbury, Massachusetts
Senior Associate in Medicine
Brigham and Women's Hospital, Boston, Massachusettes

GERALD M. POHOST, M.D.

Associate Professor of Medicine, Harvard Medical School,
Director of Nuclear Cardiology and Director of Nuclear Magnetic Resonance Research
Massachusetts General Hospital, Boston, Massachusetts

YEAR BOOK MEDICAL PUBLISHERS, INC.
Chicago • London

To Gail, Joan, and Marlene,
and to those who continue to teach us

Library of Congress Cataloging in Publication Data

Morganroth, Joel.
Noninvasive cardiac imaging.

Includes bibliographies and index.
1. Ultrasonic cardiography.
2. Radioisotope scanning. 3. Heart—Diseases—
Diagnosis. I. Parisi, Alfred F. II. Pohost,
Gerald M. III. Title. [DNLM: 1. Echocardiography.
2. Heart—Radionuclide imaging.
3. Heart diseases—Diagnosis. WG 141 M849n]
RC683.5.U5M67 1983 616.1′207543 82-11095
ISBN 0-8151-5946-3

ASSOCIATE EDITORS

CHARLES A. BOUCHER, M.D.
Assistant Professor of Medicine
Harvard Medical School
Attending Cardiologist
Massachusetts General Hospital
Boston, Massachusetts

DANIEL DAVID, M.D.
Senior Lecturer in Cardiology
Sackler School of Medicine of Tel Aviv University
Attending Cardiologist
Meir General Hospital
Tel Aviv, Israel

ROBERT D. OKADA, M.D.
Assistant Professor of Medicine
Harvard Medical School
Attending Cardiologist
Massachusetts General Hospital
Boston, Massachusetts

DANIEL A. PIETRO, M.D.
Instructor in Medicine
Harvard Medical School
Chief of Cardiology
Brockton VA Medical Center
Brockton, Massachusetts

CONTENTS

FOREWORD

IT IS IMPOSSIBLE to overemphasize the magnitude of the health care problem caused each year by cardiovascular disease. Every day an estimated 3,400 Americans, more than two each minute, suffer heart attacks. Some 25,000 children are born with defective hearts every year, and there are over 100,000 children and 1.7 million adults who suffer from rheumatic heart disease. Coronary heart disease, the leading cause of death in the United States which accounts for two thirds of all cardiovascular deaths, was responsible for nearly 640,000 deaths in 1980, of which more than 150,000 occurred in people under 65 years of age.

Diseases of the cardiovascular system account for more than 50% of all deaths in the United States each year. They rank first among all diseases in terms of Social Security disability benefits, acute hospital bed days, and limitation of activity. It has been conservatively estimated that the total economic cost of cardiovascular disorders is in excess of 60 billion dollars annually, accounting for more than one fifth of the total cost of illness in the United States.

Since 1968, however, there has been a dramatic, unprecedented decline in mortality from cardiovascular disease in this country. The decline has been confirmed as real and has been observed in all age, sex, and race groups. The causes of the decline are many and credit can be given both to improved treatment regimens and to primary prevention through life-style changes.

One of the most dramatic areas of advance in this past decade has been in the development of noninvasive diagnostic techniques.

The 1970s saw rapid progress in the diagnosis of heart disease by tests that are of low risk to patients. Included in these so-called noninvasive diagnostic techniques are echocardiography, low activity radioactive tracers, and computerized tomographic x-ray techniques. Echocardiography has provided an in vivo assessment of heart anatomy by using reflected sound waves from the heart and great vessels. It now allows a diagnosis to be made in situations that in the past were either uncertain or usually required cardiac catheterization. Several radiopharmaceuticals such as technetium 99 and thallium 201 have been used in the clinical assessment of infarct size, myocardial perfusion, and ventricular function. They permit thorough sequential observations for a more effective evaluation of a patient's course, prognosis, and responsiveness to therapeutic or potentially harmful agents. Though earlier and more exact cardiac diagnosis alone can neither prevent nor treat cardiac disease, the information these new techniques provide has made the practice of cardiology eminently more rational.

The introduction and availability of these noninvasive techniques have set the stage for improved and earlier diagnosis of atherosclerosis and coronary heart disease. Radionuclear techniques now allow the direct observation of the metabolism and segmental movement of the left ventricular wall during exercise as well as at rest. They also allow the assessment, with increasing precision, of the amount of heart muscle undergoing damage at the time of a heart attack. Echocardiography has gained prominence as a means of diagnosing and detecting heart defects in the fetus in utero and in the newborn. The same technology is now being used effectively to follow congenital disease in older children and adults. With such devices as real-time sector scanners, the spatial locations of the chambers of the heart and the major heart valves can be visualized. It has become possible to determine how well the heart valves are functioning as well as to identify chamber enlargement and responsiveness to medical regimens.

The same noninvasive instrumentation has led to an increased frequency in recognition of certain cardiomyopathies. While the causes of most cardiomyopathies remain obscure, diagnosis is easier and a number of factors have been identified as causative agents.

It is thus most timely that this text on noninvasive cardiac imaging has appeared. Drs. Morganroth, Parisi, and Pohost have edited an integrated compendium on the state of the art with these new, most promising techniques. Building from basic principles the authors have clearly and effectively contrasted the information obtainable with different techniques as well as detailed the uses and limitations of currently available methodology. Individual chapters on assessment of left ventricular function, diagnosis of cardiomyopathy, chronic and acute coronary artery disease, the different valvular heart defects, intracardiac masses, congenital heart disease, and pericardial disease clearly define the clinical applicability of these new techniques. I would recommend this book to all students of cardiology whether in school or in practice as well as to those interested in one of today's most exciting areas of biomedical engineering.

Noninvasive cardiac imaging has dramatically improved our diagnostic capabilities. In the future its even wider application promises to make the treatment of the at-risk patient as well as the evaluation of new forms of therapeutics not only safer but also more effective and efficient. One can only hope that the authors plan to update this text in the future, for there is no doubt that current techniques will be further expanded upon and that future directions such as nuclear magnetic resonance and digital subtraction radiography, described briefly in the last chapter, will soon warrant one or more full chapters of their own.

ROBERT I. LEVY
DEAN OF THE SCHOOL OF MEDICINE
TUFTS UNIVERSITY
BOSTON, MASSACHUSETTS

PREFACE

Over the last several years, as instrumentation has become more sophisticated, noninvasive cardiac tests have been utilized with ever-increasing frequency. Accordingly, a vast array of methods is available for the clinician to use in evaluation of patients with cardiovascular disease. In many cases, M-mode and two-dimensional echocardiography and radionuclide imaging can provide similar diagnostic and pathophysiologic information. The purpose of this book is to provide the clinician with a comprehensive resource to review echocardiography and nuclear cardiologic techniques and to evaluate and compare their usefulness, indications, and limitations. This monograph starts with a description of fundamental instrumentation and then proceeds systematically through the important cardiac disease categories. Although these procedures help to fuel increasing health care costs, they can be used very effectively by the knowledgeable practitioner. This book provides a careful appraisal of these noninvasive techniques and forms a basis for choosing the most appropriate and/or cost-effective test(s) in a particular clinical setting or for solving a specific clinical problem.

For each disease state, echocardiographic and nuclear cardiologic imaging information is presented and followed by editorial discussion of the clinical merits and limitations of these techniques. Finally, in the last chapter, potential future developments in noninvasive imaging are addressed.

This text is particularly suited for clinicians and cardiovascular specialists with the objective of promoting an understanding of the diagnostic and technical data that noninvasive cardiac imaging techniques can provide in the clinical setting. Because of its abundant illustrations, this text can, in many instances, substitute as an atlas for each of the topics covered. The bibliographies after each chapter are intended for use as primary reference sources in the field of cardiac imaging.

Joël Morganroth

Alfred F. Parisi

Gerald M. Pohost

PART I

Principles and Techniques of Echocardiography and Radionuclide Imaging

ECHOCARDIOGRAPHY

Alfred F. Parisi, Barbara J. Ray, and Paul F. Moynihan

PHYSICAL PRINCIPLES

ECHOCARDIOGRAPHY produces cardiac images by reflecting pulses of ultrasound from the structures of the heart and then recording the reflected sound signals. The received sound wave pattern is usually displayed in a video format; permanent records are produced by photography or by using a strip chart recorder. In order to appreciate this technique one must understand the physical properties of ultrasound and its behavior in tissues of the chest.

Sound consists of a moving series of compressions and rarefactions which represent local changes in pressure in a medium. These serial rarefactions and compressions can be represented graphically by a sine wave function (Fig 1–1). The distance between two points in the same phase of rarefaction or compression (or between two corresponding points on the sine wave pattern) defines the wavelength (λ). The number of times the sound wave achieves its pressure maximum per unit time defines the sound wave frequency (f). It follows that the velocity of propagation of a sonic wave can be given by the equation $v = f\lambda$. By definition, frequency and wavelength are inversely related at any velocity.

The frequency of sonic waves is most commonly measured in cycles per second (cps). These units of measurement are also termed Hertz (Hz), and 1 cps = 1 Hz. Audible sound encompasses frequencies between 20 and 20,000 Hz. Sound frequencies above 20,000 Hz—i.e., the upper frequency limit of normal human hearing—are by definition termed *ultrasound*.

Reflection of ultrasound from cardiac structures is the crucial phenomenon which underlies the practice of echocardiography. Several factors determine the effectiveness of this process when the heart is examined:

1. *The propagation of the ultrasonic beam to and through the heart*. If the beam fails to reach the heart or return to the transducer, no meaningful information is recorded. For practical purposes, ultrasound does not propagate through air; thus one of the most frequent difficulties encountered in the clinical practice of echocardiography is failure to obtain an adequate examination, particularly in patients with chronic obstructive pulmonary disease, in whom the heart tends to be completely surrounded by hyperinflated pulmonary tissue.

2. *The angle of the ultrasonic beam in relation to the surface of the desired target*. In clinical echocardiography the transducer used to generate the ultrasound wave is also used to detect the reflected wave. Structures perpendicular to the beam reflect ultrasound waves back to the transducer considerably more effectively than nonorthogonal targets.

3. *The ultrasound wavelength*. The smaller the wavelength, the more likely it is to be reflected from a thin target. Since wavelength and frequency are inversely related, higher frequency ultrasound has the potential for better reflection from small targets and hence has better resolution (separation of two small objects in space). However, as a corollary, since higher frequency ultrasound

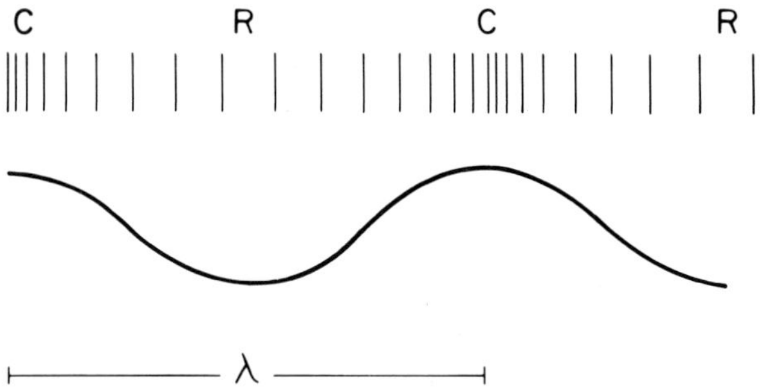

Fig 1–1.—Schematic drawing showing moving series of sonic compressions *(C)* and rarefactions *(R)* as they occur in space. The sine wave function and wavelength (λ) for these compressions and rarefactions are shown below.

is more likely to be reflected from small structures, it intrinsically does not penetrate tissue as well as ultrasound of lower frequency and hence may not propagate adequately to reach desired targets.

The ultrasound used in cardiac examinations is usually of the order of 1.5 to 5 million cps (MHz), most commonly 2.25 MHz. Ultrasound in the 3- to 5-MHz range allows better definition of cardiac structures and is commonly used in pediatric echocardiography; in adult echocardiography the lower frequency transducers are commonly used because greater depth penetration is required to traverse the adult chest and heart. However, there is a movement toward using higher frequency transducers whenever possible because of their superior resolution.

Ultrasound is emitted in pulses of extremely short duration from a special transducer; this transducer also acts as a signal receiver for reflected ultrasound waves. The active element in an echocardiographic transducer is a piezoelectric crystal. The term "piezoelectric" connotes that the crystal can transform electric energy into mechanical (sound) energy, and vice versa. Single crystals that are used in adult clinical echocardiography are commonly pulsed for a duration of 1/1,000,000 second (1 μsec); this pulsing is repeated every 1/1,000 second (1 msec). Periods of sound transmission are alternated with periods of sound reception, during which echoes reflected from structures within the heart are detected. The duration of the transmission period and the duration of the reception period differ by three orders of magnitude, since the transmission period lasts 1 μsec while the reception period embraces nearly 1 msec (999 μsec). A complete cycle of transmission and reception encompasses 1 msec. Consequently, the ultrasound beam samples cardiac structures at the rate of 1,000 times in 1 second. Ultrasound traverses the soft tissues of the chest at an average velocity of 1,540 m/second. In most patients cardiac targets are less than 15 cm from the chest wall. Thus, sampling rates of the order of 1,000 per second are eminently feasible—i.e., an individual target reflection can be recorded for each and every pulse emitted.

Ultrasound is reflected whenever tissue acoustic impedance changes. For practical purposes, this occurs at the interfaces of tissues of different density. Thus, it is possible to image the internal structure of the heart because blood, cardiac valves, myocardium, and pericardium present different tissue densities or acoustic impedances to the ultrasound beam. Moreover, the echographic information is available virtually instantaneously because of the high rate of travel of ultrasound through the chest in relation to the shallow depth of the soft tissues characterized.

INSTRUMENTATION AND TECHNIQUES

Ultrasound travels through the soft tissues of the chest at a well-defined average velocity (v = 1,540 m/sec). The time (t) between signal emission and signal reception can be accurately measured with an oscilloscope. The oscilloscope is calibrated using the distance (d) formula, $d = vt$. Thus it is possible to display the depth of tissue structures within the heart from which sound is reflected by displaying the vt product.

Several oscilloscopic techniques have been used to depict structure depth. The "amplitude" or A-mode displays the most intense echoes from cardiac surfaces as tall vertical spikes, while less intensely reflecting surfaces have lower spike amplitudes (Fig 1–2). In the A-mode, the oscilloscopic spikes oscillate rapidly back and forth along the horizontal (depth) axis with each heart beat as intracardiac targets move closer to or farther from

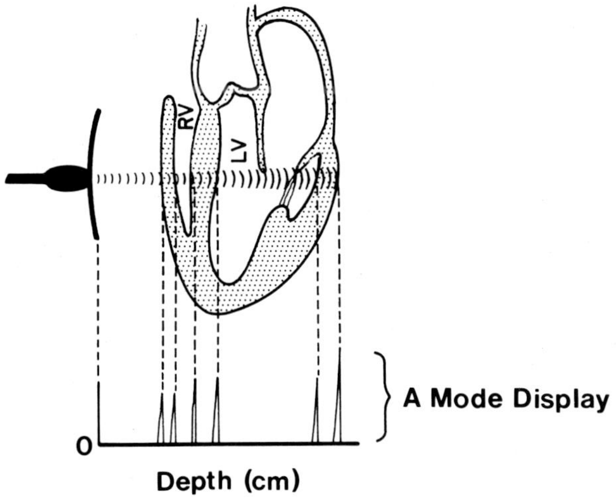

Fig 1–2.—Ultrasound reflection from the heart in A-mode display. Transducer is shown transmitting sound through cardiac structures. Reflections back to the transducer (not illustrated) are displayed below as spikes, the amplitude of which is proportional to the intensity of the reflected signal.

the transducer during the cardiac cycle. More than a decade ago, echocardiography was practiced with heavier reliance on the A-mode display; however, the A-mode does not lend itself well to producing a permanent record of the motion of intracardiac structures. In order to display motion, amplitude spikes can be converted to dots, with the brightness of the dots proportional to the amplitude of the spikes. This is known as B-mode, the "B" standing for brightness. If the B-mode dot pattern from moving intracardiac structures is presented on a sweeping oscilloscope, a time-motion or M-mode ("M" for motion) display is generated (Fig 1–3).

M-Mode Examination

Echocardiography is today most widely available and practiced using the M-mode display. In this format time is displayed on the horizontal axis and cardiac structures are displayed on the vertical axis, in direct proportion to the depth of tissues from which the sound is reflected (see Fig 1–3, *right*); the more intensely reflecting surfaces appear as darker lines. In real time the echocardiographic signals traverse the video screen from left to right and can be related to a concomitant ECG signal; a strip chart recorder is most often used to produce a permanent record. This technique permits identification of structures by anatomical continuity since new targets are encountered as the angle of the transducer is varied with respect to the heart. The effects of gradual varia-

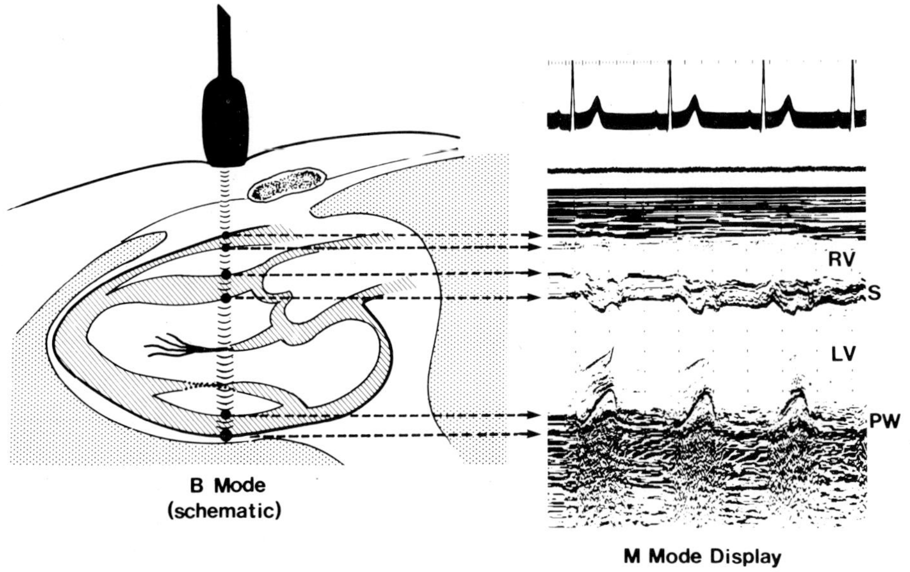

Fig 1–3.—The relationship between B-mode and M-mode displays. In the B-mode display *(left)* the size of the dots is intended to show relative brightness. The posterior pericardial echo is indicated by the largest dot and shows up as the darkest moving line on the M-mode display *(right)*. See text for details. *RV,* right ventricle; *LV,* left ventricle; *S,* septum; *PW,* posterior wall.

tions in transducer angulation can then be followed by long strip chart writeouts, so that the continuity of anatomical structures is discerned.

Figure 1–4 shows a patient undergoing an echocardiographic examination using a commercially available M-mode echocardiograph. Although the examination can be done with the subject supine, it is often facilitated if the subject assumes varying degrees of semirecumbency with some left lateral rotation. The technician's initial approach to examination is to place the transducer perpendicular to the chest wall in an intercostal space in the left parasternal region. As mentioned above, ultrasound traverses aerated tissues poorly; because of its high density, bone also reflects a great deal of ultrasonic energy—hence the usual necessity to work in a parasternal intercostal space. In the adult with a normal heart, the standard echocardiographic "window" is located in the third or fourth left intercostal space just to the left of the sternum. In this region the anterior parietal pericardium relates directly to the chest wall without intervening lung or bone. Alternative approaches from the suprasternal, supraclavicular, or subcostal areas, the cardiac apex, and other anatomical locations are often used when the parasternal approach is inadequate. A standard nomenclature has been recommended for these transducer locations (Fig 1–5)[1] and is followed throughout this monograph. Due to hyperinflated lung, patients with chronic obstructive pulmonary disease are difficult to examine from the precordium, but satisfactory recordings can often be obtained from a subcostal window. A suprasternal or supraclavicular approach in which the transducer is directed from the medial aspect of the right supraclavicular fossa toward the aortic root can also be used to determine the relative size of the aorta and right pulmonary artery and to characterize the motion of aortic valve prostheses. Views in which the transducer is placed at or near the cardiac apex can be used for a more adequate characterization of the motion of the anterior heart wall and mitral prostheses; apical views also permit a measurement which approximates the long axis of the left ventricle.

Currently, echocardiography is usually done by directing a single ultrasonic beam from the precordial region through the heart, focusing on structures easily recognized by their characteristic motion. Mitral valve and aortic root motion are usually detected readily. Once a known structure is identified, the sonic beam can be redirected toward other regions within the heart. As additional structures are imaged, their identity is established by their anatomical continuity with previously identified structures and by their characteristic motion. Structural continuity is a particularly

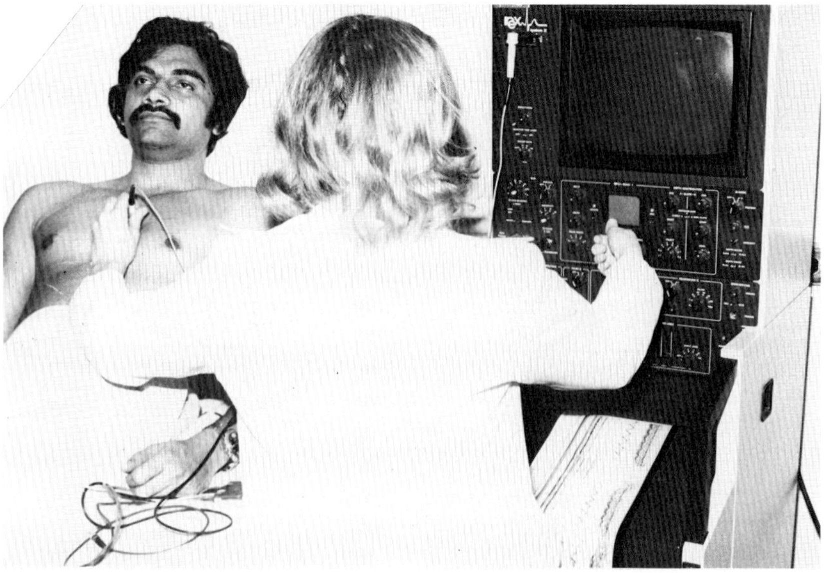

Fig 1–4.—Typical M-mode echocardiogram in progress.

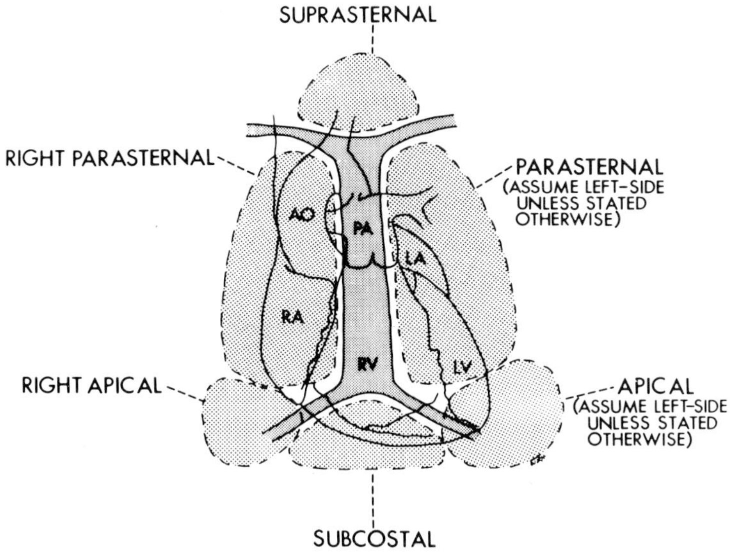

Fig 1–5.—Nomenclature for transducer location as recommended by the American Society of Echocardiography. The relationship of cardiac chambers to these surface positions is indicated on the diagram. *RA,* right atrium; *RV,* right ventricle; *PA,* pulmonary artery; *LA,* left atrium, *LV,* left ventricle; *AO,* aorta. (From Henry W.H., et al.: *Circulation* 62:212, 1980. Reproduced by permission of the American Heart Association.)

helpful guide to anatomical relations. In a typical M-mode examination, the transducer is directed in a plane which represents a diagonal section through the chest rather than a traditional sagittal, horizontal, or frontal view (Fig 1–6). In this manner, the plane of the echocardiographic beam approximates the long axis of the left ventricle, extending from the cardiac apex inferiorly and laterally to the center of the aortic root, which lies to the right, superiorly and medially. An M-mode scan in this plane from the root of the aorta to the apex of the left ventricle is shown in Figure 1–7. On a routine examination, the anterior leaflet of the mitral valve is often imaged initially. This structure lies within the upper body of the left ventricle, between the septum and posterior walls, and is one of the most readily recognizable cardiac targets because of its prominent anteroposterior swinging, which often resembles a distorted letter "M." Thereafter the echocardiographic beam is directed superiorly and medially toward the base of the heart. By this means, the interventricular septum is imaged in continuity with the anterior aortic wall, while the anterior leaflet of the mitral valve is connected to the posterior aortic wall (see Fig 1–7). Thus, the aortic root in normal subjects can be demonstrated to overlie directly the left ventricular outflow tract. As Figure 1–7 indicates, scanning from the aortic root produces a composite image in which most major left heart structures can be visualized. Aortic leaflets appear as a parallelogram within the root. As the beam is redirected inferiorly and laterally through the mitral valve region toward the cardiac apex, the left ventricular chamber tapers in its internal dimension as chordae from the mitral leaflets are traced into the thick posterior papillary muscle.

Although M-mode echocardiography offers a very narrow "ice pick" image of cardiac structure, its spatial resolution of 1–2 mm along the axis of the sound beam is the highest resolution of any widely available, noninvasive cardiac diagnostic technique. Furthermore, since this high-resolution image is obtained over short (1/1,000 second) intervals, there is also a very high degree of temporal resolution. Despite this high degree of axial and temporal resolution, however, there is no simultaneous field of view lateral to the transducer

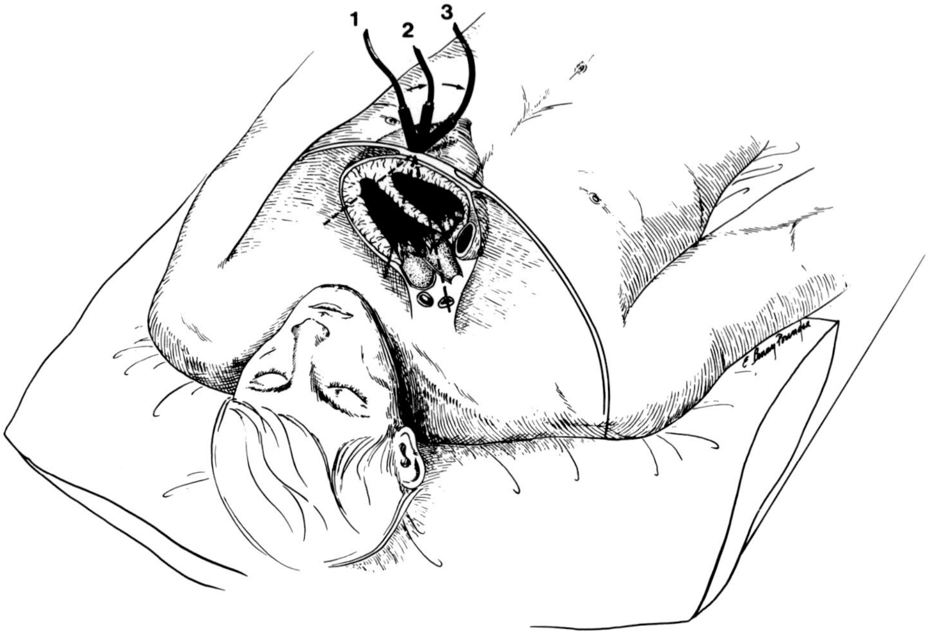

Fig 1–6.—Procedure of transducer angulation in performing an echocardiographic examination. In position 1 the ultrasound beam penetrates the base of the heart, passing through the aortic root. The transducer is then continuously angled inferiorly and laterally, passing through positions 2 and 3. An M-mode echocardiogram produced by this manipulation is shown in Figure 1–7.

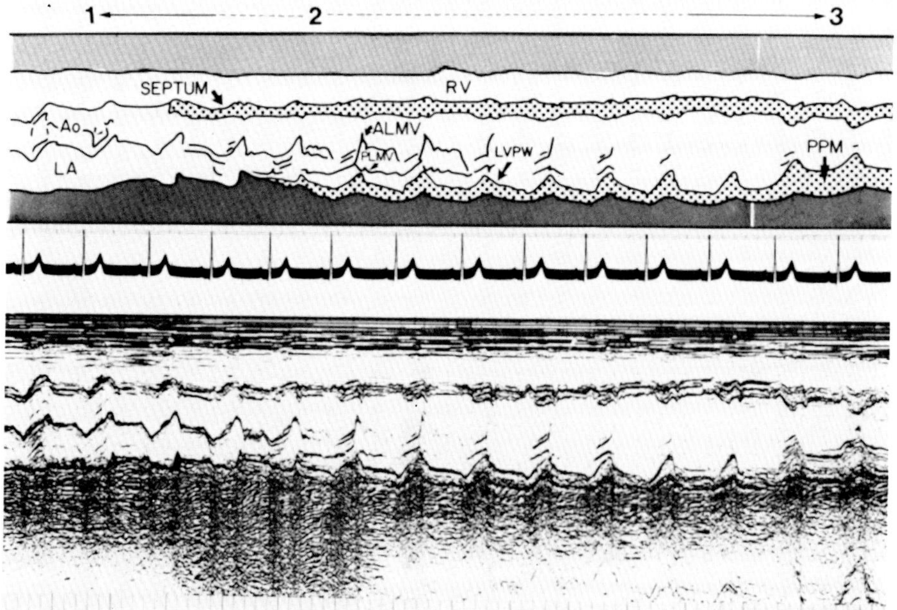

Fig 1–7.—Schematic *(top)* and actual *(bottom)* M-mode scans from the base to the apex of the heart. The numbers at the top correspond to the transducer angles shown in Figure 1–6. *ALMV,* anterior leaflet of the mitral valve; *PLMV,* posterior leaflet of the mitral valve; *LVPW,* left ventricular posterior wall; *PPM,* posterior papillary muscle.

beam. This shortcoming has prompted the development in the past few years of real-time, two-dimensional echocardiography (2DE), also known as cross-sectional echocardiography.

Two-Dimensional Echocardiography

Historically, the first two-dimensional images of the heart were produced using a B-scan technique (Fig 1–8).[2] With this approach, echographic examination of the heart was conducted in much the same way as ultrasonic examinations of the abdomen are done today. The transducer is systematically translocated across the precordium. Since the heart is a moving structure, however, a gating mechanism is required to pulse the transducer at the same relative time in successive cardiac cycles from each chest position. Over a number of cycles, an image of a "cut" of the heart can be built up on a storage oscilloscope. By selection of the appropriate time in the cardiac cycle to activate the transducer (e.g., QRS complex, T wave), a diastolic or systolic image can be constructed. Such an image represents a *retrospective average* of the preceding beats, which are displayed as dots along individual B-mode lines. This approach is time-consuming and depends heavily on the reliability of the gating mechanism. Obviously, arrhythmias such as atrial fibrillation, which involves varying cycle lengths and consequently varying diastolic and systolic image sizes, can cause difficulty with proper image construction.

Two-dimensional cardiac echograms that portray "live images," i.e., instantaneous and continuous tomographic displays of the heart's action in real time, have been produced in several ways. One of the earliest instruments achieved this goal by using a linear array of 20 miniature transducer crystals (Fig 1–9).[3] In this multicrystal echograph, each element is fired in succession. Signals received by each crystal are displayed in a corresponding line on an oscilloscope. By rapid repetition of the activation process, a live image is produced. Such a system can be used particularly well

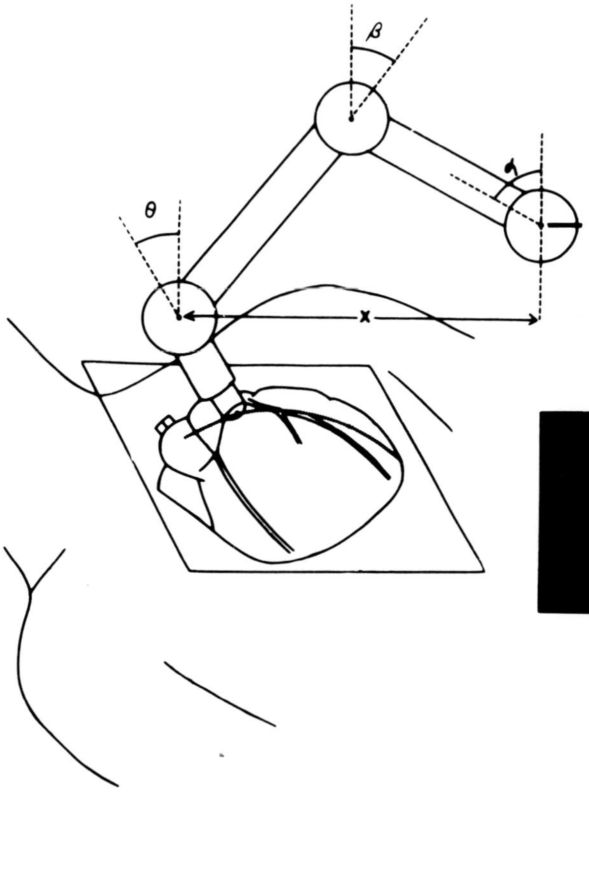

Fig 1–8.—B-mode two-dimensional ultrasonogram. *Left,* schematic of supporting mechanism for translation of the transducer. *Center,* long axis image of heart produced by this type of examination. *Right,* schematic identifying the structures traversed. (Adapted from Teichholz L.E., et al.: *N. Engl. J. Med.* 291:1220, 1974. Reproduced by permission.)

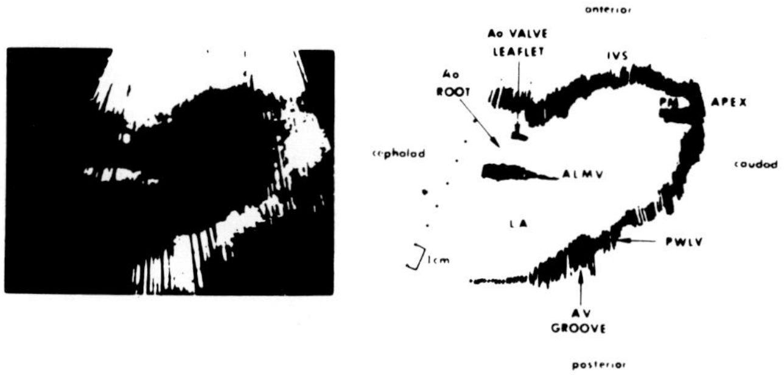

in pediatric echocardiography, wherein the transducer array completely encompasses the transverse or longitudinal dimensions of the heart. In adult echocardiography, approximately two thirds of the heart can be imaged at any one time. However, this system has very limited resolution owing to its low line density (20 lines per frame); there is also image degradation as reverberating echoes are secondarily received by transducer elements not in line with underlying anatomical structures. In addition, difficulty with transmission through calcified costal cartilages renders the information along certain lines less effective than along others.

Currently, in the United States, live two-dimensional echocardiograms are usually obtained by the use of sector scanners. In these instruments, the ultrasound beam is swept in an arc across the heart from a single point on the chest wall.[4, 5]

The most inexpensive sector scanners involve mechanical sweeping mechanisms, which are principally of two types. The earliest mechanical sector scanners used a single M-mode transducer to obtain B-mode scan lines. This was accomplished by mounting the transducer on a rapidly oscillating motor which rocked the ultrasonic crystal through a 30- to 40-degree arc on the chest wall. Through the course of this arc, the transducer can serially perform transmit-receive cycles, producing as many as 120 B-scan lines. The spatial orientation of each B-scan line is determined from the mechanical position of the transducer and is displayed in its proper position on a video screen. Since the sector subtended by the transducer can be produced 30–60 times per second, a "moving picture" is generated, in which each frame consists of a full sweep of the transducer through its arc. These oscillating mechanical systems yield high-resolution images but are limited by their narrow field of view and by the vibrations produced when the transducer is in contact with the chest wall.

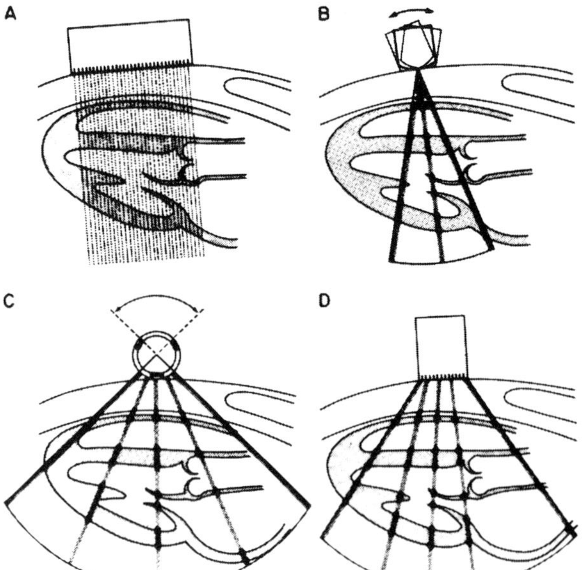

Fig 1–9.—Schematic demonstrating real-time two-dimensional echocardiographic systems as described in the text. *A,* multicrystal scanner. *B,* mechanical sector scanner with oscillating transducer. *C,* mechanical sector scanner with three-element rotary transducer. *D,* phased array sector scanner. (From DeMaria A.N., et al.: *Am. J. Cardiol.* 46:1097, 1980. Reproduced by permission.)

A rotary scanning transducer was subsequently developed in which three or four transducers cut from the same piezoelectric crystal are mounted equidistantly on the perimeter of a wheel. In a four-element rotary transducer these crystals are 90 degrees apart. The supporting wheel rotates in an oil-filled plastic housing which is placed on the chest wall. Ultrasonic signals are sequentially processed from each element as it traverses the 90 degrees of its arc closest to the chest wall. This type of transducer will produce a 90-degree sector scan without vibrating contact through the transducer to the patient. Its standoff mechanism, the oil-filled plastic housing, however, may contribute to some image degradation not encountered in the simpler oscillating system.

Live two-dimensional images can also be produced by electronic sector scanners. These instruments have small multielement (usually 32 to 64) transducers cut from the same piezoelectric crystal. Unlike the linear array scanner, in which the transducer elements are pulsed independently, the transducer array in electronic sector scanners is discharged in phased patterns, hence the term "phased array" technique. Phased array scanners take advantage of Huygen's principle, namely, multiple small wave fronts of sound will combine to form a single sound wave whose direction is determined by the component wavelets. Figure 1–10 demonstrates this principle using four selected elements from a phased array. When all four are *pulsed simultaneously* (see Fig 1–10, *center*) the new wave front propagates directly in front of the transducer face. If a small fraction of a second time delay is introduced so that elements 1 through 4 are now *pulsed sequentially from right to left* (see Fig 1–10, *left*), the net wave front will move to the left of the transducer. If the transducers are pulsed in reverse sequence (see Fig 1–10, *right*), the net wave front will be to the right of the transducer. Furthermore, by changing the time delays between activation of elements of the array, one can electronically steer the sonic beam at varying angles from the multielement transducer face. Electronic scanners have the additional potential of achieving beam focusing through appropriate computer-coordinated timing of element activation. Electronic scanners have some advantages over mechanical scanners: (1) electronic focusing offers higher potential image resolution, and (2) simultaneous M-mode and 2DE examinations are possible since the information from a selected wave front can be recorded concomitantly by time-sharing the imaging circuits. However, these instruments are more complex and consequently more expensive than mechanical scanners (Table 1–1).

TABLE 1–1.—CHARACTERISTICS OF SECTOR SCANNERS

PHASED ARRAY	MECHANICAL
Advantages	
Simultaneous single or dual M-mode	Simplicity and lower cost
Complex scan interlacing	Fewer side lobes
Dynamic focusing	
Transducer: small overall size, no moving parts	
Disadvantages	
Complexity and higher cost	Transducer: larger, subject to mechanical unreliability
Large side lobes	Simultaneous M-mode only recently available
	Accurate interlacing difficult

In practical terms, high-quality echocardiographic images have been achieved by experienced echocardiographers using either type of instrument.

In contrast to the unidimensional ultrasound beam used in M-mode units, 2DE units pass a planar beam of ultrasound through the heart and produce "slice-like" tomographic images from the orientation of the transducer beam. Two-dimensional echocardiographic images are displayed on a video screen. Both the absolute and the relative sizes of cardiac structures are readily appreciated

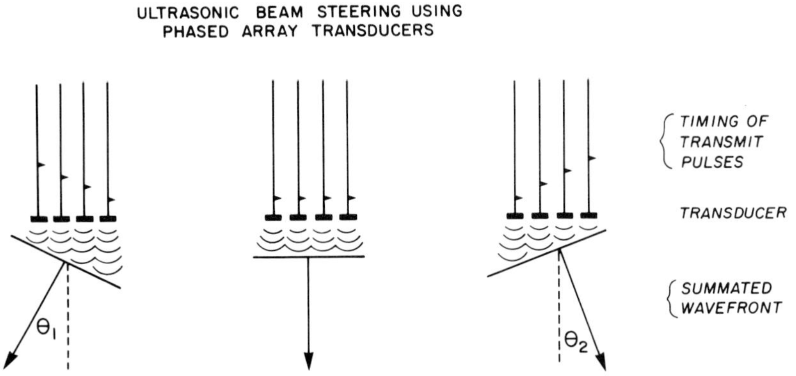

Fig 1–10.—The phased array principle is illustrated using a four-element transducer. The timing of transmitted pulses is shown by small peaks on each transducer element wire. *Left,* sonic beam propagates to the left from the midline at an angle θ_1 as the transducer elements are pulsed sequentially from right to left. *Center,* beam propagates straight ahead as each of the transducer elements is pulsed simultaneously. *Right,* beam propagates to the viewer's right as the transducer elements are temporally pulsed in reverse sequence.

from these slice-like anatomical cross-sectional images. The course of events (e.g., motion of heart structures from diastole to systole) can be further studied using videotaping systems; however, temporal resolution is not as great for 2DE as for M-mode echocardiography since it takes approximately 1/30 to 1/60 second to construct each video frame.

The information obtained about cardiac anatomy depends on the orientation of the ultrasonic sector beam. Many views of the heart and great vessels are possible with different transducer locations (e.g., parasternal, apical) and orientations (i.e., with the beam directed transversely, obliquely, or longitudinally) toward the structure of interest. The direction of the sonic beam is determined by the technician, who tilts and/or rotates the transducer to produce standard image presentations. The most common images in adults are obtained from orthogonal planes derived from parasternal and apical transducer locations (Fig 1–11).

A representative view of the normal left heart obtained from parasternal placement of the transducer with the echo beam directed to approximate the long axis of the left ventricle is shown in Figure 1–12. In most adults, the 80- to 90-degree beam is not quite wide enough to encompass the entire length of the left ventricle from the aortic root to the apex. By tilting the beam inferiorly or sliding the transducer inferolaterally to the next lower intercostal space, the apex can often be viewed. The parasternal long axis of the left heart allows examination of the size and shape of the left atrium, left ventricle, aortic root, and right ventricle, as well as the action of the mitral and aortic valves.

If the transducer is rotated 90 degrees clockwise at the same parasternal location from which the long axis of the left ventricle was imaged, a

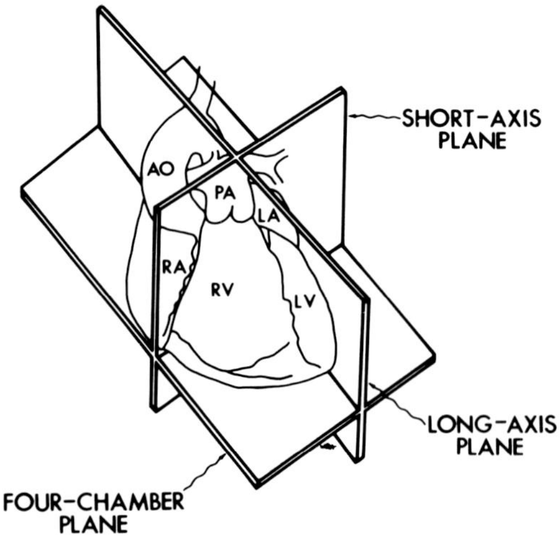

Fig 1–11.—Two-dimensional echocardiographic imaging planes with nomenclature proposed by American Society of Echocardiography. (From Henry W.H., et al.: *Circulation* 62:212, 1980. Reproduced by permission of the American Heart Association.)

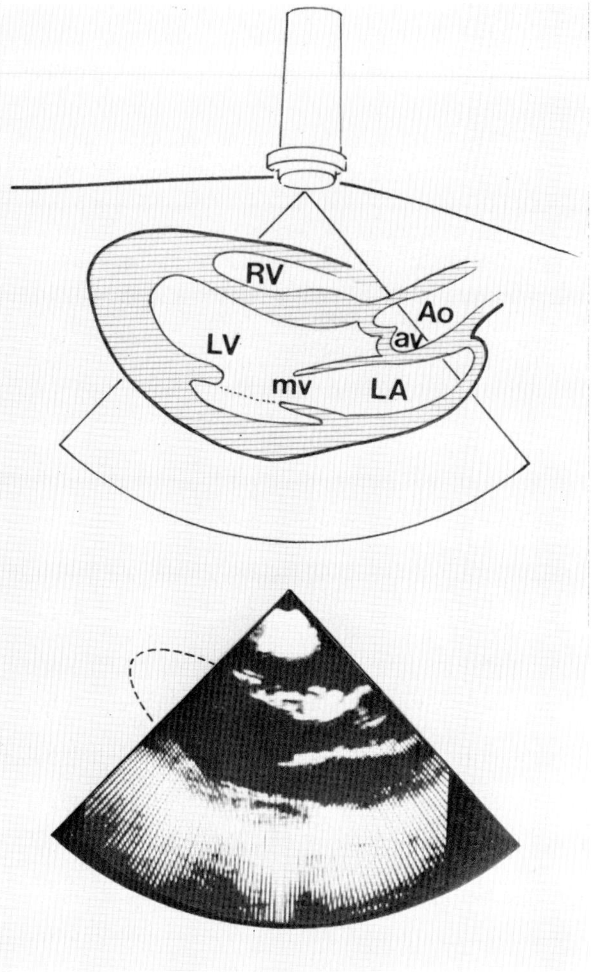

Fig 1–12.—Schematic long-axis, two-dimensional echocardiographic image *(top)* and actual still frame image *(bottom). AV,* aortic valve; *MV,* mitral valve. Other abbreviations as in previous figures.

short-axis view of the heart can be obtained. Depending on the extent of craniocaudal transducer tilt, this view may include the low or high left ventricle or the great vessels at the base of the heart (Fig 1–13). Inferiorly, the left ventricle appears as a rounded cavity indented by the protuberances of the papillary muscles. As the transducer is tilted superiorly, the view of both ventricular cavities enlarges and the leaflets of the mitral valve are displayed (opening in diastole and closing in systole) within the upper left ventricular cavity. The diastolic size of the mitral orifice can readily be appreciated in this view.

Further superior angulation of the transducer permits imaging of the aorta as it is partially encircled in front by the right ventricular outflow tract. Both atria, divided by the interatrial septum, lie behind the aortic root. This view of the base of the heart is very helpful in assessing certain congenital heart lesions, since the relation-

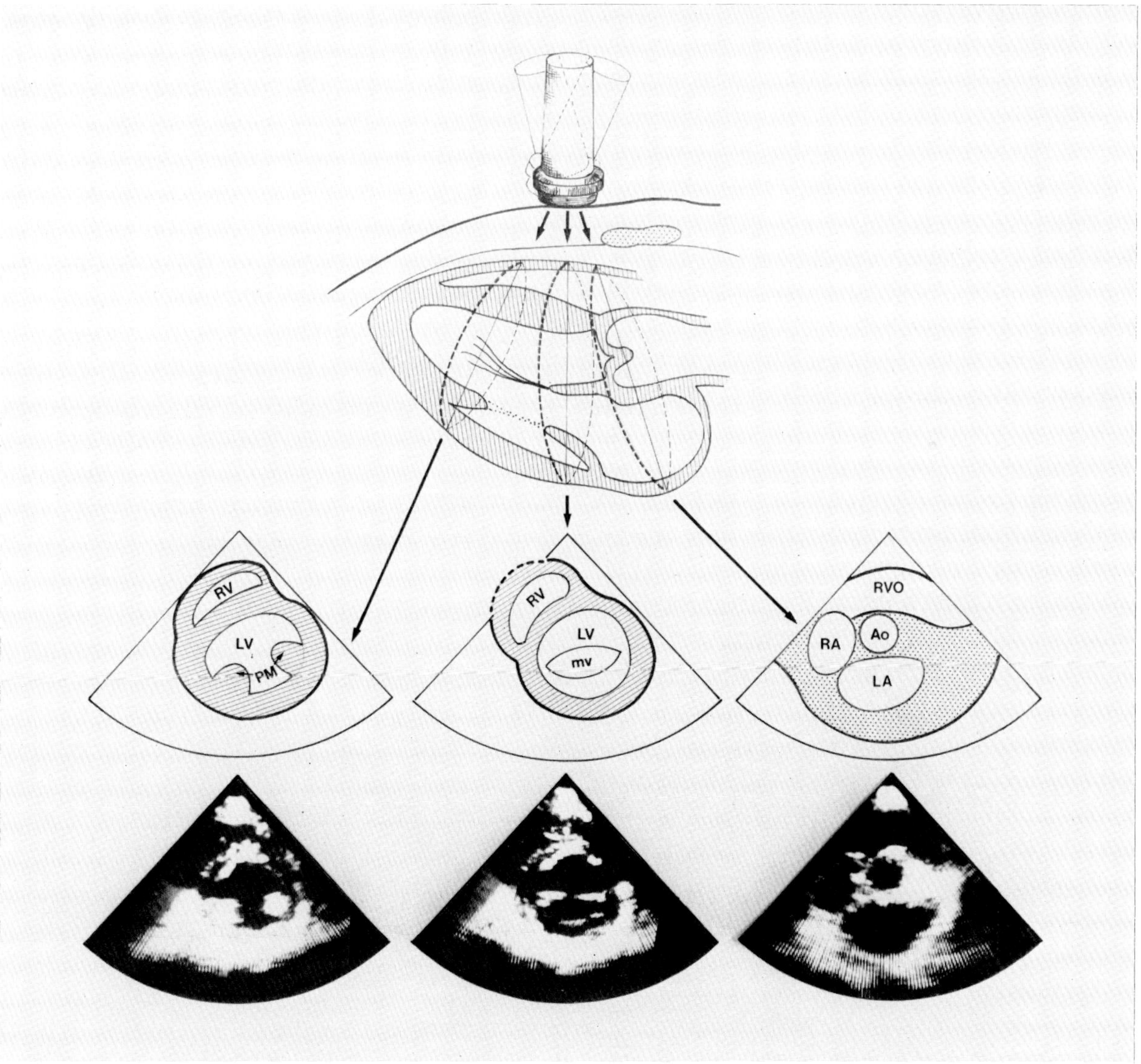

Fig 1–13.—Short-axis images of the heart. *Left,* papillary muscle *(PM)* level; *center,* mitral valve level; *right,* aortic root level. (From Parisi A.F., et al.: *J. Cardiovasc. Med.* 5:39, 1980. Reproduced by permission.)

ships of the great vessels can be established and abnormal right atrial to left atrial flow patterns can be observed after intravenous injections of fluid (see below).

Apical placement of the transducer produces a picture in which the distal portions of one or both ventricles are imaged in the near field. If the sector beam is directed toward the base of the heart at a shallow angle from the frontal body plane, a four-chamber view is obtained; both atria are seen to be separated from the ventricles by the mitral and tricuspid valves (Fig 1–14,*A*). If the transducer is then rotated at this location into a more nearly sagittal plane and the beam is directed along the long axis of the left ventricle, a view orthogonal to the four-chamber view is obtained, which displays anterior and posterior left ventricular wall motion (Fig 1–14,*B*).

Multiple variations of these views of the heart are possible by making small changes in transducer angulation from these standard orthogonal planes. For example, higher short-axis projections can be used to image the relationship of the great vessels and to identify the pulmonic bifurcation, which serves to distinguish the pulmonary artery from the aorta in evaluating congenital heart lesions. Additional transducer locations are also helpful. A subcostal transducer location not only serves as a window in patients who cannot be imaged from the parasternal area, but also gives optimal views of the hepatic veins and inferior vena caval inflow to the right heart (Fig 1–15), which cannot be obtained from parasternal and apical locations. Suprasternal transducer locations can be used to give alternate views of the great vessels, to evaluate the aortic arch (Fig 1–16), to detect dissecting aortic aneurysms, and to localize aortic coarctations.

Relationship of M-Mode Echocardiography to 2DE

In recent years, those who have had 2DE available have found it faster and easier to use than M-mode echocardiography. The latter technique, however, is still clinically useful; the advantages and limitations of each technique are summarized in Table 1–2. The inherent advantage of imaging two dimensions in space facilitates the detection of ventricular aneurysms, provides a quantitative approach to assessing the severity of valvular stenosis, and offers a rational basis for distinguishing many complex congenital heart lesions. On the other hand, M-mode echocardiograms graphically display the course of intracardiac events in time, a dimension appreciated only coarsely by 2DE. The superior temporal resolution of M-mode provides clues from time-motion analysis that are valuable for defining altered cardiac physiology; e.g., the severity of aortic regurgitation can be graded if premature closure of the mitral valve occurs, coronary disease can be detected from abnormal

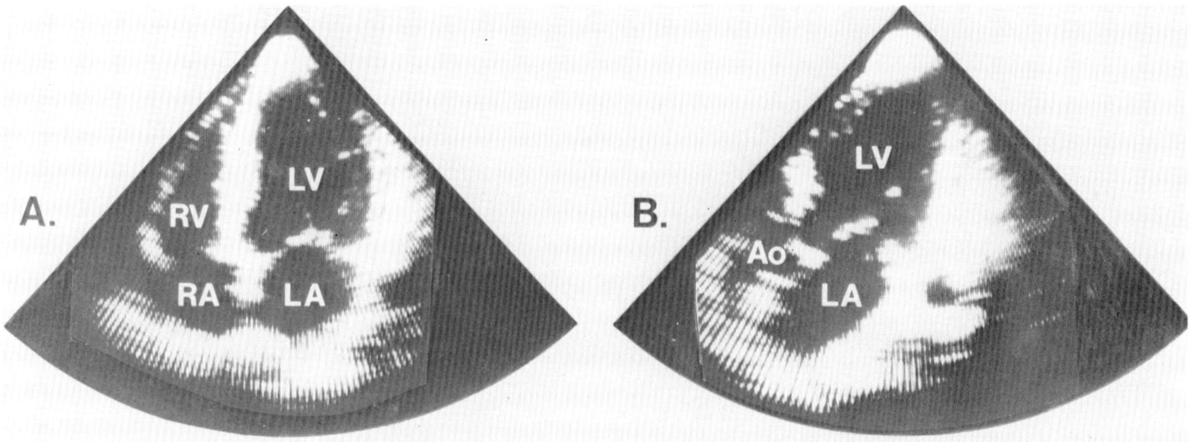

Fig 1–14.—*A*, apical four-chamber image of the heart. *B*, apical two-chamber image of the heart. (From Parisi A.F., et al.: *J. Cardiovasc. Med.* 5:39, 1980. Reproduced by permission.)

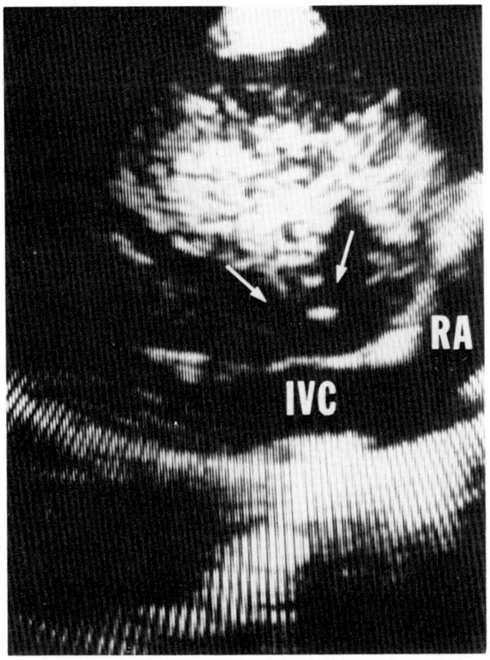

Fig 1–15.—Subcostal image of the inferior vena caval *(IVC)* inflow into the right atrium *(RA)*. The high-intensity echoes in the near field are from the liver. Hepatic veins *(arrows)* can be seen crossing toward the vena cava.

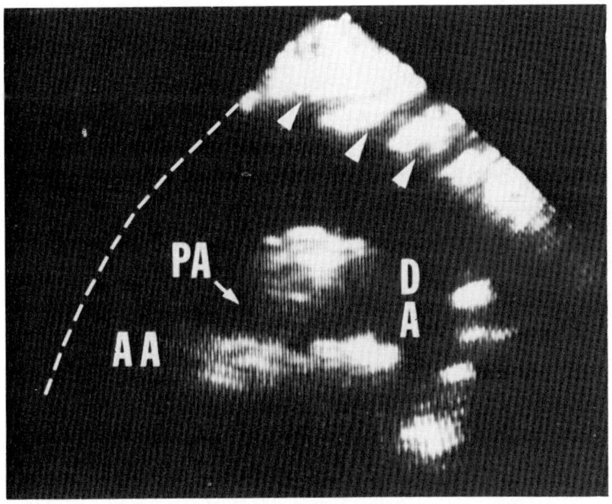

Fig 1–16.—Suprasternal image of the aortic arch from a healthy young woman. The ascending aorta *(AA)* passes over the pulmonary artery *(PA)*. The three major branches—innominate, left common carotid, and left subclavian—emerge from the arch from left to right, as indicated by *arrowheads*. The descending aorta *(DA)* proceeds inferiorly from the arch at the region of the left subclavian.

wall thickening during systole, and constrictive pericarditis can be detected from abnormally flat rather than sloping posterior left ventricular wall motion during the slow filling phase of diastole. Thus, M-mode echocardiography complements 2DE, providing temporal information and details of regional motion not possible with the latter technique. In a modern well-equipped diagnostic laboratory, both techniques are routinely used to obtain the information needed for optimal patient care.

TABLE 1–2.—Advantages and Limitations of Echocardiographic Techniques

Two-Dimensional Echocardiography	M-Mode Echocardiography
Advantages	
Better quantification of valvular stenosis Higher sensitivity in detection of ventricular aneurysms Quantification of ventricular function in irregularly shaped and/or asymmetrically contracting ventricles Ascertainment of great vessel interrelationships in congenital heart disease Ready discernment of intracardiac and pericardial masses Examination of structures (e.g., right atrium) difficult to image on M-mode Direct comparison of relative chamber size, since multiple chambers can be visualized simultaneously More complete evaluation of flow patterns after fluid injection	Enhanced temporal resolution of valve and wall motion facilitates *(a)* grading of aortic regurgitation, *(b)* detection of subtle wall motion abnormalities in coronary disease, *(c)* detection of constrictive pericarditis More consistent spatial resolution due to fixed axial imaging allows more precise assessment of regional wall function, e.g., amplitude of motion, % systolic thickening in CAD
Limitations	
Temporal resolution is limited due to low frame rates Lateral resolution is inferior to axial resolution, which introduces some image distortions	Absence of lateral imaging prolongs search for structures and makes some structures impossible to assess

INTERVENTIONS WITH ECHOCARDIOGRAPHY

Standard interventions such as dynamic and isometric exercise, drug administration, and respiratory maneuvers have all been used with either M-mode echocardiography or 2DE. However, by far the most valuable adjunct in echocardiography is the intracardiac or intravascular injection of fluids, which allows delineation of flow patterns and chamber continuity within the heart and great vessels.

Fluid Injections

In 1969, when Raymond Gramiak and associates were performing echocardiography at cardiac catheterization, they discovered that cloud-like turbulence occurred within cardiac chambers during bolus injections of indocyanine green dye.[6] Subsequent studies indicated that freshly mixed solutions of normal saline, dextrose in water, and even the patient's own blood could produce the same effect. This phenomenon initially helped to confirm the identity of ultrasonically imaged structures, e.g., at cardiac catheterization a chamber showing left ventricular pressure pulses which subsequently filled with turbulence after fluid was injected through the catheter[7] was obviously the left ventricle. It also has served to confirm structure boundaries. For example, the exact location of the right side of the interventricular septum can be confirmed after right ventricular fluid injection as the interface between chamber turbulence and the immediately posterior tissue echoes.

Ultrasonically detected intravascular turbulence is thought to be reflected from microbubbles which are produced in freshly drawn solutions. These bubbles are not visible to the naked eye, but they possess the high ultrasonic reflectivity of microscopic air-filled structures. This technique has become extremely valuable in studying diseases associated with abnormal flow patterns, particularly when used with 2DE. In a normal heart, after intravenous injection, the flowing cloud of turbulent echoes can be traced sequentially through right heart chambers into the pulmonary artery. Intravenously injected microbubbles are effectively filtered by the pulmonary microcirculation and thus are not imaged in the left-sided chambers of the heart. Congenital lesions involving abnormal right-to-left shunting are most easily detected using this approach. For example, right-to-left shunting through an atrial septal defect can be discerned by inappropriate turbulence crossing from the right to left atrium in an apical four-chamber view. Abnormal left-to-right shunting can also be detected, but with greater difficulty, from interruption of the right-sided turbulence pattern by a stream of effectively unopacified blood.

Recently, Reale has shown that fluid injections in the pulmonary capillary wedge position can traverse the pulmonary bed and flow through left ventricular structures.[8] If this method gains further acceptance it will serve as an alternative way of directly demonstrating left-to-right shunting.

Exercise

Several groups have reported recording echocardiograms during both supine and upright bicycle ergometry.[9–12] The technique is difficult to execute because of respiratory interference; long, continuous beat-to-beat recordings are not usually possible. Nevertheless, transient wall motion abnormalities have been demonstrated in patients with coronary disease and exercise-induced chest pain.[13 14]

Isometric (handgrip) exercise is readily performed in conjunction with echocardiography, but it precipitates ischemic left ventricular dysfunction much less frequently than dynamic exercise. In patients with isometrically-induced angina, however, striking transient localized wall motion defects have been noticed.[15] Early reports also indicate that isometric exercise may be useful in assessing left ventricular dysfunction in patients with aortic regurgitation.[16]

Pharmacologic Intervention

Acute pharmacologic intervention during echocardiography has been reported with a wide variety of agents. Many drugs have been studied with echo and concurrent invasive measurements and hence are not routinely employed in clinical eval-

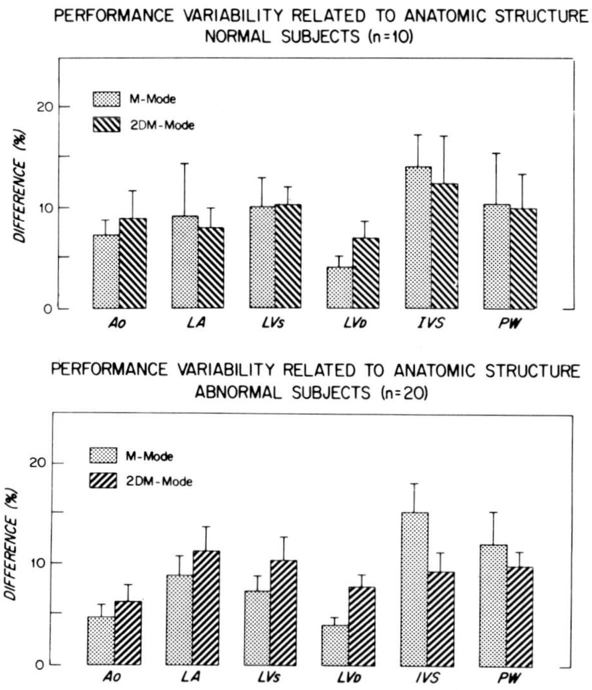

Fig 1–17.—Variability of measurements obtained from repeated M-mode examinations in healthy subjects and in patients with heart disease. Variability changed from structure to structure, being least for the left ventricular internal diastolic dimension *(LV_D)* and most for the interventricular septum *(IVS)*. Performing the examinations with two-dimensional (2DM) echocardiographic guidance improved consistency for the smallest structures—IVS and left ventricular posterior wall *(PW)*—but not for the other left heart structures. *LV_S,* left ventricular internal systolic dimension. Other abbreviations as previously defined. (From Pietro D.A., et al.: *Chest* 79:29, 1981. Reproduced by permission.)

uations. Recently emerging reports suggest that the end-systolic pressure-dimension relationship defined during methoxamine infusion may be a useful measure of ventricular function.[17] Probably the agent most often used clinically is amyl nitrite, which reduces left ventricular afterload, leading to increased left ventricular stroke volume. Like the Valsalva maneuver, amyl nitrite is useful in demonstrating left ventricular outflow obstruction in idiopathic hypertrophic subaortic stenosis (IHSS).

Echocardiograms are commonly used to evaluate the effects of chronically administered cardiovascular medications. It is essential to establish the *reproducibility* of examination findings in a given laboratory for echocardiography to be used validly in serial cardiac evaluations. Recent studies have shown that reproducibility varies with the structure under examination (Fig 1–17).[18, 19] As a rule, left ventricular internal diastolic dimensions with approximately 5% variability are among the most reproducible of any left heart measurement.

Respiratory Maneuvers

Echocardiograms can be recorded during both Valsalva and Müller maneuvers. In fact, M-mode echocardiograms have demonstrated a different

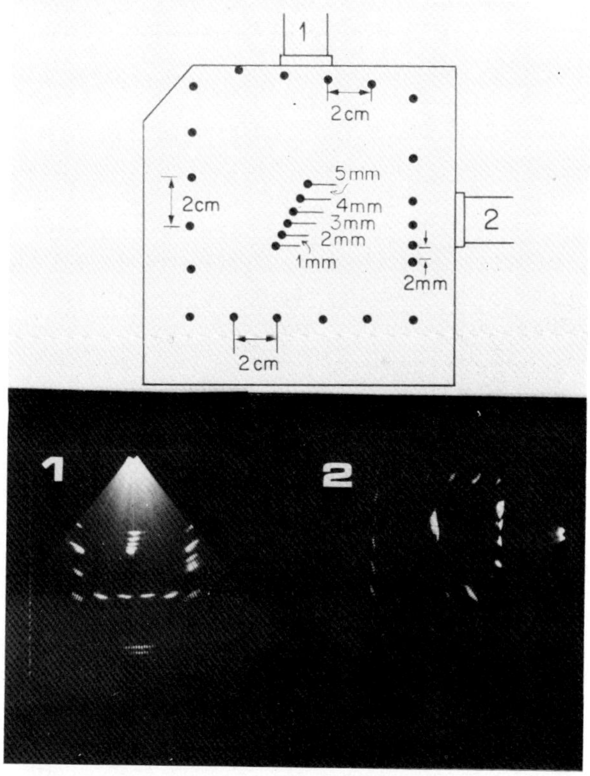

Fig 1–18.—*Top,* side view of the AIUM standard for performance of ultrasonic instruments. The black dots represent the position of wires suspended in a tank with the distances of separation specified. *Bottom, 1* and *2* represent ultrasonic images made with a real-time, phased array sector scanner with transducer positions corresponding to 1 and 2 at top. Note that reflections from the wires appear as small arcs rather than discrete dots. Imaging of the central set of wires from positions 1 and 2 demonstrates the superiority of axial over lateral resolution in this system.

ventricular response to the strain phase of the Valsalva maneuver in normal individuals (who decrease their internal dimensions during strain) and patients with dilated ventricles and heart failure (who do not decrease their internal dimensions during strain).[20] Respiratory maneuvers, like dynamic exercise, make it more difficult to record satisfactory echocardiograms. The Valsalva maneuver is often used to demonstrate potential left ventricular outflow obstruction in IHSS, and it can be used to explore the patency of a foramen ovale or detect a small atrial septal defect, since transient right-to-left shunting may occur during this intervention. Beyond these specific applications, the Valsalva maneuver does not have further current clinical application in the routine course of echocardiographic studies.

Atrial Pacing

Atrial pacing is a stress frequently used in the cardiac catheterization laboratory to evaluate left ventricular function. M-mode studies have shown that left ventricular dimensions inversely relate to paced heart rate.[21] If angina pectoris is precipitated by the pacing intervention, regional left ventricular dysfunction may be detected. This technique has not been widely accepted because it essentially adds an invasive element to the clinical echocardiographic examination. Furthermore, the logistics involved can be as time-consuming and costly as catheterization itself. Thus, for practical purposes, it is a procedure best used to resolve specific questions in selected patients.

LIMITATIONS OF ECHOCARDIOGRAPHY

By far the greatest problem in echocardiography today is the inability to obtain a complete diagnostic examination in all patients referred for study. Some views are possible in nearly every patient. Most clinical questions (e.g., "rule out pericardial effusion") can be answered more than 90% of the time, but delineation of all the important cardiac structures, particularly the endocardium of the left ventricle in its entirety, is achieved only 70%–80% of the time.[22] This problem can be

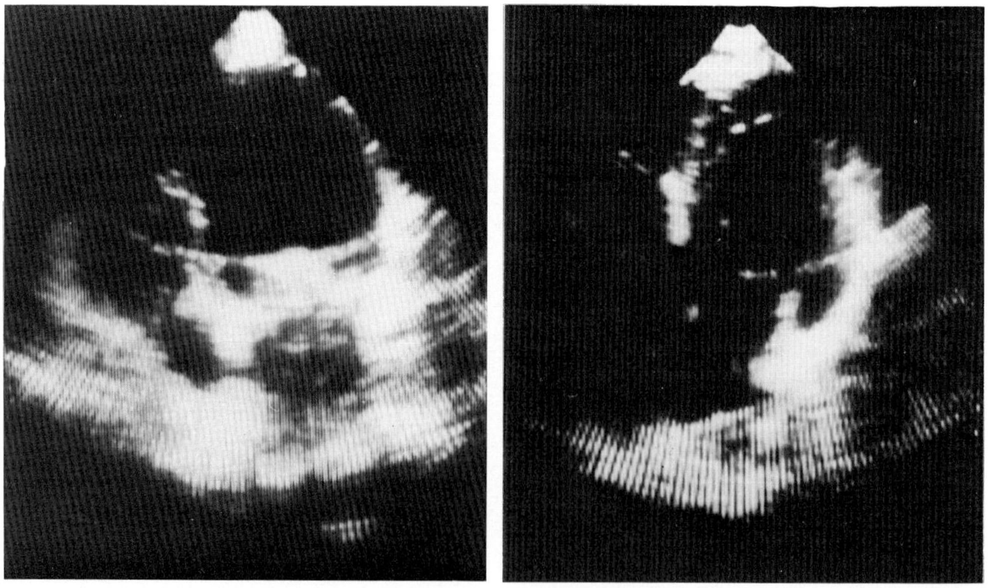

Fig 1–19.—Side lobe artifacts from a real-time imaging system; apical four-chamber views. *Left,* arc-like echo traversing both ventricles is coming from a prosthetic mitral valve. *Right,* arc-like echo enters the proximal left ventricle from its lateral wall. This echocardiogram was taken from another subject who did not have a prosthetic heart valve.

complicated by an overzealous observer, who may be tempted to render definitive interpretations on marginal or frankly inadequate studies.

Some of the commonest interpretive difficulties emanate from failure to appreciate the ultrasonic characteristics of a given instrument. All ultrasonic beams have a defined breadth and height, with minimal dimensions comparable to the size of the crystal transducer face. Beyond its focal point, the beam's cross-sectional area enlarges in direct proportion to the distance from the transducer face. In M-mode echocardiography, two laterally separated structures may appear in direct anteroposterior relationship when they fall within the same beam path. Two-dimensional techniques also produce distortions, which are greater the farther a target is from the central beam axis. In these instruments, axial resolution (1–2 mm) is superior to lateral resolution (4–5 mm) (Fig 1–18). Because of the complex nature by which two-dimensional images are generated, artifacts can sometimes appear as intracardiac masses to the casual observer. One such common artifact is a prominent side lobe, which appears as an arc-like, hazily bordered lateral extension of a prominently echo-producing intracardiac structure (Fig 1–19). With excessive gain settings on any instrument, cloud-like "noise" in cardiac cavities may also be misread as intracardiac thrombosis.

Despite these limitations, echocardiography possesses resolution which is still superior to all commonly used noninvasive techniques. In appropriately selected subjects, it is unexcelled in providing information on the anatomical and functional state of the pericardium, myocardium, valves, and cardiac chambers.

REFERENCES

1. Henry W.H., DeMaria A.N., Gramiak R.: Report of the American Society of Echocardiography Committee on Nomenclature and Standards in Two-Dimensional Echocardiography. *Circulation* 62:212, 1980.
2. Teichholz L.E., Cohen M.V., Sonnenblick E.H., et al.: Study of left ventricular geometry and function by B-scan ultrasonography in patients with and without asynergy. *N. Engl. J. Med.* 291:1220, 1974.
3. Bom N., Lancee C.T. Jr., van Zwieten G., et al.: Multiscan echocardiography: I. Technical description. *Circulation* 48:1066, 1973.
4. Griffith J.M., Henry W.L.: A sector scanner for real time two-dimensional echocardiography. *Circulation* 49:1147, 1974.
5. von Ramm O.T., Thurstone F.L.: Cardiac imaging using a phased array ultrasound system: I. System design. *Circulation* 53:258, 1976.
6. Gramiak R., Shan P.M., Karmer D.H.: Ultrasound cardiography: Contrast studies in anatomy and function. *Radiology* 92:939, 1969.
7. Feigenbaum H., Stone J.M., Lee D.A., et al.: Identification of ultrasound echoes from the left ventricle by use of intracardiac injections of indocyanine green. *Circulation* 41:615, 1970.
8. Reale A.: Contrast echocardiography: Transmission of echoes to the left heart across the pulmonary vascular bed. *Am. J. Cardiol.* 45:401, 1980.
9. Stein R.A., Michielli D., Fox E.L., et al.: Continuous ventricular dimensions in man during supine exercise and recovery. *Am. J. Cardiol.* 41:655, 1978.
10. Weiss J.L., Weisfeldt M.L., Mason S.J., et al.: Evidence of Frank-Starling effect in man during severe semisupine exercise. *Circulation* 59:655, 1979.
11. Crawford M.H., White D.H., Amon K.W.: Echocardiographic evaluation of left ventricular size and performance during handgrip and supine and upright bicycle exercise. *Circulation* 59:1188, 1979.
12. Sugishita Y., Koseki S.: Dynamic exercise echocardiography. *Circulation* 60:743, 1979.
13. Mason S.J., Weiss J.L., Weisfeldt M.L., et al.: Exercise echocardiography: Detection of wall motion abnormalities during ischemia. *Circulation* 59:50, 1979.
14. Wann L.S., Faris J.V., Childress R.H., et al.: Exercise cross-sectional echocardiography in ischemic heart disease. *Circulation* 60:1300, 1979.
15. Widlansky S., McHenry P.L., Corya B.C., et al.: Coronary angiographic, echocardiographic and electrocardiographic studies on a patient with variant angina due to coronary artery spasm. *Am. Heart J.* 90:631–635, 1975.
16. Kemper A.J., Shulman R.M., Ray B., et al.: Echocardiographic assessment of left ventricular systolic function in aortic regurgitation during isometric exercise, abstracted. *Clin. Res.* 29:213A, 1981.
17. Marsh J.D., Green L.H., Wynne J., et al.: Left ventricular end-systolic pressure-dimension and stress-length relations in normal human subjects. *Am. J. Cardiol.* 44:1311–1317, 1979.
18. Clark R.D., Korcuska K., Cohn K.: Serial echocardiographic evaluation of left ventricular function in valvular disease, including reproducibility guidelines for serial studies. *Circulation* 62:564, 1980.
19. Pietro D.A., Voelkel A.G., Ray B.J., et al.: Reproducibility of echocardiography: A study evaluating the variability of serial echocardiographic measurements. *Chest* 79:29–32, 1981.
20. Parisi A.F., Harrington J.J., Askenazi J., et al.: Echocardiographic evaluation of the Valsalva ma-

neuver in healthy subjects and patients with and without heart failure. *Circulation* 54:921–927, 1976.

21. DeMaria A.N., Neumann A., Schubart P.J., et al.: Systematic correlation of cardiac chamber size and ventricular performance determined with echocardiography and alterations of heart rate in normal persons. *Am. J. Cardiol.* 43:1, 1979.
22. Folland E.D., Parisi A.F., Moynihan P.F., et al.: Assessment of left ventricular ejection fraction and volumes by real-time, two-dimensional echocardiography: A comparison of cineangiographic and radionuclide techniques. *Circulation* 60:760–766, 1979.

RADIONUCLIDE IMAGING

Curtis A. Bakal and H. William Strauss

IT HAS BEEN estimated that more than 2,000 hospitals in the United States used cardiac nuclear imaging (CNI), in 1979 and that this number will double by 1983, when expenditures are likely to exceed $200 million.[91] Clearly, medical perception of the clinical utility of these studies has grown, in large part as a function of the improved technology. Nuclear cardiology has come a long way since 1927, when Blumgart and Weiss injected radioactive radon intravenously to determine circulation time,[14] but the continual improvement in instrumentation and pharmaceuticals will make even today's methodologies seem relatively crude in five or ten years.

Cardiac nuclear imaging studies can be broadly categorized into two groups:

1. Studies of myocardial perfusion, viability, or acute necrosis. Examples are radiolabeled palmitic acid studies, thallium 201 perfusion scans, and technetium pyrophosphate infarct imaging. These studies evaluate events within the myocardium itself.

2. Studies of cardiac function or performance. The major example is radionuclide ventriculography. Function is determined from assessing changes in activity in the blood contained within the cardiac chambers and related structures, without direct visualization of the myocardium.

Cardiac nuclear imaging techniques are safe, may be performed noninvasively, and usually entail less than 1 rad in total body radiation dose (Table 2–1). Thus, these examinations can be repeated at frequent intervals with low morbidity, if clinically necessary. Generally they can be performed on sick patients, and most can be done with portable instrumentation. Nuclear techniques do not rely heavily on the geometric assumptions of contrast ventriculography, and they are less affected than echocardiography by interference from overlying structures such as bone or surgical dressings. Nuclear cardiology differs from echocardiography in that the techniques measure primarily physiologic rather than anatomical information.

To maximize the utility of CNI in clinical practice, a few general operating principles should be followed.

1. Each study should follow a standard protocol to ensure reproducibility. Variations from this protocol may be needed, depending on the clinical situation; the imaging physician should have cardiology training to understand the clinical rationale for the study.

2. Technical evaluation of an individual study should be done before the patient leaves the imaging area, since repeated or additional views may be needed. While semiautomated computer programs are extensively used in CNI, the final assessment of technical adequacy lies with the human operator.

3. The physician must be aware of the circumstances under which the study was acquired and which may affect the data. For example, proper interpretation of such studies would require knowledge of the patient's cardiac drug regimen. To evaluate these studies appropriately, a thorough knowledge of both the radiotracers and the instrumentation used to record the studies is important.

TABLE 2–1.—Dosimetry of Diagnostic Studies

PROCEDURE	DOSE (mrad)	ORGAN
Gated blood pool scan (20 mCi ^{99m}Tc-labeled RBCs)*†	290 (.0029 Gy)	Whole body
	290–350	Gonads
	1,900	Spleen
First-pass radionuclide ventriculogram (20 mCi $Tc04^{-}$)[65]	490	Whole body
	8,000	Gut
Myocardial perfusion (1.5 mCi ^{201}Tl thallous chloride)†	390	Whole body
	510	Gonads
	3,150	Kidneys
Echocardiogram	None	
Cardiac catheterization (varies widely with fluoroscopy time)[4, 46, 94]	28,000	Skin entrance dose
	12	Gonads
	1,400	
Chest x-ray, PA and lateral[138]	80	Skin entrance dose
	0.16	Gonads, male
	0.8	Gonads, female
Abdominal KUB, AP[138]	600	Skin entrance dose
	400	Gonads, male
	140	Gonads, female

*One gray (Gy) = 100 rad.
†Calculated by Frank Castronovo, Ph.D., from reference 109.

RADIOPHARMACEUTICALS

Radiopharmaceuticals or radioactive tracers generally consist of (1) a radionuclide which emits γ-rays (photons) or x-rays, which can be detected by a scintillation camera, and (2) a ligand which determines the tracer's biodistribution. The radionuclide tag (such as technetium 99m) may be placed on a physiologic marker such as human serum albumin or red blood cells. In some cases, these moieties reside in a single atom or molecule, such as thallium 201.

Below are defined some basic terms used in nuclear physics:

Activity: The number of nuclear transformations per unit time. The Curie (Ci) equals 3.7×10^{-10} disintegrations per second (dps) and is the special unit of activity; it will soon be replaced as the standard unit by the Becquerel (Bq), which equals 1 dps. The most common fractions of the Curie used are the millicurie (mCi) and the microcurie (μCi).

Decay, radioactive: Disintegration of the nucleus of an unstable nuclide by spontaneous emission of charged particles and/or photons. γ-Rays or photons with characteristic discrete energies are emitted during nuclear decay of some nuclides; these can be detected on interaction with matter. *X-rays* emanating from the atomic orbitals are essentially the same as γ-rays and may be used for nuclear medicine imaging. *Beta-particles* with mass and charge equal to the mass and charge of electrons are not useful for imaging but add to radiation dose. A unique type of beta-particle decay occurs in certain manmade isotopes, results in emission of *positrons,* and is discussed below.

Dose: A general term denoting the quantity of radiation or energy absorbed. The *absorbed dose* is the energy imparted to tissue by ionizing radiation per unit mass of the irradiated material at the place of interest. The unit of absorbed dose is the *rad,* which equals 100 ergs/gm. The rad will soon be replaced as the standard by the gray (Gy), which equals 100 rad.

Positrons: Positively charged particles with mass equal to that of electrons. On interaction with an electron, the electron-positron pair is annihilated and produces two 511-keV photons, which leave the collision site in opposite directions. The simultaneous emission of these two photons can be detected by a panel of opposing scintillation detectors connected with electronic coincidence circuitry, and thus the collision site may be localized in space if data are collected from multiple angles.

Prototype positron emission cameras are available only at a few research centers, as are the on-site cyclotrons needed to produce most of these short-lived nuclides.[7, 49, 102]

An ideal radionuclide for scintillation camera imaging should have the following properties: (1) Photon energy in the 80-keV to 300-keV range with a minimum of beta-particulate emissions, which add to patient radiation burden, but with energy high enough to escape the body and be detected externally. (2) A physical half-life equal to or greater than the time required to perform the study but not so long as to increase the radiation dose to the patient. (3) Suitable chemical forms that are localized by and taken up in the structure under study significantly faster than in the surrounding tissues (high target-to-background ratio). (4) Produces no alteration of the physiology under investigation. (5) Has low toxicity in the chemical form used for imaging.[7, 49, 116] Though much progress has been made in the area of radiopharmacy, to date no tracer has been found that adequately satisfies all these criteria.

TABLE 2–2.—Characteristics of Technetium 99m and Thallium 201[35, 127]

	TECHNETIUM 99M	THALLIUM 201
Characteristic energy	140 keV	69–80 keV (95%–98%)* 167 keV (8%–10%) 135 keV (2%–3%)
Physical half-life (T/½)	6–10 hr	73 hr
Dosage†	20–25 mCi [SI units: 740–925 MBq]	1–2 mCi [SI units: 37–74 MBq]

*Mercury x-ray.
†Adults. In children, dosages are individualized by surface area.

The two most widely used radionuclides in nuclear cardiology are technetium 99m (^{99m}Tc) and thallium 201 (^{201}Tl). Their physical parameters are listed in Table 2–2.

INSTRUMENTATION

For effective imaging, a number of phenomena must occur.[116] The radiotracer should distribute in proportion to the function under investigation, emit a photon with sufficient energy to traverse the chest wall, and then interact with a device which will permit its localization. Image quality is therefore largely a function of target-to-background (signal-to-noise) ratio, photon attenuation, and resolution of the imaging device, which consists of a scintillation camera, collimator, and display unit, usually connected to a computer.

The Scintillation Camera

Scintillation cameras, or gamma cameras, have three components: (1) a crystal that converts the γ-ray energy to visible light; (2) a photomultiplier (PM) tube that converts this light to an electronic signal, and (3) a processing unit that amplifies the signal and selects it for recording or rejects it by means of pulse height analysis.[82] Each of these steps is basically linear, with output amplitude proportional to amplitude of energy received.

The most commonly used gamma camera is the Anger camera (Fig 2–1).[3] The detector on this instrument consists of a single thallium-activated sodium iodide crystal, generally 25–35 cm in diameter and 0.64–1.25 cm thick. This thickness has been found to minimize Compton reactions and thus best localize the position of an event; however, a crystal of this size has limited photon-stopping capabilities, so optimum efficiency is achieved in the relatively limited range of photon energy below 200 keV. The scintillation produced by interaction with the γ-ray both propagates throughout the entire crystal and traverses the crystal to the back surface, where it is sensed by the PM tube.

Current-generation Anger cameras most commonly have 37 PM tubes optically coupled to the back of the crystal and closely packed in a hexagonal array. Anger "logic" localizes a scintillation on the crystal in the following manner. Each PM tube "sees" light from an event on the crystal and produces a voltage pulse proportional to the strength of the scintillation. For example, the tube closest to the event sees the most light and therefore produces the highest voltage pulse. Anger logic

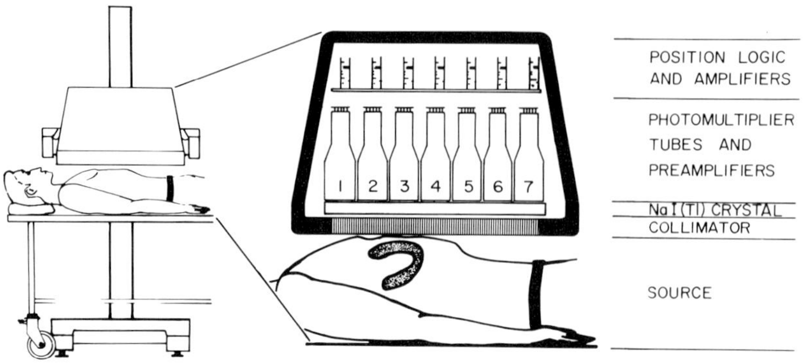

Fig 2–1.—Anger scintillation camera, schematic representation. (From Strauss H.W., et al.: *Am. J. Cardiol.* 46:1109–1116, 1980. Reproduced by permission.)

analyzes the voltages produced by the individual PM tubes and fixes the location of the event as x,y coordinates in space.[45] It may be seen, therefore, that resolution of low-energy photons is lower than that for high-energy photons since the scintillations in the crystal which reach the PM tube are less intense and, therefore, are associated with decreased certainty of positioning. The pulse height analyzer serves to further clarify the data: photons that are scattered have lost part of their energy before arriving at the radiation detector. The pulse height analyzer allows only those voltage pulse amplitudes which fall within a predetermined range to be recorded as "counts" into the data, and thus scattered photons may be screened out.[98] The pulses that pass pulse height analyses are then displayed on a cathode ray tube in a manner that replicates the regional distribution of photons emanating from the patient.

Selection of a camera for use in CNI is usually predicated on three variables: field size, intrinsic resolution, and count rate capacity. A standard 25-cm field of view is usually employed in nuclear cardiology, but 35-cm large-field cameras are not uncommon. For a given camera, as the energy window setting is widened to increase count rate, spatial resolution is adversely affected, because more scattered photons are recorded.[98] At high count rates, the Anger camera is said to have difficulty due to problems processing at high speed. This can result in apparent loss of sensitivity, where sensitivity is defined as the proportion of counts recorded to counts actually emitted by the patient. Over the past few years, sensitivity has been improving. High intrinsic spatial resolution, mobility, and applicability of the Anger camera to general nuclear medicine has popularized it for use in most types of radionuclide cardiac studies.

An alternative instrument for use in nuclear cardiology is the multicrystal scintillation camera, which features a rectangular array of 294 sodium iodide crystal detectors. Each crystal is optically coupled by light pipes to two PM tubes, one corresponding to the row and the other to the column in the array of crystals. A total of 35 PM tubes are used. Time-coincident pulses in both a row and a column PM tube identify the crystal in which the scintillation has occurred and thus localize the photon in space. Since all that is required is fast coincidence circuitry, event localization can be made significantly more rapidly than by Anger logic. Thus, the multicrystal camera is more sensitive at high count rates and is regarded by many as the instrument of choice for first-pass studies. However, spatial resolution during dynamic acquisition is obviously limited by the size of the individual crystals.[25, 143]

Minimal variations in specifications of individual PM tubes will yield a nonhomogeneous field. The uniformity of the instrument is critical in determining image quality and accurate quantitation of function and so the camera should be equipped with provisions for uniformity correction to less than 5% variation across the field, when possible.[95, 121]

Collimators

Since γ-ray and x-ray photons cannot be focused efficiently, a meaningful image can be recorded only when the source of photons entering the detector is known. A collimator is essentially a piece of lead, with a specified pattern of holes, that is placed just in front of the crystal. It is used to define the direction of photons reaching the crystal such that each photon-crystal interaction corresponds with a high degree of certainty to a defined reference point in space.

The pattern of holes as well as the width and depth of the septae between them define the field of view and spatial resolution. Multiple-hole collimators may have a parallel, converging, or diverging array of channels. There is generally a trade-off between resolution and sensitivity. While resolution is necessary for defining anatomy, sensitivity is needed to ensure statistical reliability of the data, and it also determines the length of study acquisition (inversely related to acquisition time). Parallel-hole collimators may be designated as "high-sensitivity," "high-resolution," or "all-purpose," a compromise between the other two. In practice, however, if a high-sensitivity collimator can decrease acquisition time and thus patient movement, in situations where the count rate is low it may yield a higher-resolution study. Each clinic or laboratory should determine the type of collimation needed for a particular study, since collimator labels such as "high-resolution" or "high-sensitivity" are placed by the manufacturers and specifications may vary considerably.[122, 143] The principal difference in image definition between high-resolution and high-sensitivity collimators is the rate at which resolution decreases as the object moves away from the collimator surface. This is important, since the heart is at a depth of 5 cm or more from the camera.[61] Differences at the collimator surface, where resolution is greatest for either type, are minimal. Thus, skin contact with the collimator is essential for good image quality (Fig 2–2).[45]

Parallel-hole collimation is used almost exclusively in CNI because it provides the best trade-off in spatial resolution and geometric efficiency for imaging large organs.[98] Most importantly, parallel-hole collimation yields no significant spatial distortion with depth imaging when compared with diverging- or converging-hole collimators. Since many CNI procedures, notably calculation of ejec-

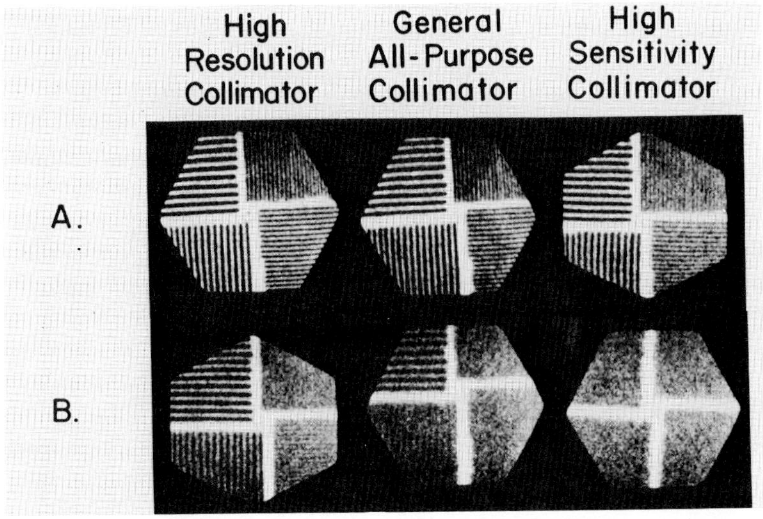

Fig 2–2.—One million-count images of 3-, 4-, 5-, and 6-mm bar phantom using a 2-mCi Tc-99m flood source and three common types of parallel-hole collimators. Note that maximal spatial resolution is achieved for all three collimators, with minimal differences between them in *row A,* with the source at the collimator face. However, noticeable differences in resolution are seen in *row B,* where the source is 7.5 cm from collimator.

tion fraction, assume a linear relationship between perceived counts and volume, non-parallel-hole collimators generally should not be used.[119, 135]

The Computer

Computer systems are used to acquire, analyze, and then display studies qualitatively as an image and quantitatively as numbers or curves. Interfaced to the gamma camera, they usually consist of a central processing unit, memory, and a terminal for data manipulation and information display. They must also have the capacity to transfer data to some form of long-term storage system. While it is possible to acquire and analyze some types of CNI data without a computer, optimally, all clinics doing CNI should use one. Computers allow the operator to perform multiple manipulations, such as count summation within defined regions of interest, background erasure, and contrast enhancement. The operator may try different approaches to data processing on the same study without destroying the original data. The images recorded by computer are as good as or better than those recorded on film.[98]

Ideally, the computer used for CNI should feature at least two disk drives, one for the program software and one for data storage, as well as a selection of data matrices (ranging from 32 × 32 to 256 × 256 pixels), with high count densities obtainable in each matrix. It must have the capacity for simultaneous easy viewing of both the cardiac image and physiologic data, such as the ECG, and must be able to process data quickly during the acquisition.[116] The system must accommodate the easy and rapid placement of a stationary pointer or outlining of a region of interest with a light pen or joystick. The computer must be able to generate time-activity curves for multiple regions of interest within an image,[33] as well as perform other manipulations such as data smoothing. There should be provision for side-by-side display of at least two studies simultaneously in either static or cinematic mode. Replay speed in the cinematic mode must be variable, since wall motion abnormalities may be perceived differently at different speeds. A full, variable gray scale of at least 256 shades should be available, since contrast enhancement is used to assess structures such as valve planes or chamber borders. The instrument must be capable of displaying images in different sizes. Optimally, an image should define a 3-degree arc on the viewer's retina; this corresponds to an image height of 5 cm when viewed at the distance of 1 meter.[117] All of these functions must be easily and continuously controllable by the operator.

Acquired data are placed into the core memory for manipulation, display, and eventual transfer to long-term storage. Storage is generally on magnetic tape or floppy disks. Disks are generally reliable, convenient, and significantly faster in accessing data than tape. But in the clinical environment, disks may be affected by dirt, dust, or even fingerprints, which may cause loss of part or all of the study. Also, disk storage is significantly more expensive than tape storage, often by a factor of three to five.[68] Some clinics use a combination of short-term floppy disk storage with transfer to tape for long-term filing.

Thus, the ability to differentiate normal structures from lesions on studies performed with modern gamma camera-computer systems depends on a number of factors, including photon energy, collimation, count density, the electronics of the display system, and the experience of the operator.

MYOCARDIAL PERFUSION STUDIES

One of the most pressing clinical problems is to identify patients with coronary artery disease prior to myocardial infarction and irreversible damage. Significant numbers of false negative and false positive exercise tolerance ECGs have engendered interest in ways to evaluate myocardial perfusion accurately and noninvasively. Today, ^{201}Tl is the agent used to noninvasively assess myocardial perfusion and to improve the results of exercise treadmill testing.[5, 16] The fundamental differences between contrast coronary arteriography, an anatomical technique, and ^{201}Tl perfusion imaging, a physiologic technique, cannot be overstated. The morphological identification of a stenosed coronary artery at catheterization may or may not have physiologic consequences on the perfusion of the heart muscle. In addition, new techniques in perfusion imaging may in the future be used for studying cardiac metabolism under a variety of pathophysiologic conditions.

Perfusion studies of the heart are predicated on the Sapirstein principle. Sapirstein noted that if a tracer is almost totally extracted by an organ and rapidly cleared from the blood by other tissues on the first pass, then the regional distribution of the tracer in the organ is flow related.[64, 100, 101] Applied to the heart, this means that uptake of the tracer is proportional to myocardial blood flow,[5] but only soon after injection, before distribution is altered by the ongoing processes of equilibrium.[113]

Early work on myocardial perfusion imaging centered on $^{43}K^{+}$ and, to a lesser degree, on ^{81}Rb. The potassium 43 ion was shown to be highly extracted by the myocardium,[73] and $^{43}K^{+}$ distribution correlated well with flow, as demonstrated by the distribution of microspheres.[92, 145] Potassium 43 ion studies also showed that perfusion through stenotic arteries at rest might become inadequate when myocardial oxygen demands are increased, such as during exercise.[124] Soon, however, interest began to move toward ^{201}Tl. This radionuclide displayed higher extraction and retention by the myocardium and was considered to be more suitable for imaging due to its low-energy x-ray and relatively lower hepatic and gastric uptake.[32, 64, 66, 114] Thallium 201 is cyclotron-produced and is commercially supplied as ^{201}Tl thallous chloride with a half-life of 73 hours, which decays by electron-capture to mercury 201. Photons useful for imaging are the 68–80 keV mercury x-rays (95%–98% abundance) and the γ-rays of 135 keV (2%–3%) and 167 keV (8%–10%).[35, 66]

After intravenous injection, 8%–10% of ^{201}Tl is extracted by the lungs before the remainder is distributed to other organs in proportion to their share of the cardiac output.[88] The myocardium receives approximately 4% of the total cardiac output, and within physiologic range it extracts 85%–88% of the ^{201}Tl presented to it on the first pass.[88, 139] Thus, the heart muscle will extract about 3%–3.5% of the injected dose.[20] Within the myocardium itself, the uptake of ^{201}Tl is linearly related to regional blood flow.[77] Myocardial ^{201}Tl extraction is probably not significantly affected by ischemia until cell death occurs.[88]

At first, ^{201}Tl perfusion images were acquired after two separate injections. The initial set of images was usually obtained immediately after injection of ^{201}Tl at peak exercise to define blood flow under conditions of stress, and the second set was acquired immediately after injection at rest, at least three days later. (The hiatus resulted from the 73-hour half-life of the tracer.) Defects in uptake seen on both sets of images were thought to represent zones of scar, while those seen on exercise scans but not on scans obtained at rest were thought to represent stress-induced ischemic zones.[78] However, it was soon shown that some ^{201}Tl defects noted at rest filled in if imaging was carried out long enough after injection, and it was believed that these represented zones of chronic underperfusion.[9, 42] Thus, it became apparent that the two-injection technique might not adequately differentiate ischemic but viable from nonviable myocardium unless delayed images were obtained. In 1977, Pohost et al. suggested that sequential imaging for 1–6 hours after a single dose of ^{201}Tl injected during exercise could differentiate between ischemia and infarction or scar.[89] They also noted that defects related to ischemia would resolve in time, calling this phenomenon "redistribution," and that defects related to scar or infarction would persist. The single-dose technique offers advantages over the double-injection method. It is probably more physiologic; it achieves a 50% reduction in radiopharmaceutical administration, thus decreasing both radiation burden and cost to the patient; it yields lower background activity than on images obtained at rest; and it requires only one patient visit.[78, 88] For these reasons, the single-injection method has become the standard procedure.

Thus, initial distribution of ^{201}Tl is closely related to regional blood flow according to the Sapirstein principle, so that defects on initial images may be related to either underperfusion and/or scar or infarction. Defects in zones of scar or infarction persist due to lack of effective flow. However, initial perfusion defects related to ischemia will resolve or redistribute with time.

Though not completely understood, the redistribution of ^{201}Tl into ischemic zones apparently occurs via the following mechanism[8, 43, 88]:

1. Blood activity rapidly falls after the first pass as ^{201}Tl is extracted by multiple organ beds.
2. Over time, there is exchange between the cardiac, the extracardiac organ, and the vascular compartments as ^{201}Tl concentration equilibrates between them.
3. Thallium 201 in the normal heart, therefore, will gradually clear in relation to the large myocardial to blood concentration gradient which is achieved within the first few passes of tracer.
4. Since blood flow and hence ^{201}Tl delivery to ischemic myocardium is reduced but these cells still efficiently extract the tracer, ischemic tissue will eventually increase ^{201}Tl concentration, but this peak will occur later than in normally perfused myocardium.

Thus, the intracellular ^{201}Tl concentration at any time depends on the initial concentration and the net difference between amounts entering and leaving the cell. According to the model above, the normal myocardium slowly releases the thallium (20%–30% clearance at 4 hours), while ischemic areas may clear more slowly or experience net accumulation of tracer (Fig 2–3). This accounts for the apparent fill-in of defects in the later images. The major determinant of clearance rate, however, is blood activity and any factors that affect blood activity clearance.[88]

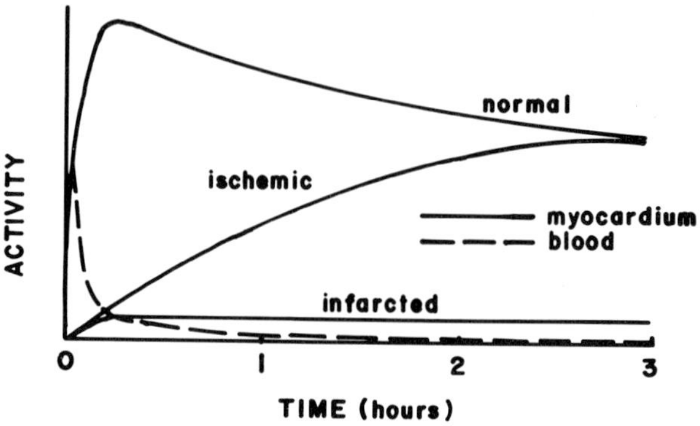

Fig 2–3.—Relative thallium activity in blood and normal and abnormal myocardium as a function of time after injection at exercise.

Acquisition of Thallium Studies

Thallium exercise studies should be acquired using the Anger camera with an all-purpose, parallel-hole collimator. The main x-ray photon peak at 68–80 keV is employed for imaging. If the instrument allows using multiple peaks, then the γ-ray 135-keV and 167-keV peaks may also be used to increase sensitivity. A dose of 1.5–2 mCi (56–74 MBq) of ^{201}Tl thallous chloride is used in adults. Ideally, the patient should be in a fasting state and beta-blockers such as propranolol should be discontinued before the examination, if possible.

Stress testing in a nuclear medicine laboratory should be done with the same precaution that prevails for (nonimaging) routine cardiology stress testing, under the continued supervision of a qualified physician certified in life support.[40, 50] A crash cart and defibrillator should be immediately available. One of any number of standard protocols (e.g., the Bruce protocol), may be used. While hemodynamic responses such as a change in heart rate or end-diastolic volume may differ somewhat among types of exercise,[40, 90, 126] these differences are clinically insignificant for many patients.[78] It is the *level* of stress that is paramount.[23] The object of exercise testing is to evoke the peak stress response, since the greater the rise in heart rate blood pressure product, the greater the likelihood of uncovering coronary artery disease.[88] The scan cannot be adequately interpreted without reviewing the ECG, blood pressure, and work load response.

The stress laboratory should be adjacent to the nuclear medicine imaging area. With an intravenous line in place, the patient exercises in either the supine or upright positions. At maximal exercise, the patient is injected with the radioisotope and is encouraged to continue exercising for an additional 30–45 seconds to allow initial distribution as well as blood clearance of the tracer.[88] If the patient develops chest pain, the dose is injected and exercise is discontinued. The patient is placed in the supine position under the camera and a postexercise ECG is obtained. (Any object on the chest wall which could attenuate the image, such as a breast prothesis or coins in a pocket, should have been removed.) The precordial leads are removed and the anterior image is obtained; next, limb leads are removed and the 50-degree and 70-degree left posterior oblique (LPO) images are acquired. It is essential that imaging begin as soon as possible after exercise, certainly no later than three minutes, since significant redistribution may occur soon after injection.[8, 104] The anterior image is generally acquired first because it exposes the largest quantity of myocardium. Women should be positioned for the low left anterior oblique (LAO) view with the torso at a 50-degree oblique angle to the table to minimize attenuation by breast tissue. Each image is collected for seven to ten minutes, which allows acquisition of 300,000 counts per frame with the standard adult dosages. These acquisition times represent an empirical compromise between length for optimal resolution and brevity for depicting transient defects before they fill in.[88] Delayed images (without exercise) are acquired 2½–4 hours later. It is critical that the delayed images be collected for the same time and in identical projections as the initial images to ensure technical adequacy of the study. Multiple views are essential, since lesions are best defined when seen either in tangent or en face.[32] A computer should be interfaced with the camera, since subtle defects are best determined by computer display.[88] If a computer is not available, an isolated gamma camera may be used and images should be collected for preset counts in order to normalize the later images to the initial views for analysis.[78, 88]

Thallium studies may be done at rest to define areas of infarction or chronic underperfusion. The rest scan is a less sensitive technique for the detection of coronary artery disease than the exercise study. Nevertheless, rest ^{201}Tl studies are extremely useful for patients who cannot exercise, for example, following acute myocardial infarction. The protocol for a rest acquisition is essentially the same as for an exercise study, except that imaging begins 15 minutes after injection of the radiopharmaceutical.

Rest ^{201}Tl scans can be obtained in the acute stages of myocardial infarction to assess infarct size and to determine if significant areas of viable myocardium are still at risk. The ability of ^{201}Tl radionuclide imaging to detect acute myocardial infarction decreases as the interval between the onset of symptoms and scanning increases.[135]

The sensitivity of ^{201}Tl detection of coronary artery disease in patients who cannot exercise can be increased by administering dipyridamole intravenously with the patient at rest.[1, 47, 78, 120] This drug is an adenosine deaminase inhibitor and causes high levels of adenosine, a potent coronary vasodilator, to accrue. Adenosine has a profound effect on the coronary bed. Arteries with fixed stenoses that do not interfere with blood flow at rest may not dilate, as much as normal vessels. Administration of ^{201}Tl at the peak effect of the drug permits identification of these differences in flow due to coronary artery disease. With continuous ECG monitoring, the patient is injected with ^{201}Tl after an infusion of a total dose of 0.56 mg/kg of dipyridamole over four to five minutes, and imaging is begun. Clinical evaluation of this technique relative to ^{201}Tl exercise testing is ongoing, and early results have been encouraging. In theory, this approach is less risky for the patient than exercise testing since it does not usually result in ischemia.

Evaluation of Thallium Studies

The evaluation of ^{201}Tl images must be both technical and substantive. Technical factors that can degrade the quality of perfusion studies include artifacts on the chest wall, which can usually be recognized by their relative positions in multiple views, and variations in camera field uniformity, which can influence image quality and even create artifacts within the myocardium that could affect study accuracy. A very extensive inferior wall defect seen in the 70-degree LAO view (or left lateral view, if used), but not visualized in the other projection may actually result from a high left hemidiaphragm and must be recognized as such. Attenuation by breast tissue may yield an artifactual defect in the anterolateral or anterior wall or in the septum. Excessive patient movement or deep respiration may cause an apparent thickening or hypertrophy of the myocardium and may mask the presence of a small perfusion defect. Generally, this artifact is seen only in the initial anterior view, which is taken immediately after exercise. Some researchers, therefore, routinely acquire repeated anterior views immediately after the high LAO exercise view. Ongoing operator involvement and evaluation during the study acquisition can help minimize some of these problems. Decreased splanchnic uptake should be evident on initial views if the level of stress attained was adequate. A radiopharmaceutical dose that infiltrates the subcutaneous tissue will alter tracer kinetics, causing poor uptake on initial views, altered redistribution, and a technically inadequate study.

The initial and delayed views should be projected side by side on the computer display. The activity concentration (counts per pixel) should be determined for the zone of myocardium that appears brightest. The values thus displayed can be used for calculating myocardial clearance rates. Poor clearance can be a consequence of globally decreased initial uptake. This may be seen with extensive three-vessel disease, in the absence of focal defects. The later images should be multiplied by the inverse of the clearance factor so that the count densities of the two sets are equalized.

Lung activity as a fraction of myocardial activity on the initial anterior image should be assessed next. Count densities of lung tissue usually do not exceed one-half the count density in the part of the myocardium with the greatest ^{201}Tl concentration. The exact mechanism for abnormally increased lung uptake is not entirely understood, but it is related in part to an elevated left atrial pressure. Its presence should alert the observer to the probability of an underlying impairment of left ventricular (LV) function.[12, 63] (This finding may be the only clue to the presence of coronary artery disease in an otherwise normal study.)

The size of the LV cavity and the thickness of its myocardium should be assessed. Significant dilation after exercise is an abnormal finding indicative of decreased functional reserve. It is important to realize that an initial ^{201}Tl "defect" may appear to fill in on later images when a dilated LV returns to normal size. This artifact is most frequently seen at the apex, which is normally thin and nonhomogeneous.[32] Myocardial thickness is readily evaluated visually and may be manually measured by pixel counting on the computer display. Increased septal to free wall ratios in the 50-degree LAO view may be seen in idiopathic hypertrophic subaortic stenosis.[26] Although the major application of ^{201}Tl imaging has been in assessment of the LV, there is evidence that ^{201}Tl studies may aid in the evaluation of the right ventricle (RV) as well. Thallium 201 has been used to assess the effects of pulmonary hypertension on the RV myocardium,[31] and it may be of value in looking at RV perfusion as well.[24] The RV is normally well seen after injection at exercise, and it is faintly visible on computer-displayed, rest-injected images. The observer should, therefore, note the thickness and perfusion pattern of the RV as well as the LV. The pattern of ^{201}Tl distribution within the LV myocardium should next be evaluated. The normal heart exhibits homogeneous distribution of the tracer. It may be necessary to view the images at a range of contrast: low contrast for the RV which

TABLE 2–3.—Evaluation of Exercise Thallium Scans

CHARACTERISTICS	COMMENTS
Technical factors	Chest wall artifacts, patient movement and positioning, attenuation by breast and diaphragm
Activity below diaphragm	Splanchnic activity (except kidney) on initial images should be absolutely decreased and decreased when compared to delayed images, if adequate stress achieved
Pulmonary activity	Lung activity ≤½ maximum myocardial activity on initial anterior view; if increased, probable LV dysfunction
Myocardial clearance	25%–40% washout of LV activity normally between initial and 3–4 hour delay images; less than 20% clearance indicates infiltrated injection, low cardiac index, or poor global perfusion, in absence of regional defects in uptake
Right ventricle	Absence on initial images suggests right coronary disease; thickened myocardium suggests RV pressure or volume overload
Left ventricle: size and myocardial thickness	Dilation with exercise suggest LV dysfunction; evaluate possibility of LVH, ASH
Left ventricle: thallium distribution	Normal distribution homogeneous Persistent defect: infarction Initial defect, redistribution: ischemia Initial defect, partial redistribution: infarction and/or severe ischemia

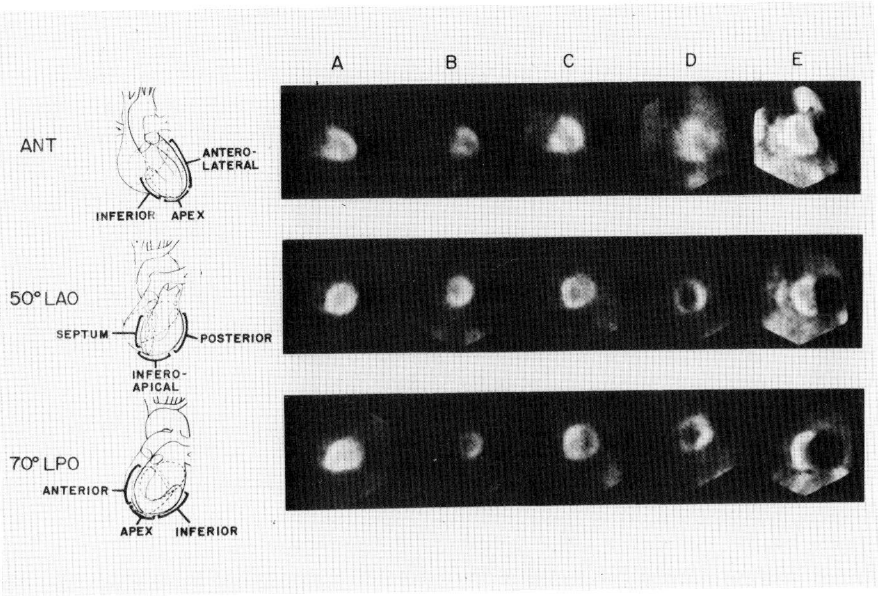

Fig 2–4.—Thallium distribution, examples from five patients. *A,* normal; *B,* defect in septum; *C,* defect in LV posterior wall; *D,* extensive defect in anterolateral, anteroseptal, and apical inferior regions (increase in pulmonary activity is seen on anterior view); *E,* large posterior pseudoaneurysm.

has a low tracer concentration and high contrast for LV evaluation.[31, 122] The need for contrast enhancement results from the low target to background rate ratios achieved with ^{201}Tl.

Perfusion defects may appear as a region of normal count density that is thinner than normal myocardium when viewed tangentially, as a full-thickness region with decreased count density, or as a combination of these patterns. Persistent defects are, by definition, stable over the course of the study. Redistribution is seen as a normalization of these defects on the delayed views and may be partial or total. Clinically significant defects usually exhibit at least a 25% decrease in counts relative to normal areas.[122] Small defects are often seen on one view, but defects involving extensive portions of the myocardium generally can be seen in multiple projections. Papillary muscles are variably seen as "hot areas" on the anterior and posterior wall. Great care must be taken in evaluating the basal aspects of the myocardium since these are normally obscured by valve planes, the aorta, and the pulmonary outflow tract (Table 2–3; Fig 2–4).

Obviously, if the initial ^{201}Tl images are entirely normal, it is not strictly necessary to obtain the delayed views. However, the range of normal on the initial study makes it possible to miss subtle changes that become apparent only when the initial and delayed views are viewed together. Therefore, it is preferable to obtain delayed views even when the initial study is apparently normal.

Despite its proven clinical utility, ^{201}Tl is not an ideal tracer for perfusion studies. Its abundant photon, at 80 keV, experiences significant soft tissue attenuation, especially those photons emanating from areas of the heart farther away from the camera in planar images.[97] This radiopharmaceutical yields low target to background ratios and is relatively expensive, costing approximately $100 per dose. Furthermore, its physical and biologic half-lives are much longer than is needed for acquiring the data. This necessitates limiting the administered dose to maintain an acceptable radiation burden while yet acquiring useful diagnostic data.

New Techniques in Perfusion Imaging

Intuitively, it would seem that tomographic techniques could improve the detection of subtle perfusion defects. In single-photon emission tomography, standard gamma-emitting radionuclides such as technetium or thallium are used. The region of interest is imaged from multiple projections and the data reconstructed from filtered back projection. An alternative to transverse section tomography is limited angle tomography, where the heart is viewed from several angles and then projected to different regions of the crystal. The data are reconstructed by computer algorithm to yield a series of images which correspond to multiple planes or sections of the heart.[132] Out-of-plane information is defocused and lesions may become more clearly delineated, at least in theory, since there is little superimposition of normally perfused myocardium over areas of decreased perfusion. These techniques require the use of specially constructed tomographic collimators and optimally should be performed using a wide-field scintillation camera. Seven-pinhole collimator tomography has shown no advantage over standard planar ^{201}Tl imaging, in large part because of lessened specificity and image distortion.[97, 131, 132] Work with the rotating slant-hole collimator continues, but significant problems remain. Interest has been shown in using positron-emitting radionuclides such as rubidium 82, rubidium 81 and gallium 68 albumin microspheres for precise location of perfusion defects.[76] However, positron-emission tomography still remains essentially a research tool with limited clinical applicability.

Quantitation techniques for ^{201}Tl imaging are also under investigation. Simple and complex interpolative background subtraction techniques have been described,[75, 130] but these are based on pericardiac activity, which may poorly reflect the activity truly emanating from behind the heart.[44, 75] The controversy over what, if any, type of background correction should be used has not been resolved. Quantitative techniques may, in some instances, improve accuracy and decrease observer variance, but in general these techniques have not added much clinical information to that obtainable by visual evaluation of ^{201}Tl images by experienced observers.

ASSESSMENT OF VENTRICULAR FUNCTION

"Radionuclide ventriculography" is the general term applied to a class of nuclear imaging techniques used to assess cardiac function. The nomenclature may also denote the specific methodology by which the radioventriculogram (RVG) is acquired; thus, an RVG may either be "gated" or "nongated." Gated scans can be acquired during the first pass of a labeled bolus through the heart or after equilibrium of the tracer within the entire vascular space (blood pool scanning). Alternatively, nongated first-pass studies can also be used to assess cardiac function. First-pass studies are often called "radionuclide angiograms."

To record a gated scan after injection of a tracer, an ECG-triggered switch, or "gate," is used to select a specific portion of the cardiac cycle during which the display oscilloscope or computer will accept data.[144] The gate concept was introduced in 1969 by Mullins and co-workers, who used it to collect a single end-diastolic image to assess ventricular volume.[74] Soon after, Strauss et al. and Zaret et al. acquired an end-diastolic image for 200–400 beats, moved the gate position relative to the R wave, and collected an end-systolic image over an additional 200–400 beats. By comparing these two static images, they were able to calculate the LV ejection fraction and assess regional wall motion.[123, 144] Introduction of high-speed computers enabled *multiple gating*. This technique allows acquisition of images through most or all of the cardiac cycle. The R wave trigger initiates recording of image data into the first frame of the computer memory for a preset time. Then data are recorded into the second frame for the same preset time, and so on. When the next R wave occurs, the gate resets, data are recorded into the first frame once again, and the entire process of recording into sequential frames is repeated (Fig 2–5). Data from corresponding parts in each cycle are added together into the computer memory until sufficient counts are recorded. The frames can then be replayed as an endless-loop cinematic display.[2, 27]

Gated acquisition yields a final study which depicts one "average" cardiac cycle. Equilibrium gated studies routinely collect data from 100 to 600 cardiac cycles. In equilibrium studies, all four

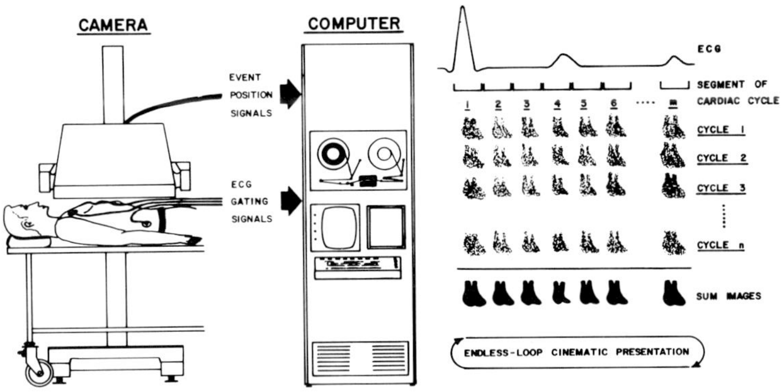

Fig 2–5.—Multigated acquisition. The computer memory is commonly divided into 14 to 32 matrices. The ECG R wave starts acquisition into the first matrix for a preset time, then into the second for the same time, and so on. The process is repeated with the next R wave. Data from multiple cycles are thus added together, and the matrices are viewed in an endless-loop cinematic display. (From Beller G.A., et al.: Radionuclide imaging, in Johnson R., Haber E., Austen G. (eds.): *The Practice of Cardiology.* Boston, Little, Brown & Co, 1980. Also from Strauss H.W., et al.: *Am. J. Cardiol.* 46:1109–1116, 1980. Reproduced by permission.)

cardiac chambers may be visualized simultaneously, and sequential observations can be performed for 4 to 10 hours on a single injection; thus, blood pool studies easily lend themselves to assessing the effects of an intervention such as a drug or exercise on cardiac function, as well as to assessment of regional wall motion on multiple views. Study quality is not severely effected by transient arrhythmias, although image quality may be degraded if more than 10%–20% of the beats are aberrant.

First-pass imaging does not depend on electrocardiographic gating. After bolus injection and a 10-ml saline flush, images of the first transit are acquired on a multicrystal camera (System 77, Baird Corp., Bedford, Mass.). Time-activity curves of right ventricular, pulmonary, and left ventricular transit are generated. This method has the major advantage of rapid acquisition and true temporal and spatial separation of right and left ventricle. Its disadvantage is that lower counts result in worse image resolution.

Blood Pool Labeling

Technetium 99m is the decay product of its parent, molybdenum 99. The daughter ^{99m}Tc can be separated at regular intervals with the use of a commercially available alumina column generator. On elution with normal saline, the technetium is separated from the column as technetium pertechnetate, while the parent nuclide remains strongly bound. Elution of the generator is generally performed on-site in the clinical radiopharmacy. Technetium 99m decays to technetium 99, with a half-life of 6.01 hours, emitting a 140-keV gamma photon.[35, 116, 127]

To record a diagnostic-quality equilibrium blood pool scan, the radiotracer must distribute uniformly throughout and stay within that vascular space for the time required to acquire the study.[53] Initially, ^{99m}Tc-labeled human serum albumin was used, in large part because the labeling procedure was relatively easy and convenient and could be done on a once-daily basis. However, significant loss of radiopharmaceutical to the extravascular space and liver uptake yielded low target to background ratios and, therefore, low-resolution images. To eliminate these problems, work began on methods to label autologous red blood cells with ^{99m}Tc. Early methods were so cumbersome that Strauss and Pitt, in 1977, were moved to declare that red cell labeling was unsuitable for routine clinical use in a busy clinic.[119] That, of course, is no longer the case. In vitro methods of technetium labeling improved[108] and then were superceded by in vivo techniques. In vivo labeling eliminated the risk of external manipulation of the patient's red cells prior to reinjection and were felt to be less complicated.[51, 86, 112] Though relatively time-consuming, the advantages of the technetium-labeled red blood cell method have led to its becoming the standard tracer for gated equilibrium studies in most nuclear cardiology laboratories.

Recently, Callahan et al.[28] developed a simple, efficient manner for red cell labeling which yields a very high target to background ratio. This "in vitro" method can achieve 95% labeling of the technetium activity to the hemoglobin beta chain of red cells. The method is given below. Adult dosages are used throughout.

1. The patient is injected with 1 mg of stannous chloride 15–20 minutes prior to labeling with the technetium pertechnetate.
2. A standard injection kit including a butterfly catheter, a 4-way stopcock, saline, alcohol sponges, and gloves are needed. In addition to the standard kit, two 2-cc single-dose vials of 10 units/cc of heparin are required. Withdraw 4 cc of heparin into a 10-cc syringe containing 4 cc of saline (this is used to foreflush).
3. Approximately 15–20 minutes after the injection of stannous chloride, the butterfly catheter with the 4-way stopcock affixed to the end is inserted into the patient's vein (preferably an antecubital vein).
4. The heparin-saline is injected through the butterfly to heparinize the catheter.
5. A syringe containing the technetium pertechnetate in a *syringe shield* is affixed to the free port on the 4-way stopcock.
6. The heparinized saline within the catheter and the patient's blood are withdrawn into the syringe containing the technetium pertechnetate. Syringe volume should be 3 cc. Withdrawing the heparinized saline and blood into the technetium syringe insures anticoagulation.
7. Following withdrawal of the patient's blood in the syringe, the catheter is again filled with heparinized saline. The butterfly catheter should remain heparinized for the duration of the incubation of technetium 99m with the RBCs to prevent thrombosis.
8. The patient's blood and technetium pertechnetate should remain in the syringe and be gently agitated for no less than 10 minutes. At this point, a standard Oldendorf injection can be performed to record a bolus flow study.
9. Following injection of the ^{99m}Tc-labeled red cells, the catheter should be removed from the patient's vein.

Acquisition of Gated Blood Pool Studies

Data are usually recorded both at rest and on exercise with a standard field-of-view camera and a low-energy, general all-purpose collimator peaked on the technetium photon energy of 140 keV with a 25% window. Autologous red blood cells labeled with 20–25 mCi of ^{99m}Tc are injected and imaging can begin almost immediately. An information density of 300 counts per pixel yields satisfactory resolution; each view can be acquired in approximately 10 minutes. (A picture element or pixel refers to the elemental data unit of the computer matrix.)

The length of each frame is determined from the patient's RR interval. Experience has shown that 16 frames per cycle provides adequate temporal resolution for clinical evaluation of regional wall motion and ejection fraction. Some laboratories use a 24- or 32-frame acquisition; high temporal resolution is particularly important for calculation of ejection and filling rates. Acquisition of the entire cycle is preferred, although sacrifice of mid-late diastole is sometimes needed to allow framing rates which are short enough ($\leq$ 60 msec) to adequately characterize both end-systole and end-diastole in the presence of a slow heart rate. The computer should simultaneously display the image, the patient's ECG, and a running total of counts accumulated so that the operator can continually evaluate image quality and gating consistency.[117]

Blood pool studies should be acquired in at least two and preferably three views to best assess regional wall motion and anatomy. The anterior and LAO views can be obtained with the patient supine, thus ensuring reproducibility and minimal patient motion,[119] while the LPO view can be acquired with the patient supported on his right side (Figs 2–6 and 2–7).

The anterior view is used to assess the right atrium, tricuspid valve plane, RV, pulmonary outflow tract, and the anterolateral and apical aspects of the LV. The 40- to 50-degree LAO view should be optimized to show uniform septal thickness and is obtained to maximally separate the left and right ventricles; it is the view generally used for calculation of the LV ejection fraction (EF). The 30-degree LPO view, in essence a "flipped" RAO image, can be obtained to best show the long axis of the LV.[117] It is also the best projection in which to assess left atrial size. While the RAO projection is used in contrast angiography, it is not optimal for equilibrium blood pool imaging with a parallel-hole collimator because RV activity is superimposed on the LV. Furthermore, the large gap

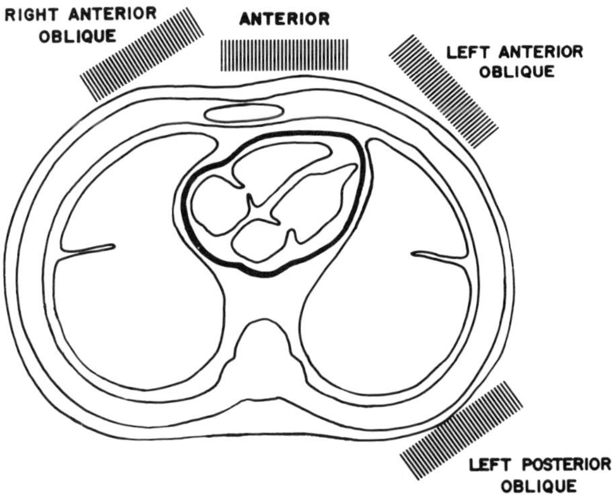

Fig 2–6.—Standard views used in radionuclide ventriculography. Transverse section through thorax looking cephalad. Positions identified on figure refer to the collimator position on the chest wall.

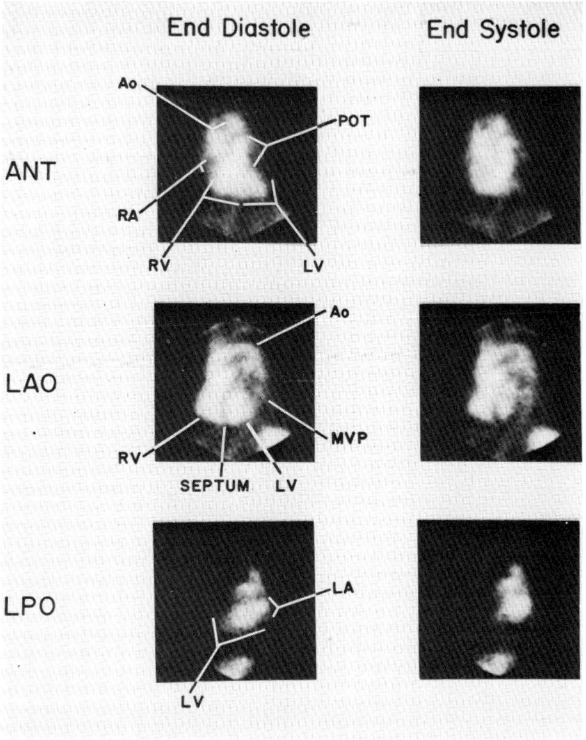

Fig 2–7.—Gated equilibrium blood pool scan in three standard views. *RA,* right atrium; *RV,* right ventricle; *MVP,* mitral valve plane; *LA,* left atrium; *LV,* left ventricle; *Ao,* aorta; *POT,* pulmonary outflow tract.

between collimator and LV in this view results in decreased resolution of LV borders.[117] To isolate the right heart, an RAO image is often acquired as a gated first-pass study, usually in conjunction with and immediately preceding the equilibrium blood pool scan.

Specific views should be individualized to the patient, especially if there is significant cardiac rotation within the chest or marked chamber enlargement. For example, significant RV dilation may displace the LV posteriorly and decrease ventricular separation on a 45-degree LAO view. In this case, a steeper LAO image should be acquired. Occasionally studies are requested for estimation of the LVEF only. Because LVEF is calculated from the LAO view exclusively, there is a temptation to do only a single-view study. This should be avoided, if possible, and at least one other view (generally the anterior) should be obtained, since an unusual anatomical pattern that is unappreciated on the single LAO view can alter the quantitative estimate of EF. Recently a slant-hole collimator has been developed to acquire gated studies in a single, caudal-tilt, modified LAO projection.[83] The clinical efficacy of this technique, especially with regard to assessment of wall motion, remains to be evaluated.

Problems and Limitations in Acquisition

Technical problems, though not frequent, may be encountered during the acquisition of the gated blood pool scan. Poor technetium labeling of the red cells may result in decreased resolution, with a poor target to background ratio and increased gastric activity. This may occur, for example, if inadequate time is left between steps of the labeling procedure, since labeling is both temperature- and time-dependent. Electrodes in the field of view may give rise to artifactual "cold" lesions or may obscure cardiac anatomy.

The gating process itself is prone to disturbance. Loose ECG leads will cause poor gating and gating to random noise, yielding a study with an artifactual decrease in heart function. Pacemaker spikes or large T waves may cause "double gating"; this problem can be corrected by moving the leads to minimize the height of the second, undesired trigger spike.

Since systole shortens proportionately less than diastole as heart rate rises, small variations in pulse rate during acquisition will not significantly affect data of interest, that is, end-diastole through end-systole. Rhythm disturbances can cause distortion of the recorded data if they are severe enough. (A significant slowing of the pulse from baseline during acquisition could theoretically cause the deletion of true end-systole, though this rarely happens in practice.) Wide swings in heart rate or irregular gating will cause an underestimation of true cardiac function. Inappropriate framing intervals can often be recognized either by a "snapping back" or apparent temporal discontinuity in the later part of the cardiac cycle as it is displayed. It is important to determine whether diffuse hypokinesis is real or results from a gating artifact caused by aberrations in heart rate. If changes in RV volume or in the right or left atrium are observed in the face of decreased LV function, then the left ventricular hypokinesis cannot be artifactual.[118]

A sudden coarsening in the image quality as the initial part of the cycle with higher counts is replaced by the portion with lower counts may signal a regular cardiac event. This problem should be suspected if a greater than 10% variation in counts per frame is seen through the cardiac cycle. Total counts per frame should remain relatively constant if the LV comprises only part of the field of view.[121]

Atrial fibrillation and multifocal premature contractions may cause irregular gating disturbances, with a gradual drop in counts through the cardiac cycle. Arrhythmia filtering can be used to delete beats not falling within a specified RR interval. However, this may prolong acquisition time significantly. Arrhythmia filtering should be used in clinical practice only rarely and is generally contraindicated during exercise gated scans, where a loss of beats is not well tolerated due to the short time available for acquisition.[117] If aberrant beats constitute more than 10% of the total, image quality will be affected, and if they constitute more than 20% of the total, consideration should be given to postponing the study until rhythm is controlled.

At the conclusion of the study, data are generally stored on film as well as on magnetic tape or floppy disk. The film should show at least the end-diastolic and end-systolic images and a subtracted "stroke volume" image in each view. In addition, the LV time-activity curve used for EF determination, the calculated EF, end-diastolic volume, heart rate, total number of beats sampled, and the number of aberrant beats should be listed.

Evaluation of the Gated Scan

Analysis of the gated scan should consist of both an assessment of the technical adequacy of the study and a substantive interpretation of the data. The technical factors that affect image quality have already been discussed. Substantive analysis is two-phased. The physician first renders a *qualitative* determination of structure and function, including the size of the chambers and great vessels, global function, regional wall motion, thickness of the free walls and septum, and a determination of whether there is increased separation between the heart and surrounding tissues due to either pericardial fluid or excessive fat. In addition, distortions of the LV shape due to false or true aneurysms should also be considered.[141, 142] For the physician to make these determinations effectively, the multigated study should be displayed cinematically at different rates, from stop motion to faster than real time, and images from previous and current studies or from multiple views within a single study should be viewed side by side for comparison. *Quantitative* analysis of function generally consists of determination of LVEF. Additional quantitative measures may include determination of RVEF, regional EF, dV/dt, quantitative wall motion, or LV volume (Table 2–4).

Calculation of Ejection Fraction

The term "ejection fraction" was introduced by Folse and Braunwald in 1962.[39] Ejection fraction has been found to have valuable diagnostic and therapeutic implications. The need for rapid noninvasive determination of the EF has been one of the prime factors in the development of nuclear cardiology as a discipline. Initially, the LVEF was obtained by applying standard biplane angiographic formulas to gated end-diastolic and end-systolic images. While this method correlated well with the LVEF measured by contrast ventriculography,[123] it was difficult and time-consuming to

TABLE 2–4.—Evaluation of Radionuclide Ventriculograms

CHARACTERISTICS OR STRUCTURES	COMMENTS
Technical factors	Quality of gating, chest wall artifacts
Gated first-pass study: RAO position	RA size and function; reflux from RA into IVC during RV systole indicates tricuspid regurgitation; calculation of RVEF; general evaluation of LV size and function
Gated equilibrium study	
Evaluation of pericardiac lucency	LV hypertrophy, pericardial effusion
Great vessels	Pulmonary outflow tract is equal to or minimally larger than aorta
Right atrium	Triangular shape with tricuspid valve plane well-defined in anterior view; periatrial fat pad often well defined; normally contracts from lateral aspect toward valve plane
Right ventricle	Thin RV myocardium not normally seen around blood pool; systole: movement of tricuspid valve, may see pulmonary outflow tract contracted; apex normally shows mild to moderate systolic movement; contractions should be synchronous; RV dysfunction generally manifested by dilation
Interventricular septum	Thickens and moves posteriorly during systole; best defined on LAO view
Left atrium	Slightly smaller than RA; normally not seen on anterior view; LA appendage variably seen on LAO view; LA size best seen on LPO view, but difficult to define normal contractions due to superimposed structures
Left ventricle	Normal myocardium seen as "halo" around blood pool; ovoid shape in anterior, LAO positions; (size equal to or slightly smaller than RV on LAO view); well defined on anterior, LAO, LPO views, but not on RAO view; contractions occur synchronously along entire perimeter, with most movement along minor axis; normally no focal regions of asynergy; evaluate for presence of aneurysm, thrombus, pseudoaneurysm; normal LVEF: 50%–65%

perform. Furthermore, the RV has complex geometry which does not approach an ellipsoid of revolution and hence does not conform well to planimetric assumptions.[53] To overcome these problems, a count-based method was developed. This method is predicated on the fact that for LV volumes of up to 300 cc, ventricular activity as measured in counts is proportional to volume.[84, 117] Thus the EF can be calculated as follows:

$$EF = SV/EDV = EDV - ESV/EDV = EDC - ESC/EDC$$

where EDC and ESC are background-corrected end-diastolic and end-systolic counts, respectively, and SV is the stroke volume.

The values for background-corrected EDC and ESV are computed by subtracting the background time-activity curve from the ventricular time-activity curve in each frame. These time-activity curves display counts (ordinate) as a function of time in the cardiac cycle (abscissa); they are derived by computer algorithm after appropriate regions of interest have been defined either manually by the operator or semiautomatically by computer algorithm. The point of maximal counts on the time-activity curve corresponds to end-diastole; this usually occurs in the first frame, where the ECG R wave is used to trigger the gate. Minimum count value is, by definition, end-systole. Left ventricular ejection fractions measured by the counts method on multiple-gated blood pool scans correlate well with those derived from contrast ventriculography.[27, 38, 134] Ejection fractions calculated by this method depend on the linear relationship of count rates or volumes rather than on quantitative or absolute values for ventricular volume. As a result, parallel-hole collimation is necessary to ensure accuracy (Fig 2–8).

Since target to background ratios in equilibrium images are on the order of 2.5–3:1, it is obvious that adjacent blood pool and vascular structures contribute a significant proportion of the total activity. This accounts for the need for background correction when calculating EF by the counts method, an operation not required when using planimetric techniques. Furthermore, the counts method is not entirely free of geometric assumptions, due to the attenuation of activity with increasing depth. At ventricular volumes of less than 300 cc this is not clinically significant, but above 500 cc the counts method is invalid.[117] However,

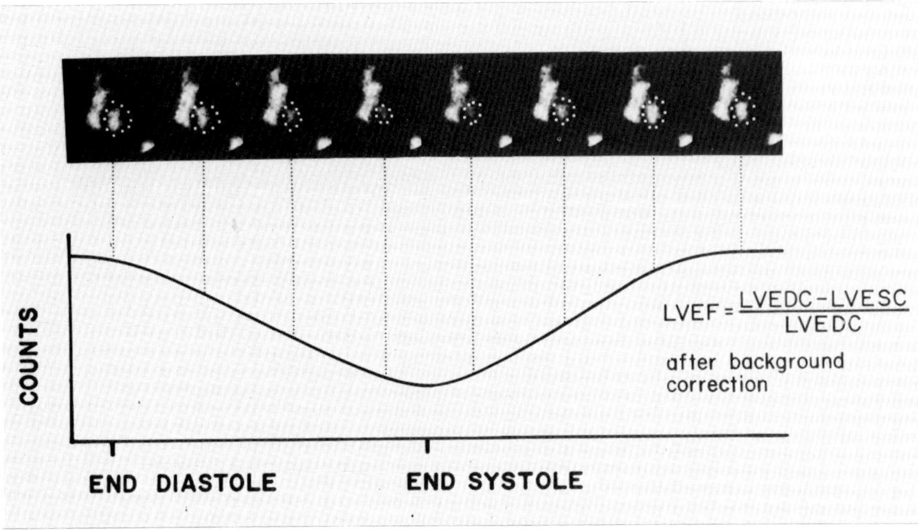

Fig 2–8.—Calculation of LVEF. In the LAO view, background subtraction is first performed. Then, variable regions of interest are located around the LV in each frame. End-diastole and end-systole occur at the maximum and minimum values of the time-activity curve generated from the counts in regions of interest.

the counts method is accurate in most situations and relatively easy to use, so it is currently the method generally accepted for clinical use.

Right ventricular ejection fraction cannot be easily calculated in the equilibrium scan, since the RV cannot be separated from neighboring chambers. Significant background counts are contributed from the LV in the anterior or RAO projections and from the RA in the LAO projection. Therefore, most clinics use gated or nongated first-pass methods for calculating RVEF. A technique for calculation of the RVEF using the 30-degree slant-hole collimator during blood pool studies has been reported.[55] This method requires application of a regression equation, and its widespread clinical utility has yet to be determined.

Left ventricular ejection fraction will be variably underestimated in the presence of an aneurysmal or otherwise asynergic area at the apex, owing to the persistence of the nonejected counts near the camera. The observer should be aware of this when interpreting the data. Although the left atrium contributes very little activity to the LV region of interest owing to its distance far from the camera and its position relative to the LV, its presence should be noted. A portion of an enlarged left atrium appendage may be inadvertently included during LV systole by the operator or by the semiautomatic region-of-interest computer algorithm, thus underestimating the LVEF.

Total counts per frame should remain relatively constant if the LV comprises only part of the total field, since blood ejected from the ventricles during systole enters the lungs and great vessels while the atria are filling. If there is a greater than 10% variation in counts per frame through the cardiac cycle due to irregular gating, then count normalization of the later low-density frames to an earlier high-density frame should be performed prior to data analysis. Failure to do so will result in a spurious elevation of EF.[121]

Generally, data are smoothed prior to EF analysis. Smoothing is a form of interpolation in which a data point is modified on the basis of the values of neighboring points; it is designed to reduce statistical fluctuations in the data and to present a more satisfying image to the observer.[68]

Calculation of Background Region of Interest

Accurate background correction of LV counts is essential. Underestimation of background counts will spuriously depress the calculated EF, while background overestimation will overestimate the true EF.

In principle, an attempt is made to select a background region of interest near the heart with a count density equal to that of the region which is directly behind the heart in the LAO view. No program has been able to do this precisely.[75] Many background correction methods have been proposed. Utilization of a background zone just posterior to the LV free wall above the spleen and away from the descending aorta is straightforward and appears to adequately correct the LV activity curve.[27, 67, 107, 116, 117, 121] With this method, the defined time-activity curve of the background region of interest should be flat. For first-pass imaging, the background is determined within the left ventricular region of interest just before the arrival of activity into the left ventricle. Some investigators have suggested that computer calculation of background activity may decrease interobserver and intraobserver variability,[107] but in practice this manual method has worked well in the hands of experienced observers.

Left Ventricular Region of Interest

The LV region of interest for count summation may be defined either manually or semiautomatically. *Variable* regions of interest are recalculated for each frame and must closely follow the LV edge as it moves through the cardiac cycle. Manual detection of the LV edge in end-diastole and end-systole is straightforward and may be the only available method if an oddly positioned or oddly shaped ventricle precludes use of semiautomated methods.

Semiautomatic computer software for LV edge detection currently employs one of two techniques, both of which are accurate and reproducible in most situations.[27, 107, 111] In both methods, the operator first manually approximates the borders of the ventricular blood pool. The computer algorithm then searches from the center of this region outward for the ventricular edge in each frame. The edge may be defined either by *gradient* analysis, which uses a second derivative of the change in counts, or by *threshold* analysis, which seeks points at a percentage of the peak counts in the ventricular center.[116] Activity within the defined region is then counted by the computer. The operator is the final judge of quality and must be prepared to recalculate a value which does not correlate well with his qualitative visual impression. Typically, about 10%–15% of semiautomatically generated LVEFs are recalculated.

An alternative to the variable region-of-interest approach is that in which the operator defines one *fixed* region of interest around the LV during end-diastole and sums the counts in this entire area throughout the cardiac cycle. It is inherently less accurate than the variable method, since the fixed region of interest will include activity from chambers other than the LV, such as the RV or left atrium, which may swing into the region of interest during systole. Thus, the fixed region-of-interest method will underestimate the true EF at rest, and it may yield a falsely blunted EF response during exercise, when heart motion within the chest may be pronounced.[27, 110, 111] Fixed ventricular region-of-interest selection should therefore be avoided.

Estimation of Ventricular Volume and Regurgitant Fraction

Left ventricular size can be estimated by viewing the heart in at least two projections. Quantitation of LV size may be accomplished using a count-based or a geometry-based method. Both techniques require images to be acquired with a parallel-hole collimator. In geometric methods, the pixel size of the instrument is first calculated using a bar phantom. The end-diastolic volume can be computed by relating the number of pixels included in the ventricular outline to real space via a geometric formula. One such approach, described by Tarolli, uses the length of the longest chords to calculate areas of the projected anterior and LAO images, correcting for nonorthagonality.[18, 117] The LV volumes can then be normalized for body surface area to yield a volume index.

Left ventricular volumes can be calculated independently of a geometric assumption about chamber shape on the equilibrium blood pool studies. Because tracer is well mixed with the blood, the number of events from an LV region of interest will be proportional to the volume of blood in the chamber. Left ventricular regions of interest are constructed in end-diastole or end-systole, or both. Left ventricular borders should be strictly defined and left atrium activity carefully excluded. Background-corrected count rates are then divided by count rates per unit volume of peripheral blood (corrected for body attenuation), and the LV volume is obtained. Usually a regression equation must be used to correct for attenuation and to determine true volume. Excellent correlation (r = .95–.98) has been reported between angiographic and counts-based radionuclide imaging technique.[90, 106]

In a normal heart, the volume of blood and hence the counts ejected from the left and right ventricles should be equal. Since stroke volume inequality is generally associated with dilation of one or more cardiac chambers, this finding should alert the operator to the possible presence of a volume-overloaded ventricle due to valvular regurgitation or shunting. Quantitative confirmation of the stroke volume difference can be obtained by manually defining and then subtracting counts of end-systolic from end-diastolic regions for each of the ventricles in the LAO view. Utilizing this approach, LV stroke counts usually exceed RV stroke counts by about 15% in normal hearts, an artifact produced by right atrial contribution to RV end-systolic activity. Thus, in practice, if the LV stroke volume counts exceed RV stroke volume counts by 15%, a volume overload of the LV is suggested. This technique appears sensitive enough to detect moderate degrees of regurgitation with high reliability if there is no concurrent RV volume overload.[96]

Regional Wall Motion

The assessment of regional wall motion increases the value of the gated blood pool scan in detecting focal diseases of the myocardium such as coronary artery disease. In the clinical setting, regional wall motion is usually determined qualitatively by the observer, although quantitative computer programs have been devised. All points on the ventricular surface should commence contraction and reach end-systole simultaneously; the anterolateral and posterolateral LV walls generally move more than the apex, septum, and inferior wall.[117] Hypokinesis may be present if approximately 20% shortening along a radius drawn from the border to the LV center does not occur.[118] By comparing wall movement to a computer-generated stationary pointer placed on the edge of the segment in question, evaluation of subtle wall motion abnormalities may be enhanced. The interventricular septum normally moves posteriorly toward the LV during systole. It may exhibit anterior or paradoxic motion in left bundle-branch block, RV overload, septal infarction, or for many years after cardiopulmonary bypass.[13]

The physician must take into account the anatomy of the individual heart under analysis. For example, a large right atrium may overlap the RV and thus obscure the RV border on the LAO view, mimicking a hypokinetic anterior RV wall. Large or even moderate-sized aneurysms may obscure surrounding anatomy. Regional wall motion can be adequately assessed only by analyzing multiple views of the heart.

Three approaches to the quantitation of regional wall motion have been described: (1) The determination of edge movement on multiple views, typically without any realignment of the long axis of the ventricle, in similar fashion to the methods devised for analysis of contrast ventriculograms. This approach has been validated against contrast studies (r = 0.8). One major factor influencing the edge detection approach is the coarseness of the matrix used to acquire data. (2) The determination of regional changes in ventricular volume, usually on the LAO view, to measure regional EF. Since this approach condenses edge data from the two perspectives into information from a single view, validation of the approach is more difficult. However, Holman and colleagues have reported a good overall correlation. (3) A variation on the volume approach is the use of a fully automated method of obtaining the data: phase and amplitude analysis. In this method, the data are analyzed without operator intervention to produce two images: one of the phase, that is, the time of onset of contraction (change in volume) within each picture element of the study, and one of the amplitude, that is, the maximal change in activity in each picture element. The amplitude image is related to regional volume change. This image can then be analyzed for regional changes in activity which are equivalent to regional volume changes.[41, 69, 70]

First-Pass Radionuclide Ventriculograms

First-pass methods, gated or nongated, are performed on the first transit of a radionuclide bolus through the heart prior to equilibration through the vascular space, and they therefore yield temporal and anatomical separation of the cardiac chambers. First-pass studies may be acquired in 10–20 seconds per view, as opposed to the 2–10 minutes needed for each projection in gated blood pool studies. Therefore, they may be of significant value in imaging the clinically ill or unstable patient or in trying to define transient physiologic events that might be lost in averaging the several hundred cardiac cycles that comprise the gated equilibrium study. On the other hand, first-pass radionuclide angiography requires a separate injection for each view. The first-pass study may be undone by even a few aberrant beats, and assessment of subtle regional wall motion abnormalities may be more difficult than in gated equilibrium studies, owing to the relatively few counts which are accumulated. Furthermore, it is often technically difficult to inject a compact bolus, especially in ill patients with few "good veins."

In clinical practice, a gated first-pass radioangiogram may be acquired immediately prior to the equilibrium blood pool study as a complement to it. When done in the 30-degree RAO projection, the first-pass study provides information about RV function not available from the equilibrium study. However, only a gross evaluation may be made about LV function, since that chamber is located at a distance from the collimator in this view (Fig 2–9).[140]

The first-pass study requiring a compact bolus injection of tagged red blood cells, less than 3–5 cc, is an absolute requirement. Such an injection can usually be accomplished via a modification of the Oldendorf technique.[81] With the patient's arm slightly elevated, a blood pressure cuff is inflated for 3 minutes to distend the distal circulation. The cuff pressure is then increased until it substantially exceeds systolic pressure (to 250 mm Hg). The tracer is then injected through a small needle into an antecubital vein, optimally the basilic vein. The cuff is removed abruptly while still inflated and the collapsing venous pool rapidly propels the bolus centrally. However, a better bolus is achieved by injecting a tracer through an indwelling cathe-

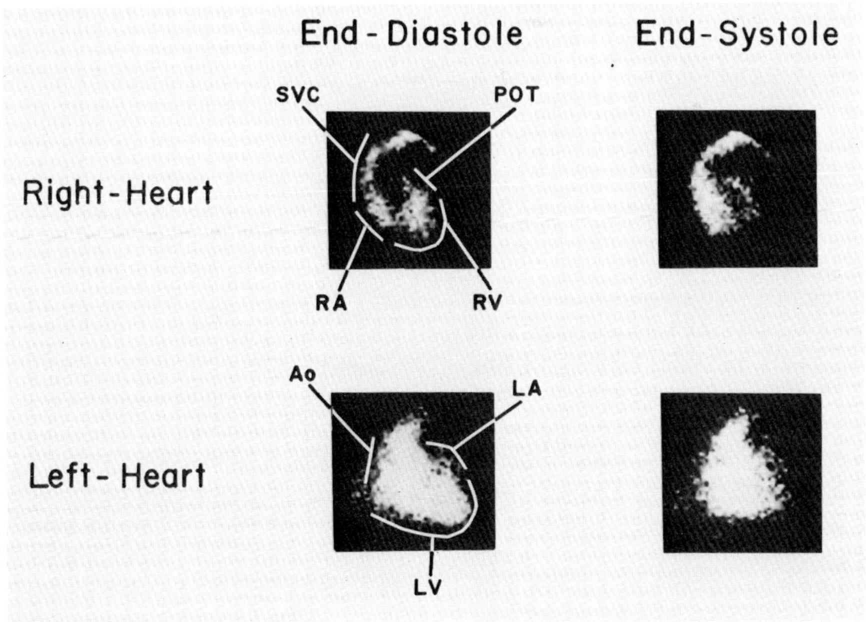

Fig 2–9.—Gated first-pass study, RAO view. *SVC,* superior vena cava; *RA,* right atrium; *RV,* right ventricle; *LA,* left atrium; *LV,* left ventricle; *POT,* pulmonary outflow tract; *Ao,* aorta.

ter, followed by a vigorous saline or dextrose flush. For a gated first-pass study, right heart image acquisition is started with the release of the cuff and is terminated when activity is seen in the lungs, generally after five or six cardiac cycles. Then acquisition of the levo phases begins as the bolus leaves the pulmonary venous circulation and traverses the left heart. This method yields two average "cardiac cycles," one each for right and left hearts.

When a peripheral injection through the superior vena caval system is used, the reflux of the "hot" tracer from the right atrium into the "cold" inferior vena cava during RV systole indicates tricuspid insufficiency. Right ventricular wall motion can be assessed and RVEF measured, since it is assumed that homogeneous mixing of tracer with the blood has occurred by the time the bolus reaches the RV.[143] Occasionally, however, the bolus may not adequately mix in the RV, resulting in poor delineation of the RV apex. This artifact may cause erroneous estimation of ventricular size and function. A discrepancy in RV size and wall motion between first-pass and equilibrium phases of a study should alert the physician to the possible occurrence of this phenomenon. In addition, it is critical that the right heart study be started and stopped with proper regard to the position of the bolus relative to each chamber. For example, contamination of the right heart phase by left heart yields an inadequate study and can occur if accumulation of the RV phase is inadvertently prolonged by even a few extra seconds. This could yield an artifactually dilated hypokinetic RV if LV function is poor.

The first-pass RAO view separates the right atrium from the RV because the tricuspid valve plane is perpendicular to the detector. Background correction is not needed when RVEF is calculated via the counts method because only a small percentage of the injected activity is in the lung. The RV end-diastolic and end-systolic borders are defined in two separate regions of interest, and the RVEF is calculated from the change in counts.

The gated first-pass method can alert the physician to the presence of an intracardiac shunt, but if such a shunt is suspected, a nongated or sequential first-transit study is preferred.

Sequential (nongated) first-pass studies can be used to study right and left heart function. In this technique, each cardiac cycle is evaluated independently and counts are accumulated in the computer as a function of space and real time.

Since long residence time in the blood pool is not needed, tracers such as Tc-DTPA or Tc sulfur colloid may be used for these studies. The radionuclide injection technique is critical, as previously noted, regardless of the tracer utilized. A tracer bolus of less than 1 cc injected through a large vein is preferred. The tracer dose of 10–25 mCi in 1 ml volume or less is briskly flushed through the intravenous catheter with 15–20 ml of saline. The adequacy of the injection should be analyzed both qualitatively and quantitatively by generating a time-activity curve of the bolus transit through the superior vena cava.

First-pass studies can be performed in any view, since individual cardiac chambers are temporally separated. Generally the anterior or 30-degree RAO position is used. However, the LPO view has been employed in the past. First-pass studies can be performed with the conventional Anger camera. However, nonlinearity of count rate response occurs at high count rates; this is most extreme during the right heart phase because of the compactness of the bolus. Although previously these "dead time" problems required application of mathematical techniques to reduce statistical uncertainty, present-generation cameras can count 80–100,000 counts per second with 20%–30% dead time losses.[11, 103] The multicrystal scintillation camera can acquire data approximately five times faster than the Anger-type instrument, but at a 1-cm or worse resolution. The multicrystal instrument can reduce the statistical fluctuation of calculated EF on first-pass studies, but definition of subtle wall motion abnormalities is a problem, owing to the low resolution of the instrument. Data are usually stored in list mode and studies are obtained at 20–50 frames per second, depending on heart rate.

Left ventricular ejection fraction is generally computed from a fixed region of interest corresponding to the end-diastolic image. Activity is analyzed only when it is seen on the LV image. Background activity must be subtracted from the fixed region of interest. Various methods of background calculation have been described. The preferred approach is the subtraction of activity directly from the right or left ventricular regions of interest immediately before the appearance of activity. No background correction is needed if tracer is injected into the right pulmonary artery and imaging is done in the RAO projection, since no activity appears in the right heart or left lung.[11, 58]

The ventricular time-activity curve will appear as a sequence of oscillations, with valleys and peaks corresponding to individual end-systoles and end-diastoles. Statistical error can be reduced either by averaging several beats or by summing three to five cycles to generate a "representative" beat. Regional wall motion can be best assessed from the summed representative cycle, either as the difference between the end-diastolic and end-systolic images or by viewing a cinematic endless-loop display of the frames. Evaluation of RV function is done similarly. Background correction may be needed in certain images if acquired in certain projections. For example, in the anterior view, there is some overlap of the right atrium and the RV; thus a background time-activity curve at the interface between right atrium and RV is generated and subtracted from the RV region of interest curve.

The EF measured from sequential first-pass studies is reproducible and correlates well with EFs obtained by contrast angiography, gated equilibrium, and gated first-pass methods.[37, 71, 128, 143] The gated first-pass technique, however, may offer better delineation of the valve planes and involve less processing time for calculating EF than the ungated first-pass method.[56]

The major drawbacks to the first-pass technique are (1) only one view may be acquired after each injection and (2) the total number of injections is limited by background accumulation, even though smaller doses are required for a first-pass than for a gated study. The problems can be partly alleviated by using multiple tracers with different clearance mechanisms. Practically, only two to three injections may be made and thus only two to three views obtained within a 24-hour period. Work on developing a technique or tracer that would eliminate these problems has accelerated. An osmium 191 → iridium 191m generator system which can deliver multiple doses of ^{191}Ir, a short-lived radionuclide ($T_{1/2}$ = 4.96 seconds), has been developed and is nearing clinical application. Repeated elutions and injections can be made in a short time with substantial reduction in patient dose and background when compared to current techniques.[29, 57] Tantalum 178 ($T_{1/2}$ = 9.3 minutes) is also being evaluated for potential applicability to radionuclide ventriculography.[54] In addition, some groups use a bifocal collimator to obtain two simultaneous views of the heart during one acquisition, but there is some distortion and slight loss of spatial resolution.[143] An $^{81}Rb \rightarrow {}^{81m}Kr$ generator system connected to a short-period infusion set has recently been described. Krypton

TABLE 2–5.—Gated Equilibrium Blood Pool and First-Pass Ventriculography

	GATED EQUILIBRIUM	FIRST-PASS: NONGATED
Acquisition time	2–10 min	10–20 sec
Instrument preferred	1. Anger camera 2. Multicrystal	1. Multicrystal 2. Anger camera
Time-activity curve	One "average" cycle	Multiple cycles in continuous real time
Chamber anatomy	Simultaneous visualization of left and right hearts	Temporal and spatial separation of left and right hearts
Injection	Multiple views or studies and imaging 4–10 hr following single injection	Reinjection needed for each view; total number of injections limited; need for compact bolus
Shunt evaluation	No direct assessment of shunting	Allows direct shunt quantification, rarely visualization
Common radiolabel	Tc 99m RBCs	TcO_4^-, Tc-sulfur colloid, Tc-DTPA, Tc 99m RBCs.
Target to background ratio	Approx. 2.5:1	3:1 for first injection; decreases with subsequent injections
Effect of transient arrhythmias	Not serious if <10% of beats aberrant	May disable study
Calculation of RVEF	−	+
Calculation of LVEF	+	+

81m ($T_{1/2}$ = 13 seconds) is continuously infused into the right heart and is exhaled very rapidly by the lungs owing to its low solubility in blood; thus, lung and left heart background activity are minimal, allowing relatively straightforward and reproducible calculation of RVEF. This technique offers promise for evaluation of right heart function, though its accuracy remains to be more fully evaluated.[61] A variation in this approach employs the injection of xenon in saline, where the tracer is cleared in the lungs. In Table 2–5 the first-pass and equilibrium techniques are compared.

ADDITIONAL APPROACHES TO EVALUATION OF CARDIAC FUNCTION

Clinically, the most useful measures of cardiac function are the EF, qualitative regional wall motion, and ventricular volumes at end-diastole and end-systole. Other parameters of LV function have been described and have found their way into clinical practice, but their utility is marginal and in some cases their reproducibility and accuracy remain to be evaluated. These parameters include LV ejection time (LVET), first third EF, and *dV/dt*.[6, 48, 105, 129]

Currently, almost all quantitative and qualitative methodologies center on the ejection phase of ventricular function, i.e., end-diastole through end-systole. However, analysis of ventricular filling or relaxation during early and mid-diastole may add useful data about cardiac function. Relaxation phase parameters are difficult to measure using current techniques because gating off the ECG R wave yields less uniform data in the latter portion of the cardiac cycle. More sophisticated types of acquisition protocols than are generally in use today will be required for the evaluation of ventricular filling and relaxation.

INTERVENTION STUDIES—THEORETICAL CONSIDERATIONS

Changes in cardiac function resulting from drug therapy or during the course of physically or pharmacologically induced hemodynamic stress can be readily determined from the radionuclide ventriculogram.[17]

Exercise radionuclide ventriculography allows noninvasive assessment of biventricular reserve in patients with conditions such as coronary artery disease, obstructive lung disease, valvular dysfunction, or cardiomyopathy.[23, 72] Some patients with significant coronary artery stenoses may have a normal EF and wall motion at rest but have dysfunction during exercise, when the imbalance between myocardial oxygen demand and supply becomes evident.[22, 67]

As in ^{201}Tl testing, one of any number of standard exercise protocols may be used; however, graded methods are preferred over fixed-load techniques. Once again, it is the level of stress which is most important, since a significant proportion of patients with heart disease will demonstrate *normal* ventricular response at inadequate stress levels. Sensitivity of detecting coronary artery disease via radionuclide ventriculography is significantly lower in patients who achieve inadequate as opposed to those who achieve adequate levels of exercise (62%–69% vs. 93%–94%).[22, 23] Interpretation of the study must include a statement about the heart rate achieved and the reason for stopping the stress test.

Exercise ventriculography may be done by either first-pass or equilibrium methods. Furthermore, since first-pass acquisition is short, on the order of 20 seconds, it seems ideal for evaluating peak exercise, which may only last a few seconds, and is suited for upright exercise. Equilibrium studies generally need a minimum of two minutes for acquisition, so imaging is usually done in the supine position to minimize patient motion. However, the equilibrium method has one major advantage over the first-pass method, namely, it can be used to acquire data almost continually throughout the rest, exercise, and recovery periods.[53] It is best to image and evaluate all stages of a graded stress test to determine the progression of global and regional function.[117] For example, an EF that increases at low work loads might decline in the final stage of exercise. Evaluation of only the initial and final points would miss the terminal blunted EF response if the final EF were still above the baseline.

EXERCISE VENTRICULOGRAPHY: PRACTICAL CONSIDERATIONS

If possible, the patient should discontinue taking medications such as beta-blockers before the stress test since these agents may limit heart rate response. A rest gated blood pool study in at least the anterior and LAO positions should be performed. Baseline ECG, heart rate, and blood pressure should be monitored throughout the study to recovery. The patient's shoulders and head should be well supported and handgrips should be used to minimize movement of the torso during exercise. While some patient motion is tolerable, excessive movement degrades image quality and causes errors in EF and regional wall motion assessment. This is most likely to happen during vigorous exercise.[110]

Following acquisition of the baseline rest study, exercise is begun on a bicycle ergometer with the collimator in the LAO position. Every three minutes, the resistance is increased by 25 watts (150 kpm) while a constant peddling rate of 55–60 revolutions per minute is maintained. The technician uses the first minute of each stage to allow heart rate to stabilize at the new level and to set a new gating interval if one is needed. This is an important step, since wild swings in heart rate during acquisition will severely distort the data.[22] The last two minutes of the exercise stage are used for acquisition. In both phantom studies and clinical practice, image quality does not significantly improve with a high-sensitivity collimator, despite the limited counts that can be accumulated in two minutes; therefore, a general all-purpose collimator is adequate.[99]

Evaluation of the studies is facilitated by a side-by-side cine display of baseline and exercise images. Significant ventricular dilation in either end-diastole or end-systole or development of regional wall motion abnormalities with exercise are abnormal findings. While there is wide variation among individual patients, failure to increase the LVEF at least 5% during peak exercise over baseline suggests cardiac disease and inadequate ventricular reserve.[110, 143] Exercise EFs are generally accurate and reproducible[21]; however, interobserver and intraobserver variability in evaluation of exercise images may be higher than that for rest studies, and it has been suggested that two separate determinations of both rest and peak exercise EFs be made.[79]

The sensitivity of the exercise radioventriculogram for detecting heart disease may be increased by analyzing changes in pulmonary blood pool activity. This can be done by obtaining count densities in comparable regions of interest over the left lung in the end-diastolic frames of both the rest and exercise studies. Okada et al. found that patients with coronary artery disease not limited to the right coronary artery usually had an increase in the exercise to rest pulmonary blood volume ratios, whereas patients with normal coronary arteries had no change in the pulmonary blood volume from rest to exercise.[86] It is likely that this finding is not specific for coronary artery disease, but rather is an indicator of decreased LV reserve due to a number of etiologies.[117]

Since acquisition during exercise must be short, only one view for each stage is obtainable. This is adequate for determining changes in EF but is not ideal for assessing regional wall motion. The development of the bifocal diverging collimator has enabled simultaneous recording of two views of the heart 50 degrees apart[19] and thus theoretically may improve detection of regional wall motion abnormalities. This technique is promising and yields results that correlate well with parallel-hole collimators, but the true marginal utility of the bifocal diverging collimator over standard techniques remains to be demonstrated. It is hoped that future developments in tomographic imaging of the heart during exercise will enable detection of localized wall motion abnormalities not well seen on planar imaging.[78, 133]

Often patients cannot exercise adequately due to shortness of breath, claudication, poor general conditioning, or specific nonconditioning of the lower extremity skeletal muscle groups.[23] In one study, only 81% of patients with coronary artery disease and 53% of "normals" achieved maximal exercise.[22] Under these circumstances, a physician might consider using either isometric handgrips[15] or cold pressor stress to achieve a greater stress stimulus.[62]

NONIMAGING APPROACHES TO CARDIAC FUNCTION

Nonimaging nuclear techniques for evaluating cardiac function are currently undergoing clinical evaluation. The nuclear probe or "stethoscope" consists of a computerized portable sodium iodide crystal affixed to a single-bore, small converging collimator, interfaced to the ECG. It can generate a real-time LV time-activity curve without gating. This instrument may be easily used at the bedside and provides beat-to-beat information on global LV performance; when ^{99m}Tc-labeled red blood cells are used, patients may be monitored continuously for several hours.[10, 136, 137] Other approaches involve the use of either single or multiple cadmium telluride detectors that can be attached to the chest wall via a beltlike or vestlike harness for continuous evaluation of LV function in ambulatory patients.[52, 115] These devices are all in the prototype stages and problems with positioning and background, and thus accuracy and reproducibility, remain. Although less expensive and certainly more portable than camera-dependent imaging, these instruments cannot give information on regional wall motion or structure. They are expected to complement rather than to supplant nuclear ventriculography.

OTHER NUCLEAR TECHNIQUES

While ^{201}Tl studies of myocardial perfusion can reliably indicate the *presence* of a myocardial infarction, ^{201}Tl imaging cannot yield information on the *age* of the infarction. Technetium pyrophosphate, a member of a class of technetium chelates widely used for bone scanning, is currently used clinically to identify the presence of acute myocardial infarction and to determine the location and extent of the infarcted area.[85]

Because many cardiovascular disorders originate at the cell level, new techniques for the study of regional myocardial metabolism are being developed that use positron-emitting computerized tomography. It is hoped, for example, that "physiologic tomography" will be able to characterize the local metabolic alterations associated with ischemia.[102] Some of these agents are listed in Table 2–6.

TABLE 2–6.—AGENTS USED IN ASSESSMENT OF REGIONAL MYOCARDIAL INTEGRITY AND METABOLISM*

AGENT	COMMENTS
Thallium 201	Persistent "cold spot" indicates infarct, age not determinable
Tc pyrophosphate	Infarct-avid agent; "hot spot" imaging; maximal tissue concentration reached in 48–72 hr; insensitive in subendocardial infarction; many circumstances yield false positive scan; difficult to interpret; clinical utility limited
Antimyosin antibodies	Infarct-avid agent; low-contrast images make interpretation difficult
Tc glucoheptonate	Infarct-avid agent; can image early during acute stages of infarction, but low-contrast images have limited clinical use
F 18 deoxyglucose	Activity reflects regional utilization rates of glucose; accuracy of myocardial glucose utilization rates await validation; positron-emitter, ? clinical applicability
C 11 palmitate	Assessment of fatty acid metabolism; positron-emitter, has been used for infarct sizing; complex FFA kinetics make measurements very difficult; ? clinical applicability

*See references 30, 34, 36, 53, 59, 60, 85, 87, 93, 102, 125.

ACKNOWLEDGMENT

Prepared in part under NHLBI grant No. HL07416-03.

REFERENCES

1. Albro P.C., Gould K.L., Westcott R.J., et al.: Noninvasive assessment of coronary stenoses by myocardial imaging during pharmacologic vasodilation: III. Clinical trial. *Am. J. Cardiol.* 42:751–760, 1978.
2. Alpert N.M., McKusick K.A., Pohost G.M., et al.: Noninvasive nuclear cinecardiography. *J. Nucl. Med.* 15:1182–1184, 1974.
3. Anger H.O., Davis D.H.: Gamma ray detection efficiency and image resolution in sodium iodide. *Rev. Sci. Instrum.* 35:693–697, 1964.
4. Ardran G.M., Hamill J., Emrys-Roberts E., et al.: Radiation dose to the patient in cardiac radiology. *Br. J. Radiol.* 43:391–394, 1970.
5. Bailey I.K., Griffith L.S.C., Rouleau J., et al.: Thallium-201 myocardial perfusion imaging at rest and during exercise: Comparative sensitivity to electrocardiography in coronary artery disease. *Circulation* 55:79–87, 1977.
6. Battler A., Slutsky R., Karliner J., et al.: Left ventricular ejection fraction and first third ejection fraction early after acute myocardial infarction and value for predicting mortality and validity. *Am. J. Cardiol.* 45:197–202, 1980.
7. Beck R.N.: Some essential characteristics of radioactive materials, in Gottschalk A., Potchen E.J., (eds.): *Diagnostic Nuclear Medicine.* Baltimore, Williams & Wilkins Co., 1976, pp. 14–21.
8. Beller G.A., Watson D.D., Achell P., et al.: Time course of thallium-201 redistribution after transient myocardial ischemia. *Circulation* 61:791–801, 1980.
9. Berger B.C., Watson D.D., Burwell L.R., et al.: Redistribution of thallium at rest in patients with stable and unstable angina and the effect of coronary bypass surgery. *Circulation* 60:1114–1125, 1979.
10. Berger H.J., Davies R.A., Batsforth A., et al.: Beat to beat left ventricular performance assessed from the equilibrium cardiac blood pool using a computerized nuclear probe. *Circulation* 63:133–142, 1981.
11. Berger H.J., Matthay R.A., Pytlik L.M., et al.: First pass radionuclide assessment of right and left ventricular performance in patients with cardiac and pulmonary disease. *Semin. Nucl. Med.* 9:275–295, 1979.
12. Bingham J.B., McKusick K.A., Strauss H.W.: Influence of coronary artery disease on pulmonary uptake of thallium-201. *Am. J. Cardiol.* 46:821–826, 1980.
13. Bingham J.B., McKusick K.A., Boucher C.A., et al.: Gamut: Paradoxical septal motion. *Semin. Nucl. Med.* 11:165–167, 1981.
14. Blumgart H.L., Weiss S.: Studies on the velocity of blood flow: VII. The pulmonary circulation time in normal resting individuals. *J. Clin. Invest.* 4:399–425, 1927.
15. Bodenheimer M.M., Banha V.S., Fooshee C.M., et al.: Detection of coronary heart disease using radionuclide determined regional ejection fraction at rest and during handgrip exercise: Correlation with coronary arteriography. *Circulation* 58:640–648, 1978.
16. Bodenheimer B., Banha V.S., Fooshee C.M., et al.: Extent and severity of coronary artery heart disease: Determination by thallous-chloride Tl-201 myocardial perfusion scanning and comparison with stress electrocardiography. *Arch. Intern. Med.* 139:630–634, 1979.
17. Borer J.S., Bachrach S.L., Green M.V., et al.: Real time radionuclide cineangiography in the non-invasive evaluation of global and regional left ventricular function during exercise in patients with coronary artery disease. *N. Engl. J. Med.* 296:839–844, 1977.
18. Boucher C.A., Bingham J.B., Osbakken M.D., et al.: Early changes in left ventricular size following correction of LV volume overload. *Am. J. Cardiol.* 47:991–1003, 1981.
19. Boucher C.A., Strauss H.W., Okada R.D., et al.: The bifocal diverging collimator: A means of simultaneous biplane imaging of the heart during equilibrium radionuclide ventriculography. *J. Nucl. Med.* 21:71–76, 1980.
20. Bradley-Moore P.R., Lebowitz E., Greene M.W.: Thallium-201 for medical use: II. Biological behavior. *J. Nucl. Med.* 16:156–160, 1975.
21. Brady T.J., Lo K., Thrall J.H., et al.: Exercise radionuclide ejection fraction: Correlation with exercise contrast ventriculography. *Radiology* 132:703–705, 1979.
22. Brady T.J., Thrall J.H., Clare J.M., et al.: Exercise radionuclide ventriculography: Practical considerations and sensitivity of coronary artery disease detection. *Radiology* 132:697–702, 1979.
23. Brady T.J., Thrall J.H., Lo K., et al.: The importance of adequate exercise in the detection of coronary heart disease by radionuclide ventriculography. *J. Nucl. Med.* 21:1125–1130, 1980.
24. Brown K.A., Boucher C.A., Strauss H.W., et al.: Serial right ventricular thallium-201 imaging following exercise: Relationship to right coronary artery disease, abstracted. *J. Nucl. Med.* 22:P-84, 1981.
25. Buddemeyer E.V., Bachrach S.L., Mitchell T.G.: Instrumentation in nuclear cardiology, in: Strauss H.W., Pitt B. (eds.): *Cardiovascular Nuclear*

Medicine, ed. 2. St. Louis, C.V. Mosby Co., 1979, pp. 3–45.

26. Bulkley B.H., Rouleau J., Strauss H.W., et al.: Idiopathic hypertrophic subaortic stenoses: Detection by thallium-201 myocardial perfusion imaging. *N. Engl. J. Med.* 293:1113–1116, 1975.
27. Burow R.D., Strauss H.W., Singleton R., et al.: Analysis of LV function from multiple gated acquisition cardiac blood pool imaging: Comparison to contrast angiography. *Circulation* 56:1024–1028, 1977.
28. Callahan R.J., Froelich J.W., McKusick K.A., et al.: A modified method for the in vivo labeling of red blood cells with Tc-99m, unpublished.
29. Cheng C., Treves S., Samuel A., et al.: A new Osmium-191—Iridium-191m generator. *J. Nucl. Med.* 21:1169–1176, 1980.
30. Cochavi S., Pohost G.M., Elmaleh D.R., et al.: Transverse-sectional imaging with Nal8F in myocardial infarction. *J. Nucl. Med.* 20:1013–1017, 1979.
31. Cohen H.A., Baird M.G., Rouleau J.R., et al.: Thallium-201 myocardial imaging in patients with pulmonary hypertension. *Circulation* 54:790–795, 1976.
32. Cook D.J., Bailey I., Strauss H.W., et al.: Thallium-201 for myocardial imaging: Appearance of the normal heart. *J. Nucl. Med.* 17:583–589, 1976.
33. Cradduck T.D., Knowles L.G.: Computers in nuclear medicine, in Rollo F.D. (ed.): *Nuclear Medicine: Physics, Instrumentation and Agents*. St. Louis, C.V. Mosby Co., 1977, pp. 453–470.
34. Dewanjee M.K., Kohn P.C.: Mechanism of localization of ^{99m}Tc-labeled pyrophosphate and tetracycline in infarcted myocardium. *J. Nucl. Med.* 17:639–646, 1976.
35. Dept. of Health, Education and Welfare: *Radiologic Health Handbook*, rev. ed. Rockville, Md., 1970.
36. Fetz R.C., Stadalnik R.C., Martin P.: Myocardial "false positive" 99mTc-pyrophosphate scintigrams. *Semin. Nucl. Med.* 11:64–65, 1981.
37. Fletcher J.W., Herbig F.K., Daley J.L., et al.: Measurement and comparison of left ventricular ejection fraction utilizing first transit and gated scintigraphy, unpublished.
38. Folland E.D., Hamilton G.W., Larson M.S., et al.: The radionuclide ejection fraction: A comparison of three radionuclide techniques with contrast angiography. *J. Nucl. Med.* 18:1159–1166, 1977.
39. Folse R., Braunwald E.: Determination of the fraction of left ventricular volume ejected per beat and of ventricular end-diastolic and residual volumes. *Circulation* 25:674–685, 1962.
40. Fortuin N.J., Weiss J.L.: Exercise stress testing. *Circulation* 56:699–712, 1977.
41. Frais M.A., Botvinick E.H., O'Connell J.W., et al.: The phase image: An accurate means of detecting and localizing abnormal foci of ventricular activation, abstracted. *J. Nucl. Med.* 22:18, 1981.
42. Gewirtz H., Beller G.A., Strauss H.W.: Transient defects of resting thallium scans in patients with coronary artery disease. *Circulation* 59:707–713, 1979.
43. Gewirtz H., O'Keefe D.D., Pohost G.M., et al.: The effect of ischemia on thallium-201 clearance from the myocardium. *Circulation* 58:215–219, 1978.
44. Goris M.L., Duspit S.G., McLaughlin P., et al.: Interpolative background subtraction. *J. Nucl. Med.* 17:744–747, 1976.
45. Gottschalk A., Hoffer P.: Stationary detectors, in Gottschalk A., Potchen E.J. (eds.): *Diagnostic Nuclear Medicine*. Baltimore, Williams & Wilkins Co., 1976, pp. 94–103.
46. Gough J.H., Davis R., Stacey A.J.: Radiation doses delivered to the skin, bone marrow and gonads of patients during cardiac catheterization and angiocardiography. *Br. J. Radiol.* 41:508–514, 1968.
47. Gould K.L., Westcott R.J., Albro P.C., et al.: Noninvasive assessment of coronary stenoses by myocardial imaging during pharmacological coronary vasodilatation: II. Clinical methodology and feasibility. *Am. J. Cardiol.* 41:279–287, 1978.
48. Hammermeister K.E., Brooks R.C., Warbasse J.R.: The rate of change of left ventricular volume in man: I. Validation and peak systolic ejection rate in health and disease. *Circulation* 49:729–738, 1974.
49. Harper P.V.: Factors which influence the choice of an isotope, in Gottschalk A., Potchen E.J. (eds.): *Diagnostic Nuclear Medicine*. Baltimore, Williams & Wilkins Co., 1976, pp. 22–25.
50. Hartley L.H.: Exercise testing procedures. Read before the Third Workshop on Nuclear Cardiology, Massachusetts General Hospital, Boston, December 7–8, 1979.
51. Hegge F.N., Hamilton G.W., Larson S.N., et al.: Cardiac chamber imaging: A comparison of red blood cells labeled with Tc-99m in vitro and in vivo. *J. Nucl. Med.* 19:129–133, 1978.
52. Hoffer P.B., Berger H.J., Steidley J., et al.: A miniature cadmium detector module for continuous monitoring of left ventricular function. *Radiology* 138:477–481, 1981.
53. Holman B.L.: Cardiac imaging in nuclear medicine. *Radiology* 133:709–716, 1979.
54. Holman B.L., Neirinckx R.D., Treves S., et al.: Cardiac imaging with tantalum-178. *Radiology* 131:525–576, 1979.
55. Holman B.L., Wynne J., Zielonka J.S., et al.: A simplified technique for measuring right ventricular ejection fraction using the equilibrium radionuclide angiogram and the slant hole collimator. *Radiology* 138:429–435, 1981.
56. Harolds J.A., Grove R.B., Bower R.D., et al.: Right

ventricular function assessed by two radionuclide techniques: A concise communication. *J. Nucl. Med.* 22:113–115, 1981.

57. Hnatowich D.J., Kulprathipanja S., Treves S.: An improved 1910s–191mIr generator for radionuclide angiocardiography. *Radiology* 123:189–194, 1977.
58. Jengo J.A., Mena I., Blaufuss A., et al.: Evaluation of left ventricular function (ejection fraction and segmental wall motion) by single pass radioisotope angiography. *Circulation* 57:326–332, 1978.
59. Khaw B.A., Beller G.A., Haber E.: Experimental myocardial infarct imaging following intravenous administration of Iodine-131 labeled antibody (Fab′ 2) fragments specific for cardiac myosin. *Circulation* 57:743–750, 1978.
60. Khaw B.A., Gold H.K., Leinbach R.C., et al.: Early imaging of experimental myocardial infarction by intracoronary administration of I-131-labeled anticardiac myosin (Fab′2) fragments. *Circulation* 58:1137–1142, 1978.
61. Knapp W.H., Helms F., Lambrecht R., et al.: Kr-81m for determination of right ventricular ejection fraction (RVEF). *Eur. J. Nucl. Med.* 5:487–492, 1980.
62. Kurb R.G., Brady T.J., Beszzi M.D., et al.: Cold pressor radionuclide ventriculography, abstracted. *Clin. Res.* 28:189A, 1980.
63. Kushner F.G., Okada R.D., Kirshenbaum H.D.: Lung thallium-201 uptake after stress testing in patients with coronary artery disease. *Circulation* 63:341–347, 1981.
64. L'Abbate A., Biagini A., Michelassi C., et al.: Myocardial kinetics of thallium and potassium in man. *Circulation* 60:776–784, 1979.
65. Lange R.C.: Introductory physics and instrumentation, in Schneider P.B., Treves S. (eds.): *Nuclear Medicine in Clinical Practice*. Amsterdam, Elsevier-North Holland Biomedical Press, 1978, pp. 1–20.
66. Lebowitz E., Greene M.W., Fairchild P., et al.: Thallium-201 for medical use. *J. Nucl. Med.* 16:151–155, 1975.
67. Leitl G.P., Buchanan J.W., Wagner H.N. Jr.: Monitoring cardiac function with nuclear techniques. *Am. J. Cardiol.* 46:1125–1132, 1980.
68. Lieberman D.E.: Computer methods: The fundamentals of digital nuclear medicine. St. Louis, C.V. Mosby Co., 1977, pp. 3–98.
69. Maddox D.E., Holman B.L., Wynne J., et al.: Ejection fraction image: A noninvasive index of left ventricular wall motion. *Am. J. Cardiol.* 41:1230–1238, 1978.
70. Maddox D.E., Wynne J., Uren R.: Regional ejection fraction: A quantitative radionuclide index of regional left ventricular performance. *Circulation* 59:1001–1009, 1979.
71. Marshall R.C., Berger H.J., Reduto L.A., et al.: Variability in sequential measures of left ventricular performance assessed with radionuclide angiocardiography. *Am. J. Cardiol.* 41:531–536, 1978.
72. Matthay R.A., Berger H.J., Davies R.A., et al.: Right and left ventricular exercise performance in chronic obstructive pulmonary disease: Radionuclide assessment. *Ann. Intern. Med.* 93:234–239, 1980.
73. McGowan R.L., Martin N.D., Zaret B.L., et al.: Diagnostic accuracy of non-invasive myocardial imaging for coronary artery disease: An electrocardiographic and angiographic correlation. *Am. J. Cardiol.* 40:6–10, 1977.
74. Mullins C.B., Mason D.T., Ashburn W.L.: Determination of ventricular volume by radioisotope angiography. *Am. J. Cardiol.* 24:72–78, 1969.
75. Narahara K.A., Hamilton G., Williams D.L., et al.: Myocardial imaging with thallium-201: An experimental model for analysis of the true myocardial and background image components. *J. Nucl. Med.* 18:781–786, 1977.
76. Nichols A.B., Moore R.H., Cochavi S., et al.: Quantification of myocardial infarction by computer-assisted positron emission tomography. *Cardiovasc. Res.* 14:428–434, 1980.
77. Nielson A.P., Morris K.G., Murdoch R., et al.: Linear relationship between the distribution of thallium-201 and blood flow in ischemic and nonischemic myocardium during exercise. *Circulation* 61:797–801, 1980.
78. Okada R.D., Boucher C.A., Strauss H.W., et al.: Exercise radionuclide imaging approaches to coronary artery disease. *Am. J. Cardiol.* 46:1188–1203, 1980.
79. Okada R.D., Kirshenbaum H.D., Kushner F.G., et al.: Observer variance in the qualitative evaluation of left ventricular wall motion and the quantitation of left ventricular ejection fraction using rest and exercise multigated blood pool imaging. *Circulation* 61:128–136, 1980.
80. Okada R.D., Pohost G.M., Kirshenbaum H.D., et al.: Radionuclide determined change in pulmonary blood volume with exercise: Improved sensitivity of multigated blood pool scanning in detecting coronary artery disease. *N. Engl. J. Med.* 301:569–576, 1979.
81. Oldendorf W.H., Kitano M., Shinizo S.: Evaluation of a simple technique for abrupt intravenous injection of radionuclides. *J. Nucl. Med.* 6:205–209, 1965.
82. Oppenheim B.E., Beck R.N.: The scintillation detector, in Gottschalk A., Potchen E.J. (eds.): *Diagnostic Nuclear Medicine*. Baltimore, Williams & Wilkins Co., 1976, pp. 63–73.
83. Parker J.A., Uren R.F., Jones A.G., et al.: Radionuclide left ventriculography with the slant hole collimator. *J. Nucl. Med.* 18:848–851, 1977.
84. Parker J.A., Secker-Walker R., Hill R., et al.: A

new technique for the calculation of ejection fraction. *J. Nucl. Med.* 13:649–651, 1972.

85. Parkey R.W., Bonte F.J., Meyer S.L.: A new method for radionuclide imaging of acute myocardial infarction in humans. *Circulation* 50:540–546, 1974.
86. Pavel D.G., Zimmer A.M., Patterson V.N.: In vivo labeling of red blood cells with 99mTc: A new approach to blood pool visualization. *J. Nucl. Med.* 18:305–308, 1977.
87. Pitt B., Thrall J.H.: Thallium-201 versus technetium-99m pyrophosphate myocardial imaging in detection and evaluation of patients with acute myocardial infarction. *Am. J. Cardiol.* 46:1215–1223, 1980.
88. Pohost G.M., Alpert N.M., Ingwall J.S., et al.: Thallium redistribution: Mechanism and clinical utility. *Semin. Nucl. Med.* 10:70–93, 1980.
89. Pohost G.M., Zir L.M., Moore R.H., et al.: Differentiation of transiently ischemic from infarcted myocardium by serial imaging after a single dose of thallium-201. *Circulation* 55:294, 1977.
90. Poliner L.R., Dehmer G.J., Lewis S.E., et al.: Left ventricular performance in normal subjects: A comparison of the responses to exercise in the upright and supine patient. *Circulation* 62:528–541, 1980.
91. Pozen M.W., Lerner D.J., D'Agostino R.B., et al.: Utilization of cardiac nuclear imaging procedures in the United States: An analysis of the extent and costs. Unpublished data, 1980.
92. Prokop E.K., Strauss H.W., Shaw J., et al.: Comparison of regional myocardial perfusion determined by ionic potassium-43 to that determined by microspheres. *Circulation* 50:978–983, 1974.
93. Pugh B.R., Buja L.M., Parkey R.W., et al.: Cardioversion and false positive technetium-99m stannous pyrophosphate myocardial scintigrams. *Circulation* 54:399–403, 1976.
94. Reuter F.G.: Physician and patient exposure during cardiac catheterization. *Circulation* 58:134–139, 1978.
95. Richardson R.L.: Anger scintillation camera, in Rollo F.D. (ed.): *Nuclear Medicine Physics, Instrumentation and Agents*. St. Louis, C.V. Mosby Co., 1977, pp. 231–270.
96. Rigo P., Alderson P.O., Robertson R.M., et al.: Measurement of aortic and mitral regurgitation by gated cardiac blood pool scans. *Circulation* 60:306–312, 1979.
97. Ritchie J.L., Williams D.L., Caldwell J.H.: Seven pinhole emission tomography with thallium-201 in patients with prior myocardial infarction. *J. Nucl. Med.* 22:107–112, 1981.
98. Rollo F.D., Harris C.C.: Factors affecting image formation, in Rollo F.D. (ed.): *Nuclear Medicine Physics, Instrumentation and Agents*. St. Louis, C.V. Mosby Co., 1977, pp. 387–485.
99. Rothendler J.A., Brown K.A., Wilson R.A., et al.: Influence of the collimator on measurement of ejection fraction in simulated gated cardiac images, abstracted. *J. Nucl. Med.* 22:P–18, 1981.
100. Sapirstein L.A.: Fractionation of the cardiac output of rats with isotonic potassium. *Circ. Res.* 4:689–693, 1956.
101. Sapirstein L.A.: Regional blood flow by fractional distribution of indicators. *Am. J. Physiol.* 193:161–168, 1958.
102. Schelbert H.R., Phelps M.E., Hoffman E.: Regional myocardial blood flow, metabolism and function assessed non-invasively with positron emission tomography. *Am. J. Cardiol.* 46:1269–1277, 1980.
103. Schelbert H.R., Verba J.W., Johnson A.D., et al.: Non-traumatic determination of left ventricular ejection fraction by radionuclide angiocardiography. *Circulation* 51:902–909, 1975.
104. Schwartz J.S., Ponto R., Carlyle P., et al.: Early redistribution of thallium-201 after temporary ischemia. *Circulation* 57:332–335, 1978.
105. Slutsky R., Battler A., Karliner J.S., et al.: First third ejection fraction at rest compared with exercise radionuclide angiography in assessing patients with coronary artery disease. *Radiology* 136:197–201, 1980.
106. Slutsky R., Karliner J., Ricci D., et al.: Left ventricular volumes by gated equilibrium angiography: A new method. *Circulation* 60:556–564, 1979.
107. Slutsky R., Pfisterer M., Verba J., et al.: Influence of different background and left ventricular assignments on the ejection fraction in equilibrium radionuclide angiography. *Radiology* 135:725–730, 1980.
108. Smith T.D., Richards P.: A simple kit for the preparation of 99mTc-labeled red blood cells. *J. Nucl. Med.* 17:126–132, 1976.
109. Snyder W.S., Ford M.R., Warner G.G., et al.: "S", absorbed dose per unit cumulated activity for selected radionuclide and organs. New York, Society of Nuclear Medicine, 1975.
110. Sorenson S.G., Caldwell J., Ritchie J., et al.: "Abnormal" response of ejection fraction to exercise in healthy subjects caused by region of interest selection. *J. Nucl. Med.* 22:1–7, 1981.
111. Sorenson S.G., Hamilton G.W., Williams D.L., et al.: R wave synchronized blood pool imaging: A comparison of the accuracy and reproducibility of fixed and computer-automated varying regions of interest for determining the left ventricular ejection fraction. *Radiology* 131:473–478, 1979.
112. Stokely E.M., Parkey E.W., Bonte F.J., et al.: Gated blood pool imaging following 99mTc-pyrophosphate imaging. *Radiology* 120:433–434, 1976.
113. Strauss H.W., Harrison K., Pitt B.: Thallium-201: Non-invasive determination of the regional distri-

bution of cardiac output. *J. Nucl. Med.* 18:1167–1170, 1977.
114. Strauss H.W., Harrison K., Langan J.K., et al.: Thallium-201 for myocardial imaging: Relation of thallium-201 to regional myocardial perfusion. *Circulation* 51:641–645, 1975.
115. Strauss H.W., Lazewatsky J., Moore R.H., et al.: The vest: A device for the continuous monitoring of cardiac function in ambulatory patients, abstracted. *Circulation* 60(suppl. II):II–246, 1979.
116. Strauss H.W., McKusick K.A., Bingham J.B.: Cardiac nuclear imaging: Principles, instrumentation and pitfalls. *Am. J. Cardiol.* 46:1109–1116, 1980.
117. Strauss H.W., McKusick K.A., Boucher C.A., et al.: Of linens and laces: The eighth anniversary of the gated blood pool scan. *Semin. Nucl. Med.* 9:296–309, 1979.
118. Strauss H.W., Pitt B.: Common procedures for the noninvasive determination of regional myocardial perfusion, evaluation of regional wall motion and detection of acute infarction. *Am. J. Cardiol.* 38:731–738, 1976.
119. Strauss H.W., Pitt B.: Gated cardiac blood pool scan: Use in patients with coronary heart disease. *Prog. Cardiovasc. Dis.* 20:207–216, 1977.
120. Strauss H.W., Pitt B.: Noninvasive detection of subcritical coronary arterial narrowings with a coronary vasodilator and myocardial perfusion imaging. *Am. J. Cardiol.* 39:403–406, 1977.
121. Strauss H.W., Pitt B.: Gated blood pool imaging: Techniques, in Strauss H.W., Pitt B. (eds.): *Cardiovascular Nuclear Medicine,* ed. 2. St. Louis, C.V. Mosby Co., 1979, pp. 126–139.
122. Strauss H.W., Pitt B.: Cardiovascular nuclear medicine, in Leiberman D.E. (ed.): *Computer Methods: The Fundamentals of Digital Nuclear Medicine*. St. Louis, C.V. Mosby Co., 1977, pp. 176–180.
123. Strauss H.W., Zaret B.L., Hurley P.J., et al.: A scintiphotographic method for measuring left ventricular ejection fraction in man without cardiac catheterization. *Am. J. Cardiol.* 28:575–580, 1971.
124. Strauss H.W., Zaret B.L., Martin N.D., et al.: Noninvasive evaluation of regional myocardial perfusion with potassium-43: Technique in patients with exercise-induced transient myocardial ischemia. *Radiology* 108:85–90, 1973.
125. TerPogossian M.M., Klein M.S., Markham J., et al.: Regional assessment of myocardial metabolic integrity in vivo by positron-emission tomography with 11C-labeled palmitate. *Circulation* 61:242–255, 1980.
126. Thadani V., Parker J.O.: Hemodynamics at rest during supine and sitting bicycle exercise in normal subjects. *Am. J. Cardiol.* 41:52–59, 1978.
127. Tran P.T., Wasnick R.: *Practical Nuclear Pharmacy*. Honolulu, Banyan Press, 1979.
128. Upton M.T., Rerych S.K., Newman G.E., et al.: The reproducibility of radionuclide angiographic measurements of left ventricular function in normal subjects at rest and during exercise. *Circulation* 62:126–132, 1980.
129. VanAswegen A., Alderson P.O., Nickoloff E.L., et al.: Temporal resolution requirements for left ventricular time-activity curves. *Radiology* 135:165–170, 1980.
130. Vogel R.A.: Quantitative aspects of myocardial perfusion images. *Semin. Nucl. Med.* 10:146–153, 1980.
131. Vogel R.A., Kirch D.L., LeFree M.T., et al.: Thallium-201 myocardial perfusion scintigraphy: Results of standard and multi-pinhole tomographic techniques. *Am. J. Cardiol.* 43:787–793, 1979.
132. Vogel R.A., Kirch D., LaFree M., et al.: A new method of multiplanar emission tomography using a seven pinhole collimator and an Anger scintillation camera. *J. Nucl. Med.* 19:648–654, 1978.
133. Vogel R.A., Kirch D.L., LaFree M.T., et al.: Gated blood pool tomography using the seven pinhole Anger camera technique. *Circulation* 59,60(suppl. II):II–29, 1979.
134. Wackers F.J., Berger H.J., Johnstone D.E., et al.: Multiple gated cardiac blood pool imaging for left ventricular ejection fraction: Validation of the technique and assessment of variability. *Am. J. Cardiol.* 43:1159–1166, 1979.
135. Wackers F.J., Sokole F.B., Samson G., et al.: Value and limitation of thallium-201 scintigraphy in the acute phase of myocardial infarction. *N. Engl. J. Med.* 295:1–5, 1976.
136. Wagner H.N. Jr., Wahe R., Nickoloff E., et al.: The nuclear stethoscope: A simple device for generation of left ventricular volume curves. *Am. J. Cardiol.* 38:747–750, 1976.
137. Wagner H.N. Jr., Rigo P., Baxter W., et al.: Monitoring ventricular function at rest and during exercise with a non-imaging nuclear detector. *Am. J. Cardiol.* 43:975–978, 1979.
138. Webster E.W., Merrill O.E.: Radiation hazards: II. Measurement of gonadal dose in radiographic examinations. *N. Engl. J. Med.* 257:811–819, 1957.
139. Weich H.F., Strauss H.W., Pitt B.: The extraction of thallium-201 by the myocardium. *Circulation* 56:188–191, 1977.
140. Winzelberg G.G., Boucher C.A., McKusick K.A., et al.: Right ventricular function in aortic and mitral valve disease: Relationship of gated first pass radionuclide angiography to clinical and hemodynamic findings. *Chest* 79:520–528, 1981.
141. Winzelberg G.G., Miller S.G., Okada R.D., et al.: Scintigraphic evaluation of false left ventricular aneurysm. *Am. J. Radiol.* 135:569–574, 1980
142. Winzelberg G.G., Strauss H.W., Bingham J.B., et al.: Scintigraphic evaluation of left ventricular aneurysm. *Am. J. Cardiol.* 46:1138–1143, 1980.

143. Zaret B.L., Berger H.J.: Techniques of nuclear cardiology, in Hurst J.W., Logue R.B., Schlant R.C., et al. (eds.): *The Heart, Arteries and Veins,* ed. 5. New York, McGraw-Hill Book Co., to be published.
144. Zaret B.L., Strauss H.W., Hurley P.J., et al.: A noninvasive scintiphotographic method for detecting regional ventricular dysfunction in man. *N. Engl. J. Med.* 284:1165–1170, 1971.
145. Zaret B.L., Strauss H.W., Martin N.D., et al.: Noninvasive myocardial perfusion with radioactive potassium. *N. Engl. J. Med.* 288:809–812, 1973.

PART II

Assessment of Left Ventricular Function

ECHOCARDIOGRAPHY

Edward D. Folland and Alfred F. Parisi

THE PUMPING FUNCTION of the left ventricle can be measured quantitatively in terms of volume and pressure. Traditionally, pressure measurements have required the use of intracardiac catheters and volume measurements have been made with high-speed x-ray contrast angiography. If frequent simultaneous measurements of volume and pressure are plotted against one another for a complete cardiac cycle, a pressure-volume loop is generated (Fig 3–1) which provides the basis for several commonly employed clinical indices of function. The measurement made at a single instant in the cardiac cycle is known as a *static measurement* or *static index*. Examples of static indices include end-diastolic volume (EDV), end-diastolic pressure (EDP), and end-systolic volume (ESV). Changes in volume or pressure over time or the rates of such changes are referred to as *dynamic indices;* examples include stroke volume (EDV − ESV), ejection fraction $\left(\frac{EDV - ESV}{EDV}\right)$, velocity of circumferential fiber shortening (Vcf), and rate of pressure rise *(dp/dt)*.

The preceding are methods of characterizing or describing the overall or *global* function of the left ventricle. Diseases which impair left ventricular function often do so in a nonuniform fashion, adversely affecting contractile function in some regions of the myocardium and sparing function in other regions. Ischemic heart disease is the prime example of a nonuniform process. The existence of such *local* or *regional* disease processes requires some means for describing the location and extent of impairment, hence the need for indices of *regional ventricular function*. Regional ventricular impairment has traditionally been evaluated by x-ray contrast angiography, both qualitatively, through visual description of regional contraction, and quantitatively, through measurement of axis shortening or area shrinkage of various segments of the angiographic silhouette from diastole to systole.

Echocardiography is well suited for imaging the endocardial borders of the left ventricular cavity in various projections throughout the cardiac cycle and therefore can provide static and dynamic measurements which relate directly to volume indices of left ventricular function. Echocardiography cannot by itself provide information directly related to pressure indices. Since volume indices have proved to be of much greater value than pressure indices in clinical practice, echocardiography has found important application in the assessment of both global and regional ventricular function.

This chapter reviews the current status of echocardiography, both M-mode and two-dimensional, in evaluating indices of global and regional left ventricular function.

GLOBAL FUNCTION: STATIC MEASUREMENTS

Left Ventricular Internal Dimensions

Measurement of left ventricular internal dimensions by M-mode echocardiography is illustrated in Figure 3–2. The transducer is positioned in the standard left parasternal location and directed through the interventricular septum and left ventricular posterior wall at the level of the chordae tendineae (see Fig 1-3). The echocardiogram shows measurement of the left ventricular internal diastolic dimension *(large arrow)* and systolic dimension *(small arrow)* during the same cardiac cycle. Historically, there has been some disagreement among investigators as to where in the cardiac cycle the internal diastolic dimension should be measured. Some have taken it to be coincident with the ECG Q wave, others have chosen the R wave, and still others have used the maximal diastolic dimension, which usually occurs at the dip in the left ventricular posterior wall due to atrial systole.[1] Based on a survey of interobserver variability, the Committee on M-Mode Standardization of the American Society of Echocardiography has recommended that left ventricular diastole be measured from the onset of the QRS complex, with the cavity dimension taken from the leading edge of the left ventricular posterior wall endocardium to the leading edge of the echo from the left side of the interventricular septum.[2] That committee found there was little difference in reproducibility of left ventricular systolic measurements, whether they were made at the peak of posterior wall motion or at the nadir of septal motion. Because the nadir of septal motion is more closely related in time to end-systole, the standard recommendation is that the systolic dimension be measured at this point, provided septal motion is normal. When septal motion is abnormal at the level of the chordae tendineae, the left ventricular systolic dimension should be measured from the peak of posterior wall motion. In adults, the normal left ventricular internal diastolic dimension ranges between 3.7 and 5.6 cm.[2] In individual patients the predicted normal left ventricular dimension is a function of body size (body surface area) and, to a lesser extent, age. Henry et al.[3] have recently published tables of normal dimensions based on measurements made using the American Society of Echocardiography criteria. Using the equations developed in this study, one can calculate the predicted normal dimensions and 95% confidence limits for a patient of any given age or size.

Left ventricular dimensions can also be measured by two-dimensional echocardiography (2DE), which offers the advantage of imaging from apical as well as parasternal windows (Fig 3–3). Because of the added freedom of projection in 2DE and the difficulties in routinely determining the area of sectional views, normal dimensions have not yet been published.

Many investigators have compared echocardiographic and angiographic measurements made in the same patients. A high degree of correlation between echocardiographic minor-axis dimensions

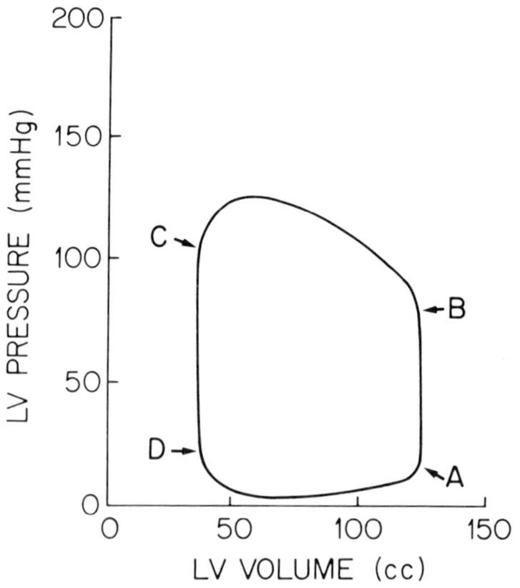

Fig 3–1.—Many aspects of left ventricular function can be succinctly summarized by a pressure-volume loop derived from simultaneous plotting of pressure and volume during the course of a single cardiac cycle. At point *A*, mitral valve closes and isovolumic contraction occurs until point *B*, where the aortic valve opens and ejection begins. At point *C*, the aortic valve closes, ejection ceases, and isovolumic relaxation takes place until mitral valve opening at point *D*. Diastolic filling occurs from point *D* to point *A*, where the cycle then repeats.

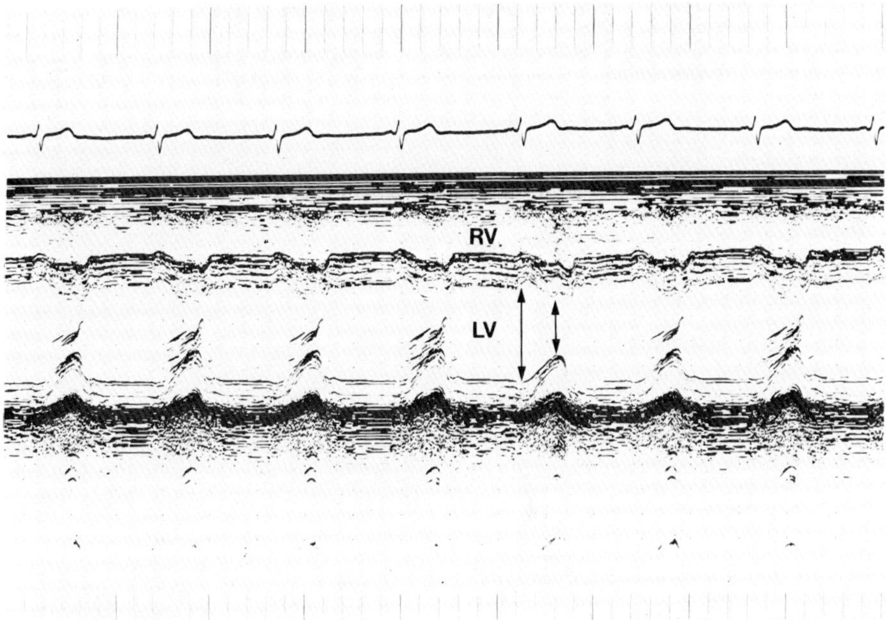

Fig 3–2.—This echocardiogram was produced by a beam orientation like the one displayed in Figure 1–3. Right ventricular *(RV)* and left ventricular *(LV)* cavities are indicated, and LV internal dimensions in diastole are denoted by the *large arrow* and in systole by the *small arrow.*

and angiographic minor-axis dimensions has been documented repeatedly.[4–6] This relationship has also been demonstrated with a high degree of correlation when long-axis measurements obtained by 2DE are included (Fig 3–4).[7–9] Regardless of whether echocardiographic and angiographic axes coincide (and there is good reason to believe they do not), the findings indicate that echocardiographic dimensions are a reliable index of left ventricular size. Indeed, of all echocardiographic measurements, left ventricular internal dimensions are subject to least interobserver variability and are the most reproducible.[2, 10] Pietro et al.[10] suggest that when serial studies are done on the same patient, a change of more than 5% in left ventricular diastolic dimensions is likely to be significant. Clark et al.[11] found similar limits of reproducibility in serial studies on patients with valvular heart disease and cited 95% confidence limits for diastolic dimension at ± 0.3 cm. Left ventricular dimensions have been shown to be particularly useful in following patients with regurgitant valvular lesions,[11–13] although there is evidence that the accuracy of the measurement decreases somewhat in larger ventricles.[9, 14]

Left Ventricular Volumes

Many attempts have been made to derive left ventricular end-diastolic and end-systolic volumes from the respective echocardiographic dimensions. These have met with variable success, depending on the patient population studied and whether M-mode echocardiography or 2DE was used.

M-mode dimensions can be used to calculate left ventricular volume through an application of the angiographic concept of the left ventricle as a prolate ellipse. The volume of such an ellipsoid may be calculated by multiplying $4/3\ \pi$ times the product of the three hemiaxes (Fig 3–5). M-mode echocardiography allows measurement of only one left ventricular dimension, the septal-posterolateral dimension, which is viewed at the level of the chordae tendineae. In order to calculate volume from this single dimension, the following assumptions must apply:

1. The individual ventricle being examined does in fact approximate the geometry of an ellipsoid, both in diastole and systole.
2. The septal-posterolateral dimension mea-

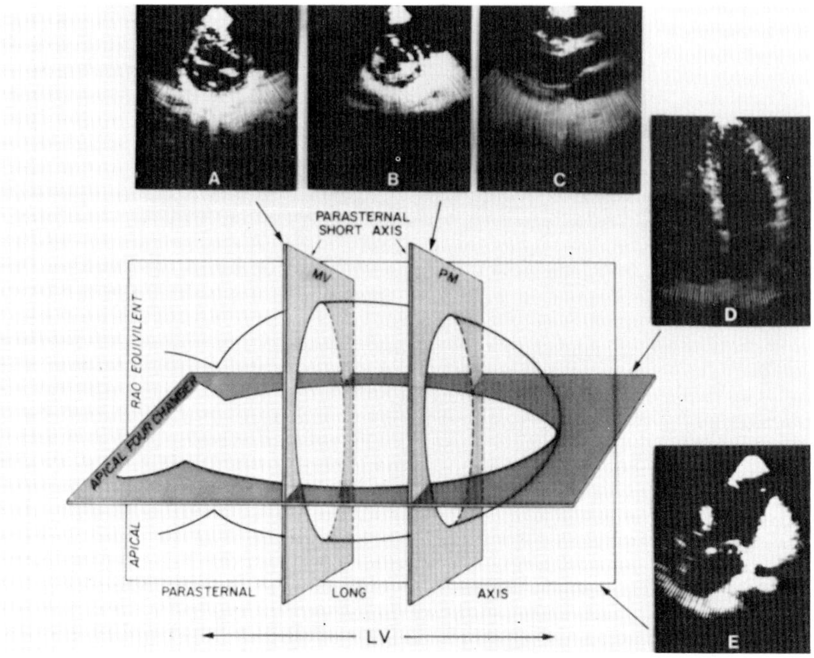

Fig 3–3.—The schematic depicts an idealized left ventricle *(LV),* which has been sectioned by five standard planes used in two-dimensional echocardiography. From the parasternal crystal position, cross section of the ventricle can be reproducibly displayed at either the mitral valve *(MV)* level **(A)** or the papillary muscle *(PM)* level **(B).** By rotating the parasternal crystal 90 degrees, the long-axis section is displayed **(C).** From the apical crystal position two standard sections are commonly employed. The four-chamber view **(D)** transects both ventricles and both atria through the mitral and tricuspid valves. By rotating the crystal 90 degrees from this position, an "RAO equivalent" view **(E)** is obtained which displays left ventricle, left atrium, and aortic root from a plane which is similar to the parasternal long-axis view. The term "RAO equivalent" derives from the similarity of this section to the right anterior oblique (RAO) view commonly employed in cineangiography.

sured coincides with the minor axis of the ellipsoid, D_1.

3. The orthogonal minor axis, D_2, is equal to the measured minor axis, D_1.

4. The major axis, L, is twice the length of the minor axes, D_1 and D_2.

If these assumptions hold true, left ventricular volume can be described by the equation:

$$V = \frac{4\pi}{3} \cdot \left(\frac{D_1}{2}\right) \cdot \left(\frac{D_2}{2}\right) \cdot \left(\frac{L}{2}\right)$$

and since $D_2 = D_1$ and $L = 2D_1$,

$$V = \frac{4\pi}{3} \cdot \left(\frac{D_1}{2}\right) \cdot \left(\frac{D_1}{2}\right) \cdot \left(\frac{2D_1}{2}\right)$$

or

$$V = \frac{\pi}{3} (D_1)^3$$

or, more simply, $V = (D_1)^3$, which is commonly known as the cube formula.[6]

Deviations from the assumptions of the cube formula are most commonly encountered in enlarged ventricles, which tend either to be spherical ($L < 2D$) or to have localized aneurysmal bulges, as in normal-sized ventricles where segmental contraction abnormalities distort the ventricle in systole. Fortuin et al.[4] have proposed regression equations to deal with the nonellipsoidal nature of larger ventricles:

$$\text{End-diastolic volume} = 0.59 \times Dd - 153$$
$$\text{End-systolic volume} = 0.47 \times Ds - 120$$

Teichholz et al.[15] have proposed a modified ellipsoid formula to compensate for this same problem:

$$V = \frac{7.0 \times D^3}{2.4 \times D}$$

Good correlations between angiographic vol-

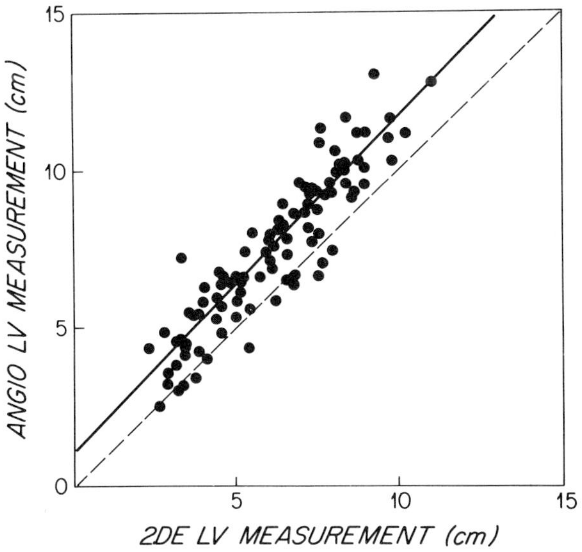

Fig 3–4.—Relationship between various left ventricular *(LV)* measurements made by two-dimensional echocardiography *(2DE)* and analogous measurements made by cineangiography *(ANGIO)* in the same patients. The *solid line* depicts the regression relationship and the *dashed line* the line of identity. There is a consistent relationship between the techniques, although echocardiography tends to underpredict angiographic dimensions. (From Parisi A.F., et al.: *Med. Clin. North Am.* 64:66, 1980. Reproduced by permission.)

umes and echo volumes have been obtained using all three formulas, provided that patients with ventricular asynergy are excluded.[4, 6, 15–17] Independent comparisons of the three methods suggest that Teichholz's method is most accurate (Table 3–1).[16, 17]

Two-dimensional echocardiography offers considerable advantage for estimation of left ventricular volume because it allows direct measurement of all three hemiaxes in the ellipsoid model and also allows application of other volume formulations, such as Simpson's rule.[18–23] Studies have shown that correlations between echocardiographic and angiographic volumes can be substantially improved by use of two-dimensional methods.[17, 18, 22, 24] Furthermore, equally good correlations (r = 0.80–0.90) with angiographic volume have been obtained, regardless of the presence of ventricular asynergy.[23, 25] In our laboratory we have estimated left ventricular volumes by 2 DE in a series of 50 patients undergoing single-plane angiography. One or more of the sections illustrated in Figure 3–3 was utilized in a series of six volume algorithms, each involving different assumptions about left ventricular geometry. Overall, the best correlations were obtained using a modified Simpson's rule formulation (Fig 3–6) and an area-length ellipsoid formulation using a biplane approach.[24] Other investigators have confirmed the validity of Simpson's rule[19, 20, 23] and area-length ellipsoid formulations.[17, 22, 25, 26] Despite the good correlations with angiographic volumes, the estimating errors of all these methods remain rather large, and appropriate judgment should be exercised in applying these estimates in any individual case. The smallest estimating errors have been published by Schiller et al.,[20] who studied 30 patients with biplane 2DE and biplane angiography. Using Simpson's rule for estimating echocardiographic and angiographic volumes, the standard error of the estimate for echocardiographic diastolic volume was 15 ml/sq m. The greatest disadvantage to quantitative 2DE is the inability to obtain technically satisfactory images in all patients and the labor involved in analyzing the studies. Most investigations to date have entailed tracing endocardial outlines on celluloid and transferring these images to digitizing computer systems. The current development of interactive, stop-action image display and automated computation systems should enhance the clinical practicability of these methods.

TABLE 3–1.—Correlation Between Angiographic and Echocardiographic Stroke Volume Using Three Common Methods

STUDY	FORMULA	N	r	SEE
Teichholz et al.[15]	$\frac{7.0 \cdot D^3}{2.4 \cdot D}$	25	0.74	18.1
Fortuin et al.[4]	EDV = $0.59 \cdot Dd - 153$ ESV = $0.47 \cdot Ds - 120$	23	0.69	18.9
Pombo et al.[6]	$(D_1)^3$	25	0.64	20.7

Adapted from Kronik et al.[16] All patients had symmetric contraction. Correlations were substantially worse in patients with asynergy.

Left Ventricular Mass

The thickness of septal and posterolateral left ventricular walls can be conveniently measured by M-mode echocardiography. Normal standards using American Society of Echocardiography criteria

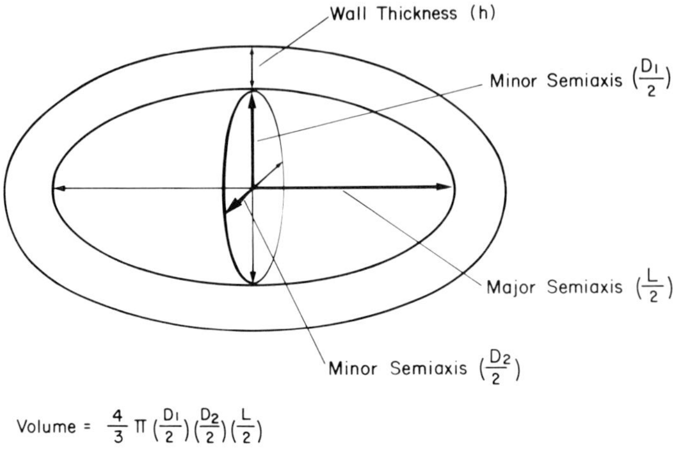

Fig 3–5.—An ellipsoid of revolution showing minor hemiaxes $D_1/2$ and $D_2/2$, major hemiaxis (L/2), and formula for volume calculation.

have been published.[2] In general, an interventricular septum (IVS) greater than 1.1 cm and posterior wall (PW) greater than 1.0 cm in thickness suggest the presence of hypertrophy. Echocardiography surpasses scalar ECG in its sensitivity for detection of true anatomical hypertrophy.[28] The mass of the left ventricle can be calculated by using the cube volume formula as follows[27, 28]:

$$V_{\text{LV wall}} = V_{\text{LV total}} - V_{\text{LV cavity}}$$
$$V_{\text{LV cavity}} = D^3$$
$$V_{\text{LV total}} = (D + PW + IVS)^3$$

therefore

$$V_{\text{LV wall}} = (D + PW + IVS)^3 - D^3$$

and

$$\text{Mass} = 1.04\,(V_{\text{wall}}) - 14\text{ gm}$$

Using this formulation, Reichek and Devereux[28] demonstrated excellent correlation ($r = 0.96$) between premortem echocardiographic mass and postmortem autopsy mass in 34 patients.

Left Ventricular End-Diastolic Pressure

Although echocardiography does not provide information relating directly to left ventricular pressure, it is possible to infer the end-diastolic pressure from the motion and timing of the mitral valve. In normal sinus rhythm in healthy subjects, mitral valve leaflet motion is smooth and continuous from the peak of atrial contraction (A wave) to the point of valve closure (C point). Furthermore, the C point occurs 40–50 msec after the onset of the ECG QRS complex (Fig 3–7). Several years ago it was noted that a plateau-like pause or "notch" (B notch) on the AC slope was a feature often associated with elevated end-diastolic pressures (see Fig 3–7).[29] Since the AC interval is influenced by atrioventricular conduction, a further refinement was attempted by subtracting the echocardiographic AC interval from the ECG PR interval. A PR − AC difference of less than .06

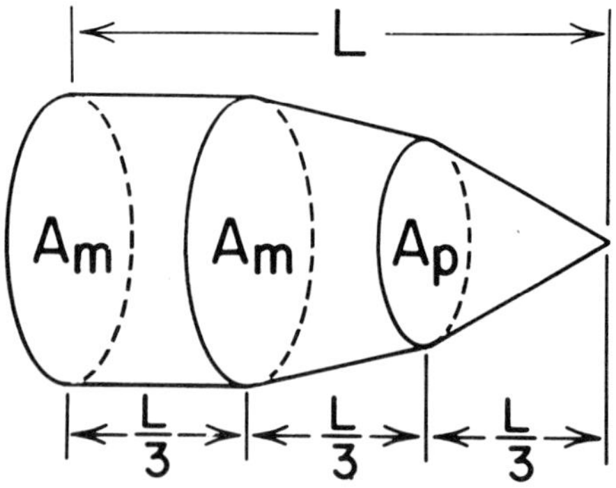

Fig 3–6.—Schematic volume model of the left ventricle using modification of Simpson's rule. The long axis of the ventricle measured from the apical view *(L)* is arbitrarily divided into thirds so that the ventricular volume is the sum of the volumes of a cylinder, truncated cone, and a cone. The areas A_m and A_p are measured from parasternal short-axis views at mitral valve and papillary muscle levels, respectively. (From Parisi A.J., et al.: *Med. Clin. North Am.* 64:68, 1980. Reproduced by permission.)

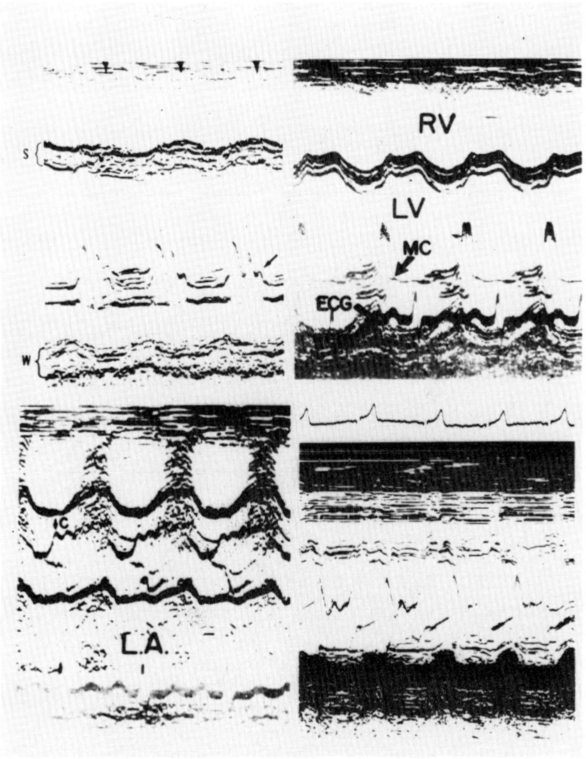

Fig 3–7.—Abnormalities of valve motion consistent with elevation of left ventricular end-diastolic pressure. *Bottom right,* normal mitral valve motion. In contrast, *top left* demonstrates notching *(arrow)* of the mitral valve closure pattern and *top right* shows premature mitral valve closure *(MC)* seen in severe aortic regurgitation. *Bottom left* demonstrates premature aortic valve cusp *(C)* opening seen in extremely severe aortic regurgitation. For comparison, normal aortic valve motion is shown in the *top left* panel of Figure 3–11.

second was suggested as an index of elevated left ventricular end-diastolic pressure[29]; however, other investigators[30, 31] have failed to confirm this relationship. Although this quantitative approach to end-diastolic pressure does not seem to be warranted, we still feel that the presence of notch on the AC slope is a worthwhile observation. When it is seen, there is almost always left ventricular failure.

In the setting of severe aortic regurgitation, the mitral valve may close prematurely due to excessive diastolic regurgitant filling from the aortic root.[32–34, 78] Left ventricular pressure rises so rapidly that it can exceed left atrial pressure even before the onset of electric left ventricular depolarization and close the mitral valve before the appearance of the ECG QRS complex. This observation, most commonly made in severe acute or subacute aortic insufficiency, indicates a left ventricular end-diastolic pressure in the range of 20–30 mm Hg (see Fig 3–7). A rare observation, seen only in most extreme forms of aortic regurgitation, is premature opening of the aortic valve (see Fig 3–7). This occurs when aortic regurgitation is so copious that there is diastolic equilibrium between aortic pressure and left ventricular pressures. This diastolic pressure equilibrium may be associated not only with premature closure of the mitral valve, but also with premature opening of the aortic valve. Premature opening of the aortic valve in the setting of aortic insufficiency usually indicates a left ventricular end-diastolic pressure of about 50 mm Hg.[33]

GLOBAL FUNCTION: DYNAMIC MEASUREMENTS

Left Ventricular Fractional Shortening

The simplest echocardiographic measure of global left ventricular contractility is the percent shortening of the left ventricular internal dimension.[4] This is derived by subtracting the systolic dimension *(Ds)* from the diastolic dimension *(Dd)* and normalizing for diastolic size by dividing by the diastolic dimension. It is usually expressed as a percent ($\%\Delta D$) and is represented by the following formula:

$$\%\Delta D = \frac{Dd - Ds}{Dd} \times 100$$

This determination assumes that the region sampled is representative of the ventricular contraction pattern as a whole; thus the formula is valid only if regional contraction abnormalities are minimal or absent. In many patients with coronary disease, areas of akinesis or hypokinesis lie distal to the usual level of sampling the left ventricle at the chordae tendineae. In these individuals, stroke volume is often maintained by increased regional motion near the base of the heart. In such instances fractional shortening of the left ventricle is likely to overpredict global left ventricular function. There is also a tendency for fractional shortening to overestimate angiographic ejection fraction in patients with valvular regurgitation. In these patients the septal-posterolateral axis may shorten excessively in relationship to the anteroposterior axis and possibly the long axis as well.

Several studies have confirmed that the normal range of $\%\Delta D$ extends from 30% to nearly 50%.[35–37] In studies comparing $\%\Delta D$ with angiographic ejection fraction, there has been acceptable correlation only in patients with symmetric contraction.[15, 16] Clark et al.[11] studied the reproducibility of $\%\Delta D$ in 15 patients with valvular disease and found the 95% confidence limit for repeated studies to be ± 5.5%.

Velocity of Circumferential Fiber Shortening (*Vcf*)

This index describes the rate of systolic shortening of the left ventricular endocardial circumference at the midventricle. Its application in M-mode echocardiography assumes that the left ventricular internal dimension is measured at midventricle. Since the circumference is πDd at end-diastole and πDs at end-systole, the absolute circumferential shortening is $\pi Dd - \pi Ds$. The difference between these two values will vary considerably with ventricular size; therefore, the expression is normalized by dividing it by the end-diastolic circumference, πDd. The *mean rate* of shortening is determined by dividing the resulting expression by the left ventricular ejection time (ET), which may be measured from the concomitant carotid pulse tracing or from the duration of echocardiographic aortic valve opening. The final expression is

$$\text{mean } Vcf = \frac{\pi Dd - \pi Ds}{\pi Dd \cdot \text{ET}}$$

which factors to

$$\text{mean } Vcf = \frac{Dd - Ds}{Dd \cdot \text{ET}}$$

which simplifies further as the left ventricular fractional shortening divided by the ejection time.[38] Peak *Vcf* can be similarly derived by extrapolation from the maximum systolic slope of posterior and septal walls. *Vcf* is subject to the same inaccuracy as $\%\Delta D$ in patients with asynergy.[39] In groups of patients having a wide range of ventricular function, mean *Vcf* measurements determined echocardiographically and angiographically have correlated reasonably.[40, 41]

Although Wilson and Reichek[42] found the echocardiographic peak *Vcf* to be a better discriminator of patients with angiographic ejection fractions below and above 55% than the echocardiographic ejection fraction or $\%\Delta D$, it remains only a qualitative indicator of left ventricular function. Likewise, mean *Vcf* has been shown to offer no practical advantage over $\%\Delta D$ in characterizing left ventricular function in patients with valvular heart disease[43] or primary myocardial disease.[38]

Left Ventricular Ejection Fraction

Ejection fraction has become the most useful single invasive index of left ventricular function because it correlates better with clinical outcome and surgical risk than other indices.[44, 45] It is the quotient of end-diastolic volume (EDV) minus end-systolic volume (ESV) divided by end-diastolic volume:

$$\text{EF} = \frac{\text{EDV} - \text{ESV}}{\text{EDV}}$$

It can be simply derived from the echocardiographic volumes discussed previously. The accuracy and clinical utility of echocardiographic EF depends on whether M-mode or 2DE studies were used for estimating volumes. The EF can be derived from M-mode echocardiography either by direct use of volumes from the formulas described earlier, or from a regression equation (EF = 1.7 × $\%\Delta D$).[36] In either case it is valid only in the absence of asynergy.[46] In our opinion, M-mode EF offers no practical advantage over the simpler $\%\Delta D$ expression of contractility.

The EF derived from 2DE volumes has been shown to have a more consistent relationship to angiographic EF, whether or not asynergy is present. Table 3–2 summarizes the methods and results of various investigators who have compared echocardiographic and angiographic EFs. In our own laboratory, a modified Simpson's rule volume algorithm (see Fig 3–6) provided reliable results

TABLE 3–2.—RELATIONSHIP OF ECHOCARDIOGRAPHIC TO ANGIOCARDIOGRAPHIC EJECTION FRACTIONS*

STUDY	METHOD	N	r	SEE	COMMENTS
		M-Mode Echocardiography			
Pombo et al.[6]	Cube formula	27	.80	.09	Mixed patient group (13/27 VHD, 3/27 IHD)
Fortuin et al.[4]	$\%\Delta D$	27	.79	.07	Mixed patient group (19/27 VHD, 1/27 IHD)
Quinones et al.[36]	Regression formula	42	.90	.08	Patients selected to have no detectable asynergy
Teichholz et al.[15]	Modified ellipsoid formula	11	.79	. . .	Patients without asynergy
		14	.37	. . .	Patients with asynergy
		Two-Dimensional Echocardiography			
Teichholz et al.[77]	B-Scan	25	.87	. . .	14/25 had asynergy
Folland et al.[18]	Modified Simpson's rule	35	.78	.10	
Parisi et al.[24]	Modified Simpson's rule	50	.80	.09	25/50 had asynergy
		25	.83	.08	25 patients only with asynergy
Carr et al.[17]	Biplane area-length	22	.93	. . .	6 had asynergy, wide spread of EFs
Schiller et al.[20]	Modified Simpson's rule	30	.87	.08	16/30 had asynergy
Chaudry et al.[76]	3-Axis Measurement	30	.73	. . .	20/30 had IHD
Nixon et al.[21]		9	.79	.04	
Ohuchi et al.[25]	Single-plane area-length	38	.88	. . .	With and without asynergy
		18	.88	. . .	Patients with asynergy

*N, number of patients; r, linear correlation coefficient; SEE, standard error of the estimate; VHD, valvular heart disease; IHD, ischemic heart disease.

in 50 patients, half of whom had angiographically documented asynergy.[24] In particular, the standard error of the estimate in our series (.09) compared favorably with the estimating error of EF measured by radionuclide angiography.[47] As in estimating volumes, the major problem with clinical use of 2DE EF is a practical one: the quantitative process is cumbersome and not technically possible in some patients.

Stroke Volume

Echocardiographic stroke volume (SV = EDV − ESV) suffers from the inherent lack of accuracy in volume estimations. Clinically, stroke volume is a less useful index than EF since it also tends to vary more widely with different physiologic circumstances such as body size, heart rate, posture, and exercise. Noninvasive determinations of cardiac output, the product of stroke volume and heart rate, are even more inaccurate, since multiplication magnifies the estimating error. Nevertheless, providing that subjects with left ventricular asynergy are excluded from analysis, fair correlations between M-mode echocardiographic stroke volume and both thermodilution and angiographic stroke volume have been published (see Table 3–1).[16]

Diminished stroke volume can sometimes be inferred from ancillary echocardiographic observations. The amplitude of M-mode echocardiographic aortic root motion is directly related to stroke volume. If used to predict stroke index determined invasively (Fick or green dye methods), there is a large estimating error; however, diminished (< 5 mm) anterior aortic motion in the adult is highly associated with a poor stroke output (Fig 3–8).[48]

The pattern of aortic leaflet motion also provides qualitative information about stroke volume. In low-output states the aortic leaflets tend to open and close less abruptly and therefore have a systolic pattern which more resembles an oval than the usual parallelogram (see Fig 3–8). Also, Jacobs et al.[49] found that the measured area between the aortic valve cusps in systole tends to decrease in direct proportion to decreased stroke volume.

E Point Septal Separation

In the normal echocardiogram the E point of mitral valve diastolic opening closely approximates the left ventricular endocardium of the septum. In patients with severe left ventricular dysfunction, considerable separation may exist between the septum and the E point. Massie et al.[50] found a negative linear correlation ($r = -0.87$)

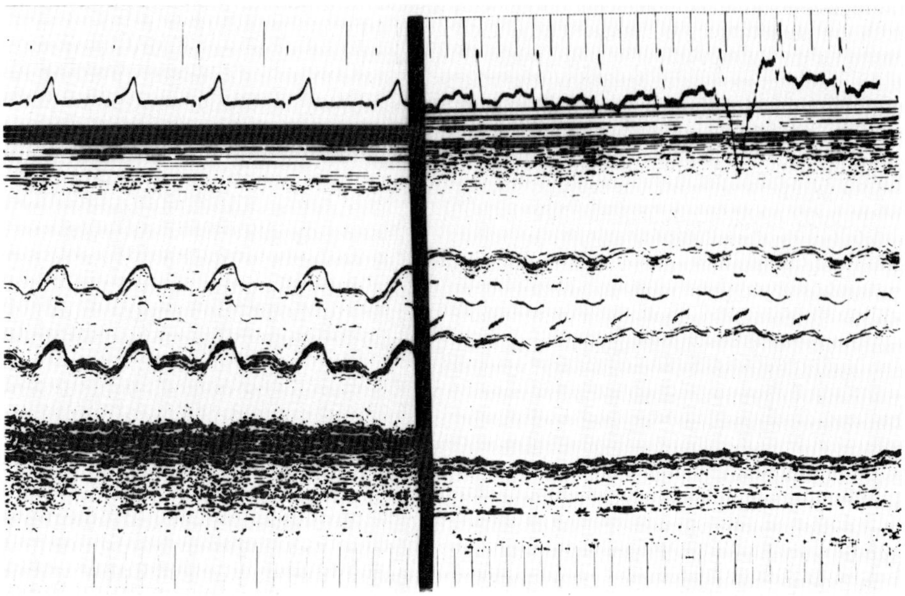

Fig 3–8.—Influence of stroke volume on aortic root and valve motion. *Left,* normal aortic root and valve motion. *Right,* diminished aortic root motion, reduced area of valve opening, and late systolic posterior drift of noncoronary cusp in a patient with severely reduced stroke volume.

between E point septal separation and angiographic ejection fraction in a large group of patients. It is usually seen in the presence of severe left ventricular dysfunction. The finding is probably a result of the combined effects of increased left ventricular size and reduced diastolic flow through the mitral valve (see Fig 3–7, *top left*).

Left Ventricular Compliance

Compliance is a term used to describe the relationship of the volume of a structure to its internal pressure. The diastolic compliance of the left ventricle is measured by recording its volume change per unit of pressure change during left ventricular filling (see Fig 3–1). Stiffness is the inverse of compliance, i.e., the pressure change per unit volume change. Diseases which lead to left ventricular hypertrophy, fibrosis, and infarction generally cause decreased left ventricular compliance; i.e., under these circumstances the ventricle is stiffer.

To measure compliance or stiffness accurately, left ventricular pressures must be recorded simultaneously with volume determination. Echocardiographic volumes can be used as a substitute for contrast angiocardiographic volumes in these circumstances.[51] The echo method avoids the possible influence of contrast agents on ventricular function. At present the use of echocardiography to measure compliance or other aspects of left ventricular function with simultaneous left heart catheterization is limited to research contexts.

A "stiff" left ventricle may be associated with slower transmitral flow rates and a decreased mitral valve diastolic E-F slope. In a series of 32 patients without mitral stenosis, Quinones et al. showed that an E-F slope of less than 60 mm/second was highly correlated with decreased left ventricular compliance.[52]

REGIONAL FUNCTION

M-Mode Echocardiography

As a means for analysis of regional left ventricular function, M-mode echocardiography is considerably restricted by its unidimensional nature and by its limitation to imaging only in the septal-posterolateral plane. Nevertheless, within the scope of these limitations, considerable information can be gleaned regarding regional myocardial function, provided that good definition of endocardial targets is obtained. Echocardiography is probably the best noninvasive modality for analysis of regional function because of its high resolution (1–2 mm), which is considerably better than that of radionuclide angiography (1 cm).[53]

The simplest measures of wall motion which can be derived from M-mode echocardiography include the *amplitude* of motion of the left side of the interventricular septum,[54, 55] the *amplitude* of motion of the posterior wall,[56] the *thickening* of both of the latter structures,[57, 58] and their *rate of motion* from end-diastole to peak systole.[59] These measurements are demonstrated schematically in Figure 3–9. The normal interventricular septum at the level of the chordae tendineae moves posteriorly 3–8 mm by end-systole; the left ventricular posterior wall moves anteriorly 9–16 mm during the same time.[57] A host of diseases and

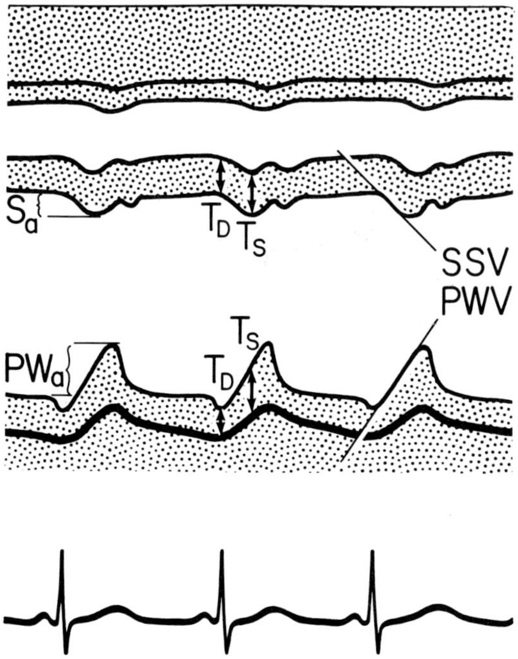

Fig 3–9.—Schematic illustrating measurement of amplitude, thickening, and rate of motion for septal and posterior walls. S_a, septal amplitude; PW_a, posterior wall amplitude; T_D, diastolic thickness; T_s, systolic thickness; *SSV,* systolic septal velocity; *PWV,* posterior wall velocity. (From Parisi A.J., et al.: *Med. Clin. North Am.* 64:71, 1980. Reproduced by permission.)

conditions can diminish the extent of normal septal motion. Most common among these is coronary artery disease in the distribution of the left anterior descending coronary artery.[54, 55] Other frequently encountered causes associated with diminished and frankly paradoxical (i.e., systolic anterior) septal motion include right ventricular volume overload (left-to-right shunts at the atrial level), tricuspid regurgitation,[60–63] hypertrophic and congestive cardiomyopathies,[57, 64] pericardial disease, including large effusions and constrictive pericarditis,[65–67] and prior open heart surgery.[68, 69] In congestive cardiomyopathy and other forms of heart disease in which there is advanced global left ventricular dysfunction, diminished septal motion is accompanied by diminished posterior wall excursions. As an isolated finding, impaired septal motion is nonspecific; however, it can often be related to a specific clinical condition when considered in the context of other findings. For example, in right ventricular volume overload states, a dilated right ventricular internal dimension almost invariably accompanies abnormal septal motion; similarly, large pericardial effusions, easily identified by echocardiography, may be accompanied by an overall swinging motion of the heart, which can explain abnormal septal motion in this setting. The amplitude of posterior wall motion is most commonly influenced by coronary disease. In patients with inferior myocardial infarctions, diminished posterior wall motion amplitude is a common finding.[57]

Exaggerated septal and posterior wall motion are found concomitantly in volume overload states (aortic regurgitation, mitral regurgitation) when the left ventricle is compensated. In coronary disease, hyperdynamic septal motion is often seen in the presence of impaired posterior wall motion, and vice versa.[70] In these instances, the contralateral wall may be conceived as performing at greater capacity in order to compensate for the opposite regional wall motion defect—a finding frequently confirmed on cineangiography.

During systolic contraction the walls of the healthy ventricle thicken (see Fig 3–9). In one study of 29 normal subjects, the average systolic thickening was 3 mm (36%) for the septum and 5 mm (47%) for the posterior wall.[57] Infarcted and actively ischemic ventricular walls fail to thicken properly. In fact, in acute infarction, the interventricular septum may actually become thinner during systole.[57] The presence or absence of abnormal septal thickening is an important observation in differentiating the several causes of abnormal septal motion. In right ventricular volume overload states the septum thickens normally, while in coronary disease septal thickening is often impaired or absent.

Two-Dimensional Echocardiography

Two-dimensional echocardiography is potentially the ideal modality for analyzing regional left ventricular wall motion. It allows visualization of left ventricular circumference in tomographic planes at continuously variable levels from three different crystal positions (parasternal, apical, and subcostal). In suitable subjects, virtually all regions of left ventricular myocardium are accessible by this high-resolution technique. As with any echocardiographic approach, it is not technically feasible in some patients, yet the capability of utilizing the apical and subcostal windows occasionally makes 2DE studies possible where M-mode echocardiography has failed.

Four specific views apply particularly to wall motion analysis because they relate well to physicians' anatomical concepts of left ventricular anatomy and because they are reproducible. These are the parasternal short- and long-axis views and apical four-chamber and two-chamber (RAO equivalent) views (Fig 3–10). The parasternal short-axis view can be reproducibly studied at two levels: mitral valve and papillary muscle (see Fig 3–3).

Heger and co-workers[71] have demonstrated excellent agreement between the location of echocardiographic left ventricular segments which were independently and qualitatively graded as abnormal and the location of electrocardiographic Q waves in 37 of 44 patients with acute infarction who were technically suitable for study. The same investigators also found that qualitative scores of echocardiographic regional asynergy correlated well with hemodynamic parameters of left ventricular function.[72]

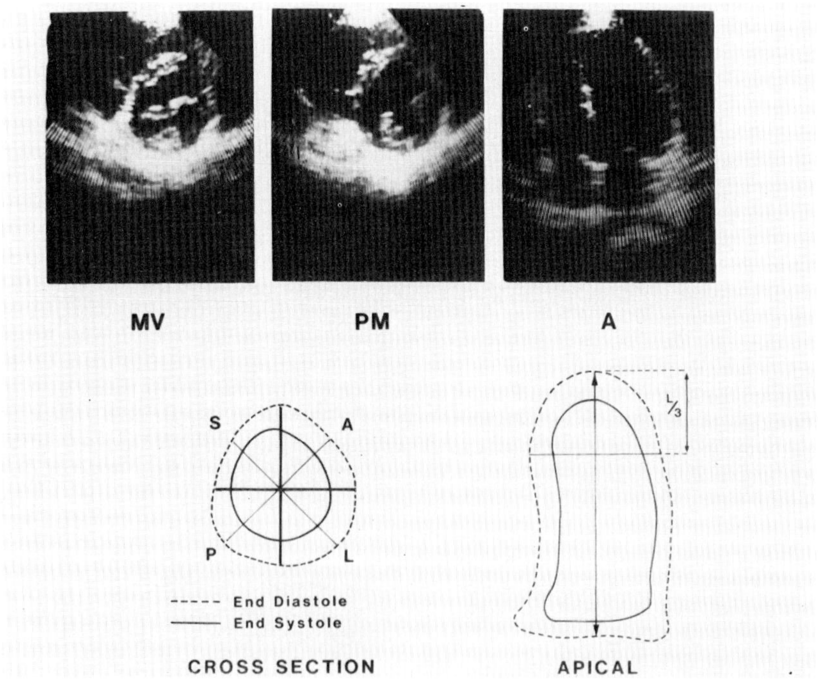

Fig 3–10.—An approach to regional wall motion analysis using systolic area shrinkage of eight wedge-shaped segments at mitral valve *(MV)* and papillary muscle *(PM)* levels of the parasternal short-axis (cross-section) view and area shrinkage of the apical segment from the apical four-chamber view *(A)*. On diagrams, *A*, anterior axis; *L*, lateral axis; *P*, posterior axis; *S*, septal axis; *L/3*, one third of long-axis length.

We have developed a quantitative approach to regional wall motion analysis in our laboratory which is based upon an eight-radian axis system at both levels (mitral valve and papillary muscle) of the parasternal short-axis view, and a longitudinal axis in the apical four-chamber view (for assessment of the apical segment) (see Fig 3–10).[73] We found percent area shrinkage of segments to be a more reproducible and less variable method of wall motion quantitation than linear axis shortening.[74] Using this approach, normal area shrinkage was defined for each of 17 segments (8 at each short-axis level and 1 apically) by analysis of studies from 10 healthy volunteers. Thirty-eight patients with documented coronary artery disease (20 with definite infarctions, 18 with angiographically normal wall motion) were similarly studied, grouped by infarction location and compared to the normal standards (Fig 3–11).[75] While values in the patients without antecedent infarction did not differ substantially from a range determined by values in the normal volunteers, values in patients with anterior and inferior infarction deviated significantly from the normal range in appropriate regions. Employing a ± 2 SD range for normality, this approach was 95% sensitive for detecting and correctly localizing infarction and 89% specific for identifying entirely normal wall motion in the study group of coronary patients.[75] Based on our studies to date, analysis of regional wall motion using 2DE short-axis cross sections is a very promising approach to evaluating regional left ventricular function.

The above approaches to wall motion require imaging of the left ventricular endocardium and following its motion during the cardiac cycle. This method is influenced by the motion of the heart as a whole, as well as by the actual contraction of

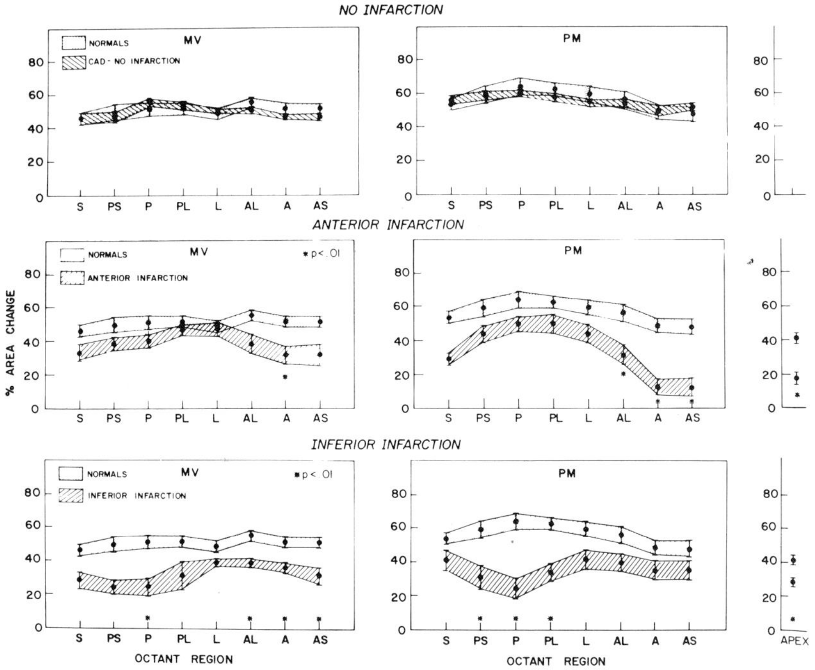

Fig 3–11.—Analysis of wall motion by the octant shrinkage method (see Fig 3–10 and text). *Finely stippled bands* represent normal area change for the various segments, ± 2 SD. *Cross-hatched bands* represent patients with coronary artery disease without infarction *(top)*, with anterior infarction *(middle)*, and with inferior infarction *(bottom)*. *MV*, mitral valve level; *PM*, papillary muscle level; *S*, septal segment; *PS*, posteroseptal segment; *P*, posterior segment; *PL*, posterolateral segment; *L*, lateral segment; *AL*, anterolateral segment; *A*, anterior segment; *AS*, anteroseptal segment. (Adapted from Parisi A.J., et al.: Quantitative detection of regional left ventricular contraction abnormalities by two-dimensional echocardiography: II. Accuracy in coronary artery disease. *Circulation* 63:761–676, 1981. Reproduced by permission of the American Heart Association.)

the segment being measured. Lieberman et al.[79] have used 2DE to study regional wall motion in dogs with experimental infarction by analyzing regional wall *thickening* rather than endocardial motion. They found that wall thickening was more precise than endocardial motion in discriminating between infarcted and noninfarcted zones of myocardium. As technical improvement in image quality allows better definition of wall thickness, this may become the optimum technique for characterizing regional myocardial function.

REFERENCES

1. Feigenbaum H.: *Echocardiography*, ed. 2. Philadelphia, Lea & Febiger, 1976.
2. Sahn D.J., DeMaria A., Kisslo J., et al.: Recommendations regarding quantitation in M-mode echocardiography: Results of a survey of echocardiographic measurements. *Circulation* 58:1072, 1978.
3. Henry W.L., Gardin J.M., Ware J.M.: Echocardiographic measurements in normal subjects from infancy to old age. *Circulation* 62:1054, 1980.
4. Fortuin N.J., Hood W.P. Jr., Sherman M.E., et al.: Determination of left ventricular volumes by ultrasound. *Circulation* 44:575, 1971.
5. Gibson D.G.: Estimation of left ventricular size by echocardiography. *Br. Heart J*. 35:128, 1973.
6. Pombo J.F., Troy B.L., Russell R.O. Jr.: Left ventricular volumes and ejection fraction by echocardiography. *Circulation* 43:480, 1971.
7. Moynihan P.F., Parisi A.F., Folland E.D., et al.: A system for quantitative evaluation of left ventricular function with two-dimensional ultrasonography. *Med. Instrum*. 14:111, 1980.
8. Parisi A.F., Moynihan P.F., Folland E.D., et al.: Quantitative analysis of left ventricular geometry assessed by two-dimensional echocardiography. *Circulation* 58:II–10, 1978.
9. Bhatt D.R., Isabel-Jones J.B., Villoria G.J., et al.: Accuracy of echocardiography in assessing left ventricular dimensions and volume. *Circulation* 57:699, 1978.
10. Pietro D.A., Voelkel A.G., Ray B.J., et al.: Reproducibility of echocardiography: A study evaluating the variability of serial echocardiographic measurements. *Chest* 79:29, 1981.
11. Clark R.D., Korcuska K., Cohn K.: Serial echocardiographic evaluation of left ventricular function in valvular disease, including reproducibility guidelines for serial studies. *Circulation* 62:564, 1980.
12. Henry W.L., Bonow R.O., Borer J.S., et al.: Observations on the optimum time for operative intervention for aortic regurgitation: I. Evaluation of the results of aortic valve replacement in symptomatic patients. *Circulation* 61:471, 1980.
13. Henry W.L., Bonow R.O., Rosing D.R., et al.: Observations on the optimum time for operative intervention for aortic regurgitation: II. Serial echocardiographic evaluation of asymptomatic patients. *Circulation* 61:484, 1980.
14. Abdulla A.M., Frank M.J., Canedo M.I., et al.: Limitations of echocardiography in the assessment of left ventricular size and function in aortic regurgitation. *Circulation* 61:148, 1980.
15. Teichholz L.E., Kreulen T., Herman M.V., et al.: Problems in echocardiographic volume determinations: Echocardiographic-angiographic correlations in the presence or absence of asynergy. *Am. J. Cardiol*. 37:7, 1976.
16. Kronik G., Slany J., Mosslacher M.: Comparative value of eight M-mode echocardiographic formulas for determining left ventricular stroke volume: A correlative study with thermodilution and left ventricular single-plane cineangiography. *Circulation* 60:1308, 1979.
17. Carr K.W., Engler R.L., Forsythe J.R., et al.: Measurement of left ventricular ejection fraction by mechanical cross-sectional echocardiography. *Circulation* 59:1196–1206, 1979.
18. Folland E.D., Parisi A.F., Moynihan P.F., et al.: Assessment of left ventricular ejection fraction and volumes by real-time, two-dimensional echocardiography: A comparison of cineangiographic and radionuclide techniques. *Circulation* 60:760–766, 1979.
19. Wyatt H.L., Heng M.K., Meerbaum S., et al.: Cross-sectional echocardiography: II. Analysis of mathematical models for quantifying volume of the formalin-fixed left ventricle. *Circulation* 61:119–125, 1980.
20. Schiller N.B., Acquatella H., Ports T.A., et al.: Left ventricular volume from paired biplane two-dimensional echocardiography. *Circulation* 60:547–555, 1979.
21. Nixon J.V., Saffer S.I.: Three-dimensional echoventriculography, abstracted. *Circulation* 57/58:II–157, 1978.
22. Silverman N.H., Ports T.A., Snider A.R., et al.: Determination of left ventricular volume in children: Echocardiographic and angiographic comparisons. *Circulation* 62:548–557, 1980.
23. Gueret P., Meerbaum S., Wyatt H.L., et al.: Two-dimensional echocardiographic quantitation of left ventricular volumes and ejection fraction: Importance of accounting for dyssynergy in short axis reconstruction models. *Circulation* 62:1308–1318, 1980.
24. Parisi A.F., Moynihan P.F., Folland E.D., et al.: Approaches to determination of left ventricular volumes and ejection fraction by real-time two-dimensional echocardiography. *Clin. Cardiol*. 2:257–263, 1979.
25. Ohuchi Y., Kuwako K., Umeda T., et al.: Real time, phased-array, cross-sectional echocardiographic evaluation of left ventricular asynergy and quantita-

tion of left ventricular function: A comparison with left ventricular cineangiography. *Japan Heart J.* 21:1–15, 1980.
26. Gehrke J., Leeman S., Raphael M., et al.: Non-invasive left ventricular volume determination by two-dimensional echocardiography. *Br. Heart J.* 37:911–916, 1975.
27. Bennett D.H., Evans D.W.: Correlation of left ventricular mass determined by echocardiography with vectorcardiographic and electrocardiographic voltage measurements. *Br. Heart J.* 36:981, 1974.
28. Reichek N., Devereux R.B.: Left ventricular hypertrophy: Relationship of anatomic, echocardiographic and electrocardiographic findings. *Circulation* 63:1391–1398, 1981.
29. Konecke L.L., Feigenbaum H., Chang S., et al.: Abnormal mitral valve motion in patients with elevated left ventricular diastolic pressure. *Circulation* 47:989, 1973.
30. Lewis J.R., Parker J.O., Burggraf G.W.: Mitral valve motion and changes in left ventricular end-diastolic pressure: A correlative study of the PR-AC interval. *Am. J. Cardiol.* 42:383, 1978.
31. Yow M.V., Reichek N.: Left ventricular end-diastolic pressure and echocardiographic mitral valve closure, abstracted. *Circulation* 52:II–51, 1975.
32. Botvinick E.H., Schiller N.B., Wickremasekaran R., et al.: Echocardiographic demonstration of early mitral valve closure in severe aortic insufficiency: Its clinical implications. *Circulation* 51:836, 1975.
33. Pietro D.A., Parisi A.F., Harrington J.J., et al.: Premature opening of the aortic valve: An index of highly advanced aortic regurgitation. *J. Clin. Ultrasound* 6:170, 1978.
34. Pridie R.B., Benham R., Oakley C.M.: Echocardiography of the mitral valve in aortic valve disease. *Br. Heart J.* 33:296, 1971.
35. McDonald I.G., Feigenbaum H., Chang S.: Analysis of left ventricular wall motion by reflected ultrasound: Application to assessment of myocardial function. *Circulation* 46:14, 1972.
36. Quinones M.A., Pickering E., Alexander J.K.: Percentage of shortening of the echocardiographic left ventricular dimension. *Chest* 74:59, 1978.
37. Stack R.S., Lee C.C., Reddy B.P., et al.: Left ventricular performance in coronary artery disease evaluated with systolic time intervals and echocardiography. *Am. J. Cardiol.* 37:331, 1976.
38. Fortuin N.J., Hood W.P. Jr., Craige E.: Evaluation of left ventricular function by echocardiography. *Circulation* 46:26, 1972.
39. Cooper R., Karliner J.S., O'Rourke R.A., et al.: Ultrasound determination of mean fiber-shortening rate in men, abstracted. *Am. J. Cardiol.* 29:257, 1972.
40. Cooper R.H., O'Rourke R.A., Karliner J.S., et al.: Comparison of ultrasound and cineangiographic measurements of the mean rate of circumferential fiber shortening in men. *Circulation* 46:914, 1972.
41. Quinones M.A., Gaasch W.H., Alexander J.K.: Echocardiographic assessment of left ventricular function. *Circulation* 50:42, 1974.
42. Wilson V.R., Reichek N.: Echocardiographic indices of left ventricular function: A comparison. *Chest* 76:441–447, 1979.
43. Rosenblatt A., Clark R., Burgess J., et al.: Echocardiographic assessment of the level of cardiac compensation in valvular heart disease. *Circulation* 54:509, 1976.
44. Nelson G.R., Cohn P.F., Gorlin R.: Prognosis in medically treated coronary artery disease: Influence of ejection fraction compared to other parameters. *Circulation* 52:408–412, 1975.
45. Hammermeister K.E., Kennedy J.W.: Predictors of surgical mortality in patients undergoing direct myocardial revascularization. *Circulation* Supplement II to volumes 49 and 50:II–112–115, 1974.
46. Henning H., Schelbert H., Crawford M.H., et al.: Left ventricular performance assessed by radionuclide angiocardiography and echocardiography in patients with previous myocardial infarction. *Circulation* 52:1069, 1975.
47. Folland E.D., Hamilton G.W., Larson S.M., et al.: The radionuclide ejection fraction: A comparison of three radionuclide techniques with contrast angiography. *J. Nucl. Med.* 18:1150, 1977.
48. Pratt R.C., Parisi A.F., Harrington J.J., et al.: The influence of left ventricular stroke volume on aortic root motion. *Circulation* 53:947, 1976.
49. Jacobs W.R., Croke R.P., Loeb H.S., et al.: Echocardiographic aortic ejection area as a reflection of left ventricular stroke volume. *J. Clin. Ultrasound* 7:369–372, 1979.
50. Massie B.M., Schiller N.B., Ratshin R.A., et al.: Mitral-septal separation: New echocardiographic index of left ventricular function. *Am. J. Cardiol.* 39:1008–1016, 1977.
51. Grossman W., Stefadous M.A., McLevrin L.P., et al.: Quantitative assessment of left ventricular diastolic stiffness in man. *Circulation* 47:567, 1963.
52. Quinones M.A., Gaasch W.H., Weisser E., et al.: Reduction in the rate of diastolic descent of the mitral valve echogram in patients with altered left ventricular diastolic pressure-volume relations. *Circulation* 49:246, 1974.
53. Borer J.S., Bacharach S.L., Green M.V., et al.: Effect of nitroglycerin on exercise-induced abnormalities of left ventricular regional function and ejection fraction in coronary artery disease. *Circulation* 57:314, 1978.
54. Gordon M.J., Kerber R.E.: Interventricular septal motion in patients with proximal and distal left anterior descending coronary artery lesions. *Circulation* 55:338, 1977.
55. Joffee C.D., Brik H., Teichholz L.E., et al.: Echocardiographic diagnosis of left anterior descending coronary artery disease. *Am. J. Cardiol.* 40:11, 1977.
56. Pernod J., Terdjman M., Kermarec J., et al.: Myo-

cardial contraction: Study by ultrasonic echography (Results in 200 normal patients). *Nouv. Presse Med.* 2:2393, 1973.
57. Corya B.C., Rasmussen S., Feigenbaum H., et al.: Systolic thickening and thinning of the septum and posterior wall in patients with coronary artery disease, congestive cardiomyopathy and atrial septal defect. *Circulation* 55:109, 1977.
58. Rasmussen S., Corya B.C., Feigenbaum H., et al.: Detection of myocardial scar tissue by M-mode echocardiography. *Circulation* 57:230, 1978.
59. Kerber R.E., Marcus M.L., Wilson R., et al.: Effects of acute coronary occlusion on the motion and perfusion of the normal and ischemic interventricular septum: An experimental echocardiographic study. *Circulation* 54:928, 1976.
60. Diamond M.A., Dillon J.C., Haine C.L., et al.: Echocardiographic features of atrial septal defect. *Circulation* 43:129, 1971.
61. Kerber R.F., Dippel W.F., Abboud F.M.: Abnormal motion of the interventricular septum in right ventricular volume overload: Experimental and clinical echocardiographic studies. *Circulation* 48:86, 1973.
62. Seides S.F., DeJoseph R.L., Brown A.E., et al.: Echocardiographic findings in isolated surgically created tricuspid insufficiency. *Am. J. Cardiol.* 35:679, 1974.
63. Tajik A.J., Gau G.T., Ritter D.G., et al.: Echocardiographic pattern of right ventricular diastolic volume overload in children. *Circulation* 46:36, 1972.
64. Cohen M.V., Cooperman L.B., Rosenblum R.: Regional myocardial function in idiopathic hypertrophic subaortic stenosis: An echocardiographic study. *Circulation* 52:842, 1975.
65. Gibson T.C., Grossman W., McLaurin L.P., et al.: An echocardiographic study of the interventricular septum in constrictive pericarditis. *Br. Heart J.* 38:738, 1976.
66. Schnittger I., Bowden R.E., Abrams J., et al.: Echocardiography: Pericardial thickening and constrictive pericarditis. *Am. J. Cardiol.* 42:388, 1978.
67. Voelkel A.G., Pietro D.A., Folland E.D., et al.: Echocardiographic features of constrictive pericarditis. *Circulation* 58:871, 1978.
68. Burggraf G.W., Craige E.: Echocardiographic studies of left ventricular wall motion and dimensions after valvular heart surgery. *Am. J. Cardiol.* 35:473, 1975.
69. Vignola P., Boucher C., Curfman G., et al.: Postoperative echocardiographic abnormal septal motion: Clinical, hemodynamic and surgical correlates, abstracted. *Circulation* 56:III–24, 1977.
70. Jacobs J.J., Feigenbaum H., Corya B.C., et al.: Detection of left ventricular asynergy by echocardiography. *Circulation* 48:263, 1973.
71. Heger J.J., Weyman A.E., Wann L.S., et al.: Cross-sectional echocardiography in acute myocardial infarction: Detection and localization of regional left ventricular asynergy. *Circulation* 60:531–538, 1979.
72. Heger J.J., Weyman A.E., Wann L.S., et al.: Cross-sectional echocardiographic analysis of the extent of left ventricular asynergy in acute myocardial infarction. *Circulation* 61:1113–1118, 1980.
73. Parisi A.F., Moynihan P.F., Folland E.D., et al.: Assessment of regional wall motion in coronary artery disease by two-dimensional echocardiography, in *Proceedings of the Third International Symposium on Echocardiography*. The Hague, Martinus Nijhoff, 1979.
74. Moynihan P.F., Parisi A.F., Feldman C.L.: Quantitative detection of regional left ventricular contraction abnormalities by two-dimensional echocardiography: I. Analysis of methods. *Circulation* 63:752-760, 1981.
75. Parisi A.F., Moynihan P.F., Folland E.D., et al.: Quantitative detection of regional left ventricular contraction abnormalities by two-dimensional echocardiography: II. Accuracy in coronary artery disease. *Circulation* 63:761–767, 1981.
76. Chaudry K.R., Ogawa S., Pauletto F.J., et al.: Biplane measurements of left ventricular volumes using wide-angle, cross-sectional echocardiography; abstracted. *Am. J. Cardiol.* 41:391, 1978.
77. Teichholz L.E., Cohen M.V., Sonnenblick E.H., et al.: Study of left ventricular geometry and function by B-scan ultrasonography in patients with and without asynergy. *N. Engl. J. Med.* 291:1220, 1974.
78. Mann T., McLaurin L., Grossman W., et al.: Assessing the hemodynamic severity of acute aortic regurgitation due to infective endocarditis. *N. Engl. J. Med.* 293:108, 1975.
79. Lieberman A.N., Weiss J.L., Jugdutt B.I., et al.: Two dimensional echocardiography and infarct size: Relationship of regional wall motion and thickening to the extent of myocardial infarction in the dog. *Circulation* 63:739–746, 1981.

RADIONUCLIDE IMAGING

Charles A. Boucher

DISEASES OF THE HEART usually impair the contraction of the ventricles, and the extent of impairment is an important determinant of clinical course and survival.[1, 2] Ventricular dysfunction is identified clinically by symptoms and signs of "congestive heart failure," e.g., dyspnea, engorged neck veins, rales, a third heart sound, cardiomegaly, and pulmonary venous hypertension on chest roentgenography. Since the development of cardiac catheterization, the ability to precisely assess ventricular function has improved markedly. Cardiac catheterization has allowed quantification of the pressures in the heart during the cardiac cycle, and the volumes and mass of the cardiac chambers can be derived on contrast angiography.[3–6] Furthermore, an assessment of regional ventricular contraction is possible.[7]

Numerous parameters of global ventricular function have been proposed. These include measures of isovolumic contraction, of the ejection phase, of the filling phase, and of the interrelationships of pressure, volume, and mass during the cardiac cycle.[8–10] Unfortunately, no single parameter is uniformly sensitive and specific, primarily because most parameters of ventricular function reflect a combination of intrinsic myocardial contractility and extrinsic factors (preload, afterload, heart rate, and adrenergic state).[4, 6, 11–16] (Preload is the extent of filling of the ventricle and is measured as end-diastolic pressure or end-diastolic volume. In accordance with the Starling principle, ejection increases as preload increases, and increasing preload therefore represents an important mechanism of compensating for impaired contractile function. Afterload is the wall tension that must be generated to eject blood. By the LaPlace relationship, systolic wall tension increases with systolic pressure and cavity size. Increases in afterload oppose ejection and are overcome by increases in preload and in the contractile state.) Despite these limitations, the ejection phase indices, particularly the ejection fraction, are most widely used because they are most easily measured, are best able to identify patients with abnormal cardiac performance, and have prognostic value for heart diseases of any etiology.

Although invasive approaches are sensitive and accurate for detecting abnormalities of ventricular function, recent developments have permitted noninvasive assessment of ventricular function. Radionuclide angiography provides safe, serial evaluation of ventricular function on an outpatient basis over time or with interventions. The current radionuclide approach employs an intravenous injection of a tracer (usually technetium 99m) to label the blood pool.[17, 18] (The technique of blood pool imaging was reviewed in detail in Chapter 2.) There are three radionuclide angiographic techniques which merit brief review here. The first two involve imaging: first-pass evaluation and multigated equilibrium evaluation. Both measure parameters analogous to those measured during cardiac catheterization, such as ejection fraction, ejection rate, and ventricular volumes. The differences between these methods are summarized in Table 4–1. The third method is a nonimaging ap-

TABLE 4–1.—First-Pass and Equilibrium Radionuclide Angiography

Advantages of the first-pass method
Rapid acquisition (5–15 cycles)
Suited to assess performance in a rapidly changing state
Temporal and anatomical separation of right and left ventricle
Pulmonary transit time may be derived
No dependence on electronic ECG gating
Adaptable to short-lived tracers
Advantages of the equilibrium method
Only one isotope injection is necessary
Suited for multiple acquisitions (multiple views or serially in the same view)
Entire blood pool is labeled, allowing visualization of relative anatomy of the cardiac chambers and noncardiac blood pools
Equilibrium condition permits a counts-based measurement of absolute ventricular volume and pulmonary blood volume
More counts may be acquired, producing higher resolution

proach that uses a probe to generate ventricular time-activity curves from which the ejection fraction and ejection rate are defined.[19–21] This method is less widely used but has the potential advantage of allowing continuous bedside monitoring, as in an intensive care unit. Regional function can be derived only with an imaging approach.

This chapter reviews the principal parameters of ventricular function that can be measured by radionuclide angiography and analyzes their physiologic significance. In addition, the effect of common interventions, such as exercise stress testing, on ventricular function in normal subjects is reviewed. Ventricular function patterns to be expected in individual cardiac disorders and the clinical utility of a radionuclide assessment of ventricular function are reviewed in separate chapters.

EJECTION FRACTION

Physiology

The ejection fraction is the ratio of the stroke volume to end-diastolic volume, or the fraction of the end-diastolic volume ejected per beat. Because it is a unitless ratio, ejection fraction values do not require calibration and are comparable from institution to institution and from technique to technique, whether invasive or noninvasive. This universality of the ejection fraction concept has enormous appeal. The normal ventricle at rest usually maintains an ejection fraction of at least 50%, and an ejection fraction below 50% defines a group of patients who are likely to have heart disease and a generally poorer prognosis.[1, 2, 22]

Because the ejection fraction is so easily measured and widely used, it is sometimes considered synonymous with ventricular function or contractility, and, if reduced, with heart failure. This is erroneous and may lead to misleading conclusions. The ejection fraction is also affected by alterations in loading conditions, such as preload and afterload. Disorders or interventions in which loading conditions are dramatically altered may produce substantial changes in the ejection fraction which may be only partly related to changes in the underlying muscle.[4, 6, 23] For example, patients with mitral valve regurgitation may have an increased ejection fraction because of increased preload and reduced afterload, whereas patients with aortic stenosis or pulmonary hypertension may have a reduced ejection fraction because of increased afterload. In both cases, the ejection fraction tends to return toward normal on correction of the abnormal loading conditions.[24] On the other hand, medicines such as beta-blockers or calcium channel blockers can affect contractile function and may also alter ejection fraction. Therefore, the ejection fraction reflects the combined effect of intrinsic myocardial contractility and extrinsic loading conditions, adrenergic state, and pharmacologic agents, and should not be used to characterize contractile function alone.

Just as ejection fraction may not be synonymous with contractility, so it may not parallel the presence or absence of heart failure (dyspnea). Although a reduced ejection fraction usually implies *myocardial* failure that may produce heart failure, congestive heart failure symptoms are actually a direct result of elevated atrial pressures (ventricular filling) and not a reduced ejection fraction (ventricular emptying). Some disorders may produce heart failure with a normal ejection fraction[25]; among them are atrioventricular valve obstruction, atrioventricular valve regurgitation, acute ventricular volume overload, high output states, restrictive disorders (e.g., pericardial effusion, constrictive pericarditis, and cardiomyopathy), and hypertrophic cardiomyopathy. The diagnostic usefulness of the ejection fraction in elucidating the cause of heart failure is evident.

Radionuclide Analysis

Both first-pass and gated equilibrium radionuclide techniques can be used to derive the ejection fraction because the blood pool activity within the right or left ventricle is proportional to the volume within the ventricle.[26–28] The change in externally detected counts during the cardiac cycle corresponds to the change in ventricular volume during the cardiac cycle. In contrast to echocardiography and contrast angiography, radionuclide imaging requires few assumptions to be made about ventricular geometry in the calculation of the ejection fraction. This is particularly important with regard to the right ventricle, because that structure does not readily conform to any single geometric shape. The accuracy of multigated equilibrium imaging depends on a second major assumption, namely, the ECG markers correctly time the cardiac cycle. This assumption appears to be valid.[27]

Although radionuclide imaging is an easy and reliable way to calculate the ejection fraction, there are errors inherent in the technique. These errors primarily relate to statistical noise and the technical limitations of nuclear imaging, including relatively low resolution, varying background activity, scatter, attenuation, and imprecision in identifying the edge of the ventricle. Although computer filtering and smoothing algorithms are routinely used in processing data, ejection fraction analysis still is not entirely automated. Operator intervention is necessary to place edges and choose background. As a result, there is intraobserver and interobserver variability in the derived values.[29, 30] Interobserver variance in the calculation of the left ventricular ejection fraction as determined from a single scan is about 0.05 at rest, and the variation in the resting ejection fraction over time is also about 0.05. Furthermore, the variance in the change in ejection fraction from rest to exercise approaches 0.10. Clearly, differences of 0.05 or less cannot be distinguished from the inherent variability of the technique, although the figures are comparable to those seen in contrast angiographic ejection fraction measurements.[31]

Radionuclide angiography has been particularly useful for measuring right ventricular ejection fraction.[32–36] Contrast right ventricular cineangiography is seldom employed in these patients, and ultrasound methods are distinctly disadvantageous because of the physical location of the right ventricle under the sternum. In addition, the geometry of the right ventricle is not suitable to an ellipsoid or any other formula. Accordingly, the use of a counts-derived ejection fraction for the right ventricle has been an important advance in understanding the impact of heart disease on the right ventricle. However, three alternative methods of calculating right ventricular ejection fraction have been reported: all are counts-based and independent of geometry and all have advantages and disadvantages. The first uses an equilibrium gated study in the left anterior oblique (LAO) view.[32] This method permits derivation of the right ventricular ejection fraction from the same images used to generate the left ventricular ejection fraction with a high count rate. However, the right ventricle in the LAO view is substantially overlapped by the right atrium, which contributes to the counts within the right ventricular region of interest. The other two methods use a first-pass approach to separate the right heart from the left heart temporally and spatially. The right anterior oblique (RAO) view or anterior view is used, which largely avoids right atrial overlap. One method involves a first-pass, beat-to-beat measurement of a bolus injection of technetium. The conventional single crystal gamma camera is of little use in this method because of the relatively low count rate from a single injection; a multicrystal camera has a higher sensitivity and may be used.[34] The third method is the gated first-pass method, which involves a gated acquisition of the cycles during the first pass of tracer through the right heart. This takes advantage of the first-pass approach and yet improves the count rate so that a right ventricular counts analysis and right heart imaging with a conventional gamma camera is possible. And because this method entails a summation of studies, it does not depend on a bolus injection. However, the method does require a full dose of tracer, and only one study may be performed in one setting. The relative advantages and disadvantages of these methods are similar to those listed in Table 4–1 for first-pass versus equilibrium imaging.

First Third Ejection Fraction

Because the ejection fraction is often normal in patients with cardiac disease, the pattern of ejection has been analyzed to derive a more sensitive parameter. The earliest abnormality in contraction in coronary heart disease occurs early in systole at the point of peak systolic wall stress.[37] For this reason, an assessment of the first third ejection fraction has been proposed as a more sensitive measure than the total ejection fraction. Using contrast angiography, Slutsky et al.[38] found that 75% of 55 patients with heart disease had a holosystolic ejection fraction within the normal range (≥ 0.56), whereas only 5% had a normal first third ejection fraction (≥ 0.28). Data were derived from contrast angiographic studies acquired at approximately 60 frames per second. Subsequent radionuclide studies have not confirmed the reliability of this approach, owing particularly to difficulty in precisely timing the first third of ejection in an acquisition which divides the cardiac cycles into only 16 frames and systole into 5–7 frames.[39–41]

Ejection Rate

In addition to the extent to which the ventricle empties in systole, the rate at which the ventricle empties may be derived.[42, 43] This is determined as the average rate of change in counts during systole, normalized to end-diastolic counts. In comparison to the ejection fraction, the ejection rate may be more sensitive to changes in contractility and the adrenergic state and less affected by heart rate. However, it is similarly altered by preload and afterload. Methodological errors in the calculation of ejection rate include those mentioned above for ejection fraction and those involved in the determination of systolic ejection time. Although the ejection time is most precisely measured from a high-fidelity pressure recording, the radionuclide ejection time is measured as the time from maximal to minimal activity in the ventricular region of interest during the cardiac cycle. Temporal precision is limited, as with the first third ejection fraction, because systole may be as short as five frames, and an error of even one frame may substantially affect the ejection time value.[39] In addition, end-systole may not be precisely defined because of "noise" in the time-activity curve and because of asynchronous contraction. Therefore, radionuclide-derived ejection time measurements are imprecise. Furthermore, the ejection time seldom varies in disease states, and so has little added value.[44] To date, there is no evidence that the ejection rate measured at rest is better than the ejection fraction as a means of separating normal subjects from diseased subjects or as a means of evaluating the effect of a complex intervention, such as exercise, on ventricular function.

VENTRICULAR VOLUMES

End-Diastolic Volume

Determination of absolute volumes gives perspective to the ejection fraction value, which is a ratio of the two absolute volumes. The end-diastolic volume is a measure of preload.[4, 6, 13] As the contractile function of the ventricle diminishes, the end-diastolic volume increases in an attempt to increase ejection (the Starling principle at work).[12] Therefore, there is usually an inverse relationship between ejection fraction and end-diastolic volume, and so few clinical situations in which an isolated end-diastolic volume value at rest is important in addition to the ejection fraction. One exception is volume overload lesions, such as aortic and mitral regurgitation.[45] A more useful application may be in the serial measurement of end-diastolic volume in the same patient over time or after an intervention. On the other hand, changes in end-diastolic volume may be small and therefore may fall within observer variability of the technique.

Absolute left ventricular end-diastolic volume may be derived from blood pool images, but the computation is considerably more difficult than for the ejection fraction.[28] Two alternative methods have been reported, the counts method and the geometric method[45–47] (Table 4–2). The counts method determines the activity within the region of interest over the left ventricle at end-diastole and derives absolute volumes by calibrating it with the activity in a known volume of blood. This method assumes that there is an equilibrium state and cannot be used with first-pass imaging. An assumed correction for attenuation of activity through the chest wall must be made. The counts method is independent of the shape of the ventricle, but it requires individualized calibration. It is also limited by errors in edge detection and variability in chest wall and blood pool attenuation. Major problems of the counts method are (1) overlap of activity in other chambers and (2) greater attenuation of blood pool activity in parts of the ventricle farther away from the camera.

The geometric method is analogous to the contrast ventriculographic method pioneered by Dodge.[4] In this method, the edge of the left ventricle is outlined and an area-length formula is used to derive volumes. This method has the advantage that the calibration is constant for a particular camera employing a parallel-hole collimator. One picture element always corresponds to the same area in a patient. The major limitations are methodological: the geometric shape assumptions and defining the edge of the left ventricle. The latter is a particular problem because of overlap of the ventricle by other cardiac chambers and the difficulty in defining the mitral and aortic valve plane. Errors in edge detection tend to be more crucial

TABLE 4–2.—Counts-Based and Geometric Radionuclide Methods of Calculating End-Diastolic Volume

Sources of error with the counts method
Scatter and background
Overlap of activity from atria and lung
Variable attenuation
Calibration of blood activity
Edge detection
Sources of error with the geometric method
Geometric assumption of ventricular shape
Edges imprecise due to low resolution and inability to separate ventricle from adjacent blood pool
Pixel field size large relative to ventricular chamber dimensions

with a geometric method because the greatest geometric volume is at the edges, whereas the highest ventricular counts are in the center of the region of interest. Nevertheless, both methods yield satisfactory correlation coefficients with left ventricular volumes derived from contrast ventriculography. Because of the assumptions necessary for either method, volume measurements are more reliable for serial studies in the same patient than for comparisons among patients. Observer error may be somewhat larger with the geometric method.[18, 48] To date, no method of deriving right ventricular end-diastolic volume is widely accepted.

Stroke Volume/Cardiac Output

End-diastolic volume multiplied by ejection fraction is the stroke volume. Stroke volume multiplied by heart rate is cardiac output, a traditional measure of cardiac performance. Although the diagnostic utility of the cardiac output generally has been surpassed by the ejection fraction, it does reflect oxygen delivery and adequacy of cardiovascular function.[3–6]

End-Systolic Volume

The end-systolic volume is determined by subtracting the stroke volume from the end-diastolic volume. End-systolic volume is usually not measured directly because the ventricle has a low number of counts at end-systole, and there is a greater likelihood that statistical errors will be introduced into the counts or geometric method. Nevertheless, the end-systolic volume is an important parameter because, unlike the ejection fraction, it is largely independent of preload.[12, 49]

End-Systolic Pressure-Volume Relationship

Recently, Sagawa and others examined the dependency of the end-systolic portion of the instantaneous pressure-volume loop on loading conditions.[50, 51] The E_{max}, or the ratio of end-systolic pressure to end-systolic volume, appears to be a measure of left ventricular function that is independent of both preload and afterload but entirely dependent on contractile state of the myocardium. For this reason, E_{max} is considered the best available indicator of global systolic function. Although difficult to measure, it has been approximated by substituting peak left ventricular pressure for end-systolic pressure. Radionuclide angiography may provide such a ratio noninvasively as the ratio of peak cuff systolic blood pressure to end-systolic volume.[52] Initially, there was hope that this might be a true contractility index. E_{max} does appear to increase appropriately with exercise and not to change with certain alterations in preload and afterload, although it does vary with other changes in afterload. Furthermore, the ratio is inversely and logarithmically related to the ejection fraction.[53] Therefore, its clinical advantage over ejection fraction remains to be demonstrated.

Although calculation of absolute volumes provides invaluable information about ventricular function, its use is generally limited to research studies. This is because the calculations are tedious to make and require extensive experience for accuracy. Furthermore, studies have indicated that the interobserver variation is as great as 20%–30%. Finally, the varying methodologies makes comparison of values from different institutions unreliable. Therefore, their clinical utility remains to be shown.

REGIONAL WALL MOTION

Besides global systolic ventricular function, noninvasive assessment of regional contraction is the other common clinical application of radionuclide angiography. Assessment of regional contraction requires an actual image of the heart and cannot be determined from ventricular time-activity curves. It is important in coronary artery disease because of the regional nature of this disorder.[7, 54]

Because conventional planar blood pool imaging evaluates the tangential edge of the ventricle, a minimum of two views is recommended. The more regions of the hearts that are assessed, the more complete the evaluation of wall motion will be.[55] At catheterization, orthogonal 30-degree RAO and 60-degree LAO views are usually obtained. First-pass studies limited to a single view (30-degree RAO or anterior) are a distinct disadvantage, if one considers the multiple views possible with equilibrium studies. At least one anterior view and one LAO view that optimizes visualization of the interventricular septum are acquired. Recently, more centers have routinely obtained a third view, a higher LAO view or a left posterior oblique view.[18, 56] This helps to define certain regions of the left ventricle, including the inferior wall, in which there is anterior overlap by the right ventricle, and the basal walls, in which there is overlap by the more apical portion of the left ventricle on the LAO view (Fig 4–1).

Exercise wall motion studies are usually performed in a single view, the anterior or 30-degree RAO view for first-pass studies and the LAO view for equilibrium studies. These particular views permit calculation of the left ventricular ejection fraction during exercise, but obtaining only one view may limit the completeness of the regional wall motion assessment during exercise. For equilibrium studies, alternatives are a caudal tilt to elongate the left ventricle, use of a biplane collimator, or continuation of the exercise long enough to acquire an anterior view at peak exercise.[57]

Wall motion may be graded qualitatively or quantitatively. Qualitative assessment involves dividing the left ventricular edge into three to six segments in each view. Each segment is then separately graded using a wall motion scoring system suggested by Herman et al.[7] Segments are graded as normal, hypokinetic, akinetic, or dyskinetic. Although this scoring system was developed to assess wall motion by contrast left ventriculography, a similar system may be used in radionuclide angiography. Our approach is a five-point scoring system in which 3 = normal motion, 2 = mild hypokinesis, 1 = severe hypokinesis, 0 = akinesis, and −1 = dyskinesis.[30] Overall interobserver variability in our laboratory is comparable to or better than that associated with left ventriculography. Only septal motion had a higher interobserver variability by scan, probably because septal structure and motion are complex and visualization of the septum may be affected by the close proximity of another large blood pool, the right ventricle.

There are three principal approaches to quantitative regional wall motion analysis.[58–61] Two are

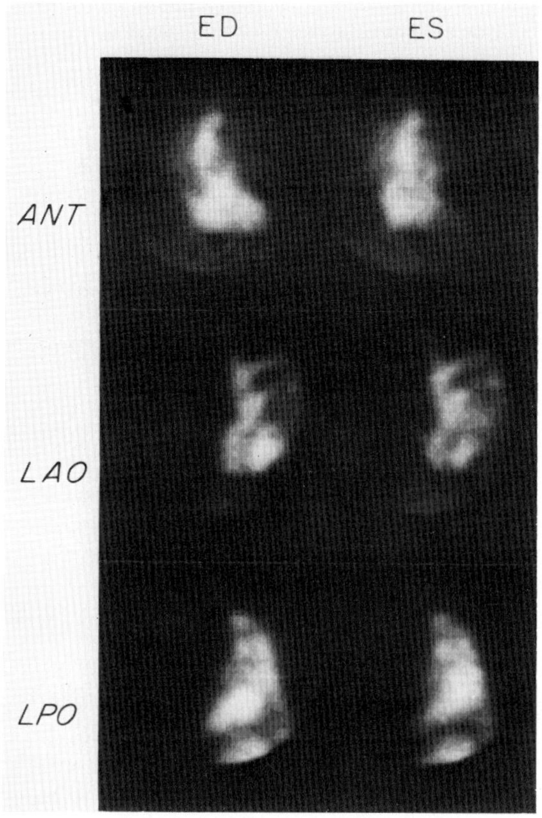

Fig 4–1.—End-diastolic *(ED)* and end-systolic *(ES)* blood pool images in three views. The anterior *(ANT)* view visualizes the anterolateral wall and apex. The left anterior oblique *(LAO)* view visualizes the septum. The left posterior oblique *(LPO)* visualizes the anterolateral wall, apex, and inferior wall and is a mirror image of a right anterior oblique view without overlap of activity from the right ventricle.

analogous to the two approaches previously mentioned for end-diastolic volume: regional ejection fraction (counts) and chord or area shortening (geometric). They have similar advantages and methodological limitations. In addition, systematic errors may be introduced into both, depending on which reference markers are used and whether the region of interest and axes remain fixed or float from end-diastole to end-systole. The third approach is a phase analysis using a temporal Fourier transformation.[62] This allows a determination of the amplitude and phase shift of ventricular contraction. It is a particularly useful way of measuring ventricular function in disorders with asynchrony such as conduction disturbances, but has not been validated or widely applied. Another parameter is the abnormally contracting segment (%ACS), the percent of the total left ventricular perimeter which is acontractile. This parameter has been utilized to assess infarct size and left ventricular aneurysms.[54] The segment may also be measured as a geometric area rather than as a perimeter.[63] Alternatively, a counts approach comparing the global ejection fraction to the contractile portion of the left ventricle has been proposed.[64]

Although radionuclide angiography permits noninvasive estimation of the severity of a wall motion abnormality, the severity of the asynergy may not necessarily correlate with the state of underlying myocardium in terms of cellular viability. A region of akinesis may be produced by irreversible infarction or severe ischemia or a combination of both. This distinction cannot be made from a wall motion assessment but may be inferred from the finding of improved motion after a premature ventricular beat after nitroglycerin administration, after revascularization, or if filling in of a perfusion defect is seen on serial thallium-201 imaging.[65, 66] In this regard, the combined use of ^{201}Tl and blood pool imaging is important.[67]

Although regional differences in contraction are the hallmark of coronary artery disease, they are not specific for the disorder. When a ventricle dilates from whatever cause, regional abnormalities may be evident. The contraction patterns in patients with a reduced ejection fraction due to idiopathic cardiomyopathy, cardiomyopathy due to coronary disease, or end-stage ventricular dysfunction associated with valvular disease often are indistinguishable.[68] The apex is often more affected than other walls, in part because of the normal thinning of apical musculature as a result of the helical fiber array in the ventricle.

RADIONUCLIDE UPTAKE IN THE LUNG

As mentioned, assessment of systolic contraction is the single best means of evaluating left ventricular function. However, measurement of left ventricular filling pressures is also an important parameter of overall cardiac compensation. The normal left heart is able to maintain an adequate cardiac output with filling pressures of 12 mm Hg or less. In diseased hearts, the filling pressure increases for a variety of reasons. In mitral valve disease, the reasons are primarily mechanical. In coronary artery disease, the exact mechanism for the elevation in left ventricular filling pressure has not been clarified; however, it is presumably due to a combination of decreased ejection with back congestion, increased preload (via use of the Starling principle) in order to maintain an adequate cardiac output, incomplete relaxation of the ventricle during ischemia, and mitral valve regurgitation due to papillary muscle ischemia.[69–73]

Although accurate measurement of left ventricular filling pressure involves right heart catheterization, radionuclide methods offer the potential of a noninvasive assessment of left atrial pressure. This is because the pulmonary circulation is sensitive to a change in left atrial pressure.[74] Radionuclide imaging provides an indirect measurement of left ventricular filling pressure owing to altered distribution of tracers in the lung. The lung extraction of ^{201}Tl appears to increase with increases in pulmonary capillary wedge pressure (Fig 4–2).[75–77] Normally, the ratio of lung activity to myocardial activity on initial postexercise images is less than 0.50 and increases above that in relation to pulmonary capillary wedge pressure. Similarly, there is a higher concentration of blood pool activity in the lung with higher pulmonary capillary wedge pressures.[78–80] These lung changes may be measured both on conventional ^{201}Tl imaging and on gated blood pool imaging because some part of the lung is always routinely imaged with the heart. Both increased lung uptake of ^{201}Tl and an elevated pulmonary blood volume on exercise reflect left ventricular decompensation with exercise, an important aspect of ventricular function which may be derived from conventional stress radionuclide imaging.

There are different approaches to the radionuclide measurement of pulmonary blood volume, depending on the kind of radionuclide method used. On first-pass studies, the pulmonary blood volume is determined indirectly by multiplying the cardiac index by the mean pulmonary transit time, using indicator dilution principles.[17] The cardiac index is the product of stroke volume index (ejection fraction times end-diastolic volume) and heart rate. Mean pulmonary transit time is mathematically derived from the time-activity curve of the tracer within a region of interest placed over the lung. This method is used to evaluate total blood volume in the lung. On equilibrium studies, the activity of pulmonary blood pool is directly measured.[79] An absolute value is not derived; rather, a ratio of activity after an intervention (usually exercise) to lung activity at rest is generated. This method evaluates the concentration of blood within the lung and not total pulmonary blood volume. Normally the ratio of lung activity at exercise to lung activity at rest is 1.06 or less; the ratio is above normal in most patients with coronary artery disease.

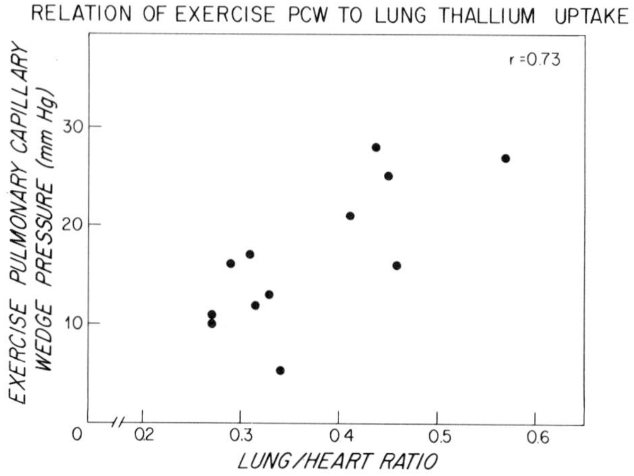

Fig 4–2.—Lung/heart activity ratio derived from the initial postexercise anterior view thallium-201 images is higher in patients with higher pulmonary capillary wedge pressures (PCW) during exercise. The 12 patients shown on the plot were exercised and imaged in the supine position during cardiac catheterization.

DIASTOLIC FILLING RATES

Although the diastolic portion of the ventricular volume curve is often ignored, it may provide useful information, particularly in ischemic heart disease. Ischemia impairs relaxation, which is an energy-requiring process. Hammermeister and Warbasse demonstrated that the relative rate of diastolic filling might be analyzed by contrast ventriculography.[81] More recently, Reduto et al. demonstrated that the first third filling fraction and filling rate could also be determined from radionuclide angiographic studies.[82] Such radionuclide studies require regular rhythm and recording of the entire portion of diastole, which may not be precisely recorded owing to the gating process. Their clinical role remains to be demonstrated.

INTERVENTIONS

Dynamic Exercise

Dynamic exercise is the most common form of stress employed in cardiac testing. Typically it is conducted using a treadmill, upright bicycle, or supine bicycle. Because coronary artery disease is the most prevalent cardiac disorder, exercise testing is frequently performed to unmask ischemia not evident at rest. The evidence for ischemia includes the development of angina, ECG abnormalities, a ^{201}Tl perfusion defect, a new regional wall motion abnormality on radionuclide angiography, or wall thinning on echocardiography. The sensitivity, specificity, and predictive accuracy of these markers of ischemia are reviewed elsewhere in this book.

Another common reason to perform dynamic exercise is to assess ventricular function and cardiovascular reserve.[44] Traditionally, cardiovascular reserve is measured as the ratio of the increase in oxygen uptake to the increase in cardiac output in relation to the change in filling pressure.[83–85] The ratio, known as the exercise factor, normally is at least 6, and the increase in cardiac output is normally achieved with no significant increase in filling pressure. Patients with reduced exercise factors are unable to increase cardiac output needs commensurate with peripheral energy needs. More recently, noninvasive rest and exercise studies using the previously mentioned radionuclide angiographic parameters have become widely used for this purpose.

In order to sustain exercise, there must be increased oxygen delivery to the working muscles.[86, 87] The adequacy of peripheral delivery of oxygen is the major limiting factor in the ability to perform on an exercise test. Although multiple factors contribute to increasing oxygen transport, including increased peripheral oxygen extraction and alterations in the regional distribution of systemic blood flow, the heart plays a crucial role in this regard. There is a threefold to fivefold increase in cardiac output with exercise as a result of an approximately twofold to threefold increase in heart rate and a smaller increase in stroke volume. The heart rate usually increases linearly with increasing workloads on a graded stress test, whereas the stroke volume increases occur primarily in the earlier stages of exercise, depending on the form of exercise.[88–92] With upright leg exercise there is peripheral venous pooling at rest. As a result, resting end-diastolic volume and stroke volume are smaller at rest than in supine studies. With exercise, there is return of this blood to the heart and a striking increase in end-diastolic volume and stroke volume. By contrast, there is little or no increase in end-diastolic volume and a smaller increase in stroke volume with supine exercise. Because ventricular volume changes differ between upright and supine exercise, the mode of exercise should always be noted.

Numerous radionuclide studies have analyzed the response of the normal heart to exercise. The rest and exercise ejection fraction and end-diastolic volume values are summarized in Tables 4–3 through 4–5. For both the left and right ventricle, the ejection fraction increases in most normal patients on either supine or upright exercise, owing to an increase in stroke volume and a decrease in end-systolic volume. The absolute increase in ejection fraction is usually 0.05; however, several studies have indicated that some normal subjects do not achieve this increase, particularly those with high resting values (≥ 0.70).[94, 97, 109] Accordingly, some workers have proposed judging the normality of a particular response by whether the values fall within a certain absolute range to be expected in normal subjects.[93] The tables suggest a remark-

TABLE 4–3.—Rest and Peak Bicycle Exercise Radionuclide Left Ventricular Ejection Fractions in Normal Subjects

STUDY (CITY)	N	RESTING VALUES Mean ± 1 SD	RESTING VALUES Lowest Value	PEAK EXERCISE VALUES Mean ± 1 SD	PEAK EXERCISE VALUES Lowest Value
Supine graded exercise					
Borer et al. (Bethesda)[93]	30	0.57 ± .05	.45	0.71 ± .09	0.55
Brady et al. (Ann Arbor)[94]	29	0.62 ± .12	. . .	0.70 ± .14	. . .
Caldwell et al. (Seattle)[95]	11	0.60 ± .05	. . .	0.63 ± .09	. . .
Slutsky et al. (San Diego)[96]	16	0.58 ± .05	.49	0.72 ± .07	0.65
Dehmer et al. (Dallas)[53]	13	0.72 ± .07	.54	0.82 ± .07	0.62
Kirshenbaum et al. (Boston)[97]	11	0.66 ± .09	.52	0.73 ± .12	0.55
Marshall et al. (Los Angeles)[98]	7	0.63 ± .05	. . .	0.73 ± .05	. . .
Upright graded exercise					
Berger et al. (New Haven)[99]	13	0.67 ± .11	. . .	0.82 ± .14	. . .
Johnson et al. (New York)[100]	11	0.68 ± .07	.52	0.76 ± .06	0.65
Jengo et al. (Torrance)[101]	8	0.65 ± .08	.56	0.81 ± .08	0.72
Poliner et al. (Dallas)[102]	7	0.72 ± .11	. . .	0.91 ± .05	. . .
Newman et al. (Durham)[103]	14	0.66 ± .09	.51	0.79 ± .08	0.64
Rerych et al. (Durham)[104]	18	0.73 ± .06	.63	0.87 ± .04	0.80
Foster et al. (Milwaukee)[105]	9	0.67 ± .09	.52	0.73 ± .07	0.62
Reduto et al. (Houston)[82]	32	0.67 ± .09	.50	0.82 ± .08	0.62
Iskandrian et al. (Philadelphia)[106]	12	0.62 ± .21	.51	0.75 ± .14	0.66

TABLE 4–4.—Rest and Peak Bicycle Exercise Radionuclide Right Ventricular Ejection Fractions in Normals

STUDY (CITY)	N	RESTING VALUES Mean ± 1 SD	RESTING VALUES Lowest Value	PEAK EXERCISE VALUES Mean ± 1 SD	PEAK EXERCISE VALUES Lowest Value
Supine exercise—equilibrium imaging					
Maddahi et al. (Los Angeles)[107]	10	0.49 ± .04	.45	0.66 ± .08	0.54
Slutsky et al. (San Diego)[108]	20	0.49 ± .0	.39	0.64 ± .12	0.43
Upright exercise—first-pass imaging					
Johnson et al. (New York)[100]	11	0.47 ± .04	.43	0.57 ± .06	0.47
Matthay et al. (New Haven)[109]	25	0.54 ± .15	.48	0.67 ± .15	0.56
Olvey et al. (Houston)[110]	10	0.53 ± .06	.45	0.63 ± .06	0.52

TABLE 4–5.—Response of Radionuclide Left Ventricular End-Diastolic Volume to Bicycle Exercise in Normals

STUDY (CITY)	N	REST (ml) Mean ± 1 SD	INCREASE WITH EXERCISE Mean, %
Supine graded exercise			
Borer et al. (Bethesda)[93]	30	Relative counts	− 3
Sorensen et al. (Seattle)[111]	9	Relative counts	+ 7
Dehmer et al. (Dallas)[53]	13	102 ± 25	+22
Slutsky et al. (San Diego)[96]	16	117 ± 21	− 1
Upright graded exercise			
Newman et al. (Durham)[103]	14	105 ± 33	+19
Rerych et al. (Durham)[104]	18	133 ± 35	+25
Poliner et al. (Dallas)[102]	7	85 ± 16	+36
Iskandrian et al. (Philadelphia)[106]	12	153 ± 86	+14

able uniformity of lower limit of normal values, whether the exercise is supine or upright or the acquisition is first-pass or equilibrium. However, the range of normal values above the lower limit is considerable. Changes in ejection rate tend to parallel changes in ejection fraction. Mean values at rest are 3.4 to 3.8 $second^{-1}$ and increase to 6.5 to 6.8 $second^{-1}$ with peak exercise.[98, 99, 105]

The increase in cardiac output with exercise is generally achieved with little or no increase in left ventricular filling pressure, and most workers agree that such preload changes do not play a major role in the normal compensation to exercise.[102] Radionuclide angiography allows further investigation into this question via the measurement of rest and exercise left ventricular end-diastolic volume and pulmonary blood volume (see Table 4–5). End-diastolic volume does not consistently increase during supine exercise, whereas it typically increases with upright exercise, largely as a result of the increase in venous return from the leg with upright exercise. The pulmonary blood volume concentration also tends to remain unchanged or to decrease with supine exercise.[79] The upper limit of exercise to rest lung activity is 1.06. In contrast, the mean total derived pulmonary blood volume tends to increase in normal subjects from 334 ml/sq m at rest to 414 ml/sq m on upright exercise.[103]

There is uniform agreement that the increase in contractility with exercise in normals is reflected in a decrease in end-systolic volume.[112, 113] As a result, the peak systolic pressure to end-systolic volume ratio dramatically increases during exercise.[52, 53] However, the range of normal values appears to vary considerably. Using supine exercise and a counts approach to volume analysis, Slutsky suggested a lower limit of normal of 2.1 at rest and 4.8 with exercise, with the normal response being +85% or more.[52] Using a similar protocol, Dehmer suggested a lower limit of normal of 4.0 at rest and 6.7 on exercise, with the normal response being +35% or more.[53] Therefore, although this parameter may approximate a true contractility index for evaluating the effect of interventions, the range of values in normal subjects may limit its use in identifying patients with heart disease.[112]

Physical fitness may affect ventricular function at rest and exercise and should be considered when analyzing individual studies.[114–117] There is improved exercise capacity with physical conditioning, but the radionuclide correlates of this are complex because both central and peripheral adjustments are involved.[104, 118] Normally, the heart of the conditioned athlete is larger and more hypertrophied. The end-diastolic volume is substantially increased for any given heart rate and, as a result, there is increased stroke volume. For this reason, the heart rate at rest is lower. At peak exercise, a larger stroke volume can be achieved at a comparable end-systolic volume, and therefore there is an improved cardiac output response to exercise. Overall, however, the improved exercise capacity is more a result of peripheral adjustments than of changes in heart size and function.

Isometric Exercise

Isometric exercise has also been used to unmask abnormal cardiac performance not evident at rest.[119–122] The usual method is to employ sustained handgrip at one third of the predetermined maximum for three minutes. Systolic and diastolic blood pressures usually increase 20 mm Hg or more, whereas the heart rate increases only 20 beats per minute. The result is a small increase in heart rate and a large increase in blood pressure in proportion to the work performed. There is little or no change in stroke volume. It has the advantage of not requiring patient motion, thereby facilitating imaging, and can be done by patients with physical limitations as a result of orthopedic or arthritic problems, peripheral vascular disease, or neuromuscular disorders. In addition, it requires less than five minutes to complete, has a simple end point, and seldom produces angina or arrhythmias. The major disadvantage to isometric exercise is that it does not produce maximal stress and there may be false negative results. Because an equilibrium state is difficult to sustain, handgrip exercise may be better suited for first-pass imaging.

In normal subjects, there is no significant change in left ventricular filling pressures, stroke volume, or ejection fraction after three minutes.[120, 122] Because stroke volume is maintained against a higher afterload, this actually represents an increase in contractile function via use of the patient's preload reserve.

Beta-Blockers

Because of the widespread use of beta-blockers such as propranolol, knowledge of the influence of propranolol on ventricular function is important. To improve the usefulness of the data acquired from radionuclide studies, patients ordinarily discontinue taking beta-blockers several days prior to the study if it is deemed safe by their physician. Because many patients have either severe angina or hypertension, it may not be clinically safe to omit these drugs, and therefore some patients must be studied during propranolol therapy. Patients who have had substantial amelioration of anginal symptoms should probably not routinely discontinue propranolol for a diagnostic imaging study.

Beta-blockers can theoretically affect ventricular function in several ways.[123, 124] Through their negative ionotropic effect, they may reduce the ejection fraction. Through their chronotropic effect, they may produce a slower heart rate for any given level of activity with little or no change in ejection fraction. If the beta-blockade causes a reduction in systemic blood pressure, there might be an increase in ejection fraction. In sum, the effect of beta-blockers on ventricular function is complex and may vary from patient to patient and from normal subjects to patients with coronary artery disease.

In 12 normal subjects studied using an upright first-pass method, propranolol administered in a dose sufficient to blunt most of the chronotropic response to 50 μg of isoproterenol caused a significant fall in heart rate and a significant increase in end-diastolic and end-systolic volume.[125] Stroke volume and blood pressure did not change significantly. Cardiac output and ejection fraction decreased significantly, the latter from $0.65 \pm .08$ to $0.57 \pm .07$ (mean $\pm$ 1 SD). By contrast, among 7 normal volunteers studied using supine equilibrium imaging, there was no effect of propranolol on resting left ventricular ejection fraction or end-diastolic volume.[98] With exercise, there was no difference in contraction in normal subjects when studied at a comparable heart rate. However, when peak exercise values were compared, patients taking propranolol had a lower heart rate, blood pressure, cardiac output, and ejection fraction. Stroke volume was not significantly different, but it occurred at higher end-systolic and end-diastolic volumes. Therefore, the influence of propranolol on left ventricular function is complex and comparisons with patients exercising off propranolol should take into account differences in heart rate, blood pressure, and workload, as well as in the adequacy of beta-blockade. It is possible that beta-blockade may cause an abnormal test result in an otherwise normal patient, and vice versa.[126]

Nitroglycerin

Numerous patients take nitrates as therapy for coronary artery disease. Therefore, the effect of nitroglycerin on left ventricular performance is important.[127-131] Nitroglycerin normally produces a small rise in heart rate and a fall in blood pressure. End-diastolic and end-systolic volumes fall, and stroke volume remains the same. As a result, the ejection fraction usually increases. Effects on normal subjects and patients with coronary artery disease are similar. The most dramatic effect of nitroglycerin, however, is on regional asynergy. Nitroglycerin produces an improvement in regional wall motion abnormalities. The effect is most dramatic when the asynergy is due to acute or chronic ischemia, but it can occur in a region of infarction as well. This is probably because the primary mechanism for the improvement is a change in loading conditions, mainly decreased afterload. Therefore, serial and interpatient analysis of ventricular function must take into consideration the effect of nitrates on ejection.

REFERENCES

1. Cohn P.F., Gorlin R., Cohn L.H., et al.: Left ventricular ejection fraction as a prognostic guide in surgical treatment of coronary and valvular heart disease. *Am. J. Cardiol.* 34:136-141, 1974.
2. Rigo P., Murray M., Taylor D.R., et al.: Hemodynamic and prognostic findings in patients with transmural and non-transmural infarction. *Circulation* 51:1064-1070, 1975.
3. Kreulen T.H., Bove A.A., McDonough M.T., et al.: The evaluation of left ventricular function in man. *Circulation* 51:677-688, 1975.
4. Dodge H.T.: Angiographic evaluation of ventricular function. *N. Engl. J. Med.* 296:551-553, 1977.
5. Sonnenblick E.H., Strobeck J.E.: Derived in-

dexes of ventricular and myocardial function. *N. Engl. J. Med.* 296:978-982, 1977.
6. Krayenbuehl H.P., Hess O.M., Turina J.: Assessment of left ventricular function. *Cardiovasc. Med.* 3:883-908, 1978.
7. Herman M.V., Heinle R.A., Klein M.D., et al.: Localized disorders in myocardial contraction: Asynergy and its role in congestive heart failure. *N. Engl. J. Med.* 277:222-232, 1967.
8. Karliner J.S., Gault J.H., Eckberg D., et al.: Mean velocity of fiber shortening: A simplified measure of left ventricular myocardial contractility. *Circulation* 44:323–333, 1971.
9. Ross J. Jr., Peterson K.L.: On the assessment of cardiac inotropic state. *Circulation* 47:435–438, 1973.
10. Peterson K.L., Skloven D., Ludbrook P., et al.: Comparison of isovolumic and ejection phase indices of myocardial performance in man. *Circulation* 49:1088–1101, 1974.
11. Ross J., Braunwald E.: The study of left ventricular function in man by increasing resistance to ventricular ejection with angiotensin. *Circulation* 29:739–749, 1964.
12. Taylor R.R., Cingotani H.E., McDonald R.H. Jr.: Relationships between left ventricular volume, ejection fraction, and wall stress. *Am. J. Physiol.* 211:674–680, 1966.
13. Rankin L.S., Moos S., Grossman W.: Alterations in preload and ejection phase indices of left ventricular performance. *Circulation* 51:910–915, 1975.
14. Quinones M., Gaasch W., Alexander J.: Influence of acute changes in preload, afterload, contractile state and heart rate on ejection and isovolumic phase indices of myocardial contractility in man. *Circulation* 53:293–300, 1976.
15. Ross J. Jr.: Afterload mismatch and preload reserve: A conceptual framework for the analysis of ventricular function. *Prog. Cardiovasc. Dis.* 43:255–269, 1976.
16. Ricci D.R., Orlick A.E., Alderman E.L., et al.: Influence of heart rate on left ventricular ejection fraction in human beings. *Am. J. Cardiol.* 44:447–451, 1979.
17. Berger H.J., Matthay R.A., Pytlik L.M., et al.: First-pass radionuclide assessment of right and left ventricular performance in patients with cardiac and pulmonary disease. *Sem. Nucl. Med.* 9:275–295, 1979.
18. Strauss H.W., McKusick K.A., Boucher C.A., et al.: Of linens and laces: The eighth anniversary of the gated blood pool scan. *Sem. Nucl. Med.* 9:290–309, 1979.
19. Wagner H.N., Rigo P., Baxter R.O., et al.: Monitoring ventricular function at rest and during exercise with a non-imaging nuclear detector. *Am. J. Cardiol.* 43:975–979, 1979.
20. Wexler J.P., Blaufox M.D.: Radionuclide evaluation of left ventricular function with non-imaging probes. *Sem. Nucl. Med.* 9:310–319, 1979.
21. Berger H.J., Davies R.A., Batsford W.P., et al.: Beat-to-beat left ventricular performance assessed from the equilibrium cardiac blood using a computerized nuclear probe. *Circulation* 63:133–142, 1981.
22. Kennedy J.W., Baxley W.A., Figley M.M., et al.: Quantitative angiocardiography: I. The normal left ventricle in man. *Circulation* 34:272–278, 1966.
23. Mason D.T.: Regulation of cardiac performance in clinical heart disease. *Am. J. Cardiol.* 32:437–448, 1973.
24. Boucher C.A., Okada R.D., Pohost G.M.: Current status of radionuclide imaging in valvular heart disease. *Am. J. Cardiol.* 46:1153–1163, 1980.
25. Johnson R.A., Boucher C.A.: Normal left ventricular ejection fraction in systemic arteriovenous fistula: Implications for the use of noninvasive methods in differential diagnosis of heart failure. *Chest* 79:607–609, 1981.
26. Ashburn W.L., Schelbert H.R., Verba J.W.: Left ventricular ejection fraction: A review of several radionuclide angiographic approaches using the scintillation camera. *Prog. Cardiovasc. Dis.* 20:267–284, 1978.
27. Green M.V., Brody W.R., Douglas M.A., et al.: Ejection fraction by count rate from gated images. *J. Nucl. Med.* 19:880–883, 1978.
28. Strauss H.W., McKusick K.A., Bingham J.B.: Cardiac nuclear imaging: Principles, instrumentation and pitfalls. *Am. J. Cardiol.* 46:1109–1116, 1980.
29. Marshall R.C., Berger H.J., Reduto L.A., et al.: Variability in sequential measures of left ventricular performance assessed with radionuclide angiocardiography. *Am. J. Cardiol.* 41:531–536, 1978.
30. Okada R.D., Kushner F.G., Kirshenbaum H.D., et al.: Interobserver and intraobserver variance in the evaluation of left ventricular regional wall motion and ejection fraction using contrast ventriculogram and rest and exercise multigated blood pool image. *Circulation* 61:128–136, 1980.
31. Cohn P.F., Levine J.A., Bergeron G.A., et al.: Reproducibility of the angiographic left ventricular ejection fraction in patients with coronary artery disease. *Am. Heart J.* 88:713–720, 1974.
32. Maddahi J., Berman D.S., Matsuoka D.T., et al.: A new technique for assessing right ventricular ejection fraction using rapid multiple-gated equilibrium cardiac blood pool scintigraphy: Description, validation and findings in chronic coronary artery disease. *Circulation* 60:581–589, 1979.
33. Slutsky R.A., Ackerman W., Karliner J.S., et al.: Right and left ventricular dysfunction in patients with chronic obstructive lung disease: Assessment by first-pass radionuclide angiography. *Am. J. Med.* 68:197–205, 1980.
34. Berger H.J., Matthay R.: Radionuclide right ven-

tricular ejection fraction. *Chest* 79:497–498, 1981.
35. Winzelberg G.G., Boucher C.A., Pohost G.M., et al.: Right ventricular function in aortic and mitral valve disease: Relation of gated first pass radionuclide angiography to clinical and hemodynamic findings. *Chest* 79:520–528, 1981.
36. Harolds J.A., Grove R.B., Bowen R.D., et al.: Right ventricular function as assessed by two radionuclide techniques. *J. Nucl. Med.* 22:113–115, 1981.
37. Holman B.L., Wynne J., Idoine J., et al.: Disruption in the temporal sequence of regional ventricular contraction: I. Characteristics and incidence in coronary artery disease. *Circulation* 61:1075–1083, 1980.
38. Slutsky R., Karliner J.S., Battler A., et al.: Comparison of early systolic and holosystolic ejection phase indexes by contrast ventriculography in patients with coronary artery disease. *Circulation* 61:1083–1090, 1980.
39. Bacharach S.L., Green M.V., Borer J.S., et al.: Left ventricular peak ejection rate, filling rate, and ejection fraction-frame rate requirements at rest and exercise. *J. Nucl. Med.* 20:189–193, 1979.
40. Slutsky R., Gordon D., Karliner J., et al.: Assessment of early ventricular systole by first pass radionuclide angiography: Useful method for detection of left ventricular dysfunction at rest in patients with coronary artery disease. *Am. J. Cardiol.* 44:459–465, 1979.
41. Battler A., Slutsky R., Karliner J., et al.: Left ventricular ejection fraction and first third ejection fraction early after acute myocardial infarction: Value for predicting mortality and morbidity. *Am. J. Cardiol.* 45:197–202, 1980.
42. Hammermeister K.E., Brooks R.C., Warbasse J.R.: The rate of change of left ventricular volume in man: I. Validation and peak systolic ejection rate in health and disease. *Circulation* 49:729–738, 1974.
43. Marshall R.C., Berger H.J., Costin J.C., et al.: Assessment of cardiac performance with quantitative radionuclide angiocardiography: Sequential left ventricular ejection fraction, normalized left ventricular ejection rate, and regional wall motion. *Circulation* 56:820–829, 1977.
44. Cohn P.F., Gorlin R.: Dynamic ventriculography and the role of the ejection fraction. *Am. J. Cardiol.* 36:529–531, 1975.
45. Boucher C.A., Bingham J.B., Osbakken M.D., et al.: Early changes in left ventricular size and function following correction of left ventricular volume overload. *Am. J. Cardiol.* 47:991–1004, 1981.
46. Slutsky R., Karliner J., Ricci D., et al.: Ventricular volumes by gated equilibrium radionuclide angiography: A new method. *Circulation* 60:556–564, 1979.
47. Dehmer G.J., Lewis S.E., Hillis L.D., et al.: Nongeometric determination of left ventricular volumes from equilibrium blood pool scans. *Am. J. Cardiol.* 45:293–300, 1980.
48. Upton M.T., Rerych S.K., Newman G.E., et al.: The reproducibility of radionuclide angiocardiographic measurements of left ventricular function in normal subjects at rest and during exercise. *Circulation* 62:126–132, 1980.
49. Borow K.M., Green L.H., Mann T., et al.: End-systolic volume as a predictor of postoperative left ventricular performance and volume overload from valvular regurgitation. *Am. J. Med.* 68:655–674, 1980.
50. Sagawa K., Suga H., Shoukas A., et al.: End-systolic pressure/volume ratio: A new index of ventricular contractility. *Am. J. Cardiol.* 40:748–753, 1977.
51. Nivatpunim T., Katz S., Scherer J.: Peak left ventricular systolic pressure/end-systolic volume ratio: A sensitive detector of left ventricular disease. *Am. J. Cardiol.* 43:969–974, 1979.
52. Slutsky R., Karliner J., Gerber K., et al.: Peak systolic blood pressure/end-systolic volume in normal subjects and patients with coronary heart disease: Assessment at rest and during exercise. *Am. J. Cardiol.* 46:813–820, 1980.
53. Dehmer G.J., Lewis S.E., Hillis L.D., et al.: Exercise-induced alterations in left ventricular volumes and the pressure-volume relationship: A sensitive indicator of left ventricular dysfunction in patients with coronary artery disease. *Circulation* 63:1008–1018, 1981.
54. Field B.J., Russel R.O., Dowling J.T., et al.: Regional left ventricular performance in the year following myocardial infarction. *Circulation* 46:679–689, 1972.
55. Cohn P.F., Gorlin R., Adams D.F., et al.: Comparison of biplane and single plane left ventriculograms in patients with coronary artery disease. *Am. J. Cardiol.* 33:1–6, 1974.
56. Freeman M.R., Berman D.S., Staniloff H.M., et al.: Improved assessment of inferior segmental wall motion by the addition of a 70° left anterior oblique view in multiple gated equilibrium scintigraphy. *Am. Heart J.* 101:169–173, 1981.
57. Boucher C.A., Strauss H.W., Okada R.D., et al.: The bifocal diverging collimator: A means of simultaneous biplane imaging of the heart during equilibrium radionuclide ventriculography. *J. Nucl. Med.* 21:71–76, 1980.
58. Leighton R.F., Wilt S.M., Lewis R.P.: Detection of hypokinesis by a quantitative analysis of left ventricular cineangiograms. *Circulation* 50:121–127, 1974.
59. Papapietro S.E., Yester M.V., Logic J.R., et al.: Method for quantitative analysis of regional left ventricular function with first pass and gated blood pool scintigraphy. *Am. J. Cardiol.* 47:619–625, 1981.

60. Maddox D.E., Wynne J., Uren R., et al.: Regional ejection fraction: A quantitative radionuclide index of regional left ventricular performance. *Circulation* 59:1001–1009, 1979.
61. Gelberg J.H., Brundage B.H., Glanz S., et al.: Quantitative left ventricular wall motion analysis: A comparison of area, chord and radial methods. *Circulation* 59:991–1000, 1979.
62. Links J.M., Douglass K.H., Wagner H.N. Jr.: Patterns of ventricular emptying by Fourier analysis of gated blood pool studies. *J. Nucl. Med.* 21:978–982, 1980.
63. Froehlich R.T., Falsetti H.L., Doty D.B., et al.: Prospective study of surgery for left ventricular aneurysm. *Am. J. Cardiol.* 45:923–931, 1980.
64. Stephens D.J., Dymond D.S., Stone D.L., et al.: Left ventricular aneurysm and congestive heart failure: Value of exercise stress and isosorbide dinitrate in predicting hemodynamic results of aneurysmectomy. *Am. J. Cardiol.* 45:932–939, 1980.
65. Pohost G.M., Alpert N.M., Ingwall J.S., et al.: Thallium redistribution: Mechanisms and clinical utility. *Sem. Nucl. Med.* 10:70–93, 1980.
66. Akins C.W., Pohost G.M., DeSanctis R.W., et al.: Selection of angina-free patients with severed left ventricular dysfunction for myocardial revascularization. *Am. J. Cardiol.* 46:695–700, 1981.
67. Okada R.D., Boucher C.A., Strauss H.W., et al.: Exercise radionuclide imaging approaches to coronary artery disease. *Am. J. Cardiol.* 46:1188–1204, 1980.
68. Bolen J.L., Alderman E.L.: Ventriculographic and hemodynamic features of mitral regurgitation of cardiomyopathic, rheumatic and non-rheumatic etiology. *Am. J. Cardiol.* 39:177–183, 1977.
69. Bristow J.D., Van Zee B.E., Judkins M.P.: Systolic and diastolic abnormalities of the left ventricle in coronary artery disease. *Circulation* 42:219, 1970.
70. Covell J.W., Ross J. Jr.: Nature and significance of alterations in myocardial compliance. *Am. J. Cardiol.* 32:449–455, 1973.
71. Mann T., Goldberg S., Mudge G.H., et al.: Factors contributing to altered left ventricular diastolic properties during angina pectoris. *Circulation* 59:14, 1979.
72. Ross J. Jr.: Acute displacement of the diastolic pressure-volume curve of the left ventricle: Role of the pericardium and the right ventricle. *Circulation* 59:32–37, 1979.
73. Johnson R.A., Daggett W.M. Jr.: Heart failure resulting from coronary artery disease, in Johnson R.A., Haber E., Austen W.G. (eds.): *The Practice of Cardiology*. Boston, Little, Brown & Co., 1980, pp. 339–369.
74. Fishman A.P.: Dynamics of the pulmonary circulation, in Hamilton W.F., Dow P. (eds.): *Handbook of Physiology*. Washington, D.C., American Physiological Society, 1963, pp. 1667–1743.
75. Boucher C.A., Zir L.M., Beller G.A., et al.: Increased lung uptake of thallium-201 during exercise myocardial imaging: Clinical, hemodynamic and angiographic implications in patients with coronary artery disease. *Am. J. Cardiol.* 46:189–196, 1980.
76. Bingham J.B., McKusick K.A., Strauss H.W., et al.: The influence of coronary artery disease on pulmonary uptake of thallium-201. *Am. J. Cardiol.* 46:821–826, 1980.
77. Kushner F.G., Okada R.D., Kirshenbaum H.D., et al.: Lung thallium-201 uptake following stress testing in patients with coronary artery disease. *Circulation* 63:341–347, 1981.
78. Nichols A., Strauss W., Moore R., et al.: Acute changes in cardiopulmonary blood volume during upright exercise stress testing in patients with coronary heart disease. *Circulation* 60:520–527, 1979.
79. Okada R.D., Pohost G.M., Kirshenbaum H.D., et al.: Radionuclide-determined changes in pulmonary blood volume with exercise. *N. Engl. J. Med.* 301:569–576, 1979.
80. Okada R.D., Osbakken M.D., Boucher C.A., et al.: Pulmonary blood volume ratio response to exercise: A noninvasive determination of exercise-induced changes in pulmonary capillary wedge pressure. *Circulation* 65:126–133, 1982.
81. Hammermeister K.E., Warbasse J.R.: The rate of change of left ventricular volume in man: II. Diastolic events in health and disease. *Circulation* 49:739–747, 1974.
82. Reduto L.A., Wickemeyer W.J., Young J.B., et al.: Left ventricular diastolic performance at rest and during exercise in patients with coronary artery disease. *Circulation* 63:1128–1137, 1981.
83. Ross J. Jr., Gault J.H., Mason D.T., et al.: Left ventricular performance during muscular exercise in patients with and without cardiac dysfunction. *Circulation* 34:597–608, 1966.
84. Braunwald E., Ross J., Sonnenblick E.: Circulatory adjustments during exercise, in Braunwald E., Ross J., Sonnenblick E. (eds.): *Mechanisms of Contraction of the Normal and Failing Heart*. Boston, Little, Brown & Co., 1967, p. 292.
85. Vatner S.F., Pagani M.: Cardiovascular adjustments to exercise-hemodynamics and mechanisms. *Prog. Cardiovasc. Dis.* 19:91–108, 1976.
86. Wasserman K., Whipp B.J.: Exercise physiology in health and disease. *Am. Rev. Resp. Dis.* 112:219–249, 1975.
87. Astrand P.-O.: Quantification of exercise capability and evaluation of physical capacity in man. *Prog. Cardiovasc. Dis.* 19:51–67, 1976.
88. Rushmer R.: Constancy of stroke volume in ventricular response to exertion. *Am. J. Physiol.* 196:745–750, 1959.

89. Bevegard S., Holmgren A., Jonsson B.: The effect of body position on the circulation at rest and during exercise with special reference to the influence on the stroke volume. *Acta. Physiol. Scand.* 49:279–285, 1960.
90. Thadani U., Parker J.: Hemodynamics at rest and during supine and sitting bicycle exercise in normal subjects. *Am. J. Cardiol.* 41:52–60, 1978.
91. Gorlin R., Cohen L., Elliott W., et al.: Effect of supine exercise on left ventricular volume and oxygen consumption in man. *Circulation* 32:361–366, 1965.
92. Sharma B., Goodwin J., Raphael M., et al.: Left ventricular angiography on exercise: A new method of assessing left ventricular function in ischemic heart disease. *Br. Heart J.* 38:59–67, 1976.
93. Borer J.S., Bacharach S.L., Green M.V., et al.: Exercise-induced left ventricular dysfunction in symptomatic and asymptomatic patients with aortic regurgitation: Assessment with radionuclide cineangiography. *Am. J. Cardiol.* 42:351–357, 1978.
94. Brady T.J., Thrall J.H., Lo K., et al.: The importance of adequate exercise in the detection of coronary heart disease by radionuclide ventriculography. *J. Nucl. Med.* 21:1125–1130, 1980.
95. Caldwell J.H., Hamilton G.W., Sorensen S.G., et al.: The detection of coronary artery disease with radionuclide techniques: A comparison of rest-exercise thallium imaging and ejection fraction response. *Circulation* 61:610–619, 1980.
96. Slutsky R., Battler A., Gordon D., et al.: The effect of nitrates on left ventricular size and function during exercise comparison of sublingual tablets and superficially applied ointment. *Am. J. Cardiol.* 45:831–840, 1980.
97. Kirshenbaum H.D., Okada R.D., Boucher C.A., et al.: Relationship of thallium-201 myocardial perfusion pattern to regional and global left ventricular function with exercise. *Am. Heart J.* 101:734–739, 1981.
98. Marshall R.C., Wisenberg G., Schelbert H.R., et al.: Effect of oral propranolol on rest, exercise and postexercise left ventricular performance in normal subjects and patients with coronary artery disease. *Circulation* 63:572–583, 1981.
99. Berger H.J., Reduto L.A., Johnstone D.E., et al.: Global and regional left ventricular response to bicycle exercise in coronary artery disease: Assessment by quantitative radionuclide angiocardiography. *Am. J. Med.* 66:13–21, 1979.
100. Johnson L.L., McCarthy D.M., Sciacca R.R., et al.: Right ventricular ejection fraction during exercise in patients with coronary artery disease. *Circulation* 60:1284–1291, 1979.
101. Jengo J.A., Oren V., Conant R., et al.: Effects of maximal exercise stress on left ventricular function in patients with coronary artery disease using first pass radionuclide angiography. *Circulation* 59:60–65, 1979.
102. Poliner L.R., Dehmer G.J., Lewis S.E., et al.: Left ventricular performance in normal subjects: A comparison of responses to exercise in the upright and supine positions. *Circulation* 62:528–534, 1980.
103. Newman G.F., Rerych S.K., Upton M.T., et al.: Comparison of electrocardiographic and left ventricular functional changes during exercise. *Circulation* 62:1204–1211, 1980.
104. Rerych S.K., Scholz P.M., Sabiston D.C. Jr., et al.: Effects of exercise training on left ventricular function in normal subjects: A longitudinal study by radionuclide angiography. *Am. J. Cardiol.* 45:244–252, 1980.
105. Foster C., Anholm J.D., Hellman C.K., et al.: Left ventricular function during sudden strenuous exercise. *Circulation* 63:592–596, 1981.
106. Iskandrian A.S., Hakki A., Kane S.A., et al.: Quantitative radionuclide angiography in assessment of hemodynamic changes during upright exercise: Observations in normal subjects, patients with coronary artery disease and patients with aortic regurgitation. *Am. J. Cardiol.* 48:239–246, 1981.
107. Maddahi J., Berman D.S., Matsuoka D.T., et al.: Right ventricular ejection fraction during exercise in normal subjects and in coronary artery disease patients: Assessment by multiple-gated equilibrium scintigraphy. *Circulation* 62:133–140, 1980.
108. Slutsky R., Hooper W., Gerber K., et al.: Assessment of right ventricular function at rest and during exercise in patients with coronary heart disease: A new approach using equilibrium radionuclide angiography. *Am. J. Cardiol.* 45:63–71, 1980.
109. Matthay R.A., Berger H.J., Davies R.A., et al.: Right and left ventricular exercise performance in chronic obstructive pulmonary disease: Radionuclide assessment. *Ann. Intern. Med.* 93:234–239, 1980.
110. Olvey S.K., Reduto L.A., Stevens P.M., et al.: First pass radionuclide assessment of right and left ventricular ejection fraction in chronic pulmonary disease. *Chest* 78:4–9, 1980.
111. Sorensen S., Ritchie J., Caldwell J., et al.: Serial exercise radionuclide angiography: Validation of count-derived changes in cardiac output and quantitation of maximal exercise ventricular volume changes after nitroglycerin and propranolol in normal man. *Circulation* 61:600–607, 1980.
112. Slutsky R., Watkins J., Peterson K., et al.: The response of left ventricular function and size to atrial pacing, volume loading and afterload stress in patients with coronary artery disease. *Circulation* 63:864–870, 1981.
113. Slutsky R.: Response of the left ventricle to stress: Effects of exercise, atrial pacing, afterload stress and drugs. *Am. J. Cardiol.* 47:357–364, 1981.
114. Saltin B., Blomqvist G., Mitchell J.H.: Response to exercise after bed rest and after training. *Circulation* 38(suppl. VII):VII-1–78, 1968.

115. Scheuer J.: Physical training and intrinsic cardiac adaptations. *Circulation* 47:677–680, 1973.
116. Letac B., Cribier A., Desplances J.F.: A study of left ventricular function in coronary patients before and after physical training. *Circulation* 56:375–378, 1977.
117. Ehsani A.A., Hagberg J.M., Hickson R.M.: Rapid changes in left ventricular dimensions and mass in response to physical conditioning and deconditioning. *Am. J. Cardiol.* 42:52–56, 1978.
118. Jensen D., Atwood J.E., Froelicher V., et al.: Improvement in ventricular function during exercise studied with radionuclide ventriculography after cardiac rehabilitation. *Am. J. Cardiol.* 46:770–777, 1980.
119. Payne R., Horwitz L., Mullins C.: Comparison of isometric exercise and angiotensin as a stress test for the evaluation of left ventricular function. *Am. J. Cardiol.* 31:428–435, 1973.
120. Bodenheimer M.M., Banka V.S., Fooshee C.M., et al.: Detection of coronary heart disease using radionuclide determined regional ejection fraction at rest and during handgrip exercise: Correlation with coronary arteriography. *Circulation* 58:640–648, 1978.
121. Flessas A.P., Connelly G.P., Handa S., et al.: Effects of isometric exercise of end-diastolic pressure, volume and function of the left ventricle in man. *Circulation* 58:839–846, 1978.
122. Peter C.A., Jones R.H.: Effects of isometric handgrip and dynamic exercise on left ventricular function. *J. Nucl. Med.* 21:1131–1138, 1980.
123. Epstein S.E., Robinson B.F., Kahler R.L., et al.: Effects of beta-adrenergic blockade on cardiac response to maximal and submaximal exercise in man. *J. Clin. Invest.* 44:1745–1753, 1965.
124. Coltart D.J., Alderman E.L., Robinson S.C., et al.: Effect of propranolol on left ventricular function, segmental wall motion and diastolic pressure-volume relation in man. *Br. Heart J.* 37:357, 1975.
125. Port S., Cobb F., Jones R.: Effects of propranolol on left ventricular function in normal men. *Circulation* 61:358–366, 1980.
126. Battler A., Ross J., Slutsky R., et al.: Improvement of exercise-induced left ventricular dysfunction with oral propranolol in patients with coronary heart disease. *Am. J. Cardiol.* 44:318–324, 1979.
127. McAnulty J.H., Hattenhauer M.T., Rosch J., et al.: Improvement in left ventricular wall motion following nitroglycerin. *Circulation* 51:140–145, 1975.
128. Borer J.S., Bacharach S.L., Green M.V., et al.: Effect of nitroglycerin on exercise-induced abnormalities of left ventricular regional function and ejection fraction in coronary artery disease. *Circulation* 57:314–320, 1978.
129. Salel A.F., Berman D.S., Denardo G.L., et al.: Radionuclide assessment of nitroglycerin influence on abnormal left ventricular segmental contraction in patients with coronary heart disease. *Circulation* 53:975–982, 1976.
130. Ritchie J.L., Sorensen S.G., Kennedy J.W., et al.: Radionuclide angiography: Noninvasive assessment of hemodynamic changes after administration of nitroglycerin. *Am. J. Cardiol.* 43:278–284, 1979.
131. Slutsky R., Curtis G., Battler A., et al.: The effect of sublingual nitroglycerin on left ventricular function at rest and during spontaneous angina pectoris assessment by a radionuclide approach. *Am. J. Cardiol.* 44:1365, 1979.

COMMENT: LEFT VENTRICULAR FUNCTION

Alfred F. Parisi

IN RECENT YEARS, multiple investigators have independently confirmed that two-dimensional echocardiography (2DE) can be used to measure the *global* ejection fraction of the left ventricle. Two-dimensional echocardiography has considerable advantage over M-mode echocardiography for determining ejection fraction since regions difficult to identify with the single-beam M-mode approach readily fall within the field of a planar two-dimensional sector scan. Two studies have directly compared determination of ejection fraction by radionuclide angiography and 2DE in the same patient subsets. In one study of 35 patients, Folland et al. found a correlation coefficient of 0.80; O'Rourke's group found a correlation coefficient of 0.9 in a subgroup of 75 patients.

As a pragmatic procedure used solely to determine left ventricular ejection fraction, radionuclide angiography at present offers both real and theoretical advantages over 2DE. First, the proportion of patients who are successfully studied by the radionuclide method approaches 100%; by contrast, the reported success in obtaining a 2DE study in which there are high-quality targets suitable for outlining the left ventricle endocardium is 60%–85%. Both radionuclide imaging and 2DE have been used in conjunction with dynamic exercise testing, which is an important intervention in assessing patients with coronary artery disease. As an intervention, however, exercise makes data acquisition with 2DE even more difficult, and there are fewer successful exercise studies than resting studies. In many radionuclide imaging laboratories, exercise ejection fraction determinations are a routine clinical procedure; in most echocardiographic laboratories, routine clinical exercise studies are the exception rather than the rule.

Second, radionuclide procedures are highly automated compared with echocardiographic analysis. To date, a generally accepted satisfactory system for target recognition using 2DE, which allows automated tracing of the endocardium, has not been developed, although there is hope that some such system will soon be available. The procedure of tracing endocardium manually, as can be done by ventriculographers with contrast angiography, is tedious and time-consuming. This process is not facilitated by videotape recording methods in which a large visual degradation takes place when a stop frame image is viewed.

Third, from a theoretical point of view, radionuclide angiography, unlike 2DE, does not depend on the fixed geometry of proposed models which are needed to derive the end-diastolic and end-systolic volumes for ejection fraction determination. By defining an area of interest, radionuclide angiography is not geometry independent, but rather possesses a flexible geometry which can be varied from patient to patient in a more realistic way than the models used with 2DE.

As a method for dealing with *regional* abnormalities of myocardial contraction, 2DE offers considerable advantage over radionuclide imaging. Because of its inherent higher spatial resolution, the ultrasound method permits a more detailed look at specific areas of the left ventricle. Also, since it is a tomographic rather than silhouetting technique, ultrasound is free of the problem of chamber superimposition, which can complicate the interpretation of radionuclide angiograms. Thus, 2DE can be used to identify, localize, and quantify the size of regional myocardial functional defects. No studies have yet directly compared the sensitivity of the two techniques for detecting regional dysfunction. In part, this delay emanates from the lack of universally accepted standard methods of approaching regional function by either technique; most likely such studies will be forthcoming in the future. If regional contraction defects fall within an M-mode beam (a process that is facilitated by having a concomitant M-mode capability on 2DE instruments), considerable detail is made available by ultrasound which cannot be provided by radionuclide flow studies. In particular, the amount of regional systolic myocardial *thickening* (or thinning in disease states), which some studies suggest is a more precise indication than regional endocardial motion, can be assessed. As experience with 2DE increases, it is likely that measurement of regional wall thickening will emerge as a standard way of assessing regional left ventricular function.

Both radionuclide angiography and ultrasound can measure time-dependent events associated with a cardiac cycle. Two-dimensional ultrasound and radionuclide angiography have similar framing rates; the latter is routinely associated with bolus injections which can be statistically defined. The net result is that measures such as pulmonary transit time can be easily measured by radionuclide angiography but not by 2DE. For precise timing of intrinsic intracardiac events, however, M-mode echocardiography offers a special advantage. Since the temporal information displayed by M-mode echocardiography occurs at the rate of a thousand frames per second, precise definition of cardiac events from which abnormalities of left ventricular function can be deduced have been recorded by M-mode echocardiography. Early closure of the mitral valve in severe aortic insufficiency, early opening of the aortic valve in extreme aortic insufficiency, and flat posterior wall motion of the left ventricle in constrictive pericarditis are but a few examples of how M-mode echocardiography is useful in this regard.

If resting left ventricular dysfunction is present, echocardiography is better able to determine its *cause* than radionuclide angiography. The higher resolution and more detailed tomographic sampling of the echocardiographic method allows greater sensitivity in detecting regional wall motion abnormalities associated with coronary artery disease. Furthermore, the specific heart valve abnormalities which underlie pressure and volume overload lesions can be directly imaged by echocardiography but, at best, only inferred from radionuclide angiography. Similar reasoning based on the comparatively high resolution of echocardiography with respect to radionuclide angiography points to echocardiographic advantages in distinguishing vegetations and mass lesions that may affect left ventricular function.

Echocardiography also provides additional dividends because in a single study it can evaluate the heart more completely than the radionuclide method. Ultrasonic examination can be used to determine the state of the pericardium, to exclude pericardial effusion, to evaluate the quality as well as the thickness (mass) and regional thickening of the myocardium, information which is not obtained on a single first-pass or gated radionuclide ventriculographic study.

In a clinical setting, when a patient with the suspected diagnosis of coronary artery disease presents with no abnormal physical findings and a resting study is sought for objective determination of ejection fraction and regional function, radionuclide ventriculography is the preferred method because of its intrinsically higher success rate. This preference should be stronger if exercise studies are desired. However, if there are associated findings that require evaluation (e.g., murmurs, cardiomegaly), echocardiography is the method of choice, since it allows exclusion of complicating findings such as pericardial effusion and can identify specifically important degrees of concomitant valvular heart disease.

If serial studies are indicated, it is unclear at present whether echocardiography or radionuclide ventriculography is the preferred technique. While the reproducibility of both techniques appears to be comparable, 2DE has not been tested in a practical setting for this purpose. Radionuclide ventriculography appears to be useful in following patients serially to detect early evidence of ventricular dysfunction, when they have received adriamycin chemotherapy. If repeated studies are needed in a short time frame, echocardiography has an important advantage over radionuclide method in that the patient will not be exposed to multiple injections of radioactive substances. Thus, in the setting of acute myocardial infarction, where interventions are being actively assessed, and the initial echocardiographic examination is adequate, the ultrasound method has important theoretical advantages. Whether or not ultrasound will prove useful in this setting will be the object of intense research during the next few years.

In summary, the relative merits and uses of 2DE and radionuclide angiography should not be judged in the abstract but in defined clinical contexts. Depending on the situation, each of these tests can be either mutually exclusive or complementary. It is the physician's skilled judgment, based on clinical data and knowledge of the limitations of these techniques, which determines whether both, either, or neither can be used to promote the care of an individual patient.

PART III

Diagnosis and Assessment of Cardiomyopathy

ECHOCARDIOGRAPHY

Joseph Soffer, Chin C. Chen, Daniel David, and Joel Morganroth

UNTIL RECENTLY, most patients who presented with congestive heart failure but no evidence of congenital, valvular, pericardial, or hypertensive disease were often presumed to have ischemic heart disease, even though they might never have had a myocardial infarction or experienced angina pectoris. With the increasing use of more sophisticated invasive and noninvasive cardiac diagnostic aids, a more accurate diagnosis can now be made. Cardiomyopathy is now diagnosed when myocardial dysfunction is present and other causes of cardiac disease are excluded by noninvasive testing or cardiac catheterization.[1]

The presenting signs and symptoms of cardiomyopathy are often nonspecific and may not be distinguishable from those of coronary, valvular, or pericardial disease. The patient may complain of classic anginal chest pain, with signs of congestive heart failure on physical examination, or have cardiomegaly on a chest radiograph or Q waves or frequent premature ventricular depolarizations on the ECG. Treatment for ischemic, valvular, or pericardial disease is specific and usually quite different from treatment for the various cardiomyopathies, so accurate diagnosis is mandatory.

The cardiomyopathies are being recognized more frequently by physicians and are a major cause of morbidity and mortality.[2] In some parts of the world, over 30% of all cardiac deaths are due to cardiomyopathy.[3] Echocardiography is a noninvasive technique which has been extremely useful in diagnosing and elucidating this diverse group of disorders.

CLASSIFICATION

The cardiomyopathies may be classified by several different schemes. One classification divides cardiomyopathies into primary and secondary types. Primary cardiomyopathy is considered to be an idiopathic disease of the myocardium that is not secondary to dysfunction of other cardiac structures, such as the valves or pericardium, nor related to a known generalized systemic disorder.[4] Secondary cardiomyopathy is diagnosed when the myocardium is involved as part of a generalized disease process, such as amyloidosis, which may affect multiple organs.

Another scheme classifies cardiomyopathies according to their numerous etiologies. However, etiologic classifications have limited utility since most cardiomyopathies are idiopathic.[1] Probably the most useful classification system is that described by Goodwin[5] and Goodwin and Oakley,[6] which divides cardiomyopathies into three types: congestive, hypertrophic, and restrictive.

Congestive cardiomyopathy is characterized by the presence of a dilated ventricle and congestive physiology. This syndrome results from injury to ventricular myocardium that is usually of unknown cause, and the syndrome is therefore called "idiopathic" or "primary congestive cardiomyopathy." A few cases are related to a known cause, and these are called "secondary congestive cardiomyopathies"; the various etiologic factors are listed in Table 5–1. In all types of congestive cardiomyopathy, the systolic pumping function of the ventricular myocardium is principally impaired,[5] resulting in diffuse ventricular hypokinesis.

Hypertrophic cardiomyopathy is characterized by thickened left ventricular walls with asymmetric hypertrophy of the interventricular septum in the genetic form. In this disorder the ventricular septum is characteristically at least 1.3 times thicker than the posterior left ventricular free wall. The major hemodynamic problem in hypertrophic cardiomyopathy is impaired left ventricular filling during diastole, which results from the thickened, poorly compliant chamber. When left ventricular outflow tract obstruction is also present, this condition is often called "idiopathic hypertrophic subaortic stenosis" (IHSS).

Restrictive cardiomyopathy may be considered a hybrid of the other two types.[7] The left ventricle exhibits a concentric increase in wall thickness and results in impaired diastolic filling, often combined with reduced systolic contractile function.

TABLE 5–1.—CLASSIFICATION OF CARDIOMYOPATHIES

CONGESTIVE CARDIOMYOPATHY
Primary or idiopathic (e.g., post partum[8])
Secondary
End-stage valvular or hypertensive heart disease
Ischemic (e.g.,[9, 10] following multiple myocardial infarctions)
Inflammatory
Infectious (e.g., viral, bacterial, rickettsial, fungal, spirochetal, parasitic[11])
Noninfectious (e.g., systemic lupus erythematosus[12])
Toxic (e.g., alcohol, adriamycin,[13] cobalt[14])
Metabolic (e.g., nutritional deficiencies such as beriberi,[15] hypophosphatemia[16])
Endocrine (e.g., myxedema)
Hematologic (e.g., sickle cell anemia,[17] polycythemia vera)
Physical agent (e.g., radiation)
HYPERTROPHIC CARDIOMYOPATHY
Primary or genetic
Secondary (e.g., resulting from chronic pressure overload such as long-standing severe hypertension)
RESTRICTIVE CARDIOMYOPATHY
Primary (e.g., idiopathic fibrosis)
Secondary
Infiltrative* (e.g., amyloidosis,[18–22] iron overload,[23] glycogen storage disease,[24] neoplasia, sarcoidosis,[25, 26] scleroderma[27–29])
Obliterative (e.g., endomyocardial fibroelastosis[30])
Neuromuscular disease* (e.g., progressive muscular dystrophy,[31, 32] Friedreich's ataxia[33, 34])

*Can also present late as a congestive cardiomyopathy.

ECHOCARDIOGRAPHY IN THE DIAGNOSIS OF CARDIOMYOPATHY

Both M-mode and two-dimensional echocardiography (2DE) are extremely useful in diagnosing and differentiating the cardiomyopathies. As detailed in Table 5–2, these disorders can be distinguished on the basis of the left ventricular chamber size, wall thickness, and wall motion. Figure 5–1 includes an M-mode echocardiogram from a patient with no cardiac disease. Left ventricular chamber size at end-diastole and at end-systole just below the mitral valve, wall thickness of the interventricular septum and the left ventricular posterior wall, and wall motion (amplitude of excursions of the interventricular septum and the left ventricular posterior wall) are easily measured.

M-mode echocardiography and 2DE have complementary roles in delineating the cardiomyopathies. M-mode echocardiography is particularly useful in quantifying left ventricular size and wall thickness. Two-dimensional echocardiography, with its more global view of left ventricular function, is superior in assessing wall motion, since spatial relationships and segmental dysfunction can be better appreciated. In fact, segmental disease seen on 2DE may be the first clue to the presence of ischemic heart disease.

CONGESTIVE CARDIOMYOPATHY

Congestive cardiomyopathy is characterized by a dilated, diffusely hypokinetic left ventricle. Most cases of congestive cardiomyopathy are idiopathic in origin, although a large number of secondary

TABLE 5–2.—ECHOCARDIOGRAPHIC DIFFERENTIATION OF THE CARDIOMYOPATHIES

CONGESTIVE CARDIOMYOPATHY
Dilated LV chamber size
Normal LV wall thickness
Diffuse decrease in LV wall motion (except in ischemic congestive cardiomyopathy, in which wall motion is usually segmentally decreased. Congestive cardiomyopathy must also be distinguished from volume overloaded states—e.g., valvular regurgitation,[35] shunts, athlete's heart syndrome,[36] pregnancy, chronic anemia[37]—in which wall motion is normal or increased.)
HYPERTROPHIC CARDIOMYOPATHY
Normal LV chamber size
Asymmetric increase in interventricular septum wall thickness
Normal LV wall motion
Dynamic LV outflow obstruction may develop during maneuvers which decrease LV size or increase LV contractility
RESTRICTIVE CARDIOMYOPATHY
Normal LV chamber size
Symmetric increase in LV wall thickness
Normal or decreased LV wall motion
NORMAL VALUES[38] ON M-MODE ECHOCARDIOGRAMS
LV internal dimension 3.7–5.6 cm
Wall thickness (interventricular septum and LV posterior wall) 0.6–1.1 cm
Posterior LV wall amplitude 0.9–1.4 cm
Interventricular septum wall amplitude 0.3–0.8 cm

etiologies may be responsible, as detailed in Table 5–1. The primary and secondary congestive cardiomyopathies have in common loss of ventricular muscle with resulting replacement by fibrous tissue. The cardiac chambers, including the atria as well as the ventricles, are dilated (Fig 5–2).

M-mode echocardiography is a useful technique in the diagnosis of congestive cardiomyopathy (Table 5–3). Figure 5–3 is an M-mode echocardiogram from a patient with a congestive cardiomyopathy and demonstrates several typical features of this disorder. The left ventricular diastolic and systolic dimensions are markedly increased, with normal wall thickness but with a marked decrease in the amplitude of motion of both the ventricular septum and left ventricular posterior wall.[35, 39, 40] The E point of the anterior mitral leaflet to the ventricular septum is increased, which suggests decreased cardiac output.[41] Other features implying a decreased cardiac output include decreased aortic wall amplitude[42] and decreased maximum aortic leaflet separation (less than 15 mm), as well as various measurements using mitral valve opening as an estimate of blood flow.[43–45]

Overall left ventricular function is significantly decreased in congestive cardiomyopathy and may be roughly quantified using M-mode echocardiography. Fractional shortening of the left ventricle is such a measurement and is determined by dividing the difference between the left ventricular diastolic and left ventricular systolic dimensions by the left ventricular diastolic dimension and multiplying by 100[46] (normal is 25%–42%). This measurement assumes that the sampled region is typical of the ventricular contraction pattern as a whole.[47] In ischemic disease, where regional contraction abnormalities often exist, this assumption is not valid.[48] Therefore, M-mode echocardiography has been found to overestimate left ventricular function in patients with prior myocardial (especially anterolateral wall) infarction.[49] In patients with diffuse left ventricular hypokinesis, fractional shortening may be a useful measurement. The left ventricular ejection fraction has been calculated

TABLE 5–3.—ECHOCARDIOGRAPHIC FEATURES OF CONGESTIVE CARDIOMYOPATHY

M-MODE FEATURES
Increased LV end-diastolic (LV_D) and end-systolic (LV_S) internal dimensions
Decreased motion of the interventricular septum (VS) (<0.3 cm) and LV posterior wall (LVPW) (<0.9 cm)
Normal thickness of LVPW and VS
Delayed closure of the mitral valve suggests increased LV_D pressure
Features suggesting decreased cardiac output:
Decreased amplitude of motion of the aortic root
Decreased aortic leaflet maximum separation (<15 mm)
Early systolic closure of the aortic valve
Decreased mitral DE slope (see Fig 5–1)
Decreased total amplitude of mitral valve motion
Quantitative indices revealing decreased overall left ventricular function
Decreased fractional shortening $[LV_D - LV_S]/LV_D \times 100$ (normal 25%–42%)
Decreased ejection fraction (calculated using any of several formulas for estimating ventricular volumes from M-mode measurements)[46, 48, 50] $[LV_D \text{ volume} - LV_S \text{ volume}]/LV_D \text{ volume} \times 100$
TWO-DIMENSIONAL FEATURES
Dilated LV
Diffuse LV hypokinesis (segmental wall motion abnormalities suggest possible ischemic heart disease)
Normal LV wall thickness
Quantitative indices revealing decreased overall LV function
Decreased calculated ejection fraction
Detect potential complications of congestive cardiomyopathy
Mural thrombus
Papillary muscle dysfunction

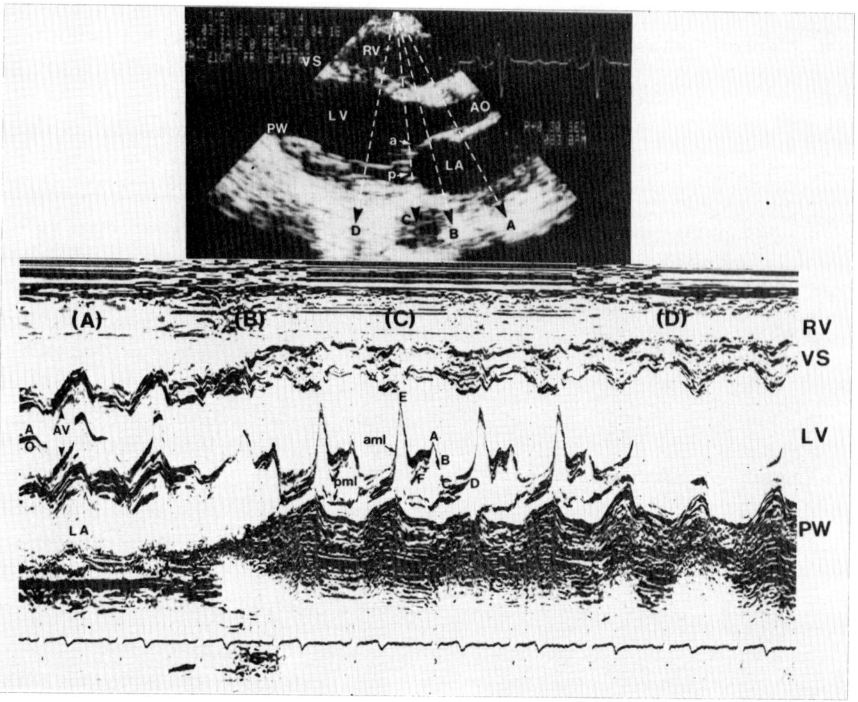

Fig 5–1.—*Top,* a representative two-dimensional echocardiographic view from the parasternal left ventricular long axis demonstrating the left ventricle *(LV),* ventricular septum *(VS),* anterior aortic wall *(AAW),* posterior aortic wall *(PAW),* aortic valve *(AV),* left atrium *(LA),* and the anterior mitral leaflet *(AL)* and posterior mitral leaflet *(PL). Bottom,* a representative M-mode echocardiogram taken from the transducer lines demonstrated by letters *A, B, C,* and *D.*

using various formulas to estimate ventricular volumes from internal dimensions, with good correlation with the angiographic ejection fraction when localized asynergy was not present.[46, 48, 50] Both the fractional shortening and estimated ejection fraction can be serially followed, and both often progressively decrease in patients with congestive cardiomyopathy.

As detailed above, M-mode echocardiography defines the major features of congestive cardiomyopathy and is usually sufficient to make this diagnosis. However, 2DE can also make significant contributions in the evaluation of patients with this disorder. Because of its similarity to conventional angiographic imaging, 2DE allows a better appreciation of overall left ventricular function. Figure 5–4 consists of end-diastolic and end-systolic frames of 2DEs from a patient with congestive cardiomyopathy. The left ventricular chambers are dilated and wall motion is diffusely decreased. Real-time viewing of 2DEs obtained in patients with congestive cardiomyopathy dramatically reveals the diffuse decrease in function and has the advantage over angiography of not depressing the ventricle further by the administration of contrast material. Two-dimensional echocardiography is superior to M-mode echocardiography in estimating ejection fraction.[51] The combination of Doppler ultrasonography with 2DE appears to be extremely promising as a noninvasive technique to estimate cardiac output.[52] Two-dimensional echocardiography is also advantageous in demonstrating regional wall motion abnormalities. Ischemic heart disease should be suspected in patients whose dilated left ventricles reveal segmental wall motion abnormalities, as shown in Figure 5–5. However, the presence of diffuse ventricular hypokinesis does not rule out the presence of ischemic heart disease as a cause of the myocardial dysfunction. We have observed that up to 25% of patients who have

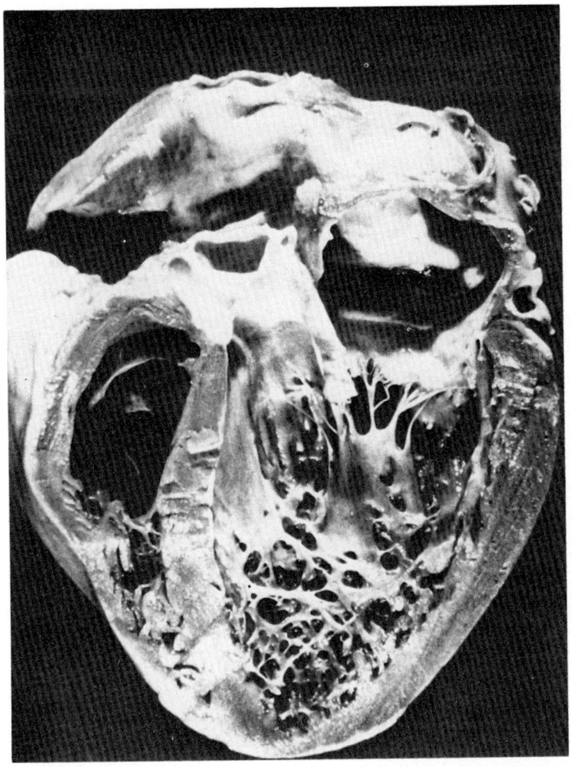

Fig 5–2.—Gross anatomical specimen of a heart from a patient with severe congestive cardiomyopathy demonstrating dilation of the atrium and ventricles. (Courtesy of Jeffrey Isner, M.D., Tufts University, Boston.)

sustained a single large anterior myocardial infarction may have diffuse left ventricular hypokinesis on 2DE performed more than six months after the infarction.

Two-dimensional echocardiography may also be useful in detailing potential complications of congestive cardiomyopathy. Figure 5–6 shows long- and short-axis 2DEs from a patient with idiopathic congestive cardiomyopathy. The left ventricle is dilated and hypocontractile. Both cross-sectional images depict the presence of a left ventricular mass compatible with clot. The apical four-chamber view is often the best view for detecting ventricular thrombi. This view may also be useful in detecting papillary muscle dysfunction,[45] which is suggested by incomplete closure of the mitral valve in systole.

Echocardiography may be helpful in following the natural history of patients with congestive cardiomyopathy. Left ventricular cavity size, wall motion, and the calculated ejection fraction are three useful parameters to follow. Serial studies may be done to determine whether improvement has resulted from various therapies. For example, echocardiography may be used to assess the beneficial effects of vasodilators in patients with congestive cardiomyopathy. It may even be used prospectively to choose which patients are likely to benefit from hydralazine therapy, as shown by

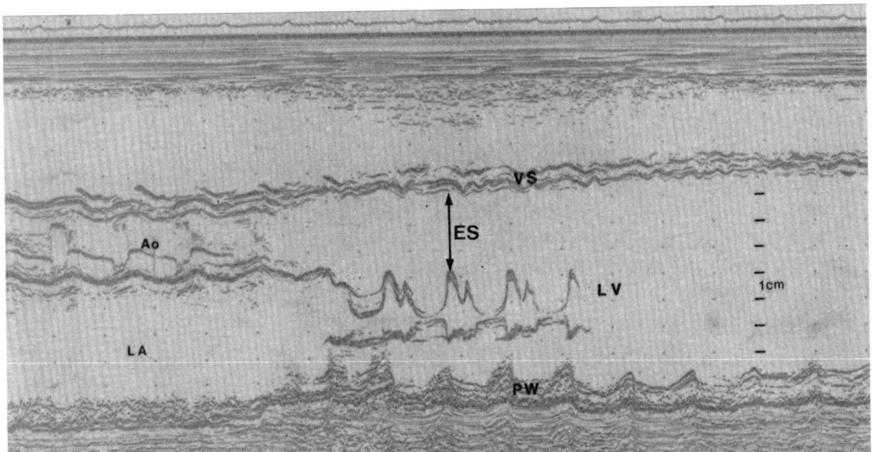

Fig 5–3.—An M-mode echocardiogram from a patient with severe idiopathic congestive cardiomyopathy detailing the characteristic features of a markedly dilated left ventricle *(LV)* and a mitral valve in which the E-septal *(ES)* distance is markedly increased, signifying marked decrease in cardiac output. The left atrium *(LA)* is markedly dilated; the aorta *(AO)* is also shown.

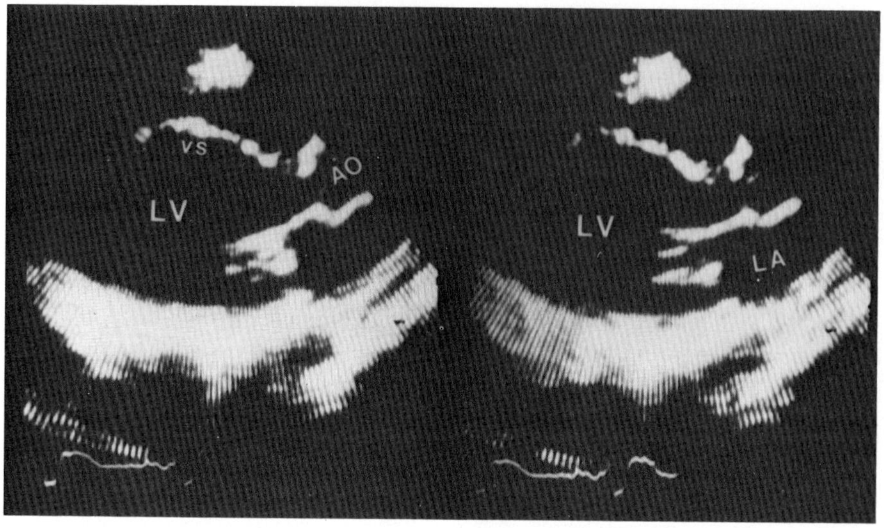

Fig 5–4.—Two-dimensional echocardiographic parasternal long-axis left ventricular views of the left ventricle *(LV)* in end-diastole *(left)* and end-systole *(right)*. Note the markedly enlarged left ventricle, which does not appear to decrease in size during systole. *VS,* ventricular septum; *AO,* aorta; *LA,* left atrium. (From Morganroth J., Chen C.C.: *Med. Clin. North Am.* 64:33–60, 1980. Reproduced by permission.)

Packer and colleagues.[53] After two to three weeks of hydralazine therapy, 15 of 24 patients with left ventricular end-diastolic diameter (LV_D) of 60 mm or greater before therapy had improved, and only 1 patient worsened. Of the 16 patients with an LV_D less than 60 mm, only 2 improved and 10 showed clinical deterioration following the institution of hydralazine.

Echocardiography has played a major role in assessing other therapies in congestive cardiomyopathy. In one study of ischemic congestive cardiomyopathy, the echocardiographically determined ejection fraction and stroke volume improved following the institution of beta-blocker therapy.[54] Surprisingly, these same two echocardiographically determined estimates of left ventricular

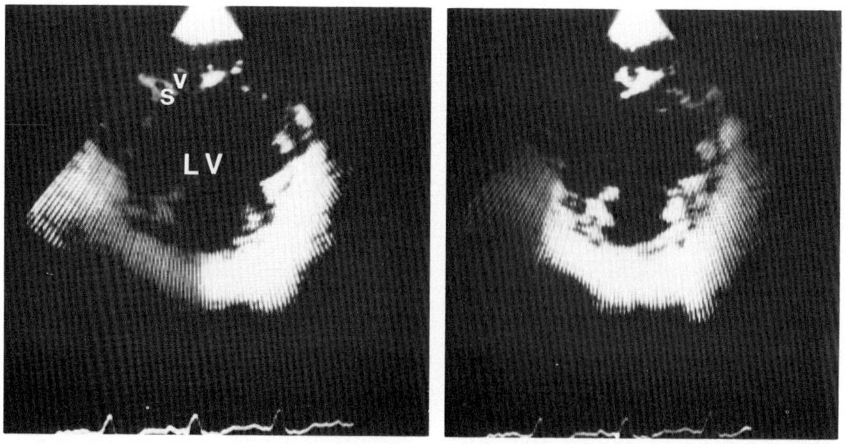

Fig 5–5.—Two-dimensional echocardiographic views of the left ventricle as seen in short axis at the level of the papillary muscles. Diastole is shown on the left and systole on the right. Note the segmental wall motion abnormality, in which there is marked hypokinesis of the entire ventricular myocardium except for the ventricular septum. *RV,* right ventricle; *VS,* ventricular septum; *PW,* posterior wall.

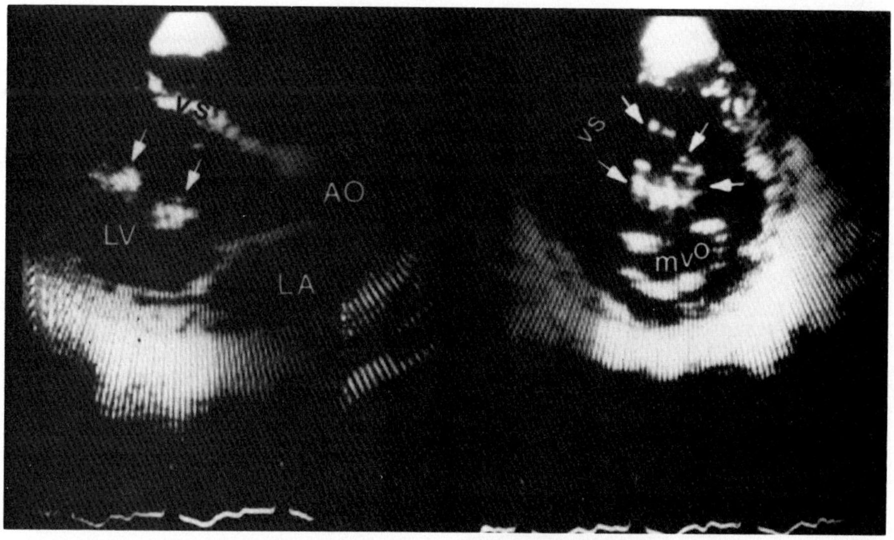

Fig 5–6.—*Left,* a two-dimensional parasternal long-axis view of the left ventricle *(LV). White arrows* point out left ventricular clot. *Right,* a short-axis view of the left ventricle at the level of the mitral valve in the same patient. *White arrows* point to location of the left ventricular clot. *LA,* left atrium; *mvo,* mitral valve orifice. (From Morganroth J., Chen C.C.: *Med. Clin. North Am.* 64:33–60, 1980. Reproduced by permission.)

function decreased following beta-blocker withdrawal in patients with idiopathic congestive cardiomyopathy,[55] establishing a possible role for this therapy.

Echocardiography may be able to detect early signs of dysfunction in cardiomyopathy, which could lead to earlier removal of potentially injurious agents or the institution of supportive drug therapy. For example, far advanced cardiac involvement in Chagas' disease leads to diffuse ventricular hypokinesis indistinguishable from idiopathic congestive cardiomyopathy. However, Acquattella and colleagues[11] have used 2DE to identify apical dysfunction with sparing of the ventricular septum in Chagas' cardiomyopathy at an earlier stage of this disease.

HYPERTROPHIC CARDIOMYOPATHY

The characteristic feature of hypertrophic cardiomyopathy is myocardial hypertrophy, usually with disproportionately greater thickening of the interventricular septum compared to the free wall. With the presence of septal hypertrophy, left ventricular outflow tract obstruction can occur when the septum opposes the anterior mitral leaflet in systole. Asymmetric septal hypertrophy can exist asymptomatically or can give rise to symptoms related to impaired left ventricular filling during diastole.

Hypertrophic cardiomyopathy was recognized pathologically in 1958 by Teare.[56] He observed that the ventricular septum was disproportionately hypertrophied compared to the left ventricular free wall. Hypertrophic cardiomyopathy was clinically recognized in the early 1960s. The first feature of hypertrophic cardiomyopathy to be highlighted was the left ventricular outflow tract obstruction, and the disease was initially called "idiopathic hypertrophic subaortic stenosis" (IHSS) in the United States, "hypertrophic obstructive cardiomyopathy" (HOCM) in Great Britain, and "muscular subaortic stenosis" in Canada.[57] Pathologic examination of hearts from patients with hypertrophic cardiomyopathy reveal a marked increase in myocardial mass with a small ventricular cavity (Fig 5–7). The degree of thickening of the interventricular septum does not predict the presence or absence of left ventricular outflow tract obstruc-

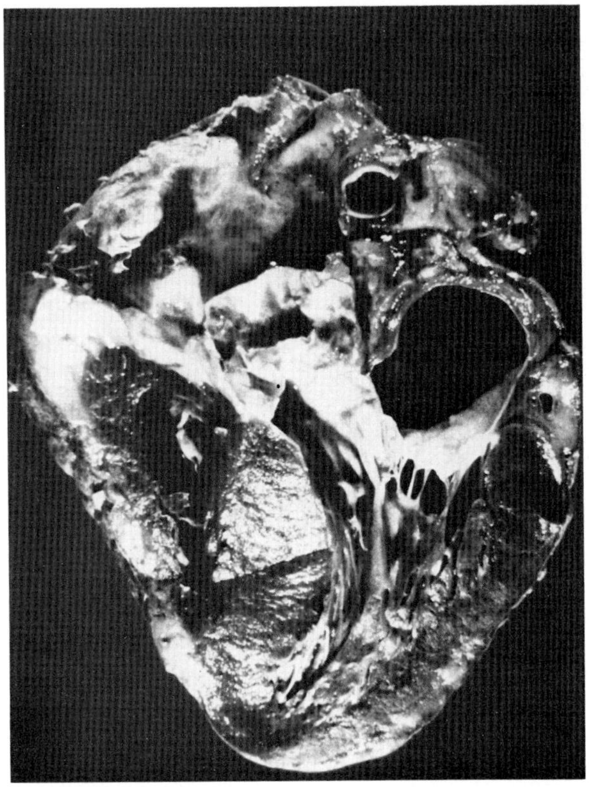

Fig 5–7.—A pathologic heart specimen from a patient with hypertrophic cardiomyopathy. Asymmetric septal hypertrophy is evident. (Photograph reproduced courtesy of Jeffrey Isner, M.D., Tufts University, Boston.)

tion.[58] The myocardial cells in the ventricular septum are disorganized, hypertrophied, and bizarrely shaped. Interestingly, in patients without outflow tract obstruction, similar bizarre cells are present extensively throughout the left ventricular free wall,[59] whereas patients with obstruction have hypertrophied cells without significant disorganization in the left ventricular free wall muscle.[60]

Hypertrophic cardiomyopathy appears to be a distinct disease entity with diverse clinical manifestations.[61] Family studies by Clark and colleagues[62] have shown that it is inherited as an autosomal dominant trait. However, there are no pathognomonic diagnostic features. Neither cellular disorganization in the ventricular septum, asymmetric septal hypertrophy, nor the presence of systolic anterior motion of the anterior mitral leaflet is pathognomonic of hypertrophic cardiomyopathy.[61] However, each finding is uncommon enough in other cardiac disorders that their combined presence is highly specific for hypertrophic cardiomyopathy. Disproportionate septal hypertrophy has been found in 10% of patients with other cardiac disorders.[61] This is often secondary to chronic pressure overload of the left or right ventricles, with resulting hypertrophy of the interventricular septum. Asymmetric septal hypertrophy has also been described in patients who sustained infarction of the free wall of the left ventricle, with resultant thinning of this wall.[63, 64] False positive asymmetric septal hypertrophy may occur in clinical states of chronic right ventricular pressure overload in which both the anterior right ventricular wall and interventricular septum hypertrophy. Extensive cellular disorganization in the interventricular septum is present in only 5% of patients with other cardiac disorders, and systolic anterior motion of the anterior mitral leaflet has been seen in only 3%[61] of this group of patients.

In an individual patient with asymmetric septal hypertrophy, there is no physical examination finding that allows accurate diagnosis of primary hypertrophic cardiomyopathy. Maron and Epstein[61] have suggested that the most practical way of diagnosing the primary form of this cardiomyopathy is to perform echocardiography on five closely related family members. Since the disorder is inherited as an autosomal trait, the probability that five first-degree relatives of a patient with hypertrophic cardiomyopathy will have normal echocardiograms is approximately 3%. Therefore, the absence of asymmetric septal hypertrophy in five first-degree relatives is strong evidence against this disorder being present on a genetic basis.

Echocardiography has had its greatest impact on the diagnosis of hypertrophic cardiomyopathy (Table 5–4). The unique ability of echocardiography to measure wall thickness has resulted in its great utility in this disorder. Numerous features of hypertrophic cardiomyopathy have been described using M-mode echocardiography. Asymmetric septal hypertrophy, as previously discussed, is a hallmark of the disorder. The interventricular septum is usually at least 18 mm thick, with the ratio of the septal to free wall thickness at least 1.3:1.0[65] or 1.5:1.0.[66] The amplitude of motion and systolic thickening of the ventricular septum are frequently decreased.[67–69] The left ventricular systolic dimension is usually small, often less than 35 mm. In over 90% of patients with IHSS, the left ventricular outflow tract is narrowed to less than 20 mm.[65] This space is defined by the ultrasonic beam traversing the midportion of the anterior mitral leaflet and is measured from the mitral C point to the interventricular septum. A most notable echocardiographic abnormality described in patients with IHSS or obstructive asymmetric septal hypertrophy is systolic anterior motion of the anterior mitral leaflet.[62–70] The anterior mitral leaflet appears to move anteriorly toward the septum in early systole and returns to its normal position at the end of systole. Henry and associates[71] have reported that the closer the anterior leaflet comes to the septum and the longer the time of contact with the septum, the greater the obstruction to left ventricular outflow. They have proposed a method of quantifying the gradient,[71] which other investigators[72, 73] have found less useful. Systolic anterior motion characteristic of genetic hypertrophic cardiomyopathy may be mimicked by exaggeration of the normal anterior systolic motion of the mitral valve, which is common when the posterior wall exhibits exaggerated motion. Chordal structures adjacent to the anterior mitral leaflet may also cause a pattern of apparent systolic anterior motion on M-mode echocardiography. Systolic anterior motion characteristic of genetic asymmetric septal hypertrophy begins after the onset of systole and abates prior to mitral valve opening.

TABLE 5–4.—ECHOCARDIOGRAPHIC FEATURES OF HYPERTROPHIC CARDIOMYOPATHY

M-MODE FEATURES
- Asymmetric septal hypertrophy. Usually the interventricular septum (VS) is $\geq$ 18 mm, with the ratio of the thickness of VS to left ventricular free wall at least 1.3–1.5:1.0.
  - False positives
    - RV pressure overload
    - LV pressure overload (10% of cases)
    - Following inferior wall infarction with posterior wall thinning
- VS with "speckled" "ground glass"[86] appearance
- Decreased VS amplitude
- Decreased LV systolic dimension (< 25 mm)
- Features suggesting LV outflow tract obstruction
  - Systolic anterior motion (SAM) of the anterior mitral leaflet
  - Aortic valve midsystolic notching
  - Narrowed LV outflow tract (<20 mm)

TWO-DIMENSIONAL ADDITIONS TO M-MODE ECHOCARDIOGRAPHY
- Substantiate the presence of true VS hypertrophy
- Identify distribution of hypertrophy
- Identify extent of texture changes in the VS
- Reveal structure(s) causing SAM

The most characteristic M-mode echocardiographic findings in patients with obstruction are aortic valve midsystolic notching and systolic anterior motion of the mitral valve with prolonged (greater than 30% of systole) contact.[74]

Figure 5–8 demonstrates many of the M-mode echocardiographic findings in hypertrophic cardiomyopathy. The ventricular septum is markedly thickened and hypocontractile. The left ventricular cavity is small and the left ventricular outflow tract is narrowed, as the mitral valve is positioned very anteriorly in the cavity. Systolic anterior motion is identified and suggests the presence of at least a provocable gradient across the left ventricular outflow tract. The combination of a narrowed left ventricular outflow space, markedly thickened interventricular septum, and systolic anterior movement of the mitral valve is virtually diagnostic of IHSS.[65] The insert in the upper right corner of Figure 5–9 shows an echocardiogram in which premature closure of the aortic valve, which is also described as midsystolic notching, is demonstrated by the black arrow. Various interventions such as the administration of amyl nitrate or a Valsalva maneuver during M-mode echocardiography may bring out systolic anterior motion of the mitral valve in a patient with provocable obstruction. Systolic anterior motion may also be more pronounced on the beat following a premature ventricular contraction because of the resulting increase in left ventricular contractility. Obstruction to right ventricular outflow may also be present in patients with hypertrophic cardiomyopathy. Echocardiography may reveal increased thickness of the right ventricular anterior wall as well as of the septum, midsystolic closure of the pulmonic valve,[75] and systolic anterior motion of the tricuspid valve.[76]

Because of its large field of view and better delineation of spatial relationships, 2DE has improved our ability to diagnose hypertrophic cardiomyopathy. As an investigative tool, it has elucidated numerous features of this disorder. Two-

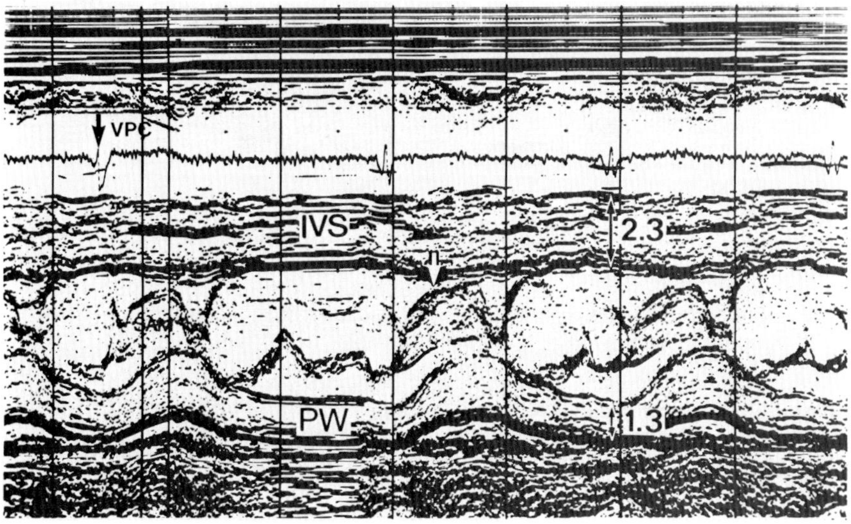

Fig 5–8.—An M-mode echocardiogram from a patient with obstructive asymmetric septal hypertrophy; the recording demonstrates a premature ventricular complex *(VPC).* Interventricular septum *(IVS)* is markedly thickened compared to the posterior left ventricular wall *(PW).* The *white arrow* points out systolic anterior motion of the mitral valve.

dimensional echocardiography may allow a technically adequate study to be done when M-mode echocardiograms of diagnostic quality cannot be obtained.[7] For example, a 2DE obtained from the apical view may give diagnostic information when M-mode echocardiography from the parasternal region is inadequate.[7] M-mode echocardiography may falsely give the impression of a thickened septum, which Fowles[77, 78] has shown to be related to anterior angulation of the septum, with an apparently abnormal thickness of the septum because of the oblique pathway taken by the single-dimensional echocardiographic beam. Wide-angle 2DE has been used to diagnose hypertrophic cardiomyopathy when the entity was not detectable by M-mode echocardiography.[79] Left ventricular hypertrophy was identified in regions through which the M-mode ultrasound beam does not usually pass (e.g., the posterior ventricular septum, anterior or lateral left ventricular free wall, and ventricular septum near the apex). Figure 5–10 (lower panel) shows a left ventricular parasternal long-axis, apical four-chamber, and apical two-chamber 2DE from a patient with hypertrophic cardiomyopathy. The marked hypertrophy of the interventricular septum is evident on all three views. Systolic anterior motion of the mitral leaflet is identified by the white arrow on the long-axis projection.

By visualizing nearly the entire interventricular septum, 2DE has elucidated the marked variability of the shape of the hypertrophied septum.[80, 81] The hypertrophy tends to be greatest in the anterolateral portion in the short-axis view and in the middle third in the long-axis view.[7] Systolic anterior motion of the mitral valve has been shown to involve not only the mitral leaflets but also the chordae tendineae and even the papillary muscles in some patients.[7, 82, 83] Distinguishing between systolic anterior motion of the chordae tendineae and the mitral leaflets may have clinical importance; the former abnormality may be an echocardiographic finding with few clinical implications,[84] whereas the latter usually implies significant left ventricular outflow tract obstruction.

Two-dimensional echocardiography has also been useful in planning and evaluating surgery for IHSS. M-mode echocardiography has been used in the operating room to help the surgeon assess wall thickness and, therefore, more optimally determine the extent of the myectomy.[85] Both M-mode echocardiography and 2DE[86, 87] can be used to identify the site of myotomy and estimate the amount of tissue removed at surgery.

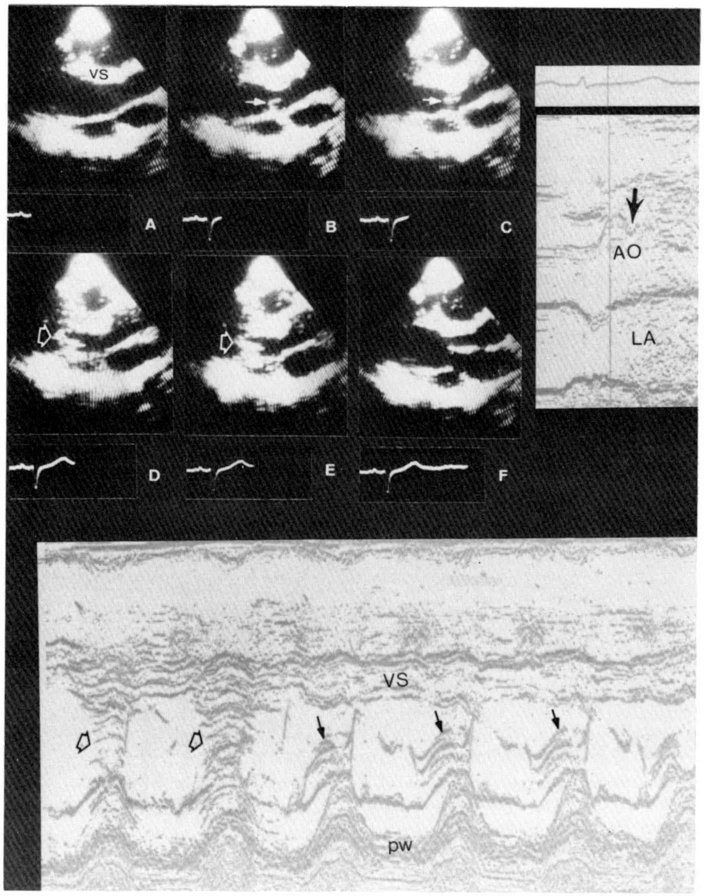

Fig 5–9.—*Top right,* an M-mode echocardiogram of the aorta *(AO)* and left atrium *(LA)* in which premature closure of the aortic valve is indicated by the *black arrow. Bottom,* systolic anterior motion of the mitral valve *(arrows). VS,* ventricular septum; *PW,* posterior wall. *Top left,* sequences A through F of the parasternal two-dimensional left ventricular long-axis view from diastole through systole. The *white arrows* depict the presence of systolic anterior motion of the mitral valve. (From Morganroth J., Chen C.C.: *Med. Clin. North Am.* 64:33–60, 1980. Reproduced by permission.

Both M-mode echocardiography and 2DE have detailed a peculiar acoustic property of the septal echoes in genetic asymmetric septal hypertrophy which has been described as "speckled" with a "ground glass texture."[86] This echo pattern is illustrated in Figure 5–11 and may be related to myocardial fiber disarray.[88]

RESTRICTIVE CARDIOMYOPATHY

Restrictive cardiomyopathy is a syndrome characterized by a stiff, poorly compliant ventricular cavity resulting either from idiopathic myocardial fibrosis or, more commonly, infiltration by various substances. These include amyloid,[18–22] iron,[23] glycogen,[24] neoplastic cells, sarcoid granulomas,[25, 26] or connective tissue as in scleroderma.[27–29] Myocardial fibrosis is often present in the neuromuscular disorders, particularly progressive muscular dystrophy[31, 32] and Friedreich's ataxia.[33, 34] The major hemodynamic abnormality is reduced diastolic ventricular compliance,[89] which is occa-

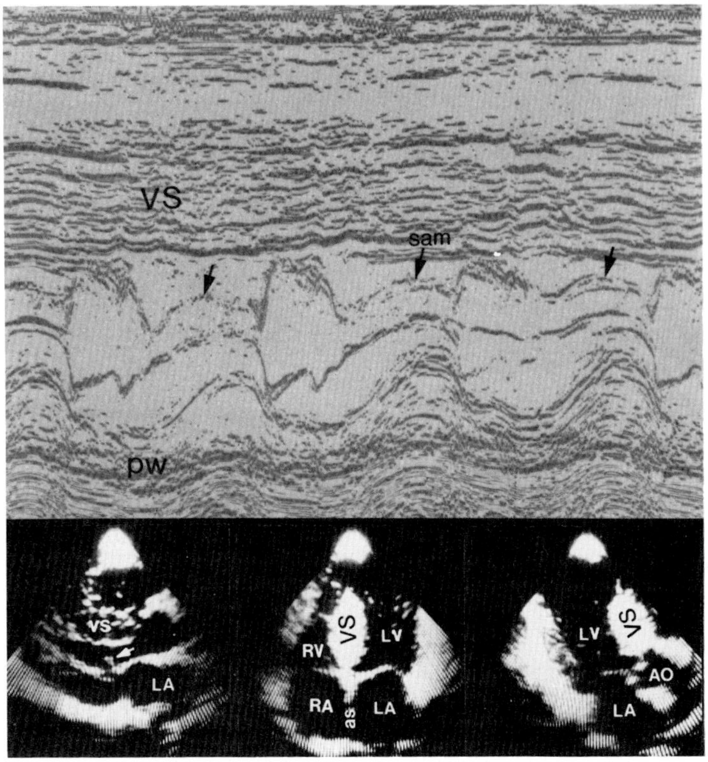

Fig 5–10.—*Bottom,* two-dimensional echocardiographic views: parasternal long-axis left ventricular view *(left),* apical four-chamber view *(middle),* and apical two-chamber view *(right).* The left ventricle *(LV),* right ventricle *(RV),* right atrium *(RA),* and left atrium *(LA)* are depicted. *VS,* ventricular septum; *AS,* atrial septum; *AO,* aorta. These views demonstrate the various configurations of the markedly hypertrophied interventricular septum in this patient with obstructive asymmetric septal hypertrophy. The *white arrow* in the long-axis view indicates systolic anterior motion, which is also indicated by the *black arrows* in the M-mode echocardiogram *(top).* (From Morganroth J., Chen C.C.: *Med. Clin. North Am.* 64:33–60, 1980. Reproduced by permission.)

sionally associated with reduced systolic pump function.[7] Similar restriction to diastolic filling is present in conditions in which the ventricular cavity is obliterated by abnormal tissue. This abnormal tissue may consist of large masses of eosinophils (as in Loeffler's eosinophilic fibroplastic endocarditis) or fibrosis and thrombus (as in endomyocardial fibroelastosis). The latter two conditions are rare outside of the tropical zones of the world.

Hemodynamically, restrictive cardiomyopathy has many similarities with constrictive pericarditis.[90] In both syndromes an early diastolic decline in the left and right ventricular pressure recordings is followed by a rapid rise to a plateau. This rapid rise and abrupt plateau in the early diastolic ventricular pressure tracing has been termed the "square root" sign. The major hemodynamic difference between those two disorders is that in restrictive cardiomyopathy there is usually greater impairment of left than of right ventricular filling, with resulting higher filling pressures in the left than in the right ventricle.[91] In constrictive pericarditis, there is usually equal diastolic pressures in the left and right ventricles. The distinction between these disorders is critical since constrictive pericarditis may be cured by surgery, whereas restrictive cardiomyopathy usually has no satisfactory therapy except for the rare case of hemochromatosis in which myocardial function may improve after removal of excess iron.[92]

Amyloid heart disease is the prototype of restrictive cardiomyopathy, and a recent study[18] de-

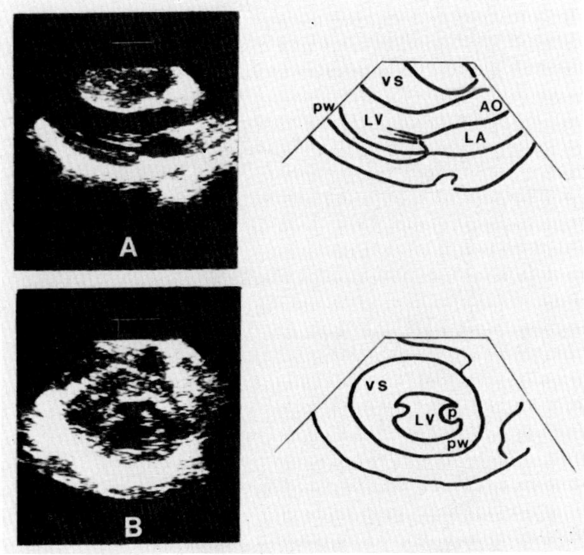

Fig 5–11.—*A,* two-dimensional echocardiographic parasternal long-axis view of the left ventricle. Accompanying diagram shows the ventricular septum *(VS),* posterior wall *(PW),* left ventricle *(LV),* aorta *(AO),* and left atrium *(LA).* Note the markedly hypertrophied ventricular septum with a "speckled" characteristic. *B,* left ventricular short-axis view at the level of the papillary muscle *(p)* in the same patient. Accompanying diagram shows the ventricular septum *(VS),* left ventricle *(LV),* and posterior wall *(PW).* Note the asymmetric septal hypertrophy.

TABLE 5–5.—ECHOCARDIOGRAPHIC FEATURES OF RESTRICTIVE CARDIOMYOPATHY

M-MODE FEATURES
Normal LV and RV cavity size
Thickened interventricular septum (VS), LV posterior wall (LVPW), and RV anterior wall (RVAW)
Normal to decreased motion of VS, LVPW, and RVAW with frequent decreased systolic thickening
TWO-DIMENSIONAL FEATURES
Normal ventricular cavity size
Thickened VS, LVPW, and RVAW (RVAW thickening better appreciated on 2DE than on M-mode echocardiogram)
Thickened valve leaflets
Thickened interatrial septum

tailed the echocardiographic features of this disorder (Table 5–5). M-mode echocardiograms were obtained on 26 patients and revealed a normal left ventricular chamber size in all and thickened ventricular walls (septum in 88%, posterior wall in 77%, and right ventricular anterior wall in 79%) with decreased systolic thickening, most prominent in the ventricular septum (96%) (Fig 5–12). Two-dimensional echocardiography in 13 patients provided additional information (Fig 5–13). A characteristic "granular sparkling" appearance of the thickened myocardium was seen in 92% of the patients and was believed to be related to the

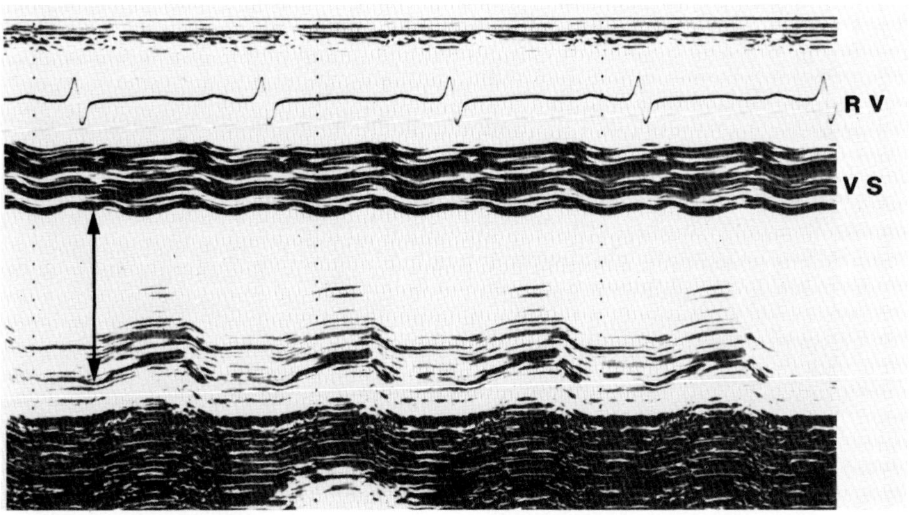

Fig 5–12.—An M-mode echocardiogram from a patient with restrictive cardiomyopathy demonstrates concentric left ventricular hypertrophy with equal thickness of the ventricular septum *(VS)* and posterior wall *(PW).* There is hypokinesis of the ventricular septum; note its granular appearance.

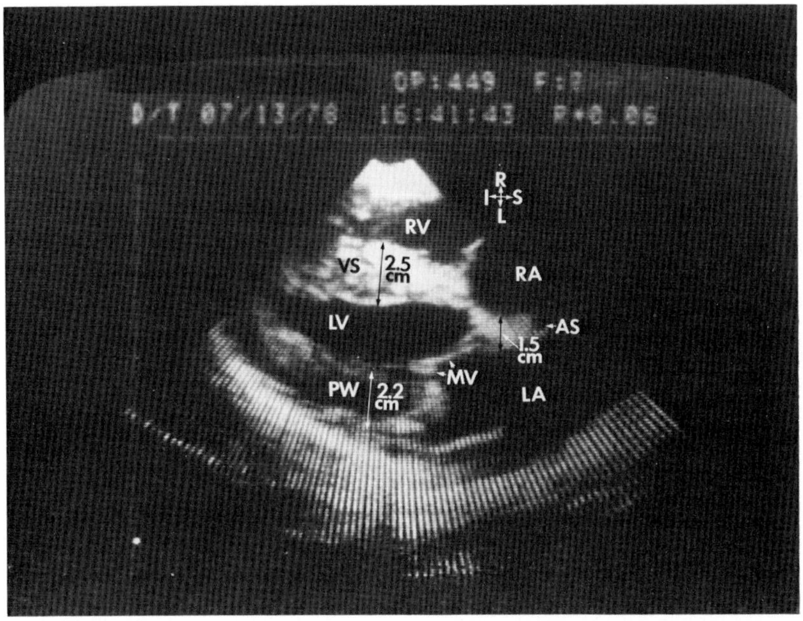

Fig 5–13.—A two-dimensional echocardiographic view of the parasternal long-axis left ventricular *(LV)* view. The ventricular septum *(VS)* and posterior wall *(PW)* demonstrate marked thickening in a concentric pattern. *MV,* mitral valve; *LA,* left atrium; *AS,* atrial septum; *RA,* right atrium; *RV,* right ventricle. Note that the *AS* is also hypertrophied and the *VS* has a granular appearance. (From Siqueira-Filho A.G., et al.: *Circulation* 63:188–196, 1981. Reproduced by permission of the American Heart Association.)

amyloid deposition. Of the 13 patients studied, 5 had increased papillary muscle thickness, 4 had thickened valves, and 3 had a thickened interatrial septum. Two-dimensional echocardiography provided a better appreciation of the right ventricular anterior wall, which was felt to be thickened in 85% of patients. The combination of findings on 2DE, including thickened left and right ventricular walls with a normal or small left ventricular cavity and mildly enlarged left atrium, along with the granular sparkling appearance of the myocardium, was felt to be virtually diagnostic of cardiac amyloidosis.[18] However, further studies will need to be done to substantiate this impression.

REFERENCES

1. Perloff J.K.: The cardiomyopathies: Current perspectives. *Circulation* 44:942–949, 1971.
2. Wynne J., Braunwald E.: The cardiomyopathies and myocarditities, in Braunwald E. (ed.): *Heart Disease: A Textbook of Cardiovascular Medicine*. Philadelphia, W.B. Saunders Co., 1980, p. 1438.
3. Burch G.E., DePasquale N.P.: Recognition and prevention of cardiomyopathy: Subcommittee on cardiomyopathy. *Circulation* 42:A-47, 1970.
4. Fowler N.D.: Classification and differential diagnosis of the myocardiopathies. *Prog. Cardiovasc. Dis*. 7:1–16, 1964.
5. Goodwin J.F.: Congestive and hypertrophic cardiomyopathies. *Lancet* 1:731–739, 1970.
6. Goodwin J.F., Oakley C.M.: The cardiomyopathies. *Br. Heart J*. 34:545–552, 1972.
7. DeMaria A.N., Bommer W., Lee G., et al.: Value and limitations of two-dimensional echocardiography in assessment of cardiomyopathy. *Am. J. Cardiol*. 46:1224–1231, 1980.
8. Brockington I.F.: Postpartum hypertensive heart failure. *Am. J. Cardiol*. 27:650–658, 1978.
9. Raftery E.B., Banks D.C., Oram S.: Occlusive disease of the coronary arteries presenting as primary congestive cardiomyopathy. *Lancet* 2:1147–1150, 1969.
10. Schuster E.H., Bulkley B.H.: Ischemic cardiomyopathy: A clinicopathologic study of fourteen patients. *Am. Heart J*. 100:506–512, 1980.
11. Acquattella H., Schiller N.B., Puigbo J.J., et al.: M-mode and two-dimensional echocardiography in chronic Chagas' heart disease: A clinical and pathologic study. *Circulation* 62:787–799, 1980.
12. Borenstein D.G., Fye W.B., Arnett F.C., et al.: The myocarditis of systemic lupus erythematosus: Association with myositis. *Ann. Intern. Med*. 89:619–624, 1978.

13. Bristow M.R., Thompson P.D., Martin R.P., et al.: Early anthracycline cardiotoxicity. *Am. J. Med.* 65:823–832, 1978.
14. Alexander C.S.: Cobalt beer cardiomyopathy. *Am. J. Med.* 53:395–416, 1972.
15. Kozam R.L., Esquerra O.E., Smith J.J.: Cardiovascular beriberi. *Am. J. Cardiol.* 30:418–422, 1972.
16. Darsee J.R., Nutter D.O.: Reversible severe congestive cardiomyopathy in three cases of hypophosphatemia. *Ann. Intern. Med.* 89:867–870, 1978.
17. Gerry J.L., Baird M.G., Fortuin N.J.: Evaluation of left ventricular function in patients with sickle cell anemia. *Am. J. Med.* 60:1968–1972, 1976.
18. Siqueira-Filho A.G., Cunho C.L.P., Tajik A.J., et al.: M-mode and two-dimensional echocardiographic features in cardiac amyloidosis. *Circulation* 63:188–196, 1981.
19. Kyle R.A., Bayrd E.D.: Amyloidosis: Review of 236 cases. *Medicine* 54:271–299, 1975.
20. Rakowski I.T., Boughiner O.R., Sole M.J., et al.: The echocardiographic diagnosis of amyloid cardiomyopathy, abstracted. *Circulation* 54(suppl. II):II–84, 1976.
21. Giles T.D., Le'on-Galindo J., Burch G.E.: Echocardiographic findings in amyloid cardiomyopathy. *South. Med. J.* 71:1393–1396, 1978.
22. Child J.S., Levisman J.A., Abbasi A.S., et al.: Echocardiographic manifestations of infiltrative cardiomyopathy: A report of seven cases due to amyloid. *Chest* 70:726–731, 1976.
23. Henry W.L., Nienhuis A.W., Wiener M., et al.: Echocardiographic abnormalities in patients with transfusion-dependent anemia and secondary myocardial iron deposition. *Am. J. Med.* 64:547–555, 1978.
24. Rees A., Eibi F., Minhasi K., et al.: Echocardiographic evidence of outflow tract obstruction in Pompe's disease (glycogen storage disease of the heart). *Am. J. Cardiol.* 37:1103–1106, 1976.
25. Lorell B., Alderman E.C., Mason J.W.: Cardiac sarcoidosis. *Am. J. Cardiol.* 42:143–146, 1978.
26. Silverman K.J., Hutchins G.M., Bulkley B.H.: Cardiac sarcoid: A clinicopathologic study of 84 unselected patients with systemic sarcoidosis. *Circulation* 58:1204–1211, 1978.
27. Gottdiener J.S., Moutsopoulos H.M., Decker J.L.: Echocardiographic identification of cardiac abnormality in scleroderma and related disorders. *Am. J. Med.* 66:391–398, 1979.
28. Eggebrecht R.F., Kleiger R.E.: Echocardiographic patterns in scleroderma. *Chest* 71:47–51, 1971.
29. Smith J.W., Clements P.J., Levisman J., et al.: Echocardiographic features of progressive systemic sclerosis (PSS): Correlation with hemodynamic and post-mortem studies. *Am. J. Med.* 66:28–33, 1979.
30. Hess O.M., Turina M., Senning A., et al.: Pre- and postoperative findings in patients with endomyocardial fibrosis. *Br. Heart J.* 40:406–415, 1978.
31. Goldberg S.J., Feldman L., Reinecke C., et al.: Echocardiographic determination of contraction and relaxation measurements of the left ventricular wall in normal subjects and patients with muscular dystrophy. *Circulation* 62:1061–1069, 1980.
32. Amhad M., Sanderson J.E., Dubowitz V., et al.: Echocardiographic assessment of left ventricular function in Duchenne's muscular dystrophy. *Br. Heart J.* 40:734–740, 1978.
33. Van der Houwaert L.G., Dumoulin M.: Hypertrophic cardiomyopathy in Friedreich's ataxia. *Br. Heart J.* 38:1291–1298, 1976.
34. St. John Sutton M.G., Olakatun A.Y., Tajik A.J., et al.: Left ventricular function in Friedreich's ataxia: An echocardiographic study. *Br. Heart J.* 44:309–316, 1980.
35. Levisman J.A.: Echocardiographic diagnosis in mitral regurgitation and congestive cardiomyopathy. *Am. Heart J.* 93:33–39, 1977.
36. Morganroth J., Maron B.J.: The athlete's heart syndrome: A new perspective. *Ann. N.Y. Acad. Sci.* 301:931–942, 1977.
37. Lewis B.S., Rachmilewitz E.A., Amitai N., et al.: Left ventricular function in β-thalassemia and the effect of multiple transfusions. *Am. Heart J.* 96:636–645, 1978.
38. Feigenbaum H.: *Echocardiography,* ed. 3. Philadelphia, Lea & Febiger, 1981, p. 550.
39. Corya B.C., Feigenbaum H., Rasmussen S., et al.: Echocardiographic features of congestive cardiomyopathy compared with normal subjects and patients with coronary artery disease. *Circulation* 49:1153–1159, 1974.
40. Ghafour A.S., Gutgesell H.P.: Echocardiographic evaluation of left ventricular function in children with congestive cardiomyopathy. *Am. J. Cardiol.* 44:1332–1338, 1979.
41. Child J.S., Krivokapich J., Perloff J.K.: Effect of left ventricular size and geometry on mitral e-point to septal separation, abstracted. *Circulation* 62(suppl. III):III–186, 1980.
42. Rasmussen S., Corya B.C., Lovelace E., et al.: Forward stroke volume derived from aortic valve echograms, abstracted. *Clin. Res.* 27:672A, 1979.
43. Rasmussen S., Corya B.C., Feigenbaum H., et al.: Stroke volume calculated from the mitral valve echogram in patients with and without ventricular dysnergy. *Circulation* 58:125–133, 1978.
44. Scheele W., Kraus R., Allen H.N., et al.: Use of M-mode echocardiography to determine stroke volume, abstracted. *Am. J. Cardiol.* 43:411, 1979.
45. Fischer J.C., Chang S., Konecke L.L., et al.: Echocardiographic determination of mitral valve flow, abstracted. *Am. J. Cardiol.* 29:262, 1972.
46. Fortuin N.J., Hood W.P., Jr., Sherman M.E., et al.: Determination of left ventricular volumes by ultrasound. *Circulation* 44:575–584, 1971.
47. Paris A.J., Moynihan P.F., Folland E.D.: Echocardiographic evaluation of left ventricular function. *Med. Clin. North Am.* 64:61–81, 1980.

48. Teichholz L.E., Kreulen T., Herman M.V., et al.: Problems in echocardiographic volume determinations: Echocardiographic-angiographic correlations in the presence or absence of asynergy. *Am. J. Cardiol.* 37:7–11, 1976.
49. Henning H., Schelbert A., Crawford M.I., et al.: Left ventricular performance assessed by radionuclide angiocardiography and echocardiography in patients with previous myocardial infarction. *Circulation* 52:1069–1075, 1975.
50. Pombo J.F., Troy B.L., Russel R.O. Jr.: Left ventricular volumes and ejection fraction by echocardiography. *Circulation* 43:480–490, 1971.
51. Carr K.W., Engler R.L., Forsythe J.R., et al.: Measurement of left ventricular ejection fraction by mechanical cross-sectional echocardiography. *Circulation* 59:1196–1206, 1979.
52. Magnin P.A., Stewart J.A., Myers S., et al.: Combined doppler and phased-array echocardiographic estimation of cardiac output. *Circulation* 63:388–392, 1981.
53. Packer M., Meller J., Medria N., et al.: Importance of left ventricular chamber size in determining the response to hydralazine in severe chronic heart failure. *N. Engl. J. Med.* 303:250–255, 1980.
54. Verdin A., Wikstrand J., Wilhelmusson C., et al.: Left ventricular function and beta-blockade in chronic ischaemic heart failure. *Br. Heart J.* 44:101–107, 1980.
55. Swedberg K., Hjalmarsun A., Waagstein F., et al.: Adverse effects of beta-blockage withdrawal in patients with congestive cardiomyopathy. *Br. Heart J.* 44:134–142, 1980.
56. Teare D.: Assymmetrical hypertrophy of the heart in young adults. *Br. Heart J.* 20:1–8, 1958.
57. Morganroth J., Chen C.C.: Noninvasive diagnosis of the cardiomyopathies. *Med. Clin. North Am.* 64:33–60, 1980.
58. Roberts W.C., Ferrans V.J.: Pathologic anatomy of the cardiomyopathies: Idiopathic dilated and hypertrophic types, infiltrative types and endomyocardial disease with and without eosinophilia. *Hum. Pathol.* 6:287–342, 1975.
59. Henry W.L., Clark C.E., Roberts W.C., et al.: Differences in the distribution of myocardial abnormalities in patients with obstructive and non-obstructive asymmetric septal hypertrophy (ASH): Echocardiographic and gross anatomic findings. *Circulation* 50:447–455, 1974.
60. Maron B.J., Ferrans V.J., Henry W.L., et al.: Differences in distribution of myocardial abnormalities in patients with obstructive and non-obstructive asymmetric septal hypertrophy (ASH): Light and electron microscopic findings. *Circulation* 50:436–446, 1974.
61. Maron B.J., Epstein S.E.: Hypertrophic cardiomyopathy: Recent observations regarding the specificity of three hallmarks of the disease: Asymmetric septal hypertrophy, septal disorganization and systolic anterior motion of the anterior mitral leaflet. *Am. J. Cardiol.* 45:141–154, 1980.
62. Clark C.W., Henry W.L., Epstein S.E.: Familial problems and genetic transmission of idiopathic hypertrophic subaortic stenosis. *N. Engl. J. Med.* 289:709–714, 1972.
63. Henning H., O'Rourke R.A., Crawford M.H., et al.: Inferior myocardial infarction as a cause of asymmetric septal hypertrophy: An echocardiographic study. *Am. J. Cardiol.* 41:817–822, 1978.
64. Stern A., Kessler K.M., Hammer W.J., et al.: Septal-free wall disproportion in inferior infarction: The echocardiographic differentiation from hypertrophic cardiomyopathy. *Circulation* 58:700–706, 1978.
65. Shah P.M.: Echocardiography in the diagnosis of hypertrophic obstructive cardiomyopathy. *Am. J. Med.* 62:830–835, 1977.
66. Abbasi A., MacAlpin R.N., Eber L.M., et al.: Left ventricular hypertrophy diagnosed by echocardiography. *N. Engl. J. Med.* 289:118–121, 1973.
67. Tajik A.J., Giuliani E.R.: Echocardiographic observations in idiopathic hypertrophic subaortic stenosis. *Mayo Clin. Proc.* 49:89–97, 1974.
68. Rossen R.M., Goodman D.J., Ingham R.E., et al.: Ventricular systolic septal thickening and excursion in IHSS. *N. Engl. J. Med.* 291:1317–1319, 1974.
69. Maron B.J., Henry W.L., Roberts W.C., et al.: Comparison of echocardiographic and necropsy measurements of ventricular wall thickness in patients with and without disproportionate septal thickening. *Circulation* 55:341–346, 1977.
70. Doi Y.L., McKenna W.J., Gehrke J., et al.: M-mode echocardiography in hypertrophic cardiomyopathy: Diagnostic criteria and prediction of obstruction. *Am. J. Cardiol.* 45:6–14, 1980.
71. Henry L.W., Clark C.E., Glancy D.C., et al.: Echocardiographic measurement of the left ventricular outflow gradient in idiopathic hypertrophic subaortic stenosis. *N. Engl. J. Med.* 288:989–993, 1973.
72. Rossen R.M., Goodman D.J., Ingham R.E., et al.: Echocardiographic criteria in the diagnosis of idiopathic hypertrophic subaortic stenosis. *Circulation* 50:747–751, 1974.
73. King J.F., DeMaria A.N., Miller R.R., et al.: Markedly abnormal mitral valve motion without simultaneous interventricular pressure gradient due to uneven mitral-septal contact in idiopathic hypertrophic subaortic stenosis. *Am. J. Cardiol.* 34:360–366, 1974.
74. Gilbert B.W., Pollick C., Adelman A.G., et al.: Hypertrophic cardiomyopathy: Subclassification by M-mode echocardiography. *Am. J. Cardiol.* 45:861–872, 1980.
75. Cardiel E.A., Alonso M., Delcan J.L., et al.: Echocardiographic sign of right-sided hypertrophic obstructive cardiomyopathy. *Br. Heart J.* 40:1321–1324, 1978.

76. Brik H., Meller J., Bahler A.S., et al.: Systolic anterior motion of the tricuspid valve in idiopathic hypertrophic subaortic stenosis. *J. Clin. Ultrasound* 6:121, 1978.
77. Fowles R.E., Martin R.P., Popp R.L.: Erroneous diagnosis of asymmetrical septal hypertrophy due to angled interventricular septum, abstracted. *Am. J. Cardiol.* 43:348, 1979.
78. Fowles R.E., Martin R.P., Popp R.L., Apparent asymmetric septal hypertrophy due to angled interventricular septum. *Am. J. Cardiol.* 46:386–392, 1980.
79. Maron B.J., Gottdiener J.S., Bonow R.O., et al.: Hypertrophic cardiomyopathy with unusual locations of left ventricular hypertrophy undetectable by M-mode echocardiography: Identification by wide-angle two-dimensional echocardiography. *Circulation* 63:409–418, 1981.
80. Taylor R.D., Child J.S., Shah P.M.: Variations in septal hypertrophy in hypertrophic obstructive cardiomyopathy (HOCM), abstracted. *Am. J. Cardiol.* 43:348, 1979.
81. Tajik A.J., Seward J.B., Hagler D.J.: Detailed analysis of hypertrophic obstructive cardiomyopathy by wide-angle two-dimensional sector echocardiography, abstracted. *Am. J. Cardiol.* 43:348, 1979.
82. Gehrke J.: New observations on systolic anterior motion of mitral valve leaflets in hypertrophic cardiomyopathy. *Br. Heart J.* 38:314, 1976.
83. Rodger J.C.: Motion of mitral apparatus in hypertrophic cardiomyopathy with obstruction. *Br. Heart J.* 38:732–737, 1976.
84. Kotler M.N., Mintz G.S., Segal B.L., et al.: Clinical uses of two-dimensional echocardiography. *Am. J. Cardiol.* 45:1061–1082, 1980.
85. Syracuse D.C., Gaudiani V.A., Kosti D.G., et al.: Intra-operative intracardiac echocardiography during left ventriculomyotomy and myectomy for hypertrophic subaortic stenosis, abstracted. *Circulation* 58(suppl. II):I–23, 1978.
86. Martin R.P., Rakowski H., French J., et al.: Idiopathic hypertrophic subaortic stenosis viewed by wide-angle phased-array echocardiography. *Circulation* 59:1206–1217, 1979.
87. Schapira J.N., Stemple D.R., Martin R.P., et al.: Single and two-dimensional echocardiographic visualization of the effects of septal myectomy in idiopathic hypertrophic subaortic stenosis. *Circulation* 58:850–860, 1978.
88. Feigenbaum H.: *op. cit.*, p. 456.
89. Benotti J.R., Grossman W., Cohn P.F.: Clinical profile of restrictive cardiomyopathy. *Circulation* 61:1206–1212, 1980.
90. Meaney E., Shabetai R., Bhargava V., et al.: Cardiac amyloidosis, constrictive pericarditis and restrictive cardiomyopathy. *Am. J. Cardiol.* 38:547–556, 1976.
91. Shabetai R., Meaney E.: Hemodynamics of cardiac restriction and tamponade. *Br. Heart J.* 37:780, 1975.
92. Easley R.M. Jr., Schreiner B.F. Jr., Yu P.N.: Reversible cardiomyopathy associated with hemochromatosis. *N. Engl. J. Med.* 287:866–867, 1972.

RADIONUCLIDE IMAGING

Mark R. Goldman and Gerald M. Pohost

THE TERM "cardiomyopathy" is used by physicians to distinguish diseases of the heart muscle from other forms of cardiac failure. All cardiomyopathies share a common feature: the reduced ability to maintain adequate systemic perfusion with normal filling pressures. Although cardiomyopathies may be grouped into categories reflecting function[1] or etiology,[2] for the purpose of this chapter, the functional classification, including congestive (dilated), restrictive, and hypertrophic cardiomyopathy, will be used. The clinical presentation of these disease states may overlap and differentiation of the functional type of cardiomyopathy may be difficult. Additionally, other forms of heart disease such as heart failure due to repeated infarction may simulate cardiomyopathy.

The judicious use of radionuclide techniques can assist the physician in differentiating the functional type of cardiomyopathy, quantifying the degree of ventricular impairment, and assessing the efficacy of therapeutic interventions.[3] The gated blood pool or radionuclide angiographic scan allows determination of ejection fraction, ventricular size, wall motion, and septal thickness and configuration. This single study generally is sufficient for the classification of the functional type of cardiomyopathy and further workup may proceed. Thallium 201 myocardial perfusion imaging is useful for detecting diseases that replace (e.g., fibrosis) or displace (e.g., tumor) myocardium. It is of particular value in distinguishing congestive cardiomyopathy from heart failure due to coronary artery disease. Myocardial imaging with ^{201}Tl may also depict the septal abnormalities of hypertrophic cardiomyopathy. Radionuclide techniques, used together with other noninvasive techniques such as echocardiography, add an important dimension to the diagnosis, management, and follow-up of patients with cardiomyopathy.

CONGESTIVE (DILATED) CARDIOMYOPATHY

Congestive (or dilated) cardiomyopathy is the most common form of cardiomyopathy. Clinically the condition is characterized by left- and right-sided heart failure, although symptoms of left ventricular failure usually predominate. While the clinical presentation and course of the disease may be quite variable,[5] pathologically the ventricles are dilated and often have mural thrombi.[6] The stroke volume is reduced and the heart, in an effort to maintain the cardiac output, increases its rate. However, the cardiac output is often diminished. The chest x-ray film demonstrates cardiomegaly, usually with evidence of pulmonary vascular redistribution. The ECG is generally not helpful, showing only nonspecific repolarization abnormalities or bundle-branch block. The differentiation of congestive cardiomyopathy from heart failure due to coronary disease may be aided by evidence of previous myocardial infarction on the ECG.

The gated blood pool scans of patients with

congestive cardiomyopathy typically demonstrate biventricular dilation and diminished wall motion. The left ventricle is usually more affected than the right. The left ventricular ejection fraction is commonly less than 0.3 and may be as low as 0.1. The atria and pulmonary artery may be dilated as well. A gated blood pool scan from a patient with congestive cardiomyopathy is shown in Figure 6–1. Patients with heart failure due to coronary artery disease and repeated myocardial infarctions may have gated blood pool scans virtually indistinguishable from the scans of patients with congestive cardiomyopathy.[7] A differentiating feature may be the reasonably normal motion of the basal septum and anterobasal wall in coronary disease as opposed to a global reduction in wall motion seen in cardiomyopathy.[8] Occasionally the scan may be misleading. Thallium perfusion imaging is often useful in this setting.

Myocardial perfusion imaging with ^{201}Tl in patients with congestive cardiomyopathy reveals biventricular dilation with normal or diffusely reduced homogeneous uptake (Fig 6–2). Heart failure due to coronary artery disease and myocardial infarction is usually associated with large (>40%) circumferential defects in the thallium image in any projection (Fig 6–3).[8] While some patients with congestive cardiomyopathy may have defects on ^{201}Tl imaging, those defects are almost always less than 20% circumferentially. Thallium scanning may therefore aid in determining whether congestive heart failure is due to cardiomyopathy or to coronary artery disease, and it is for this purpose that ^{201}Tl perfusion imaging is most useful in suspected congestive cardiomyopathy.

Although cardiac ultrasound, with its high spatial and temporal resolution, can be used to evaluate ventricular size and function, it may be dif-

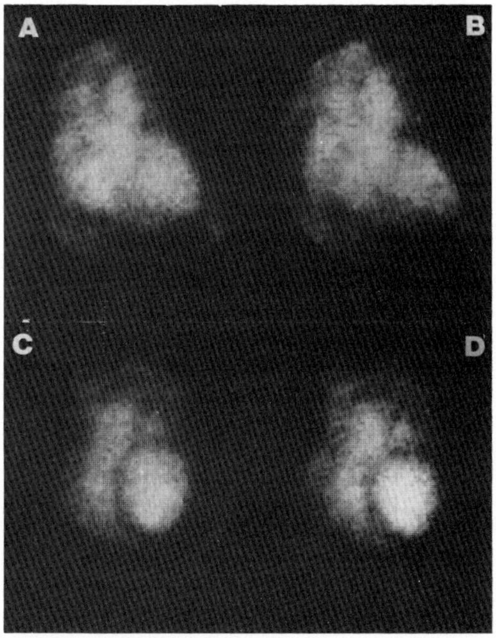

Fig 6–1.—Anterior *(upper)* and left anterior oblique *(lower)* views at end-diastole *(left)* and end-systole *(right)* of the gated blood pool scan of a patient with congestive cardiomyopathy. Note the generalized cardiomegaly and marked reduction of left ventricular contraction. *A,* anterior end-diastolic image; *B,* anterior end-systolic image; *C,* LAO end-diastolic image; *D,* LAO end-systolic image.

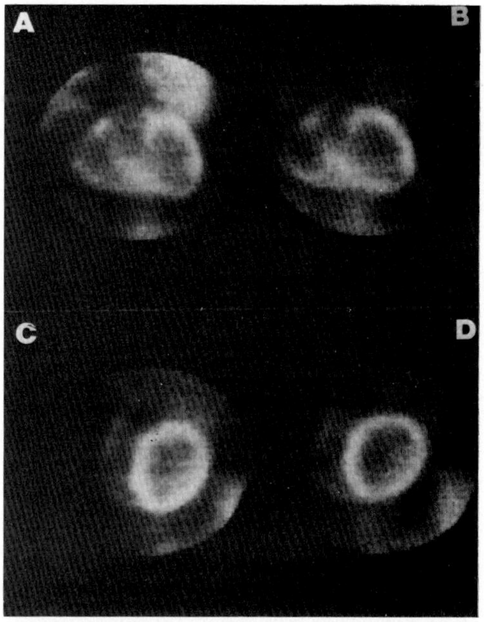

Fig 6–2.—Anterior *(upper)* and left anterior oblique *(lower)* projections of exercise *(left)* and delayed *(right)* thallium 201 perfusion scans of a patient with congestive cardiomyopathy (same patient as in Fig 6–1). There is thallium uptake throughout the myocardium, despite the severe wall motion abnormalities. Note the increased pulmonary thallium activity during exercise and the increase in left ventricular size. *A,* anterior exercise image; *B,* anterior delayed image; *C,* LAO exercise image; *D,* LAO delayed image.

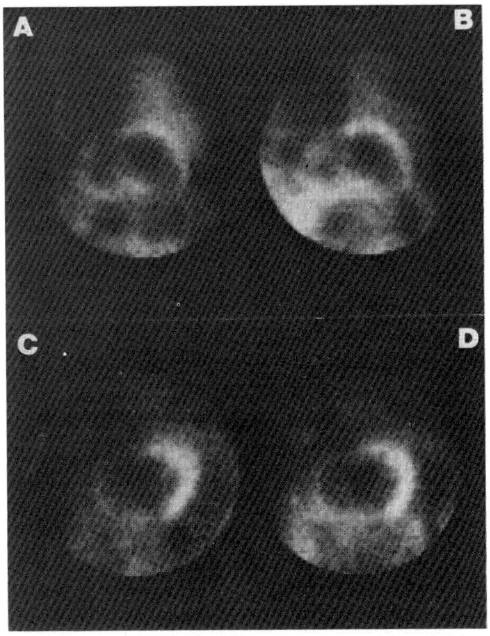

Fig 6–3.—Anterior *(upper)* and left anterior oblique *(lower)* projections of exercise *(left)* and delayed *(right)* thallium 201 perfusion scans of a patient with severe coronary artery disease and the clinical presentation of congestive cardiomyopathy. Note the large thallium perfusion defect involving the septum and inferoapical areas. Note again the increased pulmonary thallium activity during exercise. *A,* anterior exercise image; *B,* anterior delayed image; *C,* LAO exercise image; *D,* LAO delayed image.

ficult to distinguish congestive cardiomyopathy from severe coronary artery disease using the one-dimensional display.[9] The two-dimensional format appears to offer significant advantages over the one-dimensional approach, and as Folland et al. have shown,[10] the ejection fraction obtained using two-dimensional echocardiography correlates reasonably with those obtained by cineangiography and radionuclide techniques. Wall motion abnormalities are also detectable using two-dimensional ultrasound.[11] A potential disadvantage of echocardiography is the inability to obtain good studies in patients with unusual chest configurations or pulmonary disease. Radionuclide techniques, however, can be performed on all patients, regardless of size, and in multiple oblique projections.

The gated blood pool scan can be used to follow the course of congestive cardiomyopathy or to assess the efficacy of therapeutic interventions. Radionuclide angiography has been used to assess doxorubicin cardiotoxicity serially in patients with malignant disease and was more sensitive than traditional criteria.[12] Additionally, exercise gated blood pool scanning may allow detection of early left ventricular dysfunction in patients with congestive cardiomyopathy, even when the scan at rest is normal.[13]

RESTRICTIVE CARDIOMYOPATHY

Restrictive cardiomyopathy, the rarest of the cardiomyopathies, is characterized by signs and symptoms of right- and left-sided heart failure. Neck vein distention with rapid X and Y descent and pulsus paradoxus may be present. Unlike congestive cardiomyopathy, the heart is normal in size and radiographic evidence of left ventricular failure may be absent. The ECG generally is nonspecifically abnormal or may show bundle-branch block. Pathologically, the heart reveals an infiltrative process or endomyocardial fibrosis. There may be a predominance of eosinophils in the cardiomyopathy associated with hypereosinophilia. Physiologically, the distinguishing feature of restrictive cardiomyopathy is poor ventricular compliance, resulting in inadequate ventricular filling despite high diastolic atrial pressures.

The usefulness of the gated blood pool scan in restrictive cardiomyopathy is in visualizing ventricular size which, in contrast to what is seen in congestive cardiomyopathy, is normal. Systolic wall motion may be mildly depressed or normal. In diastole, the ventricle may fill rapidly in each diastole and fail to fill further, even with atrial systole.

An extremely difficult problem is the differentiation between restrictive cardiomyopathy and constrictive pericarditis. The clinical presentations may be identical. Several distinguishing points, although not totally specific, are worth mentioning. Infiltrative cardiomyopathy is often associated with an increased ventricular wall thickness, and ^{201}Tl perfusion imaging may detect this. Echocardiography may also demonstrate increased wall thickness.[14] Diastolic posterior wall flatness, if detectable by ultrasound, is believed by Voelkel et al.[15] to be characteristic of pericardial disease. Despite the use of available noninvasive techniques, it may be impossible in some situations, to determine whether the patient has restrictive cardiomyopathy or constrictive pericarditis, and right ventricular or pericardial biopsy, or both, may be necessary.

HYPERTROPHIC CARDIOMYOPATHY

Early confusion regarding the spectrum of hypertrophic cardiomyopathy primarily reflected the terminology used by various investigators to describe different features of the disease. Braunwald et al.[16] used the term "idiopathic hypertrophic subaortic stenosis (IHSS)," while Brent et al.[17] used the expression "muscular subaortic stenosis." Goodwin et al.[18] favored the term "hypertrophic obstructive cardiomyopathy," highlighting the myocardial disease. "Hypertrophic cardiomyopathy" is a general term encompassing hearts with and without outflow tract obstruction. Clinically, patients with hypertrophic cardiomyopathy may present with typical heart failure, syncope, chest pain, or palpitations. Physical examination may reveal a murmur reminiscent of mitral regurgitation or an outflow murmur increasing with Valsalva's maneuver and decreasing with squatting. The chest x-ray film may be normal or show cardiomegaly. The ECG may show left ventricular hypertrophy and/or a "pseudo-infarct" pattern due to regional ventricular hypertrophy. Pathologically, the hallmark of the disease is left ventricular hypertrophy, generally asymmetric, with the septum thickened disproportionately.[19–22] Left ventricular outflow obstruction, when it occurs, is caused by the hypertrophic septum combined with abnormal systolic anterior motion of the anterior leaflet of the mitral valve.[23, 24] There may be mitral regurgitation with or without outflow obstruction. Heart failure results from reduced left ventricular compliance, outflow obstruction, and mitral regurgitation.

Cardiac ultrasound is very useful in diagnosing hypertrophic cardiomyopathy and is the most commonly used noninvasive technique employed for this purpose. Asymmetric septal hypertrophy can usually be detected easily and for a time was thought to be pathognomonic for the disease. This finding, however, is not specific and may be seen in patients with right ventricular hypertrophy.[25] Systolic anterior motion of the anterior leaflet of the mitral valve (SAM) can be detected with echocardiography and was thought to be diagnostic of hypertrophic cardiomyopathy with obstruction.[26] A number of reports have indicated that SAM is not specific either.[27–30] Furthermore, Maron et al.[31] have demonstrated, using two-dimensional ultrasound, that some patients with hypertrophic cardiomyopathy have localized left ventricular hypertrophy in unusual regions.

Radionuclide techniques are useful in the diagnosis of hypertrophic cardiomyopathy. The gated blood pool scan allows delineation of the interventricular septum in the 40- to 50-degree left anterior oblique (LAO) projection. The normal end-diastolic LAO image is characterized by a curvilinear concavity of the septum toward the left ventricle. Pohost et al.[32] have shown that the end-diastolic LAO images reveal disproportionate upper septal thickening in about 50% of patients with hypertrophic cardiomyopathy (Fig 6–4). Loss of the normal septal concavity toward the left ventricle is found in 73% but is not specific, as it is also found in association with aortic stenosis and occasionally in patients with no organic heart disease. Left ventricular cavity obliteration may be part of the spectrum of hypertrophic cardiomyopathy and may be observed in the anterior projection of the gated blood pool scan.

Hypertrophic cardiomyopathy may be evaluated with thallium perfusion imaging. Asymmetric septal hypertrophy may be detectable.[33] Although greater basal septal thickness relative to posterior wall thickness was believed to be an indicator of left ventricular outflow obstruction, Mews et al.[34] have shown that the gated ^{201}Tl scan in patients with hypertrophic cardiomyopathy demonstrates disproportionate upper septal thickening at end-diastole similar to that observed at end-diastole in the gated blood pool scan.

Radionuclide techniques provide important in-

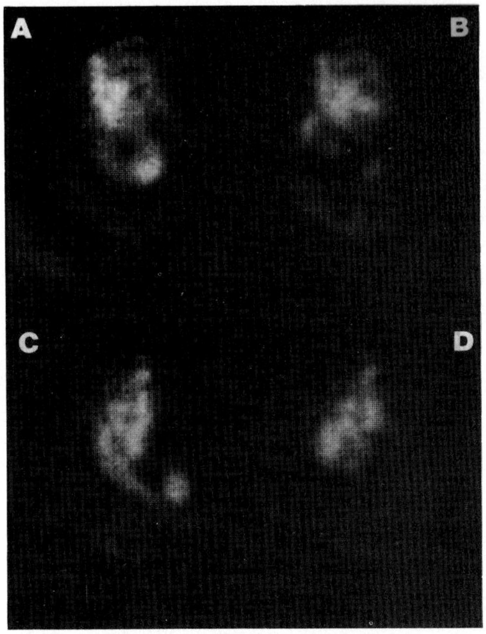

Fig 6–4.—Anterior *(lower)* and 50-degree left anterior oblique *(upper)* views at end-diastole *(left)* and end-systole *(right)* of the gated blood pool scan of a patient with hypertrophic cardiomyopathy. Note the disproportionate upper septal thickening in the left anterior oblique end-diastolic frame *(A)*. Note also the near cavity obliteration at end-systole. *A,* LAO end-diastolic frame; *B,* LAO end-systolic frame; *C,* anterior end-diastolic frame; *D,* anterior end-systolic frame.

formation useful in the diagnosis, classification, and management of patients with cardiomyopathy. These studies may be easily obtained in all patients. The gated blood pool scan, because it allows assessment of ventricular size, wall motion, and septal configuration, allows classification of the cardiomyopathy by functional group—congestive, restrictive, or hypertrophic. Thallium 201 perfusion imaging adds further information and is especially useful in differentiating congestive cardiomyopathy from severe coronary artery disease and in depicting septal abnormalities in hypertrophic cardiomyopathy. The careful application of radionuclide techniques together with traditional clinical tools and other noninvasive techniques such as ultrasound may allow diagnosis of cardiomyopathy and eliminate the need for invasive tests in many patients.

REFERENCES

1. Goodwin J.F.: Clarification of the cardiomyopathies. *Mod. Concepts Cardiovasc. Dis.* 41:41–46, 1972.
2. Hudson R.E.B.: The cardiomyopathies: Order from chaos. *Am. J. Cardiol.* 25:70–77, 1970.
3. Pohost G.M., Fallon J.T., Strauss H.W.: The role of radionuclide techniques in patients with myocardial disease, in Brest A.N. (ed.): *Cardiovascular Clinics*. Philadelphia, F.A. Davis., 1979, pp. 149–630.
4. Strauss H.W., McKusick K.A., Boucher C.A., et al.: Of linens and laces: The eighth anniversary of the gated blood pool scan. *Semin. Nucl. Med.* 9:296–309, 1979.
5. Oakley C.M.: Clinical recognition of the cardiomyopathies. *Circulation* 34,35(suppl. II):II–152–167, 1974.
6. Roberts W.C., Ferrans V.J.: Pathological aspects of certain cardiomyopathies. *Circulation* 34,35(suppl. II):II–128–144, 1974.
7. Johnson R.A., Daggett W.M.: Heart failure resulting from coronary artery disease, in Johnson R. (ed.): *Practice of Cardiology*. Boston, Little, Brown & Co., 1980, pp. 339–369.
8. Bulkley B.H., Hutchins G.M., Bailey I., et al.: Thallium-201 imaging and gated cardiac blood pool scans in patients with ischemic and congestive cardiomyopathy: A clinical and pathological study. *Circulation* 55:753–761, 1977.
9. Corya B.C., Feigenbaum H., Rasmussen S., et al.: Echocardiographic features of congestive cardiomyopathy compared with normal subjects and patients with coronary artery disease. *Circulation* 49:1153–1159, 1974.
10. Folland E.D., Parisi A.F., Moynihan P.F., et al.: Assessment of left ventricular ejection fraction and volumes by real-time, two-dimensional echocardiography: A comparison of cineangiographic and radionuclide techniques. *Circulation* 60:760–766, 1979.
11. Heger J.J., Weyman A.E., Wann L.S., et al.: Cross-sectional echocardiography in acute myocardial infarction: Detection and localization of regional left ventricular asynergy. *Circulation* 60:531–538, 1979.
12. Alexander J., Dainiak N., Berger H.J., et al.: Serial assessment of doxorubicin cardiotoxicity with quantitative radionuclide angiocardiography. *N. Engl. J. Med.* 300:278–283, 1979.
13. Leon M.B., Borer J.S., Bachrach S.L., et al.: Detection of early cardiac iron overload. *N. Engl. J. Med.* 301:1143–1148, 1979.
14. Borer J.S., Henry W.L., Epstein S.E.: Echocardiographic observations in patients with systemic infiltrative diseases involving the heart. *Am. J. Cardiol.* 39:184–188, 1977.
15. Voelkel A.G., Pietro D.A., Folland E.D., et al.:

Echocardiographic features of constrictive pericarditis. *Circulation* 58:871–875, 1978.
16. Braunwald E., Morrow A.G., Cornell W.P., et al.: Idiopathic hypertrophic subaortic stenosis: Clinical, hemodynamic and angiographic manifestations. *Am. J. Med.* 29:924–945, 1960.
17. Brent L.B., Aburano A., Fisher D.L., et al.: Familial muscular subaortic stenosis: An unrecognized form of idiopathic heart disease, with clinical and autopsy observations. *Circulation* 21:167–180, 1960.
18. Goodwin J.F., Hollman A., Cleland W.P., et al.: Obstructive cardiomyopathy simulating aortic stenosis. *Br. Heart. J.* 22:403–414, 1960.
19. Teare D.: Asymmetrical hypertrophy of the heart in young patients. *Br. Heart J.* 20:1–8, 1958.
20. Abbasi A.S., MacAlpin R.N., Eber L.M., et al.: Echocardiographic diagnosis of idiopathic hypertrophic cardiomyopathy without outflow obstruction. *Circulation* 46:897–904, 1972.
21. Henry W.L., Clark C.E., Epstein S.E.: Asymmetric septal hypertrophy (ASH): Echocardiographic identification of the pathognomonic anatomic abnormality of IHSS. *Circulation* 47:225–233, 1973.
22. Epstein S.E., Henry W.L., Clark C.E., et al.: Asymmetric septal hypertrophy. *Ann. Intern. Med.* 81:650, 1974.
23. Braunwald E., Lambrew C.T., Rockoff S.D., et al.: Idiopathic hypertrophic subaortic stenosis: I. A description of the disease based on an analysis of 64 patients, abstracted. *Circulation* 30 (suppl. IV):IV–3, 1964.
24. Henry W.L., Clark C.E., Griffith J.M., et al.: Mechanism of left ventricular outflow obstruction in patients with asymmetric septal hypertrophy. *Am. J. Cardiol.* 35:337–345, 1975.
25. Tater W.E., Allen H.D., Sahn D.J., et al.: The asymmetrically hypertrophied septum: Further differentiation of its causes. *Circulation* 53:19–27, 1976.
26. Shah P.M., Gramiak R., Kramer D.H.: Ultrasound localization of left ventricular obstruction in hypertrophic obstructive cardiomyopathy. *Circulation* 40:3–11, 1969.
27. Mintz G.S., Kotler M.N., Segal B.L., et al.: Systolic anterior motion in the absence of asymmetric septal hypertrophy. *Circulation* 57:256–263, 1978.
28. Maron B.J., Gottdiener J.S., Roberts W.C., et al.: Left ventricular outflow obstruction due to systolic anterior motion of the anterior mitral valve leaflet in patients with concentric left ventricular hypertrophy. *Circulation* 57:527–533, 1978.
29. Crawford M.H., Groves B.M., Horowitz L.D.: Dynamic left ventricular outflow tract obstruction and systolic anterior motion of the mitral valve in the absence of asymmetric septal hypertrophy. *Am. J. Med.* 67:703–708, 1978.
30. Gardin J.M., Talano J.V., Stephanides M.S., et al.: Systolic anterior motion in the absence of asymmetric septal hypertrophy: A buckling phenomenon of the chordae tendineae. *Circulation* 63:181–188, 1981.
31. Maron B.J., Gottdiener J.S., Bonow R.O., et al.: Hypertrophic cardiomyopathy with unusual locations of left ventricular hypertrophy undetectable by M-mode echocardiography. *Circulation* 63:409–418, 1981.
32. Pohost G.M., Vignola P.A., McKusick K.A., et al.: Hypertrophic cardiomyopathy: Evaluation by gated cardiac blood pool scanning. *Circulation* 55:92–99, 1977.
33. Bulkley B.H., Rouleau J., Strauss H.W., et al.: Idiopathic hypertrophic subaortic stenosis: Detection by thallium-201 myocardial perfusion imaging. *N. Engl. J. Med.* 293:1113–1116, 1975.
34. Mews G.C., Pohost G.M., Vignola P.A., et al.: Hypertrophic cardiomyopathy: Improved radionuclide detection by gated Tl-201 imaging, abstracted. *Circulation* 58(suppl. II):II–236, 1978.

COMMENT: CARDIOMYOPATHIES

Joel Morganroth

THE DIFFERENTIATION of cardiomyopathies into congestive, hypertrophic, and restrictive states with their attendant etiologic considerations has clarified our understanding of these disorders and enabled directed management. The "prevalence" of cardiomyopathy has apparently increased markedly in the last several years, undoubtedly because of physicians' improved ability to recognize and define these conditions through noninvasive cardiac testing.

ETIOLOGIC DETERMINATION

Echocardiography has become the best diagnostic tool to evaluate patients with cardiac symptoms arising from disorders of the ventricular myocardium. It precisely identifies the different pathophysiologic types of cardiomyopathy for which criteria are now well established. The greatest impact of echocardiography has been on the identification and clarification of inherited hypertrophic cardiomyopathy: echocardiography helped delineate its spectrum, genetic pattern, and clinical forms. Unfortunately, the differentiation of primary from secondary forms of cardiomyopathy cannot be made by echocardiograph alone.

Radionuclide techniques are easily done and provide additional useful information in the evaluation of patients with cardiomyopathy. They are indicated in patients in whom the echocardiographic diagnosis is equivocal or unavailable. Gated blood pool scanning can be used to differentiate congestive from hypertrophic states. Thallium 201 perfusion imaging is particularly useful in distinguishing patients with congestive cardiomyopathy due to an ischemic condition (coronary artery disease) from those with primary myocardial dysfunction.

CLINICAL AND PROGNOSTIC CONSIDERATIONS

Congestive Cardiomyopathy

Patients with congestive cardiomyopathy may present with subtle clinical or physical signs and symptoms or ECG abnormalities. The use of echocardiography in patients presenting with, for example, new onset atrial fibrillation, a ventricular arrhythmia, or dyspnea on exertion may identify the presence of an unexpected congestive cardiomyopathy as the etiology of these symptoms. Estimation of the severity and extent of left ventricular dimensional and functional changes may provide valuable criteria for the response to vasodilator therapy and the use of such agents as beta-blockers. The detection of complications such as left ventricular thrombi or an important pericardial effusion may also help guide management. The use of thallium perfusion to suggest coexisting coronary artery disease has important therapeutic ramifications in patients in whom revascularization may improve left ventricular function. Obviously, the differential diagnosis of congestive cardiomyopathy from ischemic heart disease with left ventricular aneurysm formation is an important consideration.

Radionuclide cineangiography may also be used in a similar fashion in these patients, but nuclear imaging techniques should be used when echocardiography is equivocal or not available. Echocardiography or radionuclide angiography, or both, can be used to assess acquired cardiomyopathy due to conditions such as adriamycin therapy. The potential value of exercise gated blood pool scanning to detect left ventricular dysfunction in early cardiomyopathy before abnormalities in the resting study are defined is now being explored.

Hypertrophic Cardiomyopathy

Echocardiography is an important diagnostic tool in the identification of hypertrophic cardiomyopathy in patients with subtle cardiac symptoms. As in mitral valve prolapse, echocardiography has had a major impact on the understanding of the prevalence, genetic mode of transmission, clinical state, and management of this disorder. The classification and separation of patients with left ventricular outflow tract obstruction who may most benefit from surgical myotomy and myectomy from those with diffuse hypertrophic cardiomyopathy is well established. The presence of asymmetric septal hypertrophy in response to secondary hypertrophic states, as in chronic renal failure, hypertension, and aortic valvular stenosis, has limited the ability of echocardiography to be pathognomonic in this condition. However, it remains the diagnostic standard for hypertrophic cardiomyopathy and can be used in family studies to determine whether or not the condition is inherited. Radionuclide angiography and thallium perfusion studies can provide diagnostic information in this condition as well as assess left ventricular functional reserve; they are indicated when echocardiographic data are equivocal or unavailable.

Restrictive Cardiomyopathy

The identification of restrictive cardiomyopathy by echocardiography and its differentiation from the other forms of cardiomyopathy has been established. The differentiation of restrictive cardiomyopathy from constrictive pericarditis using echocardiographic criteria remains difficult. Echocardiographic demonstration of thickened pericardium without left ventricular hypertrophy and pericardial effusion may be useful in this differential diagnosis. Thallium 201 perfusion imaging can also be useful, particularly when echocardiographic data are equivocal.

PROGNOSIS

Insufficient data have been accumulated to allow us to predict the natural history of patients with cardiomyopathy solely on the basis of echocardiographic or radionuclide imaging parameters. Serial echocardiographic examination for the purpose of identifying differences in left ventricular function as measured by left ventricular diameter and ejection fraction is likely to become important. Lack of progression of left ventricular dysfunction or even gradual improvement would suggest a better prognosis than the reverse. Such measurements can also be obtained serially with radionuclide imaging techniques, which we recommend using as a secondary approach.

PART IV

Chronic Coronary Artery Disease

ECHOCARDIOGRAPHY

Daniel David, Chin C. Chen, and Joel Morganroth

THE ANATOMICAL LOCALIZATION and determination of the severity of coronary obstruction, as well as the impact of such a lesion on myocardial function, are the three most important factors in the evaluation of a patient with coronary artery disease. Obstructive disease in the coronary arteries can be detected by (1) the direct observation of the actual narrowing of the coronary arterial lumen and (2) the indirect detection of the consequences of the ischemic process, which produces an alteration in myocardial function. Alterations in myocardial wall motion patterns can be subdivided into the acute wall motion changes that accompany an acute ischemic event and the chronic myocardial changes, such as late results of myocardial necrosis (e.g., scar formation as well as ventricular structure and shape changes) (Fig 7–1). The acute ischemic changes in myocardial function and the postmyocardial infarction ventricular structural changes are discussed elsewhere in this volume. This chapter provides an overview of the present and possible future use of echocardiography in the noninvasive detection of arteriosclerotic coronary lesions and in the evaluation of the patient with chronic myocardial changes emanating from a remote myocardial infarction.

DIRECT VISUALIZATION OF THE CORONARY ARTERIES

The two-dimensional echocardiographic (2DE) evaluation of coronary anatomy is currently limited to visualization of the left main and proximal left and right coronary arteries. This seemingly small anatomical area plays an important role, especially in the evaluation of patients with proximal left coronary artery disease. The importance of the noninvasive diagnosis of such disease stems from the fact that coronary artery bypass graft surgery for symptomatic left main coronary artery stenosis can prolong life.[1, 2] It is well accepted that there is no anamnestic or clinical feature specific for left main coronary artery disease, including a markedly positive treadmill test.[3–5] Therefore, the prompt identification of left main coronary artery disease in patients with ischemic cardiac symptoms becomes an important therapeutic challenge to the cardiologist.[6, 7] Furthermore, detection of left main coronary artery disease prior to cardiac catheterization may minimize the risk of angiography in such patients.[6, 7]

Weyman et al.[8] were the first to report the noninvasive direct visualization of the left main coronary artery in man using 2DE. Their study population included 15 normal subjects, 15 patients with coronary artery disease but no obstruction of the left main coronary arteries, 3 patients with 75% obstruction of the left main coronary artery, and 1 patient with a large aneurysm of the distal left main coronary artery. The anatomical position of the left main coronary artery has a fixed relation to the surrounding structures. It lies superior to the upper border of the left ventricle and inferior to the ascending portion of the pulmonary artery. Therefore, using a 30-degree sector scanner in the short-axis projection, the authors scanned the aortic root

TWO-DIMENSIONAL ECHOCARDIOGRAPHIC DETECTION
OF CORONARY ARTERY DISEASE

- DIRECT
  - Localization of coronary obstructive processes by direct visualization of the coronary arteries
- INDIRECT
  - Demonstration of the results of myocardial ischemia
    - Acute left and right ventricular regional wall motion abnormalities
    - Chronic myocardial structural changes (necrosis, fibrosis, scar formation)
    - Detection of complications due to remote myocardial ischemia or infarction:
      - Rupture of the intraventricular septum
      - Papillary muscle involvement
      - Global cardiac enlargement
      - Aneurysm and pseudoaneurysm
      - Pericardial tamponade

Fig 7–1.—Impact of coronary artery disease on the heart as potentially detected by echocardiography.

area in a superior-inferior arc until the left main coronary artery was visualized (Fig 7–2). The left main coronary artery appeared as two parallel sets of echoes originating from the aortic root. The echo-free space between these two linear echoes represented the arterial lumen (see Fig 7–2,B). In each of the three patients with left main coronary artery disease studied by Weyman et al.,[8] a luminal narrowing demonstrated by echocardiography correlated with an almost complete oblitera-

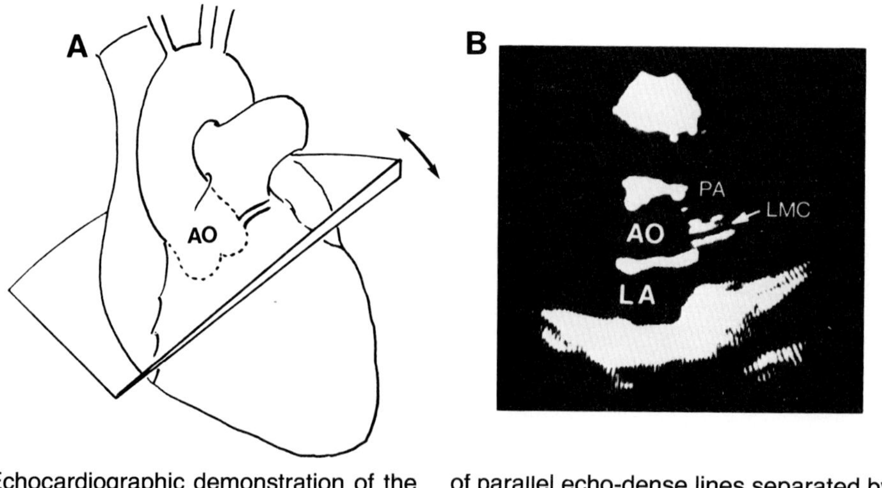

Fig 7–2.—Echocardiographic demonstration of the left main coronary artery *(LMC)* by means of the short-axis approach. The transducer is angled to view the aortic root *(AO)*. A superior-inferior scanning motion is performed **(A)** until the LMC is demonstrated as a pair of parallel echo-dense lines separated by a lumen that connects to the aortic root **(B)**. The continuous echo-free luminal demonstration of the LMC indicates a normal and patent left main coronary artery.

tion of the lumen demonstrated by angiography. An aneurysm of the left main coronary artery in one patient was also depicted. The authors stressed the importance of imaging the origin of the left main coronary artery in the aortic root and the luminal continuity between the two vessels. For this purpose a number of still frames were required to account for the cardiac movement in and out of the ultrasonic beam. Since the patients included in this study were preselected, no information on the sensitivity and specificity of this method in detecting left main coronary artery obstructions could be gained (Table 7–1). The possibility of demonstrating aneurysmal dilations of the left main coronary artery was also used by other authors to evaluate children with mucocutaneous lymph node syndrome.[9, 10] This disease is characterized by the formation of aneurysms in the main coronary arteries, complicated by thrombosis and myocardial infarction. Yoshikawa et al.,[9] using the previously described short-axis view, demonstrated both the left and right coronary ostia in all 37 patients. The left main coronary artery was visualized in 29 of 37 patients, and the proximal portion of the right coronary artery was visualized in 17. Coronary aneurysms were detected in 5 patients and were localized in both the left and the right coronary arteries. Two-dimensional echocardiography may therefore be used as a screening method to determine the presence or absence of aneurysmal dilations of the left main coronary artery in these patients. Caldwell et al.[11] were also able to demonstrate the right coronary artery in children with anomalous left coronary artery syndrome.

The technique described by Weyman et al.[8] was used by Chandraratna and Aronow[12] for the noninvasive visualization of the left main coronary artery in 123 patients with coronary artery disease. Their overall rate of success in visualizing the left main coronary artery was 58%. Left main coronary obstruction was found in all 9 patients with an angiographically proved left main luminal narrowing of more than 50%. Two-dimensional echocardiography was accurate in establishing the patency of the left main coronary artery in 95% of patients with normal angiography (see Table 7–1).

Ogawa et al.[13] used a different anatomical approach, the apical four-chamber view, to visualize the left main coronary artery. The transducer was placed at the area of the cardiac apex while the patient was in the left lateral decubitus position and the echocardiographic beam was directed toward the base of the heart perpendicular to the plane of the ventricular and atrial septa (Fig 7–3,A). The transducer was initially angled slightly posteriorly so that the beam passed through the plane of the mitral and tricuspid valves and then was angled slightly anteriorly until the aorta and left main coronary artery were imaged; no mitral valve tissue was identified. The transducer position was then altered slightly clockwise with increased rejection of low-frequency echoes until the left main coronary artery was imaged as a parallel set of echoes with a lumen-free space contiguous with the lumen of the aorta (Fig 7–3,A and B). Frame-by-frame review of the videotape after recording of the initial data was necessary since the left main coronary artery moves with each cardiac cycle. Their data indicated a slightly higher rate of success (77%) in visualization of the left main coronary artery, and the accuracy of the diagnosis of normal and abnormal vessels was also improved (see Table 7–1). It is further emphasized that when both visualization techniques (short-axis and apical four-chamber view) were combined, the visualization success rate increased to 93%.[13]

The apical four-chamber view was also used by

TABLE 7–1.—Two-Dimensional Visualization of the Left Main Coronary Artery (LMCA)

STUDY	NO. (%) OF LMCA DETECTION	DIAGNOSIS OF LMCA OBSTRUCTION	DIAGNOSIS OF NORMAL LMCA	FALSE POSITIVE FINDINGS*	FALSE NEGATIVE FINDINGS*
Weyman et al.[8]	33/33 (100%)	3/3 (100%)	30/30 (100%)	. . .	. . .
Chandraratna and Aranow[12]	71/123 (58%)	9/9 (100%)	59/62 (95%)	3/62	. . .
Ogawa et al.[13]	27/35 (77%)	2/2 (100%)	23/25 (92%)	2/25	. . .
Chen et al.[14]	52/73 (71%)	12/16 (75%)	34/36 (94%)	2/36	4/16
Rogers et al.[16]	90/100 (90%)	50/53 (94%)	24/37 (65%)	13/37	3/53

*Most false positives and false negatives were due to anatomical aberrations.

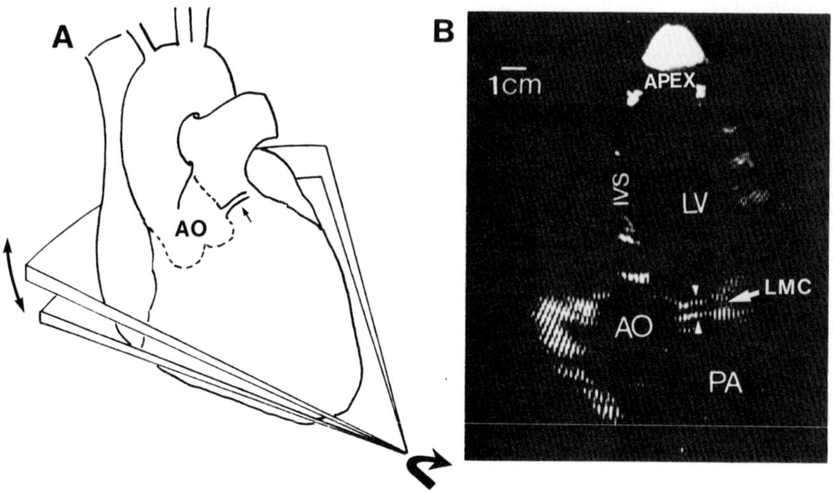

Fig 7–3.—Echocardiographic demonstration of the left main coronary artery *(LMC)* by means of the apical four-chamber view. A slight anteroposterior scanning motion combined with a clockwise rotation **(A)** brings the LMC into focus as a structure composed of two parallel echo-dense lines separated by a lumen that is located between the left ventricular cavity *(LV)* and the pulmonary artery *(PA)* and that connects to the aortic root *(AO)* **(B).**

Chen et al.[14, 15] to study the distribution of increased echo densities in the walls of the left main coronary artery. The integrity of the arterial lumen was also used as major criterion for the diagnosis of coronary obstructive disease. Of a total of 73 patients, adequate visualization of the left main coronary artery was possible in 52 (71%). Thirty-six of the 52 patients did not show significant lesions (greater than 50% luminal narrowing on angiography). Of those 36, 2DE confirmed a patent left main coronary artery in 34 (94%) (see Figs 7–2,B and 7–3,B). Results in the remaining 2 patients were false positive. Sixteen of the 52 patients (31%) had a significant left main coronary artery obstruction on angiography. In 12 (75%) of those 16, luminal irregularities and/or asymmetric echo densities were diagnostic markers for the echocardiographic diagnosis of left main coronary artery lesions (Fig 7–4). The remaining 4 patients (representing false negative diagnoses) had markedly elongated left main coronary arteries with obstructions located near the bifurcation, which could not be visualized in these patients.

Rogers et al.,[16, 17] looking for high-intensity echoes emanating from arteriosclerotic lesions located in the left coronary system, reported overall data compatible with the previously discussed studies (see Table 7–1). It is of interest that only 11 patients in their study had documented lesions located in the left main coronary artery; in the rest of the patients the coronary obstructions were localized in the proximal left anterior descending coronary artery (34 patients) and in the left anterior descending distal to the first septal perforator (5 patients).[17] The feasibility of echocardiographic demonstration of more distal arteriosclerotic lesions farther down in the left coronary system was further confirmed by Rink et al.[18] These observations are also in accordance with the in vitro visualization of the left coronary artery system as performed by Rogers et al.[19] Using a computer-aided method to improve picture resolution and to provide repeated visualization of the left main coronary artery in a given time during the cardiac cycle, Rink et al.[20] reported marked improvement in the diagnosis of left main coronary artery disease.

Thus, judging by the data available to date, 2DE may be used to visualize directly and noninvasively the left main coronary artery and proximal portions of the left anterior descending and left circumflex coronary artery in a relatively high percentage (60%–90%) of cases. The combination of the various echocardiographic approaches and the definition of high-intensity echoes emanating from the arterial walls seems to offer a high sen-

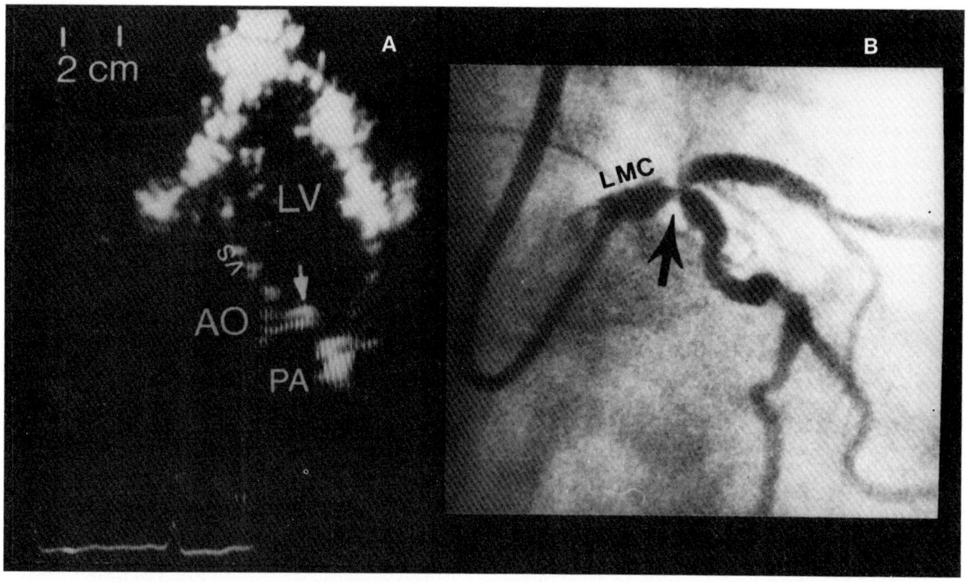

Fig 7–4.—**A,** a two-dimensional apical four-chamber view of a patient with a high-grade obstruction of the left main coronary artery *(LMC)*. The arterial lumen is almost obliterated by an echo-dense structure (atherosclerotic plaque). **B,** the corresponding angiographic picture. *LV,* left ventricular cavity; *VS,* interventricular septum; *AO,* aortic root; *PA,* pulmonary artery. (From Chen C.C., et al.: *Circulation* 62:288–293, 1980. Reproduced by permission of the American Heart Association.)

sitivity and specificity in the diagnosis and localization of arteriosclerotic lesions in the proximal left coronary system. With increasing interest in identifying subjects with left main and proximal left anterior descending coronary artery disease, further investigations of 2DE techniques and criteria aimed at the noninvasive evaluation of this problem are warranted.

ECHOCARDIOGRAPHIC DETECTION OF REMOTE MYOCARDIAL ISCHEMIA

Chronic myocardial hypoperfusion due to high-grade obstruction of a coronary artery or tissue property changes due to healed myocardial infarction result in abnormal wall motion patterns. Echocardiography is a noninvasive means of detecting, localizing, and evaluating the extent of myocardial damage in these patients. The specific M-mode echocardiographic and 2DE features of chronic myocardial ischemia are presented below.

M-Mode Echocardiography

The characteristic M-mode echocardiographic features of chronic myocardial ischemia and remote infarction are thinning of the affected wall and diminished systolic excursion (<3 mm) (Fig 7–5,A and B), whereas scar formation that follows myocardial infarction is characterized by relatively dense echoes in the effected region. (Fig 7–5,C) In the early 1970s, Jacobs et al.[21] noted echocardiographically detectable marked wall motion abnormalities in 18 of 20 patients with ECG and angiographic evidence of myocardial infarct. These abnormal wall motion patterns, defined as diminished or impaired excursions or paradoxic movement of the infarcted wall, were distinctive to those patients and were not found in normal subjects or in patients with nontransmural infarctions. It is of interest that in this study, all patients showing echocardiographic septal motion abnormalities had significant lesions in the left anterior descending coronary artery. However, in 8 patients with significant left anterior coronary artery obstruction, echocardiographic septal motion pattern was judged normal. Dortimer et al.[22] studied 56 consecutive

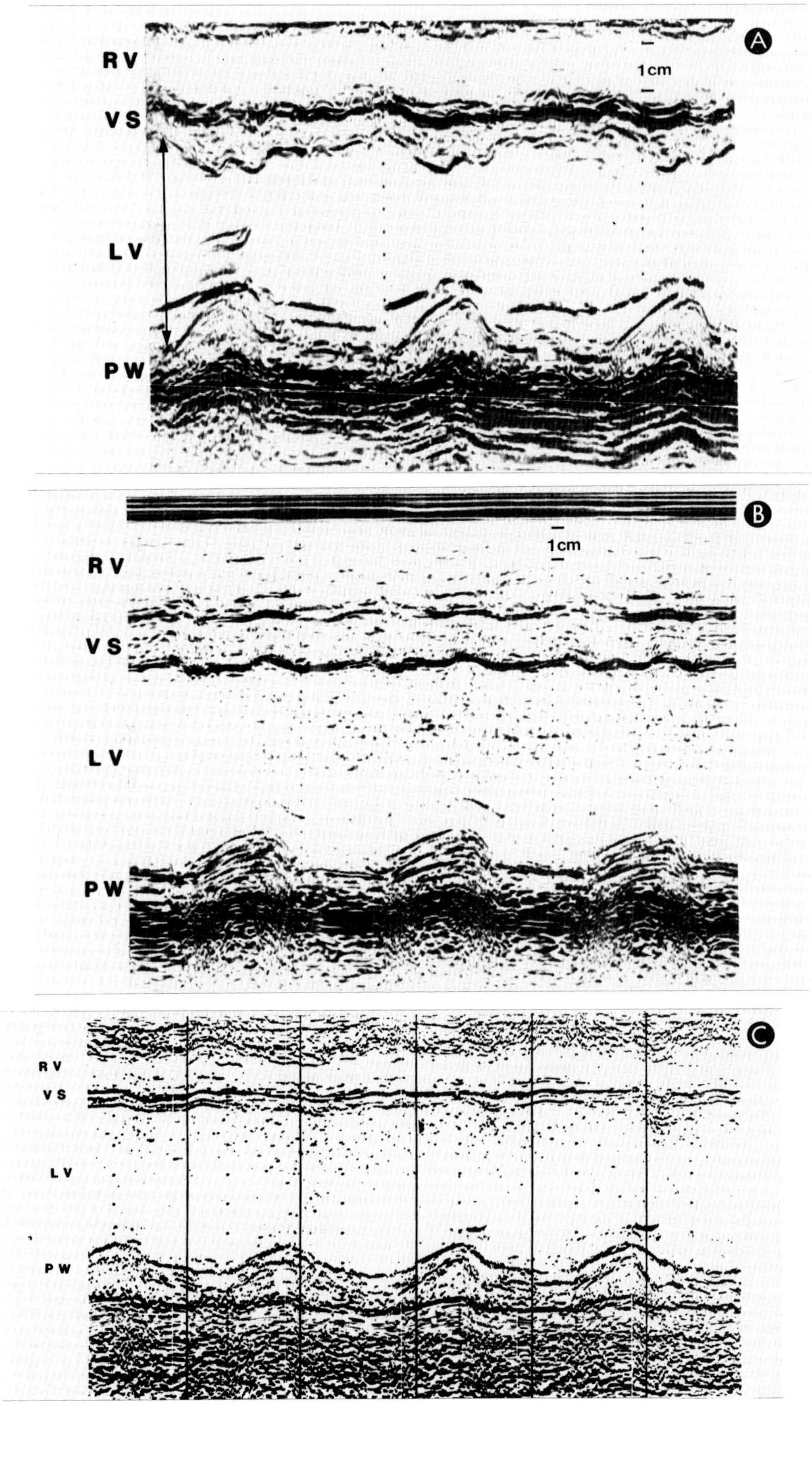
A
RV
1cm
VS
LV
PW
B
1cm
RV
VS
LV
PW
C
RV
VS
LV
PW

patients with anginal syndrome during angina-free periods and compared the results in a blinded fashion to the results of angiography. Twenty-eight (80%) of the 35 patients with significant obstructions of the left anterior descending coronary artery showed a decrease in septal motion, whereas only 14 (52%) of 27 patients with posterior vessel disease had diminished motion of the posterior wall. By combining echocardiographically determined left ventricular function and wall motion parameters with systolic time intervals, Stack et al.[23] could improve the noninvasive evaluation of patients with prior myocardial infarction. Gordon and Kerber,[24] studying patients with left anterior coronary artery disease, found that in all 17 patients with normal left anterior coronary arteries, systolic septal excursion exceeded 3 mm; however, only 12 of 26 patients had reduced septal motion (<2 mm). A subgroup of these patients who had proximal left anterior coronary obstruction had a higher incidence of decreased systolic septal motion (9/16). The same study[24] showed poor correlation between echocardiographically determined septal motion and ECG signs of remote infarction. By comparing M-mode echocardiographic, angiographic, and radionuclide imaging data, Kolibash et al.[25] studied the mechanism of abnormal regional wall motion in 25 patients with critical (>70%) lesions of the left anterior descending coronary artery. Twelve of these 25 patients had abnormal echocardiographic septal motion; of these, 8 had a past history of myocardial infarction. The remaining 13 patients showed normal septal motion on echocardiography; however, 5 of them had a previous history of myocardial infarct. Using intracoronary injection with radioactively labeled microaggregated albumin particles, Kolibash et al. showed that 10 of 12 patients with abnormal septal motion had absent resting septal perfusion. Of the 13 patients with normal septal motion, only 2 had abnormal septal perfusion. The authors concluded that in patients with severe left anterior descending coronary artery stenosis, the presence of abnormal septal motion on echocardiography strongly suggests marked abnormal septal perfusion as the cause of wall motion abnormalities. This method, however, could not clearly differentiate patients with old myocardial infarction from patients with a chronic ischemic process. Joffe et al.[26] studied 77 patients admitted for angiography for the evaluation of an anginal syndrome. Only 2 of 38 without left anterior descending disease had abnormal septal motion, whereas 17 of 39 patients with left anterior descending coronary artery disease had abnormal septal motion. The degree of septal motion depression correlated well with the location of the angiographically determined coronary obstruction, whereby more proximal obstructions resulted in a more profound depression of septal motion. Although the authors did not specify the number of patients with remote myocardial infarction, the echocardiographic demonstration of resting M-mode echocardiographic segmental ventricular septal motion abnormalities seemed quite specific for the presence of left anterior descending coronary artery disease.

Two-Dimensional Echocardiography

The use of 2DE to characterize regional areas of abnormal contraction is beginning to evolve. The information derived from M-mode techniques, such as diastolic thinning, failure of systolic thickening, and ventricular dimensional changes, has only lately been applied to 2DE (Fig 7–6). Using a computer-aided approach, Parisi et al.[27, 28] and Moynihan et al.[29] have used 2DE to quantify regional left ventricular wall motion abnormalities. There were three main groups of patients: normal volunteers, patients with coronary artery disease but without remote myocardial infarction, and patients with prior myocardial infarction electrocardiographically confirmed by abnormal Q waves on their ECGs. End-diastolic short-axis outlines of the

Fig 7–5.—M-mode echocardiographic features of myocardial infarction involving the intraventricular septum *(VS)*. **A,** the normal contractile pattern of the VS. **B,** chronic ischemia results in a hypokinetic septum that has retained normal diastolic dimensions but lost its systolic thickening ability. **C,** a remote septal infarction has created a marked thinning and akinesis of the VS. Note the marked echo-dense structures in the VS which correspond to scar tissue formation. *RV,* right ventricle; *LV,* left ventricle; *PW,* left ventricular posterior wall.

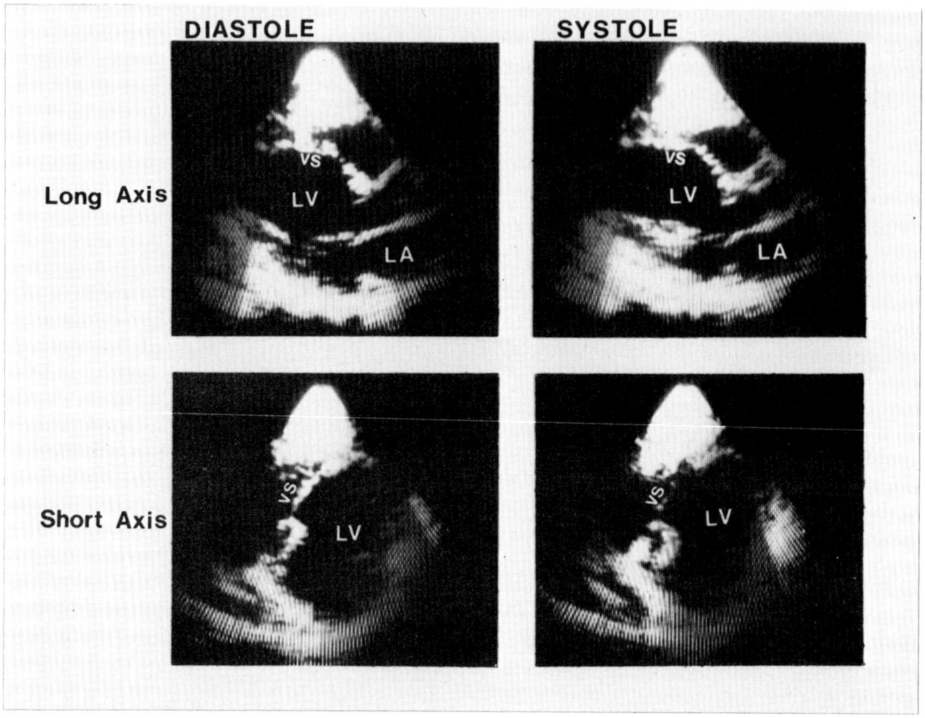

Fig 7–6.—Two-dimensional long-axis *(top)* and short-axis *(bottom)* echocardiographic views of the left ventricle *(LV)* of a patient with a remote anteroseptal myocardial infarction. The interventricular septum *(VS)* is thin, and the accumulation of fibrous scar tissue causes high echo reflectivity. In systole the septum is seen to move paradoxically. *LA,* left atrium.

ventricle at both mitral valve and papillary muscle level were traced with a light pen digitizing system using the onset of the ECG QRS complex as a marker of end-diastole. Similarly, end-systolic frames were traced using the first high-frequency component of the second heart sound as an indicator of end-systole. Thereafter, a computer algorithm was devised to divide the diastolic outline of the ventricle into posterior and anterior halves of equal area. The midpoint of this initial diastolic axis was symmetrically bisected by a series of radii. This created a radial axis system of eight chords and their enclosed areas, which allowed for segmental evaluation of the ventricle either by chord shortening or regional area shrinkage (Fig 7–7). Thirty-two patients were evaluated once the normal range of contraction was established from 10 normal volunteers. Twenty patients with coronary artery disease but without remote infarction had no differences in their contraction pattern from the group of volunteers. In contrast, 6 patients with anterior infarction showed a pattern of impaired regional motion in the anterior and anteroseptal regions, while 6 patients with inferior infarction showed an impairment in wall motion in posterior and lateral regions. When a parallel analysis with angiograms was conducted using abnormal ECG Q-waves as evidence for infarction and for the region in which wall motion abnormalities should occur, 2DE proved as sensitive as angiography for the detection of regional contraction defects. These observations confirmed that 2DE can be used systematically to study regional wall motion abnormalities in patients with remote as well as acute myocardial infarction. Similar results have been reported by Kan et al.[30]

Thus, echocardiography seems to constitute a relatively reliable noninvasive technique permitting the identification of chronic ischemic processes that affect the contractile properties of the myocardium. From the studies discussed above, chronic regional wall motion abnormalities detected by echocardiography warrant the diagnosis of a significant reduction of blood flow to the visualized region. However, this finding does not in itself permit differentiation between a region with chronically impaired blood flow caused by a high-grade obstruction of the coronary artery and a region that underwent in the past a necrotic event. Two-dimensional echocardiography ultimately has the potential not only of identifying the presence of wall motion abnormalities, but also of quantifying their extent on a global basis and assessing their potential reversibility.

IDENTIFICATION OF COMPLICATIONS FOLLOWING MYOCARDIAL INFARCTION

Many of the complications that result from an ischemic event can be identified echocardiographically. Among these are acute papillary muscle dysfunction or rupture, the acute rupture of the ventricular septum, and the formation of true or false aneurysms. Enlargement of the ventricular cavity and a global decrease in systolic excursions may indicate the development of cardiac failure, while the echocardiographic detection of pericardial fluid may be a warning sign of imminent tamponade. Detailed analysis of the echocardiographic detection of these and other complications is presented elsewhere in this volume.

ECHOCARDIOGRAPHIC EVALUATION OF TISSUE PROPERTIES

The reflection pattern of ultrasonic waves obeys the general principles of geometric optics. Absorption attenuation, refraction, and reflection are the main determinants of this phenomenon. The intensity of the reflected wave beam that is used for sonographic viewing depends on, among other factors, the absorptive and reflective properties of the target tissue. A more reflective tissue will give a brighter echocardiographic image than a tissue with lower reflective properties.

Myocardial infarction and damage result in an increased number of collagen fibers, a decrease in the amount of contractile myocardial tissue, and the gradual transformation of a necrotic lesion into a fibrotic scar formation. These changes in tissue construction result in changes in echo-reflective properties, which can conceivably be identified by echocardiography and may be of diagnostic value (see Fig 7–5,C). Mimbs et al.[31-33] demonstrated in vitro a significant decrease in ultrasonic attenuation in the acute ischemic myocardium (15 minutes to 24 hours after coronary ligation). In contrast, in the chronic infarction, a marked increase in ultrasonic attenuation and backscatter due to the increased collagen content of the infarcted tissue could be seen. Similar experimental results were reported by other investigators.[34, 35] Rasmussen et al.[36] used M-mode echocardiography to identify, retrospectively, scar tissue in 182 patients who subsequently died or underwent bypass surgery and/or ventricular resection. Their criteria for the existence of myocardial scar formation were (1) mid-diastolic myocardial thickness of less than 7 mm and increased echo density as compared to the opposing or adjacent myocardium, and (2) a regional myocardial thinning of more than 30%. Scar tissue observed during surgery or on pathologic specimens was found in 53 patients. In 48 of these patients, the echocardiographic determination of scar formation was correct. Five did not show echocardiographic signs of scar tissue. In 129 patients no pathologic or surgical evidence of scar tissue was found. In 125 of those patients the echocardiographic diagnosis was correct; in the remaining 4 the echocardiogram was falsely interpreted as showing a scar formation. The authors concluded, therefore, that M-mode echocardiography is both sensitive and specific in the detection of myocardial scar tissue. Nieminen et al.,[37] reviewing the usefulness of M-mode echocardiography in the diagnosis of myocardial infarction, also mentioned the increase in echo reflectivity of myocardial scar tissue.

The increased reflectivity of arteriosclerotic lesions in the walls of the left coronary artery was used by Rogers et al.[17] Using 2DE, these authors developed a technique for the identification of high-intensity echoes reflected from the left coronary

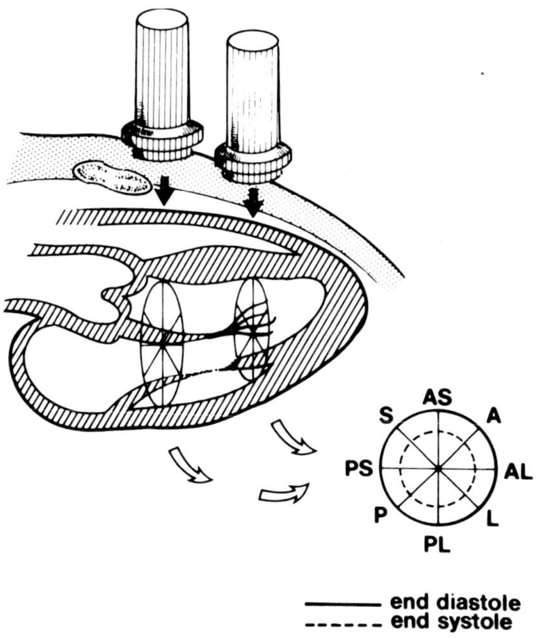

Fig 7–7.—Schematic drawing illustrating two-dimensional echocardiographic short-axis views of the left ventricle. Insert shows diastolic and systolic outlines of the left ventricle at either level as a pair of outlines that approximate concentric circles. The axis system used for analysis is superimposed. Regional function of the left ventricle can be characterized with the use of either segmental areas or chords. *A,* anterior; *AL,* anterolateral; *AS,* anteroseptal; *L,* lateral; *P,* posterior; *PL,* posterolateral; *PS,* posteroseptal; *S,* septal. (From Parisi A.F., et al.: *Am. J. Cardiol.* 46:1205–1214, 1980. Reproduced by permission.)

artery system. By this method of tissue differentiation, they were able to diagnose significant obstructive arterial lesions in the left coronary artery system with a high degree of precision (see Fig 7–4). In a similar manner Chen et al.[15] used the high-intensity echoes reflected from arteriosclerotic processes in the walls of the left coronary artery system to enhance the diagnosis of coronary artery obstruction.

The importance of this new approach in distinguishing between viable and scar tissue lies, in part, in the evaluation of the viability of the affected myocardium. Thus, the unusually thin echodense and noncontractile region, which is probably comprised mostly of scar tissue, is unlikely to have its function restored by bypass surgery, while a poorly contracting area of myocardium of normal diastolic thickness and wall character may indeed recover its function after its blood supply is restored. The potential of echocardiography in this regard will be the subject of explorations within the next few years.

REFERENCES

1. Campeau L., et al.: Left main coronary artery stenosis: Influence of aortocoronary bypass surgery on survival. *Circulation* 57:1111–1115, 1978.
2. Loop F.D., et al.: Atherosclerosis of the left main coronary artery: Five-year results of surgical treatment. *Am. J. Cardiol.* 44:195–201, 1979.
3. Cohen M.V., Gorland R.: Main left coronary artery disease: Clinical experience from 1964–1974. *Circulation* 52:275–285, 1975.
4. Plotnick G.D., et al.: Clinical indicators of left main coronary artery disease in unstable angina. *Ann. Intern. Med.* 91:149–153, 1979.
5. Bartel A.G., et al.: Graded exercise stress test in angiographically documented coronary artery disease. *Circulation* 49:348–356, 1974.
6. Conte C.R., et al.: Left main coronary artery stenosis: Clinical spectrum, pathophysiology and management. *Prog. Cardiovasc. Dis.* 22:73–106, 1979.
7. Levine P., et al.: Left main coronary artery disease: Clinical arteriographic and hemodynamic appraisal. *Am. J. Cardiol.* 30:791–796, 1972.
8. Weyman A.E., et al.: Non-invasive visualization of the left main coronary artery by cross-sectional echocardiography. *Circulation* 54:169–174, 1976.
9. Yoshikawa J., et al.: Cross-sectional echocardiographic diagnosis of coronary artery aneurysms in patients with the mucocutaneous lymph node syndrome. *Circulation* 59:133–139, 1979.
10. Hiraishi S., Yashiro K., Kusano S.: Non-invasive visualization of coronary arterial aneurysm in infants and young children with mucocutaneous lymph node syndrome with two-dimensional echocardiography. *Am. J. Cardiol.* 43:1225–1233, 1979.
11. Caldwell R.L., et al.: Cross-sectional echocardiographic differentiation of anomalous left coronary artery from primary myocardopathy. *Circulation* 57,58:II–202, 1978.
12. Chandraratna P.A.N., Aronow W.S.: Left main coronary artery patency assessed with cross-sectional echocardiography. *Am. J. Cardiol.* 46:91–94, 1980.
13. Ogawa S., et al.: A new approach to visualize the left main coronary artery using apical cross-sectional echocardiography. *Am. J. Cardiol.*, to be published.
14. Chen C.C., et al.: Differential density and luminal irregularities as criteria to detect disease in left main coronary artery by apex phased array cross-sectional echocardiography. *Am. J. Cardiol.* 43:386, 1979.

15. Chen C.C., et al.: The detection of left main coronary artery disease by apical cross-sectional echocardiography. *Circulation* 62:288–293, 1980.
16. Rogers E.W., et al.: Possible detection of coronary atherosclerosis by cross-sectional echocardiography. *Circulation* 57,58(suppl. II):II–56, 1978.
17. Rogers E.W., et al.: Possible detection of arteriosclerotic coronary calcifications by two-dimensional echocardiography. *Circulation* 62:1046–1052, 1980.
18. Rink L.D., et al.: Detection of proximal left anterior descending coronary artery obstruction with two-dimensional echocardiography. *Circulation* 62(suppl. III):III–33, 1980.
19. Rogers E.W., et al.: Evaluation of left coronary anatomy in vitro by cross-sectional echocardiography. *Circulation* 62:782–787, 1980.
20. Rink L.D., et al.: Improved echocardiographic technique for examining the left main coronary artery. *Am. J. Cardiol.* 45:435, 1980.
21. Jacobs J.J., et al.: Detection of left ventricular asynergy by echocardiography. *Circulation* 48:263–271, 1973.
22. Dortimer A.C., et al.: Distribution of coronary artery disease prediction by echocardiography. *Circulation* 54:724–729, 1976.
23. Stack R.S., et al.: Left ventricular performance in coronary artery disease evaluated with systolic time intervals and echocardiography. *Am. J. Cardiol.* 37:331–339, 1976.
24. Gordon M.J., Kerber R.E.: Interventricular septal motion in patients with proximal and distal left anterior descending coronary artery lesions. *Circulation* 55:338–341, 1977.
25. Kolibash A.J., et al.: Relationship between abnormal echocardiographic septal motion and myocardial perfusion in patients with significant obstruction of the left anterior descending artery. *Circulation* 56:780–785, 1977.
26. Joffe C.D., et al.: Echocardiographic diagnosis of left anterior descending coronary artery disease. *Am. J. Cardiol.* 40:11–16, 1977.
27. Parisi A.F., et al.: Assessment of regional wall motion in coronary artery disease by two-dimensional echocardiography, in Lancee C.T. (ed.): *Echocardiology*. The Hague, Martinus Nijhoff, 1979, pp. 125–129.
28. Parisi A.F., et al.: Echocardiography in acute and remote myocardial infarction. *Am. J. Cardiol.* 46:1205–1214, 1980.
29. Moynihan P.F., Feldman C.L., Parisi A.F.: Comparison of methods for quantitative evaluation of left ventricular function with two-dimensional echocardiography, abstracted. *Clin. Res.* 27:566A, 1979.
30. Kan G., et al.: Correlation of two-dimensional echocardiography with coronary arteriography and electrocardiogram in anterior wall infarction. *Circulation* 62(suppl. III):III–186, 1980.
31. Mimbs J.W., et al.: Detection of myocardial infarction in vitro based on altered attenuation of ultrasound. *Circulation* 41:192–198, 1977.
32. Mimbs J.W., et al.: Changes in ultrasonic attenuation indicative of early myocardial ischemic injury. *Am. J. Physiol.* 236:H-340–344, 1979.
33. Mimbs J.W., O'Donnell M., Miller J.G.: Increased collagen deposition in zones of infarction: A potential cause of increased echocardiographic density. *Circulation* 57,58(suppl. II):II–233, 1978.
34. Dines K.A., et al.: Quantitation of changes in myocardial fiber-bundle spacing with acute infarction using pulse-echo ultrasound signals, abstracted. *Circulation* 60(suppl. II):II–17, 1979.
35. Franklin T.D., et al.: Differentiation of a-mode ultrasound signals from normal and ischemic myocardium by multivariate discriminant analysis of waveform parameters, abstracted. *Am. J. Cardiol.* 45:403, 1980.
36. Rasmussen S., et al.: Detection of myocardial scar tissue by M-mode echocardiography. *Circulation* 57:230–237, 1978.
37. Nieminen M.S., Heikkila J.: Accuracy and usefulness of echoventriculography in acute myocardial infarction. *Acta Med. Scand. Suppl.* 627:152–163, 1978.

RADIONUCLIDE IMAGING

Robert D. Okada

MYOCARDIAL RADIONUCLIDE IMAGING encompasses several new techniques for the diagnosis and functional evaluation of patients with ischemic heart disease. This chapter describes the techniques used for patients with known or suspected coronary artery disease. Myocardial radionuclide imaging in patients with acute myocardial infarction or complications of acute myocardial infarction is discussed in chapter 10.

THALLIUM 201 MYOCARDIAL RADIONUCLIDE IMAGING

Stress Thallium 201 Radionuclide Imaging

Early myocardial perfusion imaging utilized radioisotopes of potassium (^{42}K, ^{43}K), its analogs (cesium 129), and rubidium 81. In 1973, Zaret and associates reported the use of potassium 43 to obtain exercise myocardial perfusion scans.[1] In 1974, Berman and associates used rubidium 81 for exercise myocardial imaging and reported improved diagnostic accuracy for coronary artery disease using this technique compared to conventional ECG stress testing.[2] Subsequently, thallium 201 (^{201}Tl) was suggested as a myocardial perfusion imaging agent based on its lower photon energies and greater myocardial concentration compared to potassium 43, rubidium 81, and cesium 129.[3] In 1976, Ritchie and associates reported the use of ^{201}Tl perfusion imaging during exercise as a noninvasive test for coronary artery disease.[4]

Study Procedures

Early ^{201}Tl exercise studies utilized separate injections of ^{201}Tl during exercise and at rest. The patient first exercised, was injected with ^{201}Tl during exercise, and then was imaged. Defects on images obtained immediately after exercise were interpreted as due to scar or exercise-induced ischemia. Patients with defects returned at least 72 hours later for a second ^{201}Tl injection at rest, with repeated imaging. If a defect was no longer present, the initial defect was interpreted as due to transient exercise-induced ischemia. A persistent defect was interpreted as scar. This technique had several shortcomings, among them a double radiation dose to the patient, the necessity of two patient visits, the doubled expense for the radioisotope, and high background activity in initial ^{201}Tl images obtained at rest. Furthermore, our laboratory has demonstrated that initial defects on ^{201}Tl images obtained at rest may be due to ischemia or scar.[5]

In 1977, our laboratory reported the disappearance of initial myocardial ^{201}Tl defects over a two-hour period following transient ischemia in dogs.[6] The same phenomenon was subsequently observed in patients who developed transient ischemia during exercise.[6] The phenomenon was called "^{201}Tl redistribution" and became the basis for the current technique for exercise ^{201}Tl imaging. Using this technique, a 12-lead ECG is obtained and a peripheral intravenous line is placed. Patients exercise following a graded protocol, either upright on a treadmill or supine using a bicycle. The ECG is monitored during exercise and the patient exercises until symptom limited by chest pain, dyspnea, or leg fatigue. About 45 seconds prior to the anticipated end of exercise, 1.5–2.0 mCi of thallous-201 chloride is injected intravenously and the patient is encouraged to continue exercising for 45 seconds. In our laboratory, images are obtained in the anterior and 50-degree and 70-degree left anterior oblique projections immediately after termination of exercise (initial images) and three to four hours later (delayed images). A medium-sensitivity collimator, an Anger scintillation camera interfaced to an imaging computer, and a 20%–30% energy window encompassing the 68- to 80-keV x-ray emissions of ^{201}Tl are utilized. Images are collected for a preset time ranging from six to ten minutes. A minimum of 300,000 counts is collected in the initial images.

Several tomographic techniques have been proposed for improving the spatial resolution of ^{201}Tl images. One widely used technique is the seven-pinhole emission tomography reported by Vogel and associates.[7] The data are projected by the pinholes onto seven different regions of the camera crystal. A computerized addition-multiplication algorithm is used to reconstruct the raw data into multiple plane images. Planar resolution is reported to be 1.0 cm, with a depth resolution of 1.5 cm.[8]

In addition to exercise, variations in the type of stress may be introduced, such as pacing and cold pressor response. However, pacing requires an invasive procedure for the placement of a temporary transvenous pacing wire. Furthermore, a recent report has questioned the adequacy of tachycardiac stress alone for stress ^{201}Tl radionuclide imaging.[9] More recently, the cold pressor response has been used with ^{201}Tl imaging.[10] The hand is immersed in ice water for a variable amount of time (usually one minute) and ^{201}Tl is injected toward the end of the immersion period. Immediately after the hand is removed from the water, ^{201}Tl images are obtained in the standard fashion.

Interpretation of Studies

Thallium 201 images are usually interpreted qualitatively. Cook and associates have described the appearance of normal ^{201}Tl images.[11] In our laboratory, images are displayed on a computer screen, with the initial and delayed images side by side for comparison. The left ventricular wall is divided into the following segments: (1) anterolateral, apical, and inferior segments on the anterior projection, (2) septal, apical-inferior, and posterior segments on the 50-degree left anterior oblique projection, and (3) anterior, apical-lateral, and posterolateral segments on the 70-degree left anterior oblique projection (Fig 8–1). Each segment is subjectively graded as 2 (normal activity), 1.5, 1.0 (reduced activity), 0.5, or zero (minimal activity). A transient defect is defined as an increase of one or more grades between the initial

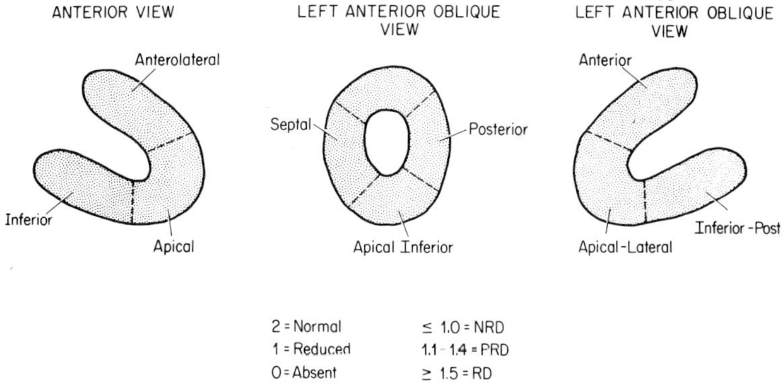

Fig 8–1.—Division of left ventricular myocardium into segments for assessment of ^{201}Tl myocardial images. Activity is not assessed in the superior segment of the left anterior oblique projection since it is normally reduced or absent in this area.

and delayed images and is interpreted as transient ischemia occurring during exercise. A persistent defect, interpreted as scar, is defined as an initial and delayed score of 1.0 or less for any segment not involving the apex. Segments involving the apex can normally have reduced activity because of myocardial thinning and are considered to have a persistent defect if initial and delayed scores are 0.5 or less. Figure 8–2 shows examples of transient and persistent ^{201}Tl defects. The appearance of a normal ^{201}Tl image in patients without coronary artery disease is described by Cook and associates.[11] It should be noted that a change in heart size or geometry between two images can give the appearance of a changing defect without an actual change in tracer distribution.[12]

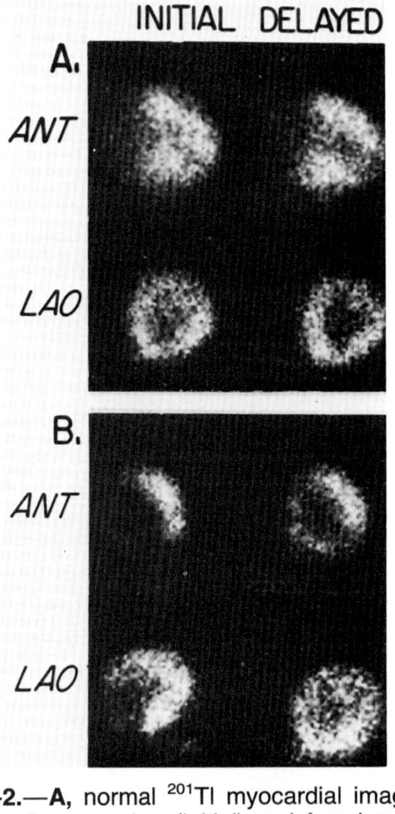

Fig 8–2.—A, normal ^{201}Tl myocardial images immediately after exercise *(initial)* and four hours later *(delayed).* Note homogeneous distribution of tracer except in the apical and apical-inferior segments, where activity can normally be slightly lower. **B,** abnormal ^{201}Tl myocardial images. Note inferior and apical defects on the initial anterior *(ANT)* view and septal and apical-inferior defects on the initial left anterior oblique view *(LAO).* There is complete redistribution into the septal and apical-inferior segments (transient defect), partial redistribution into the inferior segment, and no redistribution into the apical defect (persistent defect). (From Okada R.D., et al.: *Am. J. Cardiol.* 46:1188–1204, 1980. Reproduced by permission.)

Sensitivity of Stress ^{201}Tl Radionuclide Imaging for Coronary Artery Disease

Electrocardiographic exercise testing has been the most widely used, noninvasive technique for assessing patients with possible coronary artery disease. However, the sensitivity of the test for coronary artery disease ranges from approximately 60% to 64% and greatly depends on the level of stress achieved by the patient.[13] Although reasonably specific for coronary artery disease (specificity, 89%–93%),[12] the ECG exercise test may yield false positive results or may be difficult to interpret in patients with pre-excitation syndromes, electrolyte imbalance, carbohydrate loading, resting ST-T wave changes, interventricular conduction abnormalities or bundle-branch block, left or right ventricular hypertrophy, previous myocardial infarction, hyperventilation, or effects from various drugs such as digitalis. Because of these limitations, a number of investigators have examined the diagnostic accuracy of stress ^{201}Tl imaging for coronary artery disease. Table 8–1 summarizes a number of studies on exercise ^{201}Tl imaging. The overall sensitivity and specificity of stress ^{201}Tl imaging were 82% and 91%, respectively, in 1,897 patients. When studies that did not report exercise ECG results were excluded, the sensitivity and specificity of stress ^{201}Tl imaging were 82% and 91%, respectively, compared to a 60% sensitivity and 81% specificity of the exercise ECG test. Stress ^{201}Tl imaging was significantly more sensitive ($P < .0001$) and specific ($P < .05$) for coronary artery disease than exercise ECG.

The improved sensitivity of stress ^{201}Tl imaging compared to ECG stress testing is partially due to the many reasons for nondiagnostic ECG stress tests. Stress ^{201}Tl imaging has been reported to be useful in patients with nondiagnostic ECG stress tests due to previous myocardial infarction, pre-excitation syndrome, bundle-branch block, ventricular hypertrophy, drug effects, and hyperventilation. Botvinick and associates studied 19 pa-

TABLE 8–1.—SENSITIVITY AND SPECIFICITY OF THALLIUM 201 EXERCISE TEST VERSUS EXERCISE ELECTROCARDIOGRAPHY*

			THALLIUM 201		ELECTROCARDIOGRAPHY	
YEAR	STUDY (CITY)	N	Sensitivity	Specificity	Sensitivity	Specificity
1976	Klein et al. (London, Ont.)[18]	144	59/73	69/71	61/73	63/71
1976	Peterson et al. (San Diego)[19]	25	16/17	4/8	12/17	5/8
1977	Bailey et al. (Baltimore)[14]	83	46/63	20/20	26/63	20/20
1977	Ritchie et al. (Seattle)[20]	101	58/76	23/25	50/76	21/25
1977	Lenaers et al. (Belgium)[21]	70	52/55	14/15	. . .	. . .
1977	Rosenblatt et al. (San Francisco)[22]	18	14/15	3/3	6/8 (7 ND)	2/2 (1 ND)
1978	Okada et al. (Tucson)[8]	49	27/33 (6 ND)	9/10 (1 ND)	23/27 (11 ND)	3/4 (7 ND)
1978	Carrillo et al. (Detroit)[23]	55	34/39	16/16	21/39	12/16
1978	Verani et al. (Iowa City)[24]	82	38/48	33/34	42/48	21/34
1978	Turner et al. (Chicago)[25]	64	23/34	29/30	25/34	23/30
1978	Ritchie et al. (multiple centers)[26]	190	115/148	37/42	62/148	37/42
1978	Bodenheimer et al. (Philadelphia)[27]	45	21/32	13/13	15/32†	. . .
1978	Johnstone et al. (New Haven)[28]	33	18/26	7/7	. . .	. . .
1979	McCarthy et al. (New York)[29]	128	81/95	26/33	61/95	30/33
1979	Pohost et al. (Boston)[15]	209	140/161	36/48	103/161	37/48
1979	Dash et al. (San Francisco)[16]	96	66/81	15/15	30/81	12/15
1979	Verani et al. (Houston)[30]	58	38/46	12/12	30/46†	. . .
1979	Vogel et al. (Denver)[17]	65	31/42	22/23	. . .	. . .
1979	Meller et al. (New York)[31]	55	23/28	23/27	. . .	14/24 (3 ND)
1979	Hecht et al. (Los Angeles)[36]	56	46/46	8/10	32/46	7/10
1979	Caldwell et al. (Seattle)[32]	39	30/33	6/6	. . .	. . .
1979	Borer et al. (Bethesda)[33]	53	35/43	9/10	. . .	. . .
1979	Verani et al. (Houston)[34]	38	17/21	17/17	. . .	. . .
1979	Kirshenbaum et al. (Boston)[35]	61	43/50	10/11	32/50	11/11
1980	Schicha et al. (Germany)[37]	80	58/60	18/20	. . .	. . .
	Total	1897	1129/1365 (.83)	479/526 (.91)	631/1044 (.60)	318/393 (.81)

*ND, nondiagnostic or technically inadequate studies. Sensitivity = number of true positive results divided by number of patients with disease. Specificity = number of true negative results divided by number of patients without disease. Ellipses indicate data were not reported.

†Does not include rest Q waves.

tients with abnormal ST segments at rest.[38] Twelve of 14 patients with coronary artery disease had abnormal stress ^{201}Tl scans, whereas 5 of 5 without coronary artery disease had normal stress ^{201}Tl scans. Iskandrian and associates performed stress ^{201}Tl radionuclide imaging on 65 patients with inconclusive exercise ECGs due to either submaximal exercise or ST segment abnormalities at rest.[39] The sensitivity and specificity of stress ^{201}Tl imaging in this population were 70% and 97%, respectively (Fig 8–3). We have also found that stress ^{201}Tl imaging is not as critically dependent on the level of exercise achieved as is stress ECG. In 227 patients, we found no significant difference in the sensitivity of stress ^{201}Tl imaging for those patients who achieved 85% or more of predicted maximal heart rate and those who did not.[15]

The sensitivity of stress ^{201}Tl imaging is reported to decrease in patients taking propranolol and those who have a negative stress ECG,[15] and in the presence of coronary collateral vessels. However, Berger and associates, using stress ^{201}Tl imaging, found that coronary collateral vessels neither protect against exercise-induced hypoperfusion nor affect the occurrence of ^{201}Tl redistribution.[40] The sensitivity of stress ^{201}Tl imaging is greater for left main coronary artery disease and increases with the increasing number and severity of coronary artery stenoses.[16] Tomographic approaches to stress ^{201}Tl imaging have also been reported to increase the sensitivity for coronary artery disease. Vogel and associates reported an improved sensitivity (95%) using multipinhole tomography and quantitative interpretation compared to standard planar imaging (74%). Specificity was high for both techniques.[17] More recently, how-

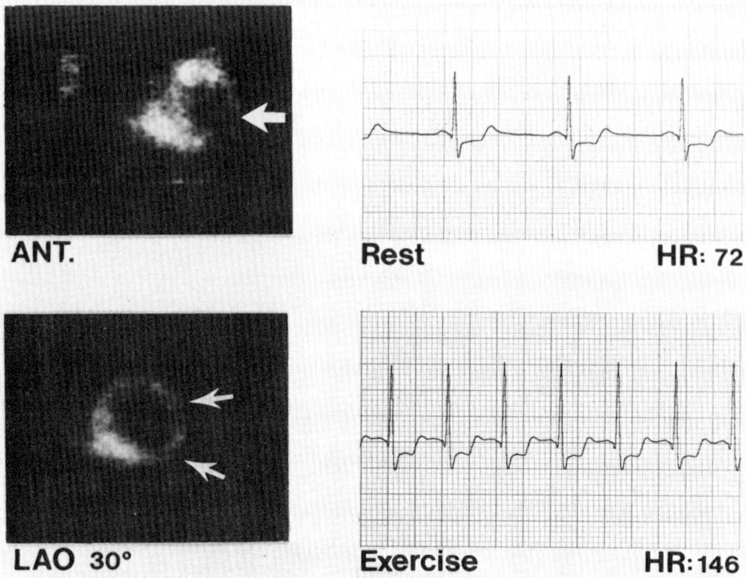

Fig 8–3.—Exercise and delayed ECGs and ^{201}Tl myocardial perfusion scans from a woman with chest pain and two-vessel coronary artery disease. Electrocardiographic lead V demonstrates ST segment depression at rest. The ^{201}Tl scan shows a perfusion defect in the anteroseptal region *(arrows)* during exercise. *LAO,* left anterior oblique projection. (From Iskandrian A.S., et al.: *Am. J. Cardiol.* 46:553–558, 1980. Reproduced by permission.)

ever, the relative contributions of tomography and quantitation toward the improved sensitivity have been examined. Much of the improved sensitivity of the quantitative tomography may be due to the quantitative process alone.[41] Other investigators have found quantitative techniques helpful for the interpretation of stress ^{201}Tl studies (Fig 8–4).[42] At present, quantitative techniques have not been shown definitely to improve the diagnostic accuracy of stress ^{201}Tl imaging. However, this approach may be valuable when experienced observers are not available.

We have studied the interobserver variance for the interpretation of segmental ^{201}Tl image scores and the changes in such scores between initial and delayed images.[43] The left ventricle was divided into six segments and graded by four independent observers on a scale of zero (minimal activity) to +2 (normal activity). Interobserver variance was determined for each segment. For a change in ^{201}Tl activity between exercise and delayed images, the interobserver variance was greatest for the apical and apical-inferior segments, intermediate for the inferior and septal segments, and least for the anterolateral and posterior segments (Fig 8–5). The sensitivity of stress ^{201}Tl imaging for coronary artery disease was found to improve significantly when the scores were interpreted using criteria derived from the interobserver variance analysis rather than arbitrary criteria. The diagnostic accuracy was increased further by averaging the scores of multiple observers and by interpreting these averaged scores by a single set of criteria applied to all six ventricular segments.

Specificity of Stress ^{201}Tl Imaging for Coronary Artery Disease

As can be ascertained from Table 8–1, stress ^{201}Tl studies are more specific than stress ECG studies for coronary artery disease. We have found stress ^{201}Tl imaging to be quite specific in patients with false positive ECG stress test results without a history of myocardial infarction. Others have

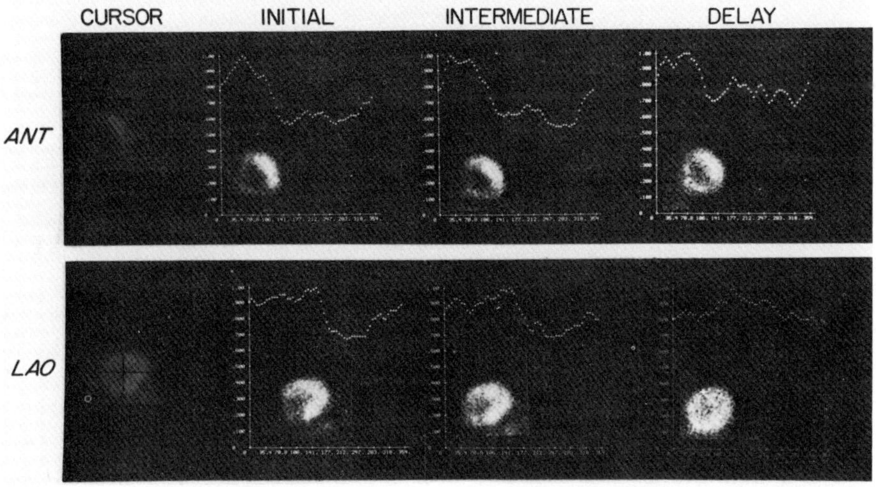

Fig 8–4.—Quantitation of myocardial ^{201}Tl distribution. Images at left show position of the cursors, which have been set by the operator at the center of the ventricular cavity, starting at 12 o'clock and proceeding clockwise. The program constructs radial lines from the center to the periphery and plots the maximal picture element counts on the *xy* graph. This figure demonstrates quantitation of the transient and persistent defects in the patient whose myocardial perfusion images are shown in Figure 8–2. (From Okada R.D., et al.: *Am. J. Cardiol.* 46:1188–1204, 1980. Reproduced by permission.)

found stress ^{201}Tl imaging helpful in asymptomatic patients with false positive ECG stress test results.[44] On the other hand, the less than perfect reported specificity of stress ^{201}Tl imaging for coronary artery disease may be due to a number of factors: (1) The specificity is reduced in study populations that include patients with subcritical coronary artery stenosis (30%–45% luminal diameter narrowing). We have found that about half of such patients have a positive stress ^{201}Tl test result.[45] Xenon 133 washout studies have demonstrated inequality of perfusion in these patients during hyperemia, and thus the stress ^{201}Tl study may be a true reflection of the hemodynamic state. (2) Preliminary results from one group of investigators have demonstrated a high incidence of abnormal right ventricular myocardial biopsy specimens from patients with positive stress ^{201}Tl studies and normal coronary arteries.[46] Positive stress ^{201}Tl test results in such patients may be due to abnormal myocardial cell integrity rather than abnormal perfusion. (3) Positive stress ^{201}Tl study results have been reported in patients with aortic stenosis, presumably due to exercise-induced subendocardial ischemia.[47] (4) Positive stress ^{201}Tl study results have been reported in patients with myocardial bridges,[48] coronary artery anomalies,[49] and idiopathic hypertrophic subaortic stenosis.[50] Recent reports have not substantiated the early reports of positive stress ^{201}Tl imaging in patients with mitral valve prolapse. We have found that in patients with negative stress ECG tests, there is

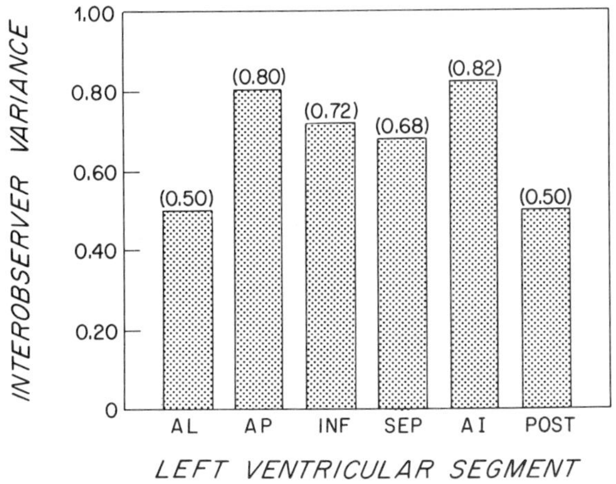

Fig 8–5.—Interobserver variance in the scoring of changes in left ventricular segmental ^{201}Tl activity and exercise and delayed images, expressed as 2 SD (scoring system from 0 to +2). Left ventricular segments are anterolateral *(AL)*, apical *(AP)*, inferior *(INF)*, septal *(SEP)*, apical-inferior *(AI)*, and posterior *(POST)*. (From Okada R.D., et al.: *Am. J. Cardiol.* 46:619–624, 1980. Reproduced by permission.)

a significantly lower specificity in female (56%) than in male (81%) subjects and in patients taking propranolol (53%) than in those who were not (82%).[15] Some of the low specificity in female subjects may be attributable to image artifacts due to breast attenuation.

Functional Information From Stress ^{201}Tl Imaging

We have observed increased lung ^{201}Tl activity on initial poststress images in patients with coronary artery disease. We have quantified lung ^{201}Tl activity by expressing it as a percentage of maximum myocardial ^{201}Tl activity (lung ^{201}Tl index) (Fig 8–6).[51] In 10 control patients, the mean initial lung ^{201}Tl index was 37.6% (Fig 8–7). In 29 patients with double- and triple-vessel coronary artery disease, the mean initial lung ^{201}Tl index was significantly elevated at 53.5%. An abnormal lung ^{201}Tl index was found to be highly specific for coronary artery disease, although not highly sensitive. We have also found that a qualitatively determined increase in ^{201}Tl lung activity is related to (1) a greater number of myocardial segmental ^{201}Tl defects, (2) increased severity and extent of coronary artery disease, (3) a greater prevalence of prior myocardial infarction, (4) a lower angiographic ejection fraction at rest, and (5) an exercise-induced increase in pulmonary capillary wedge pressure.[52]

We have also found that the amount of ^{201}Tl redistribution between initial and delayed poststress ^{201}Tl images correlates with the frequency and severity of wall motion abnormalities.[53] Sixteen patients had only transient ^{201}Tl defects suggesting exercise-induced ischemia; the mean left ventricular ejection fraction fell significantly during exercise (Fig 8–8). Eight patients had only persistent defects suggesting myocardial scar; the mean left ventricular ejection fraction was unchanged during exercise. Seventeen patients with no defects had a significant exercise-induced increase in left ventricular ejection fraction. Thus, only transient defects reliably predicted worsening left ventricular function during exercise. Other investigators have shown that transient ^{201}Tl defects in asynergic segments are associated with reversibility of the asynergy after a premature ventricular contraction.[54]

Other Considerations

Stress ^{201}Tl imaging has been used in angina-free patients with severe congestive heart failure to detect areas of ischemic myocardium and to distinguish between ischemic myocardium and scar as a cause for akinesis of left ventricular segments.[55] Myocardial revascularization in these patients with silent ischemia resulted in considerable clinical improvement in heart failure symptoms. Postoperative stress ^{201}Tl imaging demonstrated resolution of prior transient defects.

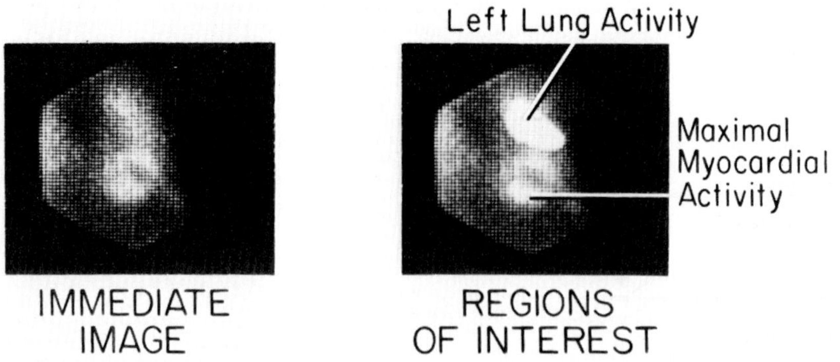

Fig 8–6.—Representative ^{201}Tl images of a patient with coronary artery disease and increased lung uptake in the anterior projection immediately after maximal supine stress testing. *Right,* regions of interest used in calculation of the lung/heart ratios. The patient had significant three-vessel coronary artery disease. The lung ^{201}Tl index for this patient was 62%. (From Kushner F.G., et al.: *Circulation* 63:341–347, 1981. Reproduced by permission of the American Heart Association.)

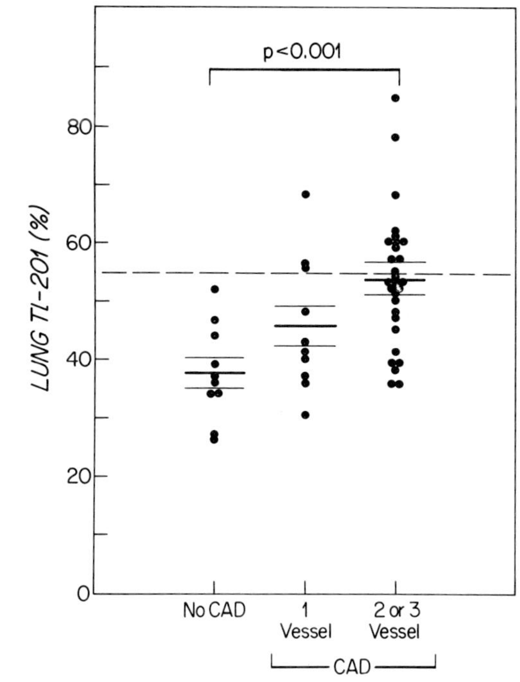

Fig 8–7.—Initial lung ^{201}Tl index (lung thallium activity/maximal myocardial thallium activity × 100%) for patients with or without significant coronary artery disease *(CAD). Thick bars* indicate mean and *thin bars* indicate SEM; *dashed line* indicates lung ^{201}Tl index of 54.5% (normal mean + 2 SD). (From Kushner F.G., et al.: *Circulation* 63:341–347, 1981. Reproduced by permission of the American Heart Association.)

The location of perfusion defects on stress ^{201}Tl imaging correlates with the location of coronary artery stenoses. Dunn and associates reported a good correlation between septal, anteroseptal, and anterior wall ^{201}Tl defects and left anterior descending coronary artery disease.[56] Defects in the inferior, posteroinferior, and posterior segments correlated with either right or left circumflex coronary artery disease. Rigo and associates have found that (1) anterior and septal wall defects are specific for left anterior descending disease, (2) inferior wall defects are specific for right coronary artery disease, and (3) proximal lateral wall defects are specific for circumflex artery disease.[57] Apical defects are not specific for any major coronary artery.

Stress ^{201}Tl imaging with submaximal exercise has been used several weeks after a myocardial infarction to identify patients with multivessel disease (two or more significantly stenotic coronary arteries) and residual jeopardized myocardium. Turner and associates have found that either transient stress ^{201}Tl defects or a positive conventional ECG exercise test result correlate with multivessel disease and residual jeopardized myocardium, with a combination of both positive being the most specific.[58] Stress ^{201}Tl imaging has also been used late after myocardial infarction to detect multivessel disease. Dunn and associates studied 40 patients with multivessel disease and found that 37

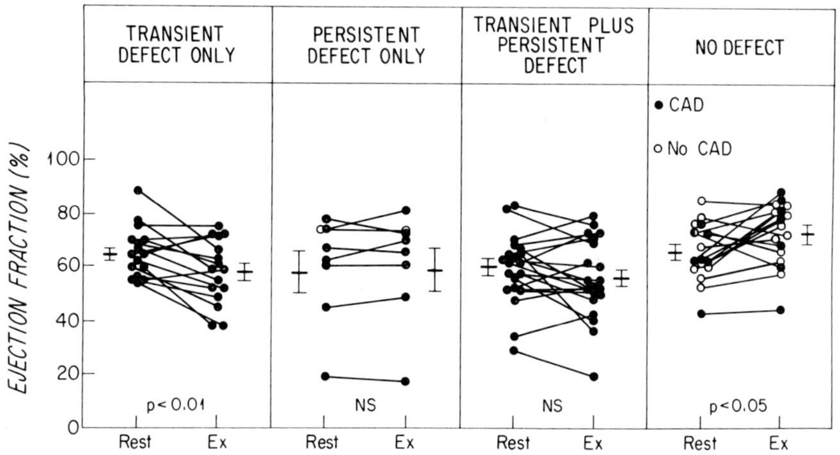

Fig 8–8.—Rest and exercise left ventricular ejection fractions, classified by the results of ^{201}Tl imaging. Means are represented by *bars,* showing ± SEM; *P* values represent comparison between rest and exercise means within the same subgroup. (From Kirshenbaum H.D., et al., *Am. Heart J.* 101:734–741, 1981. Reproduced by permission.)

(85%) had ^{201}Tl defects in more than one vascular area.[59] Of the 37, 92% had multivessel disease.

Stress ^{201}Tl imaging has been used as an indicator of graft patency following coronary artery bypass surgery. When postoperative perfusion improved compared to preoperative values, Ritchie and associates found graft patency in each case.[60] Grafts were patent in 87% of patients with no new perfusion defects postoperatively, compared to 54% of patients with a new perfusion defect postoperatively. Greenberg and associates[61] found that stress ^{201}Tl imaging was sensitive (77%) and specific for postoperative coronary artery stenoses (either graft stenosis or ungrafted native vessel), gave excellent localizing information, and added to the diagnostic accuracy of stress ECG. Others have found that either no postoperative improvement in a preoperative stress ^{201}Tl defect or the development of a new rest ^{201}Tl defect postoperatively is associated with a high incidence of graft occlusion (73% and 86%, respectively).[62] It should be noted that failure of regional myocardial perfusion to improve postoperatively does not preclude alleviation of angina.

Thallium 201 Imaging With Dipyridamole

The idea of performing myocardial perfusion imaging after administration of a coronary vasodilator such as dipyridamole was based on the properties of such agents to increase flow to normal areas in excess of the flow to areas supplied by stenosed vessels. Furthermore, such a technique is theoretically safer than exercise testing, since dipyridamole does not increase myocardial oxygen demands as much as exercise and does not use ischemia as a diagnostic end point. Gould found that myocardial perfusion imaging during dipyridamole-induced coronary vasodilation was a better way to identify moderate coronary stenoses in dogs than perfusion imaging during exercise.[63] Strauss and Pitt used ethyl adenosine–induced coronary vasodilation and produced ^{201}Tl image perfusion defects in dogs with subcritical coronary artery stenoses.[64] In patients, dipyridamole ^{201}Tl radionuclide imaging is performed as follows: A 19-gauge butterfly needle is placed in a large forearm or antecubital vein, since injection of dipyridamole into a smaller vein often results in localized burning discomfort. With the patient supine on a tilt table, the dipyridamole infusion is begun at an infusion rate of 0.142 mg/kg/minute for four minutes. The blood pressure and ECG are recorded at one-minute intervals. Two minutes after termination of the infusion, the table is tilted to approximately 70 degrees, which often results in a small fall in blood pressure. Thallium 201 (1.5–2.0 mCi) is given intravenously, the patient is again placed supine, and imaging is begun. An occasional patient may develop angina pectoris or other side effects which can be treated with aminophylline, a dipyridamole antagonist. The ^{201}Tl myocardial perfusion images obtained after dipyridamole administration are of equal or better quality than those obtained after exercise. The diagnostic accuracy of ^{201}Tl imaging after dipyridamole is comparable to that after exercise. We have found the dipyridamole ^{201}Tl study to be highly sensitive (93%) and specific (85%) for coronary artery disease (Fig 8–9).[65] Furthermore, when initial and delayed images were analyzed, 97% of persistent defects were associated with either hypokinetic or akinetic wall motion at rest, while only 9% of transient defects were associated with akinesis at rest. Thus, the dipyridamole ^{201}Tl study can be

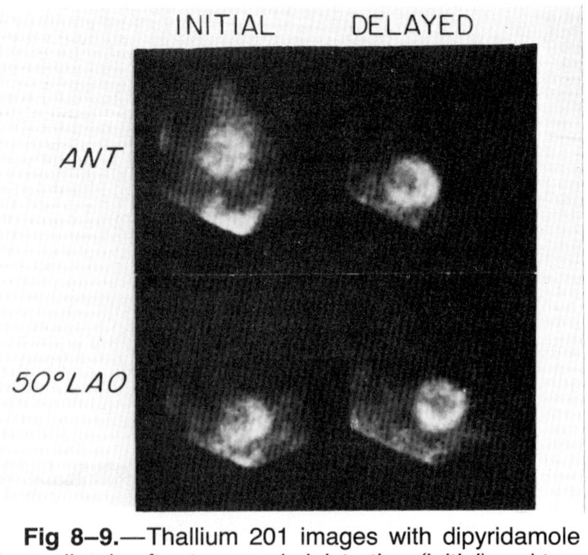

Fig 8–9.—Thallium 201 images with dipyridamole immediately after tracer administration *(initial)* and two hours later *(delayed)*. The initial 50-degree left anterior oblique *(LAO)* image shows a septal perfusion defect that has resolved at the time of the delayed images.

used to detect coronary artery disease and assess myocardial viability.

Thallium 201 Imaging at Rest

Rest ^{201}Tl scan defects were originally reported to correlate with ECG and ventriculographic evidence of myocardial scar from previous infarctions. Rest ^{201}Tl imaging was also found to be useful in localizing and quantifying the extent of prior myocardial infarction.[66] Defects were found to be larger in patients with transmural than with nontransmural infarctions. Small infarctions were often not detected by ^{201}Tl imaging. Although rest ^{201}Tl defects are usually due to myocardial scar, severe resting ischemia can also produce defects. Wackers and associates reported that 63% of patients with unstable angina have rest ^{201}Tl defects during pain-free intervals.[67] Furthermore, rest ^{201}Tl defects were seen more frequently in patients with a complicated course. Gewirtz and associates found that initial rest ^{201}Tl defects due to ischemia often demonstrated ^{201}Tl redistribution on delayed images (Fig 8–10).[5] Transient rest ^{201}Tl defects were found in patients with stable but severe coronary artery disease and were found to correlate with normal or only mildly abnormal left ventricular wall motion. Patients with transient rest ^{201}Tl defects usually demonstrate improvement in initial ^{201}Tl uptake after myocardial revascularization. Transient rest ^{201}Tl defects are also seen in patients with variant angina during an episode of pain.[68]

Rest ^{201}Tl imaging has been used noninvasively to differentiate patients with ischemic cardiomyopathy from those with idiopathic congestive cardiomyopathy. In a study by Bulkley and associates, rest ^{201}Tl images in patients with ischemic cardiomyopathy revealed defects of greater than 40% of the image circumference, whereas studies in patients with idiopathic congestive cardiomyopathy showed defects of less than 20% of the image circumference.[69]

Abnormal rest ^{201}Tl images are seen in patients with an anomalous left coronary artery arising from the pulmonary artery. There is improvement in the ^{201}Tl scan defects after medical therapy for heart failure and after surgical treatment of the anomalous coronary artery. Rest ^{201}Tl imaging has also been used to distinguish patients with an anomalous left coronary artery from those with congestive cardiomyopathy. An anomalous left coronary artery from the pulmonary artery produces localized abnormalities of ^{201}Tl uptake, whereas congestive cardiomyopathy is characterized by homogeneous ^{201}Tl uptake.

The use of rest ^{201}Tl radionuclide imaging in patients with acute myocardial infarction is discussed in chapter 12.

BLOOD POOL IMAGING

Rest Blood Pool Imaging

In 1927, Blumgart and Weiss used a radionuclide technique to measure pulmonary circulation time in normal subjects.[70] Radon was injected into one arm vein, and the time elapsing until appearance of the radionuclide in the opposite arm artery was noted. In 1948, Prinzmetal and associates monitored the transit of a radiotracer through the heart chambers using an external radiation de-

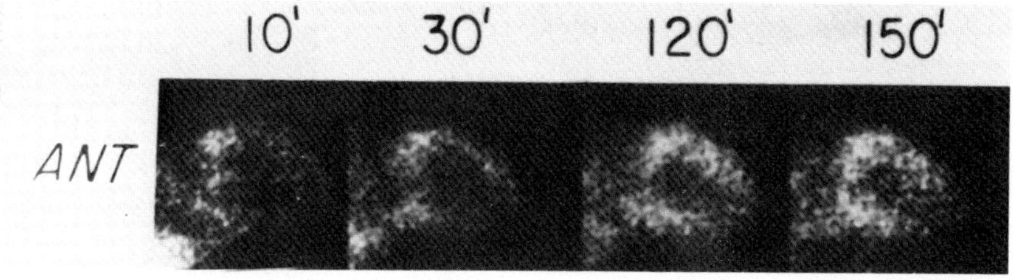

Fig 8–10.—Serial ^{201}Tl images obtained after tracer administration at rest in a patient with chronic stable angina pectoris. By 150 minutes, ^{201}Tl has redistributed to the anterior and inferior walls.

tector.[71] In 1969, Mason and associates used a bolus injection of radiopharmaceutical and rapid sequential visualization of the heart using a gamma camera to study ventricular function (first-pass technique).[72] An end-diastolic image of the heart was obtained by Mullins and associates using R-wave triggering.[73] In 1971, Zaret and associates used ECG gating to obtain both end-systolic and end-diastolic cardiac images.[74] Multigated images obtained at several points (12–64) in the cardiac cycle now allow real-time cinematic display of cardiac motion (gated equilibrium blood pool technique).

Gated Equilibrium Blood Pool Study Procedure

In our laboratory, patients are given 3 mg of stannous pyrophosphate intravenously, then 20 mCi of technetium 99m pertechnetate to complete in vivo red blood cell labeling. Red blood cells can also be labeled in vitro. Patients are then imaged in multiple projections, usually the anterior, left anterior oblique, and left posterior oblique projections. The left anterior oblique projection maximally separates the right and left ventricular chambers (usually 40- to 50-degree left anterior oblique). We use a conventional Anger scintillation camera, a high-resolution parallel-hole collimator, and a commercially available portable imaging computer. A commercially available ECG physiologic synchronizer is used for gating. Some of the variables in the equilibrium blood pool study technique are discussed in a recent review by Ashburn and associates.[75] One important variation is the list mode acquisition technique.[76] List mode acquisition collects all data and stores them in a computer as a function of time. During processing, cycles of nearly uniform length are selected from the total data and are gated. In contrast, the standard gated acquisition technique divides up the cardiac cycle before computer storage, regardless of the cycle length. Thus, list mode acquisition may improve image resolution in situations where heart rate is irregular or changes during the study. However, the list mode technique requires considerable computer storage capacity.

First-Pass Blood Pool Study Procedure

After placement of a peripheral intravenous catheter, 10–20 mCi of ^{99m}Tc-pertechnetate is injected, followed by 15–20 ml of normal saline flush. Sequential images are recorded at short intervals (usually 0.05 second) during the first 20–60 seconds after isotope injection. Various laboratories use different camera projections, including the straight anterior, left anterior oblique, left posterior oblique, and right anterior oblique projections. The right anterior oblique is the most frequently described projection. Usually, only one study can be obtained over a short time because of the relatively long half-life of ^{99m}Tc. The rapid whole body clearance of ^{99m}Tc-diethylenetriamine penta-acetic acid partially overcomes this obstacle. The use of a multicrystal scintillation camera markedly increases the acquisition count rate and thus the statistical reliability. The development of shorter-lived radiopharmaceuticals may make possible serial studies at shorter intervals.

A general description of ventricular function measurements using blood pool imaging techniques was provided in chapter 2.

Clinical Utility of Blood Pool Imaging Techniques

The uses of blood pool imaging techniques in the diagnosis and evaluation of various complications and consequences of acute ischemic coronary artery disease, including septal rupture, left ventricular aneurysm, and mitral regurgitation, were discussed in chapter 4.

As discussed in chapter 2, right and left ventricular ejection fraction, mean circumferential fiber shortening velocity, systolic ejection rates, and relaxation times can be assessed using blood pool imaging techniques. In addition to these indices of ventricular performance, blood pool imaging provides information on chamber sizes, ventricular volumes, and regional wall motion (Fig 8–11). We have compared the interobserver variances for the qualitative determination of regional wall motion on the resting gated blood pool image and the contrast ventriculogram.[77] The interobserver variances for the resting blood pool image were at least comparable to those for the contrast ventriculogram for every segment except the septum (Fig 8–12).

Patients with coronary artery disease may have no abnormalities on resting blood pool imaging. However, in those with an antecedent myocardial infarction, regional wall motion abnormalities can

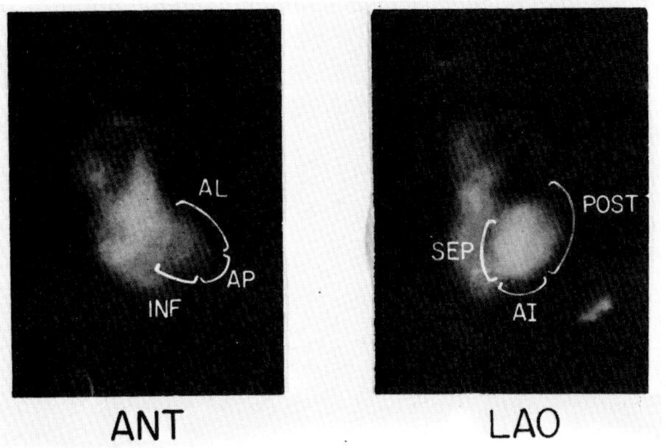

Fig 8–11.—Segmental division of the left ventricular blood pool for regional wall motion assessment. *AI,* apical-inferior segment; *AL,* anterolateral segment; *ANT,* anterior view; *AP,* apical segment; *INF,* inferior segment; *LAO,* left anterior oblique view; *POST,* posterior segment; *SEP,* septal segment. (From Okada R.D., et al.: *Am. J. Cardiol.* Reproduced by permission.)

be demonstrated.[78] Approximately 75% of documented remote myocardial infarctions are detected as wall motion abnormalities on blood pool images.[79] However, small infarctions (< 20 creatine kinase-gram equivalents) are only detectable as wall motion abnormalities in approximately 45% of cases. Wall motion abnormalities correlate with the site of ^{201}Tl perfusion defects in these patients.

Resting blood pool studies are helpful in screening patients for possible coronary artery bypass surgery. Patients with markedly reduced global left ventricular ejection fractions are high surgical risks. Additionally, good wall motion in the face of significant coronary artery disease implies jeopardized but viable myocardium, a situation amenable to coronary artery bypass surgery. The detection of jeopardized but viable myocardium is improved by administering nitroglycerin. An improvement in regional wall motion dyssynergy after nitroglycerin suggests a reversible wall motion abnormality due to myocardial ischemia.[80] The effects of pharmacologic agents on global ventricular function in patients with coronary artery disease have been studied using blood pool imaging.[81] Finally, the effects on left ventricular function of intra-aortic balloon pumping in patients with unstable angina have been assessed by blood pool imaging. Intra-aortic balloon pumping was found to enhance the contraction of ischemic myocardium and to improve ventricular function by reducing end-diastolic and end-systolic volumes.[82]

Exercise Radionuclide Angiography

Borer and associates first described the use of radionuclide angiography in conjunction with exercise stress testing for the diagnosis of coronary artery disease.[76] Normal subjects had an exercise-induced increase in left ventricular ejection fraction, whereas patients with coronary artery disease had no such improvement. Furthermore,

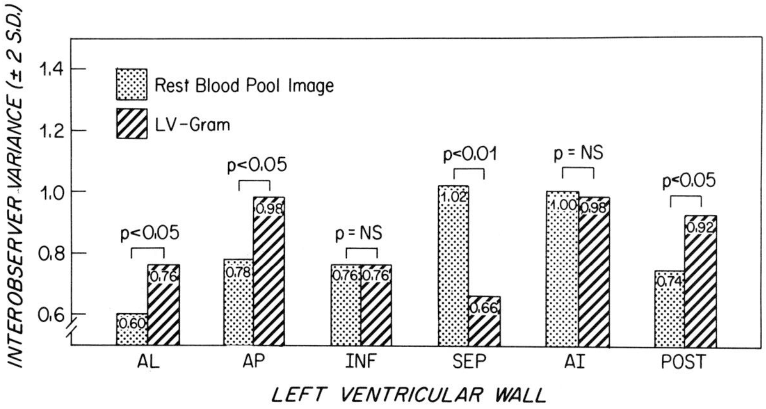

Fig 8–12.—Interobserver variance in the evaluation of left ventricular regional wall motion using the contrast left ventriculogram (LV-Gram) and the rest multigated blood pool image, expressed as ± 2 SD (five-point scoring system). Left ventricular walls are anterolateral *(AL),* apical *(AP),* inferior *(INF),* septal *(SEP),* apical-inferior *(AI),* and posterior *(POST).* (From Okada R.D., et al.: *Circulation* 61:128–136, 1980. Reproduced by permission of the American Heart Association.)

patients with coronary artery disease developed new regional wall motion abnormalities on exercise.

Exercise Technique

In our laboratory, patients exercise in the supine position using a bicycle ergometer. The table is specially equipped with handgrips and shoulder restraints to minimize patient motion. After rest image acquisition using a standard gamma camera, exercise is initiated at 150 kpm/minute and increased by 150 kpm/minute every three minutes. Electrocardiographic leads II, III, and AVF are recorded continuously and 12-lead ECGs and cuff blood pressure are recorded every three minutes. Multigated blood pool images are acquired in the left anterior oblique view during the final two minutes of each three-minute exercise interval. Exercise continues until angina, leg fatigue, or dyspnea occurs.

Other laboratories may use a different camera type, exercise interval duration, exercise position, acquisition technique, and first-pass technique. The high accuracy reported by Borer and associates may be partially due to list mode acquisition.[76] The list mode acquisition technique collects all data as it occurs, then uses only data from uniform cardiac cycles to form the image. This technique improves image quality, especially during graded exercise when heart rate and cycle length are changing. Poliner and associates have shown that the left ventricular ejection fraction response to exercise is accentuated in the upright compared to the supine position.[83]

In our laboratory, rest and peak exercise radionuclide angiograms are displayed side by side in a cinematic mode. The left ventricular wall is divided into six segments (see Fig 8–11). Regional wall motion is scored on a five-point scale: −1 = dyskinesis, 0 = akinesis, +1 = moderate to severe hypokinesis, +2 = mild hypokinesis, +3 = normal wall motion. An exercise-induced fall in wall motion score of one point or more or a rest wall motion score less than 1.5 is sufficient criterion for coronary artery disease. In addition, failure of the left ventricular ejection fraction to increase by at least 5% with exercise is considered evidence for coronary artery disease (Figs 8–13 and 8–14). The normal increase in ejection fraction with exercise has been shown to be due to a decrease in end-systolic volume. The abnormal decrease in

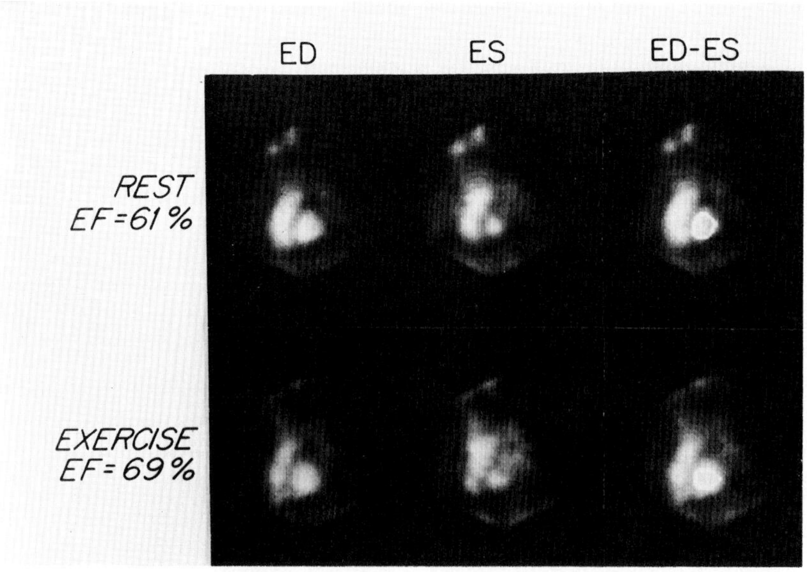

Fig 8–13.—Exercise radionuclide angiography study demonstrating normal ejection fraction *(EF)* response to exercise. *ED*, end-diastolic frame; *ED-ES*, end-diastolic frame with superimposition of end-systolic left ventricular blood pool outline; *ES*, end-systolic frame. (From Okada R.D., et al.: *Am. J. Cardiol.* 46:1188–1204, 1980. Reproduced by permission.)

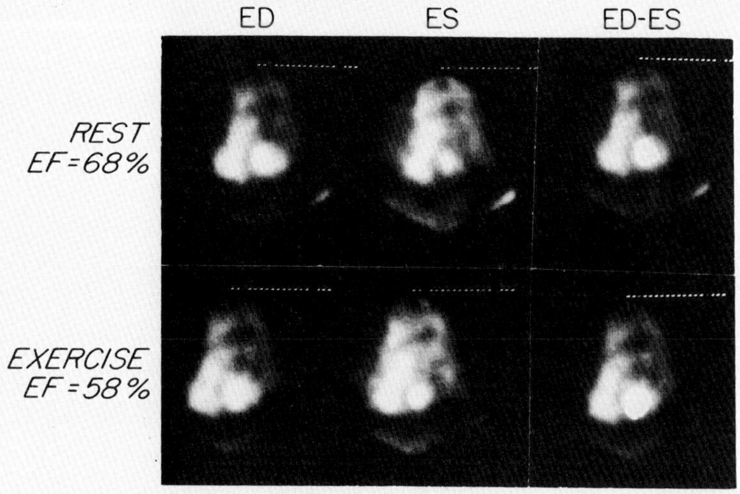

Fig 8–14.—Exercise radionuclide angiography study demonstrating abnormal ejection fraction *(EF)* response to exercise. Abbreviations as in Figure 8–13. (From Okada R.D., et al.: *Am. J. Cardiol.* 46:1188–1204, 1980. Reproduced by permission.)

ejection fraction in patients with coronary artery disease has been shown to be due to an increase in end-systolic volume.

Sensitivity of Radionuclide Angiography

Table 8–2 demonstrates the results of several studies examining the diagnostic accuracy of exercise radionuclide angiography for coronary artery disease. In 499 patients, the overall sensitivity and specificity were 89% and 90% respectively. The ECG stress test had a sensitivity and specificity of 64% and 98%, respectively, in a subset of patients. The improved sensitivity of exercise radionuclide angiography may be due to a lower ischemic threshold for contractile changes compared to electric changes. Using simultaneous exercise radionuclide angiography and ECG stress testing, Upton and associates have shown that abnormalities of left ventricular function frequently develop before angina pectoris or ECG changes.[89] Others have shown a similar sequence in an animal model.[90] Table 8–3 lists factors which have been reported to alter the sensitivity of exercise radionuclide angiography. Although propranolol has been reported to ameliorate the exercise-induced left ventricular dysfunction in patients with coronary artery disease, other workers have found no difference in diagnostic accuracy in patients on and off propranolol.[91] Although isometric stress has been reported to decrease sensitivity, Sonnemaker and associates have used handgrip stress successfully in conjunction with radionuclide angiography.[92]

Right ventricular ejection fraction response to exercise can be assessed by either the first-pass or the gated blood pool technique. Several studies have demonstrated an exercise-induced increase in right ventricular ejection fraction in normal subjects.[93–96] However, the dependence of the right ventricular ejection fraction response on both the presence of right coronary artery disease and the left ventricular response to exercise is debated. Maddahi and associates have demonstrated a significant association only between the right ventricular ejection fraction and the presence of right coronary artery disease,[94] whereas Berger and associates have found only the left ventricular response to exercise to be important.[93] Johnson and associates and Slutsky and associates have found

TABLE 8–2.—SENSITIVITY AND SPECIFICITY OF EXERCISE RADIONUCLIDE ANGIOGRAPHY VERSUS EXERCISE ELECTROCARDIOGRAPHY

			EXERCISE RADIONUCLIDE ANGIOGRAPHY		EXERCISE ECG	
YEAR	STUDY (CITY)	N	Sensitivity	Specificity	Sensitivity	Specificity
1978	Rerych et al. (Durham)[84]	60	29/30	27/30	23/30	. . .
1979	Borer et al. (Bethesda)[85]	84	60/63	21/21	43/63	20/21
1979	Berger et al. (New Haven)[86]	73	52/60	13/13	33/60	13/13
1979	Jengo et al. (Torrance)[87]	19	11/11	8/8	7/11	. . .
1979	Caldwell et al. (Seattle)[32]	39	. . .	. . .	. . .	. . .
1979	Borer et al. (Bethesda)[33]	53	40/43	10/10	. . .	. . .
1979	Verani et al. (Houston)[34]	38	11/21	16/17	. . .	. . .
1979	Kirshenbaum et al. (Boston)[35]	61	38/50	6/11	32/50	11/11
1980	Newman et al. (Duke)[88]	72	55/57	11/15	. . .	. . .
Total		499	296/333 (.89)	112/125 (.90)	138/214	44/45

both the presence of right coronary artery disease and an abnormal left ventricular response to exercise to blunt the normal right ventricular response to exercise.[95, 96]

Specificity of Radionuclide Angiography

Any condition which adversely affects left ventricular functional reserve, such as volume overload, pressure overload, and restrictive states, would be expected to produce an abnormal ejection fraction response to exercise. The following conditions are among those that have been reported to cause an abnormal response: aortic stenosis, aortic regurgitation, mitral regurgitation, mitral valve prolapse, idiopathic hypertrophic subaortic stenosis, chronic obstructive pulmonary disease, β-thalassemia and iron overload, cystic fibrosis, chest pain syndrome with normal coronary arteries, propranolol, and advanced age.

TABLE 8–3.—EXERCISE RADIONUCLIDE ANGIOGRAPHY AND CORONARY ARTERY DISEASE: FACTORS AFFECTING SENSITIVITY

Decreased sensitivity
Inadequate stress
Depressed ejection fraction at rest
Coronary artery collateralization
Propranolol
Nitrates
Isometric stress
Increased sensitivity
ECG evidence of ischemia
Left main coronary artery stenosis
Increasing number of diseased vessels
No change in sensitivity
Cardiac rehabilitation program
Digitalis

Pulmonary Blood Volume Ratio

The ratio of pulmonary blood volume at rest to that on exercise has been determined from exercise radionuclide angiography.[91] The pulmonary blood volume ratio was determined by placing a region of interest over the left lung in the rest and exercise left anterior oblique end-diastolic frames (Fig 8–15). The counts obtained at rest divided into the counts obtained during exercise was the pulmonary blood volume ratio. In the study population of 54 patients, the exercise radionuclide angiogram had a sensitivity for coronary artery disease of 90% with and 64% without the inclusion of the pulmonary blood volume ratio criterion. There was no change in specificity using the pulmonary blood volume ratio.

Observer Variance in the Evaluation of Regional Wall Motion and Ejection Fraction

We have recently determined the interobserver variance for qualitative regional wall motion assessment by radionuclide angiography.[77] Regional wall motion was scored on the five-point scale by three independent observers. Results were analyzed by a two-way analysis of variance and expressed as ± 2 SD. Figure 8–16 demonstrates these variances for the left anterior oblique rest and exercise radionuclide angiograms. Interobserver variances were significantly higher in inter-

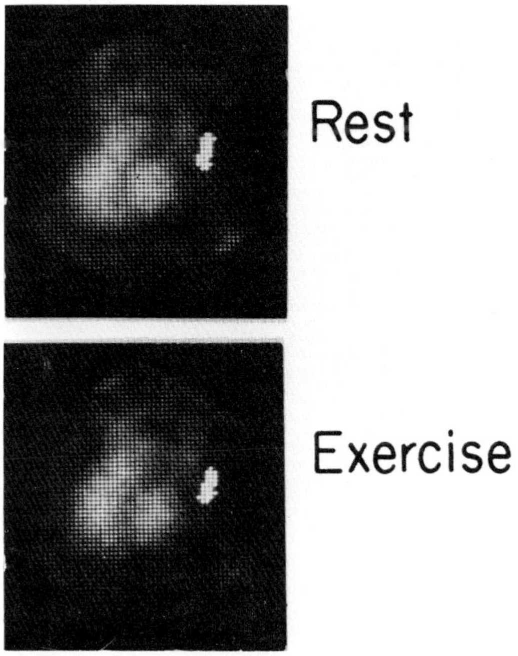

Fig 8–15.—End-diastolic frames for multigated blood pool images in the left anterior oblique projection at rest and during exercise. The regions of interest have been included. The ratio of pulmonary blood volume during exercise to that at rest was 1.16 in this patient, who had substantial coronary artery disease. Notice that the exercise-induced increase in pulmonary activity is not apparent from a visual comparison of the images obtained at rest and during exercise. (From Okada R.D., et al.: *N. Engl. J. Med.* 301:569–576, 1979. Reproduced by permission.)

preting the exercise radionuclide angiograms, especially angiograms of the septum. Interobserver and intraobserver variances in left ventricular ejection fraction determination were also calculated, with values as follows: ± 5.8% and ± 6.0%, respectively, for the rest radionuclide angiogram, ± 9.2% and ± 9.6% for the exercise radionuclide angiogram, and ± 11.0% and ± 11.4% for a change in ejection fraction between rest and exercise (Fig 8–17). However, when a single observer determined the ejection fraction twice for both the rest and exercise studies, and then compared the averaged rest ejection fraction with the averaged exercise ejection fraction, intraobserver variance was reduced to ± 4.6%. Thus, to minimize the error due to observer variance, exercise-induced changes in ejection fraction should be determined by comparing averaged ejection fractions derived from at least two determinations. Upton and associates have reported good reproducibility for rest and exercise left ventricular ejection fraction determinations using first-pass techniques.[97]

Exercise Radionuclide Angiography Versus Exercise Thallium Study

Several studies have attempted to compare the diagnostic accuracy of these two techniques for coronary artery disease.[33–35] When the results from several of these studies were combined (total of 401 patients), the exercise ^{201}Tl study had a sensitivity of 82% and a specificity of 95%. Exercise radionuclide angiography had a sensitivity of 85% and a specificity of 85%. Although the sensitivities were comparable, exercise radionuclide angiography had a significantly lower specificity ($P < .05$ by χ^2 analysis). The lower specificity is probably due to the many conditions other than coronary artery disease that adversely affect ventricular re-

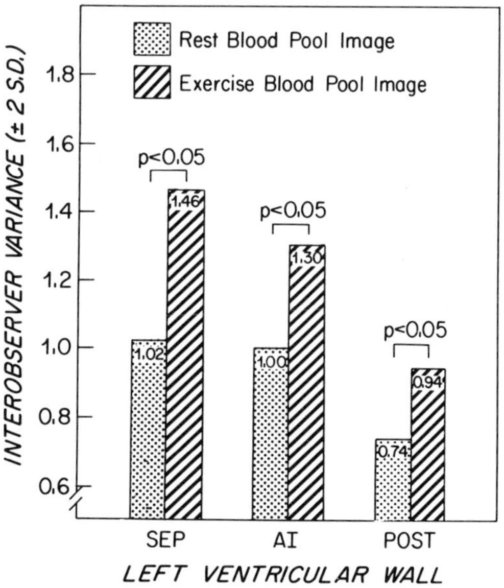

Fig 8–16.—Interobserver variance in the evaluation of left ventricular regional wall motion using the rest and exercise multigated blood pool images, expressed as ± 2 SD (five-point scoring system). Left ventricular walls are septal *(SEP)*, apical-inferior *(AI)*, and posterior *(POST)*. (From Okada R.D., et al.: *Circulation* 61:128–136, 1980. Reproduced by permission.)

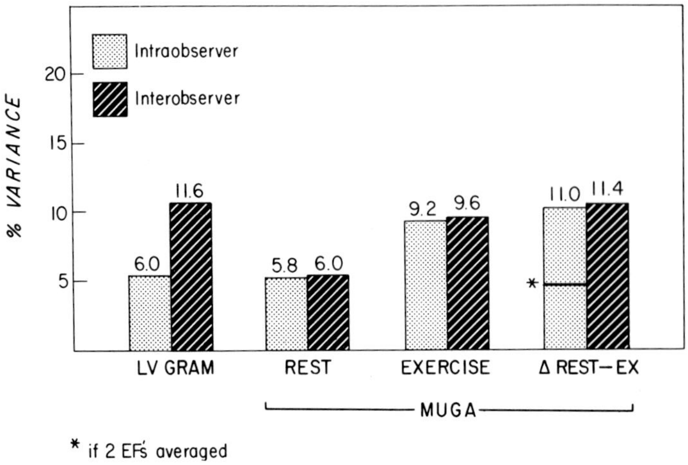

Fig 8–17.—Intraobserver and interobserver variance in the calculation of the left ventricular ejection fraction from rest and exercise gated blood pool studies and from contrast left ventricular angiography. LV-Gram, left ventriculogram; *MUGA,* multigated blood pool study.

serve function. Despite the lower specificity, additional factors must be considered when deciding what is an appropriate test in an individual patient. Table 8–4 lists several relative strengths and weaknesses of the two techniques.

Cold Pressor Test

The cold pressor test has been previously described as a stimulus known to produce vasoconstriction mediated through activation of alpha-adrenergic receptors. The test consists of immersing one hand in ice water for at least one minute. Recently it has been proposed as a substitute for exercise in conjunction with radionuclide angiography. However, preliminary reports vary on the usefulness of the test for detecting coronary artery disease. Sensitivities have ranged from 33% to 97% and specificities from 80% to 100%.[98, 99] The criteria for a normal and abnormal ejection fraction response to the cold pressor test have not been defined.

OTHER CARDIAC IMAGING TECHNIQUES

Radioactive Particles

The use of radioactive particles to estimate regional myocardial blood flow in animals was first described by Ueda and associates.[100] When injected into the coronary circulation, these microparticles were distributed in proportion to flow and were trapped in capillary beds. The heart was excised, cut into small pieces, then counted to determine the distribution of flow. Quinn and associates performed cardiac imaging using a standard gamma camera before and after canine coronary artery occlusion using radioiodinated macroaggregated albumin (MAA) injected into the ascending aorta.[101] Perfusion images of canine myocardium before and after coronary occlusion were thus obtained. Animal studies have demonstrated no adverse hemodynamic effects when particle size and number are controlled. Endo and associates obtained perfusion images in man after a direct injection of ^{131}I-labeled MAA into the left main coronary artery.[102] They proposed that the technique be used in conjunction with contrast coronary angiography to define the hemodynamic significance of coronary artery stenoses. Since that early study, human studies have utilized either human albumin microspheres (HAM) or MAA. The radioisotope has been either ^{99m}Tc, ^{113m}In, ^{123}I, or ^{131}I. Imaging is performed with a standard gamma camera. Rest studies have been performed in one

TABLE 8–4.—STRENGTHS AND WEAKNESSES OF EXERCISE ^{201}Tl IMAGING AND EXERCISE RADIONUCLIDE ANGIOGRAPHY

EXERCISE ^{201}Tl IMAGING	EXERCISE RADIONUCLIDE ANGIOGRAPHY
Strengths	Weaknesses
No definite need for computer	Definite need for computer
Detects ischemia which may precede wall motion abnormality	Detects abnormal left ventricular systolic function which occurs after ischemia
Can be performed in conjunction with routine treadmill exercise ECG	Need special supine exercise table with bicycle ergometer and gating device
May be more specific for coronary artery disease	May be less specific for coronary artery disease
Weaknesses	Strengths
^{201}Tl must be acquired commercially within several days of scheduled test	Technetium is generator produced and readily available
^{201}Tl is expensive compared to technetium	Technetium is inexpensive compared to ^{201}Tl
Expertise needed for qualitative interpretation	Ejection fraction calculation is semiautomated
Functional consequences of perfusion abnormality unknown	Detects functional consequences of ischemia

of two ways. In one technique, two thirds of the radioisotope is injected into the left main coronary artery and one third into the right coronary artery. Unfortunately, the distribution of coronary flow is not exactly two to one. Thus, inhomogeneities in isotope distribution may occur in the absence of coronary artery disease. In the second technique one radioisotope is injected into one coronary artery and a second radioisotope is injected into the other. Composite images are then produced by computer processing. Both techniques suffer from the possibility of unequal streaming of the HAM or MAA into either the left anterior descending or left circumflex coronary arteries after injection into the left main coronary artery. Finally, the radioactive particle technique is invasive, requiring cardiac catheterization. The technique does appear to be associated with minimal morbidity when properly performed.

Radioactive particle image defects at rest in patients with coronary artery disease correspond to left ventricular contraction abnormalities and prior evidence of myocardial infarction. Gould and associates[103] have assessed coronary flow reserve after injection of sodium diatrizoate. With 1-μ incremental constriction of the coronary artery in dogs, they found that resting flow measurements did not decrease until there was 85% stenosis, whereas hyperemia after sodium diatrizoate injection decreased with 30%–45% stenosis. Radioactive particle scanning in these dogs demonstrated perfusion abnormalities in the region of the coronary stenosis. In normal subjects, these investigators found uniform myocardial radioactive particle distribution before and after hyperemia. Patients with significant coronary artery disease but without previous myocardial infarction had inequalities in flow distribution during coronary hyperemia.

Diffusible Tracers

Absolute regional and mean myocardial blood flows can be derived after injection of diffusible tracers into the coronary arteries. The most commonly employed tracers are radioactive gases such as xenon 133 and krypton 81m. Both are chemically inert and physiologically inactive. The technique involves dissolving the radioactive gas in saline, then infusing the saline directly into the coronary artery. Global myocardial tracer activity can be monitored using a standard gamma camera.[104] Alternatively, regional myocardial tracer activity can be monitored using either a multicrystal gamma camera or a single-crystal gamma camera with compartmental regional blood flow analysis.[105] The initial distribution of the tracer is proportional to regional myocardial blood flow. The myocardial clearance rate of the tracer is monoexponential. The monoexponential decay constant can then be used in the Kety formula to calculate absolute myocardial blood flow.[106]

Xenon 133 has a one- to two-minute biologic half-life. This short half-life is primarily due to 95%

or greater first-pass extraction from the lungs. Therefore, expired air is radioactive and must be collected. The 81-keV gamma radiation is used for external imaging. Krypton 81m has an ultrashort half-life of 13 seconds, which allows sequential experiments over a short period. The 190-keV gamma radiation is used for imaging.

Xenon 133 perfusion studies have demonstrated homogeneous myocardial activity in normal subjects and in patients with chest pain and normal coronary arteries.[107] However, mean left ventricular flow rates have been shown to be reduced in patients with two- and three-vessel coronary artery disease.[108] Patients with subcritical and single-vessel coronary artery disease had no significant reduction in mean flows. Regional myocardial blood flow rates have been shown to be depressed throughout the myocardium in patients with multivessel disease, and depressed locally in patients with localized disease.[104] The adequacy of coronary collateral vessels in patients with coronary artery disease has been assessed using injections of ^{133}Xe at rest and during contrast agent–induced hyperemia.[109] Increases in flow during hyperemia were greater in patients with angiographically high-grade noncompromised collateral vessels than in those with lesser-grade collateral vessels. Maseri and associates[110] have demonstrated perfusion defects in patients with coronary artery disease when the tracer was infused during pacing stress.

Myocardial perfusion imaging and blood flow calculations using diffusible tracers are not widely used since the technique requires cardiac catheterization and can be complicated by several technical difficulties. These technical difficulties are related to (1) the inability to distinguish endocardial from epicardial flow, (2) myocardial fat uptake, (3) cardiac motion, and (4) tracer recirculation. Furthermore, changes in myocardial wall thickness during pacing-induced ischemia may alter tracer distribution on the images without an actual change in myocardial tracer activity.

Imaging With Positron-Emitting Radionuclides

Positron-emitting radionuclides are those with an excess of nuclear protons. The positron camera consists of multiple detectors arranged in a multicrystal array opposite to one another. Various cameras employ either opposing heads that rotate around the patient or rings of opposing detectors in which the patient is rotated. When an emitted positron interacts with an orbiting electron, the annihilation of the two particles produces two γ-rays (511-keV) that travel in 180-degree opposite directions. The opposing radiation detectors are used to detect the two γ-rays. Only simultaneous or coincident events are recorded. Thus, the origin of the two γ-rays can be determined along the axis between the two detectors, thereby allowing tomographic reconstructions.

The advantages of positron imaging are several: (1) Most of the positron-emitting radionuclides have a short half-life. Thus, the patient radiation dose is lowered and multiple sequential studies can be obtained. (2) The basic constituents of organic compounds, such as carbon, nitrogen, and oxygen, can be labeled, thus allowing study of myocardial metabolism. (3) The technique is tomographic in nature. (4) There is no attenuation with depth, since each coincident event is a result of two photons traveling the same distance, no matter how far the detector is from the source.

The positron imaging technique has not found widespread clinical applicability for the following reasons: (1) Positron imaging cameras are relatively expensive compared to standard gamma cameras. (2) Because of the short radionuclide half-lives, an on-site cyclotron must be available for many of the tracers. (3) Beta particles produced by positron-emitting radionuclides increase the radiation dose to the patient. (4) The myocardial uptake of metabolically active, labeled agents is determined by perfusion as well as by metabolic factors, making a pure analysis of metabolism difficult.

Patient myocardial perfusion imaging using positron-emitting radionuclides has been performed using rubidium 82.[105] However, the extremely short half-life of 75 seconds makes tomography difficult. Oxygen 15-labeled water, a freely diffusible tracer, has been used to quantitate myocardial blood flow in a manner similar to that using xenon 133.[111] The technique involves invasive cardiac catheterization.

The use of positron-emitting radionuclides to label metabolic substrates has been a unique ap-

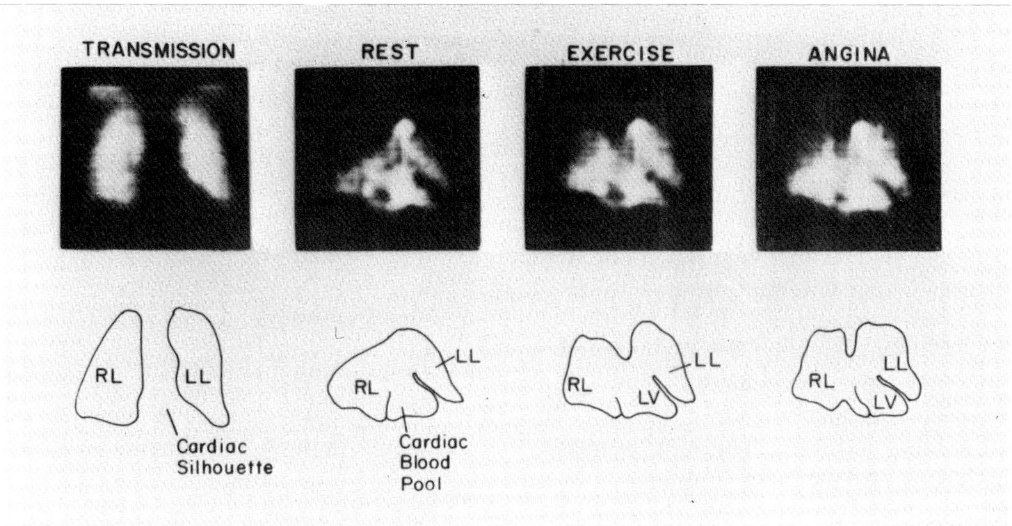

Fig 8–18.—Serial positron images of the chest obtained during rest, exercise, and angina in a 62-year-old man with severe triple-vessel coronary artery disease. During exercise the ^{11}C-carboxyhemoglobin blood label increased over the lung fields, indicating an acute increase in pulmonary blood volume. The cardiac blood pool increased concomitantly, indicating acute left ventricular dilation. The transmission image was obtained with a gallium 68 plane source for correction of chest wall attenuation and for positioning of the patient's chest. *RL,* right lung; *LL,* left lung; *LV,* left ventricle. (From Nichols A.B., et al.: *Circulation* 60:520–530, 1979. Reproduced by permission.)

plication. Nitrogen 13-labeled ammonia defects have been shown to correspond to regions of ischemia and/or infarction in patients. In one series of patients, 24 of 31 stenoses were detected using positron imaging with ^{13}N-labeled ammonia and dipyridamole.[112] Weiss and associates have used carbon 11-labeled palmitate to study fatty acid metabolism in normal and ischemic myocardium.[111] Technical problems with this technique arise from the difficulty in distinguishing uptake related to fatty acid oxidation from uptake related to storage into triglyceride pools.

Nichols and associates used inhaled carbon 11-monoxide and positron imaging to study the effect of exercise-induced myocardial ischemia on cardiopulmonary blood volume in patients with coronary artery disease.[113] Regional ^{11}C activity was measured over the lungs during rest and exercise (Fig 8–18). Pulmonary blood volume increased 18.7% over the upper lung fields and 15% over the lower lung fields at peak exercise for patients developing angina pectoris and ST segment depression. Pulmonary blood volume did not change with exercise for patients without angina or ST segment depression. The increase in pulmonary blood volume response to exercise occurred only in patients with multivessel coronary artery disease and was thought to be due to ischemia-induced left ventricular dysfunction.

REFERENCES

1. Zaret B.L., Strauss H.W., Martin N.D., et al.: Noninvasive regional myocardial perfusion with radioactive potassium. *N. Engl. J. Med.* 288: 809–812, 1973.
2. Berman D.S., Salel A.F., DeNardo G.L., et al.: Noninvasive detection of regional myocardial ischemia using rubidium-81 and the scintillation camera: Comparison with stress electrocardiography in patients with arteriographically documented coronary stenosis. *Circulation* 52:619–626, 1975.
3. Lobowitz E., Green M.W., Fairchild R., et al.: Thallium-201 for medical use. *J. Nucl. Med.* 16:151–155, 1975.
4. Ritchie J.L., Trobaugh G.B., Williams D.L., et al.: Myocardial imaging with thallium-201 at rest and exercise: Correlation with coronary anatomy and exercise electrocardiography. *Circulation* 53, 54(suppl. 2):II–216, 1976.
5. Gewirtz H., Beller G.A., Strauss H.W., et al.: Transient defects of resting thallium scans in pa-

tients with coronary artery disease. *Circulation* 59:707–713, 1979.
6. Pohost G.M., Zir L.M., Moore R.H., et al.: Differentiation of transiently ischemic from infarcted myocardium by serial imaging after a single dose of thallium-201. *Circulation* 55:294–302, 1977.
7. Vogel R.A., Kirch D.L., LeFree M.T., et al.: A new method of multiplanar emission tomography using a 7-pinhole collimator and an Anger scintillation camera. *J. Nucl. Med.* 19:648–654, 1978.
8. Okada R.D., Raessler K.L., Woolfenden J.M., et al.: Sensitivity and specificity in the detection of coronary artery disease: Clinical value of the thallium-201 stress tests. *Int. J. Nucl. Med. Biol.* 5:211–221, 1978.
9. Vrobel T.R., Madison J.D., Schwartz J.S., et al.: Insensitivity of thallium-201 imaging in detecting pacing-induced myocardial ischemia (abstracted). *Circulation* 59,60(suppl. 2):II–172, 1979.
10. Ahmad M., Dubiel J.P., Haibach H., et al.: Cold pressor thallium-201 myocardial scintigraphy in detection of coronary artery disease: An alternative to exercise scintigraphy, abstracted. *Am. J. Cardiol.* 47:444, 1981.
11. Cook D.J., Bailey I., Strauss H.W., et al.: Thallium-201 for myocardial imaging: Appearance of the normal heart. *J. Nucl. Med.* 17:583–589, 1976.
12. Gewirtz H., Grotte G.H., Strauss H.W., et al.: The influence of left ventricular volume and wall motion on myocardial images. *Circulation* 59:1172–1177, 1979.
13. Rifkin R.D., Hood W.B.: Bayesian analysis of electrocardiographic exercise stress testing. *N. Engl. J. Med.* 297:681–686, 1977.
14. Bailey I.K., Griffith L.S.C., Rouleau J., et al.: Thallium-201 myocardial perfusion imaging at rest and during exercise. *Circulation* 55:79–87, 1977.
15. Pohost G.M., Boucher C.A., Zir L.M., et al.: The thallium stress test: The qualitative approach revisited. *Circulation* 59,60(suppl. 2):II–149, 1979.
16. Dash H., Massie B.M., Botvinick E.H., et al.: The noninvasive identification of left main and three-vessel coronary artery disease by myocardial stress perfusion scintigraphy and treadmill exercise electrocardiography. *Circulation* 60:276–283, 1979.
17. Vogel R.A., Kirch D.L., LeFree M.T., et al.: Thallium-201 myocardial perfusion scintigraphy: Results of standard and multi-pinhole tomographic technique. *Am. J. Cardiol.* 43:787–793, 1979.
18. Klein G.J., Kostuk W.J.: Diagnostic accuracy of noninvasive stress myocardial perfusion scanning. *Circulation* 53,54(suppl. 2):II–204, 1976.
19. Peterson K., Tsuji J., Schelbert H., et al.: Improved diagnosis of coronary artery disease during exercise test using a computer processed thallium-201 image. *Circulation* 53,54(suppl. 2):II–207, 1976.
20. Ritchie J.L., Trobaugh G.B., Hamilton G.W., et al.: Myocardial imaging with thallium-201 at rest and during exercise. *Circulation* 56:66–71, 1977.
21. Lenaers A., Block P., van Thiel E., et al.: Segmental analysis of T1-201 stress myocardial scintigraphy. *J. Nucl. Med.* 18:509–516, 1977.
22. Rosenblatt A., Lowenstein J.M., Kerth W., et al.: Post-exercise thallium-201 myocardial scanning: A clinical appraisal. *Am. Heart J.* 94:463–470, 1977.
23. Carrillo A.P., Marks D.S., Pickard D., et al.: Correlation of exercise thallium-201 myocardial scan with coronary arteriograms and the maximal exercise test. *Chest* 73:321–328, 1978.
24. Verani M.S., Marcus M.L., Razzak M.A., et al.: Sensitivity and specificity of thallium-201 perfusion scintigrams under exercise in the diagnosis of coronary artery disease. *J. Nucl. Med.* 19:773–782, 1978.
25. Turner D.A., Battle W.E., Deshmukh H., et al.: The predictive value of myocardial perfusion scintigraphy after stress in patients without previous myocardial infarction. *J. Nucl. Med.* 19:249–255, 1978.
26. Ritchie J.L., Zaret B.L., Strauss H.W., et al.: Myocardial imaging with thallium-201: A multicenter study in patients with angina pectoris or acute myocardial infarction. *Am. J. Cardiol.* 42:345–350, 1978.
27. Bodenheimer M.M., Banka V.S., Fooshee C., et al.: Relationship between regional myocardial perfusion and the presence, severity, and reversibility of asynergy in patients with coronary heart disease. *Circulation* 58:789–795, 1978.
28. Johnstone D.E., Sands M.J., Reduto L.A., et al.: Comparison of exercise radionuclide ventricular performance and thallium-201 myocardial perfusion in coronary artery disease. *Circulation* 57,58(suppl. 2):II–132, 1978.
29. McCarthy D.M., Blood D.K., Sciacca R.R., et al.: Single-dose myocardial perfusion imaging with thallium-201: Application in patients with nondiagnostic electrocardiographic stress tests. *Am. J. Cardiol.* 43:899–906, 1979.
30. Verani M.S., Jhingran S., Attar M., et al.: Post-stress redistribution of thallium-201 in patients with coronary artery disease, with and without prior myocardial infarction. *Am. J. Cardiol.* 43:1114–1122, 1979.
31. Meller J., Goldsmith S.J., Rudin A., et al.: Spectrum of exercise thallium-201 myocardial perfusion imaging in patients with chest pain and normal coronary angiograms. *Am. J. Cardiol.* 43:717–723, 1979.
32. Caldwell J., Sorensen S., Ritchie J., et al.: Exercise radionuclide ventriculography and thallium imaging: Comparison of sensitivity and specificity, abstracted. *Am. J. Cardiol.* 43:432, 1979.
33. Borer J.S., Bacharach S.L., Green M.V., et al.: Sensitivity of stress radionuclide cineangiography and stress thallium perfusion scanning in detecting coronary artery disease, abstracted. *Am. J. Cardiol.* 43:431, 1979.
34. Verani M.S., Del Ventura L., Miller R.R.: Radionuclide ventriculograms during dynamic and

isometric exercise in coronary artery disease: Comparison with exercise thallium-201 scintigrams, abstracted. *Clin. Res.* 27:211A, 1979.

35. Kirshenbaum H.D., Okada R.D., Kushner F.G., et al.: The relation of global left ventricular function with exercise to T1-201 exercise scintigrams, abstracted. *J. Nucl. Med.* 20:687, 1979.
36. Hecht H.S., Blumfield D.E., Mirell S.J.: Superiority of the single-dose exercise and redistribution thallium-201 scan to the electrocardiogram in the diagnosis of myocardial ischemia and infarction, abstracted. *Clin. Res.* 27:174A, 1979.
37. Schicha H., Rentrop P., Facorro L., et al.: Predictive value of thallium scintigraphy in coronary artery disease. *Clin. Cardiol.* 3:184–187, 1980.
38. Botvinick E.H., Taradash M.R., Shames D.M., et al.: Thallium-201 myocardial perfusion scintigraphy for the clinical clarification of normal, abnormal, and equivocal electrocardiographic stress tests. *Am. J. Cardiol.* 41:43–51, 1978.
39. Iskandrian A.S., Wasserman L.A., Anderson G.S., et al.: Merits of stress thallium-201 myocardial perfusion imaging in patients with inconclusive exercise electrocardiograms: Correlation with coronary arteriograms. *Am. J. Cardiol.* 46:553–558, 1980.
40. Berger B.C., Watson D.D., Taylor G.J., et al.: Effect of coronary collateral circulation on regional myocardial perfusion assessed with quantitative thallium-201 scintigraphy. *Am. J. Cardiol.* 46:365–370, 1980.
41. Vogel R., Alderson P., Berman D., et al.: A multicenter comparison of standard and 7-pinhole tomographic T1-201 scintigraphy, abstracted. *Circulation* 62(suppl. III):III–9, 1980.
42. Maddahi J., Garcia E., Berman D., et al.: Quantitative analysis of stress and redistribution T1-201 myocardial scintigrams improves detection and evaluation of extent of coronary artery disease, abstracted. *J. Nucl. Med.* 21:51, 1980.
43. Okada R.D., Boucher C.A., Kirshenbaum H.K., et al.: Improved diagnostic accuracy of thallium-201 stress test using multiple observers and criteria derived from interobserver analysis of variance. *Am. J. Cardiol.* 46:619–624, 1980.
44. Berman D.S., Amsterdam E.A., Joye J.A., et al.: Thallium-201 stress myocardial scintigraphy: Application in asymptomatic patients with positive exercise electrocardiograms, abstracted. *Am. J. Cardiol.* 41:380, 1978.
45. Mews G.C., Zir L.M., Strauss H.W., et al.: A critical look at "subcritical" coronary stenosis with T1-201. *Circulation* 58(suppl. 2):II–181, 1978.
46. Losse B., Kuhn H., Krönert H., et al.: Exercise thallium-201 myocardial perfusion imaging in patients with normal coronary angiogram and ventriculogram. *Circulation* 60(suppl. 2):II–148, 1979.
47. Bailey I.K., Come P.C., Kelly D.T., et al.: Thallium-201 myocardial perfusion imaging in aortic valve stenosis. *Am. J. Cardiol.* 40:889–899, 1977.
48. Ishimori T., Raizner A.E., Verani M.S., et al.: Documentation of ischemic manifestations in patients with myocardial bridges. *Clin. Res.* 27:176, 1979.
49. Moodie D.S., Cook S.A., Gill C.C., et al.: Thallium-201 myocardial imaging in young adults with anomalous left coronary artery arising from the pulmonary artery. *J. Nucl. Med.* 21:1076–1079, 1980.
50. Hanrath P., Montz R., Mathey D., et al.: Comparison between thallium-201 myocardial scintigraphy, myocardial lactate metabolism and coronary angiography in hypertrophic obstructive cardiomyopathy. *Circulation* 57,58(suppl. 2):II–130, 1978.
51. Kushner F.G., Okada R.D., Kirshenbaum H.K., et al.: Lung thallium-201 uptake following stress testing in patients with coronary artery disease. *Circulation* 63:341–347, 1981.
52. Boucher C.A., Zir L.M., Beller G.A., et al.: Increased pulmonary uptake of thallium-201 during exercise myocardial imaging: Clinical, hemodynamic and angiographic implications in patients with coronary artery disease. *Am. J. Cardiol.* 46:189–196, 1980.
53. Kirshenbaum H.D., Okada R.D., Boucher C.A., et al.: Relationship of thallium-201 myocardial perfusion pattern to regional and global left ventricular function with exercise. *Am. Heart J.* 101:734–741, 1981.
54. Massie B.M., Botvinick E.H., Brundage B.H., et al.: Relationship of regional myocardial perfusion to segmental wall motion. *Circulation* 58:1154–1162, 1978.
55. Akins C.W., Pohost G.M., DeSanctis R.W., et al.: Selection of angina-free patients with severe left ventricular dysfunction for myocardial revascularization. *Am. J. Cardiol.* 46:695–700, 1980.
56. Dunn R.F., Freedman B., Bailey I.K., et al.: Exercise thallium imaging: Location of perfusion abnormalities in single-vessel coronary disease. *J. Nucl. Med.* 21:717–722, 1980.
57. Rigo P., Bailey I.K., Griffith S.C., et al.: Value and limitations of segmental analysis of stress thallium myocardial imaging for localization of coronary artery disease. *Circulation* 61:973–981, 1980.
58. Turner J.D., Schwartz K.M., Logic J.R., et al.: Detection of residual jeopardized myocardium 3 weeks after myocardial infarction by exercise testing with thallium-201 myocardial scintigraphy. *Circulation* 61:729–737, 1980.
59. Dunn R.F., Freedman B., Bailey I.K., et al.: Noninvasive prediction of multivessel disease after myocardial infarction. *Circulation* 62:726–734, 1980.
60. Ritchie J.L., Narahara K.A., Trobaugh G.B., et al.: Thallium-201 myocardial imaging before and after coronary revascularization: Assessment of regional myocardial blood flow and graft patency. *Circulation* 56:830–836, 1977.

61. Greenberg B.H., Hart R., Botvinick E.H., et al.: Thallium-201 myocardial perfusion scintigraphy to evaluate patients after coronary bypass surgery. *Am. J. Cardiol.* 42:167–176, 1978.
62. Kolibash A.J., Call T.D., Bush C.A., et al.: Myocardial perfusion as an indicator of graft patency after coronary artery bypass surgery. *Circulation* 61:882–887, 1980.
63. Gould K.L.: Noninvasive assessment of coronary stenoses by myocardial perfusion imaging during pharmacologic coronary vasodilatation: I. Physiologic basis and experimental validation. *Am. J. Cardiol.* 41:267–278, 1978.
64. Strauss H.W., Pitt B.: Noninvasive detection of subcritical coronary arterial narrowings with a coronary vasodilator and myocardial perfusion imaging. *Am. J. Cardiol.* 39:403–406, 1977.
65. Leppo J., Boucher C.A., Okada R.D., et al.: Utility of serial thallium imaging following dipyridamole, abstracted. *Am. J. Cardiol.* 47:483, 1981.
66. Niess G.S., Logic J.R., Russell R.O., et al.: Usefulness and limitations of thallium-201 myocardial scintigraphy in delineating location and size of prior myocardial infarction. *Circulation* 59:1010–1019, 1979.
67. Wackers F.J., Lie K.I., Liem K.L., et al.: Thallium-201 scintigraphy in unstable angina pectoris. *Circulation* 57:738–742, 1978.
68. Maseri A., Parodi O., Severi S., et al.: Transient transmural reduction of myocardial blood flow demonstrated by thallium-201 scintigraphy as a cause of variant angina. *Circulation* 54:280–288, 1976.
69. Bulkley B.H., Hutchins G.M., Bailey I., et al.: Thallium-201 imaging and gated cardiac blood pool scans in patients with ischemic and idiopathic congestive cardiomyopathy. *Circulation* 55:753–760, 1977.
70. Blumgart H.L., Weiss S.: Studies on the velocity of blood flow: VII. The pulmonary circulation time in normal resting individuals. *J. Clin. Invest.* 4:399–425, 1927.
71. Prinzmetal M., Corday E., Bergman H.C., et al.: Radiocardiography: A new method for studying blood flow through chambers of the heart in human beings. *Science* 108:340–341, 1948.
72. Mason D.T., Ashburn W.L., Harbert J.C.: Rapid sequential visualization of the heart and great vessels in man using the wide field Anger scintillation camera. *Circulation* 39:19–28, 1969.
73. Mullins C.B., Mason D.T., Ashburn W.L.: Determination of ventricular volume by radioisotope angiography. *Am. J. Cardiol.* 24:72–78, 1969.
74. Zaret B.L., Strauss H.W., Hurley P.J., et al.: A noninvasive scintiphotographic method for detecting regional ventricular dysfunction in man. *N. Engl. J. Med.* 284:1165–1170, 1971.
75. Ashburn W.L., Schelbert H.R., Verba J.W.: Left ventricular ejection fraction: A review of several radionuclide angiographic approaches using the scintillation camera. *Prog. Cardiovasc. Dis.* 20:267–284, 1978.
76. Borer J.S., Bacharach S.L., Green M.V., et al.: Rapid evaluation of left ventricular function during exercise in patients with coronary artery disease. *Circulation* 53,54(suppl. 2):II–6, 1976.
77. Okada R.D., Kirshenbaum H.D., Kushner F.G., et al.: Observer variance in the qualitative evaluation of left ventricular regional wall motion and the quantitation of left ventricular ejection fraction using rest and exercise multigated blood pool imaging. *Circulation* 61:128–136, 1980.
78. Marshal R.C., Berger H.J., Costin J.C., et al.: Assessment of cardiac performance with quantitation radionuclide angiocardiography: Sequential left ventricular ejection fraction, normalized left ventricular ejection rate, and regional wall motion. *Circulation* 56:820–829, 1977.
79. Tiefenbrunn A.J., Biello D.R., Geltman E.M., et al.: Gated cardiac blood pool imaging and thallium-201 myocardial scintigraphy for detection of remote myocardial infarction. *Am. J. Cardiol.* 47:1–6, 1981.
80. Salel A.F., Berman D.S., DeNardo G.L., et al.: Radionuclide assessment of nitroglycerin influence on abnormal left ventricular segmental contractions in patients with coronary artery disease. *Circulation* 53:975–982, 1976.
81. Marshal R., Berger H.J., Reduto L.A., et al.: Assessment of cardiac performance with quantitative radionuclide angiography: Effects of oral propranolol on global and regional left ventricular fraction in coronary artery disease. *Circulation* 58:808–814, 1978.
82. Nichols A.B., Pohost G.M., Gold H.K., et al.: Left ventricular function during intra-aortic balloon pumping assessed by multigated cardiac blood pool imaging. *Circulation* 58(suppl. 2):176–183, 1978.
83. Poliner L.R., Dehmer G.H., Lewis S.E., et al.: Left ventricular performance in normal subjects: A comparison of the responses to exercise in the upright and supine positions. *Circulation* 62:528–534, 1980.
84. Rerych S.K., Scholz P.M., Newman G.E., et al.: Cardiac function at rest and during exercise in normals and in patients with coronary heart disease. *Ann. Surg.* 187:449–464, 1978.
85. Borer J.S., Kent K.M., Bacharach S.L.: Sensitivity, specificity, and predictive accuracy of radionuclide cineangiography during exercise in patients with coronary artery disease. *Circulation* 60:572–580, 1979.
86. Berger H.J., Reduto L.A., Johnstone D.E., et al.: Global and regional left ventricular response to bicycle exercise in coronary artery disease. *Am. J. Med.* 66:13–21, 1979.
87. Jengo J.A., Oren V., Conant R.: Effects of maximal exercise stress on left ventricular function in

patients with coronary artery disease using first pass radionuclide angiography. *Circulation* 59:60–65, 1979.

88. Newman G.F., Rerych S.K., Upton M.T., et al.: Comparison of electrocardiographic and left ventricular functional changes during exercise. *Circulation* 62:1204–1211, 1980.
89. Upton M.T., Rerych S.K., Newman G.E., et al.: Detecting abnormalities in left ventricular function during exercise before angina and ST-segment depression. *Circulation* 62:341–349, 1980.
90. Scheuer J., Brachfeld N.: Coronary insufficiency: Relations between hemodynamic, electrical and biochemical parameters. *Circ. Res.* 18:178–189, 1966.
91. Okada R.D., Pohost G.M., Kirshenbaum H.D., et al.: Radionuclide-determined change in pulmonary blood volume with exercise: Improved sensitivity of multigated blood-pool scanning in detecting coronary-artery disease. *N. Engl. J. Med.* 301:569–576, 1979.
92. Sonnemaker R.E., Floyd J.L., Ayerdi E., et al.: Ejection fraction response to exercise.: A comparative study of isometric and dynamic exercise. *Circulation* 59,60(suppl. 2):II–7, 1979.
93. Berger H.J., Johnstone D.E., Sands J.M., et al.: Response of right ventricular ejection fraction to upright bicycle exercise in coronary artery disease. *Circulation* 60:1292–1300, 1979.
94. Maddahi J., Berman D.S., Matsuoka D.T., et al.: Right ventricular ejection fraction during exercise in normal subjects and in coronary artery disease patients: Assessment by multiple-gated equilibrium scintigraphy. *Circulation* 62:133–140, 1980.
95. Slutsky R., Hooper W., Gerber K., et al.: Assessment of right ventricular function at rest and during exercise in patients with coronary artery disease: A new approach using equilibrium radionuclide angiography. *Am. J. Cardiol.* 45:63–71, 1980.
96. Johnson L.L., McCarthy D.M., Sciacca R.R., et al.: Right ventricular ejection fraction during exercise in patients with coronary artery disease. *Circulation* 60:1284–1291, 1979.
97. Upton M.T., Rerych S.K., Newman G.E., et al.: The reproducibility of radionuclide angiographic measurements of left ventricular function in normal subjects at rest and during exercise. *Circulation* 62:126–132, 1980.
98. Wynne J., Holman B.L., Mudge G.H., et al.: Clinical utility of cold pressor radionuclide ventriculography in coronary artery disease, abstracted. *Am. J. Cardiol.* 47:444, 1981.
99. Kurtz R.G., Besozzi M.C., Brady T.J., et al.: Cold pressor radionuclide ventriculography. *J. Nucl. Med.* 21:P4, 1980.
100. Ueda H., Kaihara S., Ueda K., et al.: Regional myocardial blood flow measured by I-131 labelled macroaggregated albumin (I-131 MAA). *Jpn. Heart J.* 6:534–538, 1965.
101. Quinn J.L., Serratto M., Kezdi P.: Coronary artery bed photoscanning using radioiodine albumin macroaggregates. *J. Nucl. Med.* 7:107–113, 1966.
102. Endo M., Yamazaki T., Konno S., et al.: The direct diagnosis of human myocardial ischemia using ^{131}I-MAA via the selective coronary catheter. *Am. Heart J.* 80:498–506, 1970.
103. Gould K.L., Hamilton G.W., Lipscomb K., et al.: Method for assessing stress-induced regional malperfusion during coronary arteriography: Experimental validation and clinical application. *Am. J. Cardiol.* 34:557–564, 1974.
104. Ross R.S., Ueda K., Lichtlen P.R., et al.: Measurement of myocardial blood flow in animals and man by selective injection of radioactive inert gas into the coronary arteries. *Circ. Res.* 15:28–41, 1964.
105. Cannon P.J., Haft J.I., Johnson P.M.: Visual assessment of regional myocardial perfusion utilizing radioactive xenon and scintillation photography. *Circulation* 40:277–288, 1969.
106. Kety S.S.: Blood-tissue exchange methods: Theory of blood-tissue exchange and its application to measurement of blood flow. *Methods Med. Res.* 8:223–227, 1960.
107. Cannon P.J., Dell R.B., Dwyer E.M. Jr.: Measurement of regional myocardial perfusion in man with xenon-133 and a scintillation camera. *J. Clin. Invest.* 51:964–977, 1972.
108. Cannon P.J., Schmidt D.H., Weiss M.B., et al.: The relationship between regional myocardial perfusion at rest and arteriographic lesions in patients with coronary atherosclerosis. *J. Clin. Invest.* 56:1442–1454, 1975.
109. Cohn P.F., Maddox D.E., Holman B.L., et al.: Effect of coronary collateral vessels on regional myocardial blood flow in patients with coronary artery disease: Relation of collateral circulation to vasodilatory reserve and left ventricular function. *Am. J. Cardiol.* 46:359–364, 1980.
110. Maseri A., L'Abbatte A., Pesola A., et al.: Regional myocardial perfusion in patients with atherosclerotic coronary artery disease at rest and during angina pectoris induced by tachycardia. *Circulation* 55:423–433, 1977.
111. Weiss E.S., Siegel B.A., Sobel B.E., et al.: Evaluation of myocardial metabolism and perfusion with positron-emitting radionuclides. *Prog. Cardiovasc. Dis.* 20:191–206, 1977.
112. Schelbert H.R., Wisenberg G., Gould K.L., et al.: Detection of coronary artery stenosis in man by positron emission computed tomography and N-13 ammonia, abstracted. *Circulation* 60:II–60, 1979.
113. Nichols A.B., Strauss H.W., Moore R.H., et al.: Acute changes in cardiopulmonary blood volume during upright exercise stress testing in patients with coronary artery disease. *Circulation* 60:520–530, 1979.

COMMENT: CORONARY ARTERY DISEASE

Gerald M. Pohost

WITH THE ADVENT of medical and surgical therapeutic approaches that can ameliorate symptoms and increase longevity in patients with coronary artery disease, noninvasive detection and evaluation of the extent of disease have become important applications of both echocardiography and radionuclide imaging. The diagnostic evaluation of patients with possible coronary artery disease is best undertaken by considering which of the following subclassifications is represented: (1) chronic ischemic heart disease, such as a stress-related chest pain syndrome; (2) acute ischemic heart disease, such as acute myocardial infarction or unstable angina; and (3) complications of acute or chronic ischemic heart disease, such as left ventricular aneurysm or papillary muscle dysfunction. First, let us review the functional consequences of coronary artery disease and the imaging study which is most appropriate to detect that consequence.

The primary process, that of coronary arterial narrowing due to atherosclerosis, can occasionally be assessed by echocardiography when it is localized to the proximal vessels. The secondary process, that of ischemia, is initiated by a reduction in regional blood flow or an inadequate rise in regional blood flow when myocardial metabolic requirements increase in response to a stress. Such changes in regional blood flow can be assessed noninvasively using radionuclide myocardial perfusion imaging. There are no other noninvasive approaches to assess regional myocardial perfusion. The tracer (e.g., thallium 201) can be used to assess myocardial flow distribution at rest, during exercise, or during infusion of dipyridamole to induce myocardial hyperemia.

When blood flow is inadequate to sustain myocardial metabolic demand, the myocardial phosphocreatine level falls rapidly and regional myocardial function begins to deteriorate. Regional myocardial function can be assessed by echocardiography (two-dimensional studies are far superior to M-mode), by radionuclide cineangiography, by digital subtraction angiography (DSA) after an intravenous dose of a radiopaque contrast medium, or by gated proton nuclear magnetic resonance (NMR) tomography (see chap. 25). In the future it may be possible to monitor the concentration of myocardial high-energy phosphates such as phosphocreatine using NMR approaches.

In the case of assessment of regional wall motion at rest, two-dimensional echocardiography (2DE) is probably the first imaging study to be recommended in view of the following advantages: high resolution, ability to assess both wall excursion and thickening, ability to assess wall motion beat by beat, somewhat lower cost, and nonionizing radiation. However, the technical difficulty and limited perspective of echocardiography make it less than optimal for assessing global ventricular performance. Radionuclide cineangiography (RNA), using either the multigated acquisition blood pool study or the first-pass approach, is useful for evaluating global and regional wall motion with substantially lower spatial resolution than with echocardiography. However, the radionuclide approaches are best for evaluating global ventricular function (ejection fraction). RNA uses changes in radioactivity within the chamber that do not depend on ventricular geometry, and they provide information on the entire ventricular chamber, not just a series of ice pick views or a set of planes through the chamber. Further, it is technically easier to perform radionuclide cineangiography than echocardiography. High-resolution cineangiography of the ventricles now can be done after intravenous radiopaque contrast medium injection, using DSA. This approach, while producing high-resolution ventriculographic imagery for the assessment of regional and global function (which will be analyzed by geometry-independent densitometry in the future), has two disadvantages. It requires an expensive addition to an existing fluoroscopic system, and it requires the intravascular injection of contrast medium. Currently there is little justification for using DSA as the first approach, since other, less invasive ultrasound and radionuclide methods are adequate.

When regional or global ventricular function is to be assessed during exercise, echocardiography is less desirable than radionuclide cineangiography, owing to technical difficulty. In addition to some appreciation of changes in regional wall motion, radionuclide imaging allows the physician to assess the exercise-related changes in left ventricular ejection fraction, in right ventricular ejection fraction, and in pulmonary blood volume reflecting changes in left atrial pressure. Radionuclide studies are technically adequate in almost all patients, while echocardiography is technically adequate in about 80% of patients.

Shortly after wall motion becomes abnormal, the next step in the sequence of abnormalities that take place during ischemic insult is change in ECG repolarization. Thus, significant ST segment depression that occurs with anginal chest pain is virtually diagnostic of coronary artery disease, although it does not indicate the extent of disease.

Persisting ischemic insult leads to xmarked adenosine triphosphate reduction with a consequent increase in the inorganic phosphate level and, ultimately, irreversible myocardial injury. Such injury is associated with loss of cell membrane integrity and resultant loss of intracellular constituents, such as inorganic phosphate and enzymes, and intracellular access to larger extracellular molecular species, such as protein. Thallium 201 studies in fetal mouse heart organ culture suggest that thallium begins to be released from myocardial cells as soon as irreversible damage occurs. Accordingly, quantitative analysis of serial myocardial images after an intravenous dose of ^{201}Tl might provide insight into myocardial viability. Other experimental methods which may ultimately provide early clinical insight into myocardial viability include measurement of changes in ultrasound attenuation, evaluation of proton NMR relaxation parameters, and assessment of myocardial high-energy phosphate levels using ^{31}P NMR methods. Presently, the most realistic of these approaches is evaluation of proton NMR relaxation parameters. Data on stroke induced by middle cerebral artery occlusion in cats demonstrate that ischemic necrosis of brain tissue can be detected as soon as two hours after occlusion (see chap. 25). Finally, 12–24 hours after infarction, technetium 99m stannous pyrophosphate uptake can be visualized by gamma camera radionuclide imaging.

EVALUATION OF PATIENTS WITH CHRONIC STABLE CHEST PAIN

The first problem to be addressed in patients with chronic chest pain is the diagnosis of its etiology. A history of typical Heberden's angina or of well-documented myocardial infarction is virtually diagnostic of coronary artery disease. Obviously, risk factors such as age, sex, family history, hypertension, increased cholesterol levels, diabetes, or smoking should be considered in estimating the likelihood of coronary artery disease before any test is performed. Next, the rest ECG must be evaluated. Significant Q waves are reasonably specific for coronary artery disease. In addition, ST-T waves must be evaluated. If repolarization is abnormal due to digitalis therapy, left ventricular hypertrophy, left bundle-branch block, or similar problems, an exercise ECG will be difficult to interpret and another study might be necessary. If the repolarization phase on the ECG is reasonably normal, it is most appropriate for diagnostic purposes to obtain an exercise ECG. If the exercise ECG is positive and chest pain is reproduced, the diagnosis of coronary artery disease is reasonably assured. If chest pain is absent and the ECG is negative at a near-maximal level of exercise, fixed coronary artery disease is unlikely. If the diagnosis is still in question, as might be the case if the ECG is positive but there is no chest pain or vice versa, a radionuclide study is the next appropriate study. Since ^{201}Tl imaging appears more specific than but equally as sensitive as radionuclide cineangiography, the exercise or dipyridamole ^{201}Tl study should be performed next. If the patient is unlikely to achieve 85% or more of peak predicted heart rate with exercise stress (due to lack of fitness, propranolol therapy, or disability), a dipyridamole ^{201}Tl study is probably superior to exercise testing; otherwise an exercise stress test is preferred. If the result of the ^{201}Tl study is ambiguous, radionuclide cineangiography should be performed. In expert hands, stress echocardiography, although technically difficult, might provide satisfactory results.

More important than the problem of diagnosis is the prognosis: What is the probability that the patient will have a catastrophic coronary event such as myocardial infarction or sudden death? Although complete data are not yet available, the radionuclide approaches appear to have substantial predictive power. In patients that have had a previous myocardial infarction, the risk appears to be strongly related to resting left ventricular ejection fraction, which is best determined noninvasively by radionuclide cineangiography. In patients that have had no previous myocardial infarction, data from our laboratory suggest that the number of transient (ischemic) ^{201}Tl defects is an excellent predictor of risk. Data from others suggest that the extent of left ventricular functional deterioration during exercise radionuclide cineangiography has similar predictive power. Thus, prognosis appears to be related to the extent of myocardial damage (or survival) in patients with previous myocardial infarction and to the extent of myocardium at risk in patients without previous myocardial infarction. Since the echocardiogram has a more limited window than the radionuclide studies, it is unlikely to provide a measure of the global extent of disease in the asymmetric coronary artery pathologic process.

EVALUATION OF PATIENTS SUSPECTED OF HAVING ACUTE ISCHEMIC HEART DISEASE

Similarly, there are two components to the evaluation of patients presenting with acute chest pain: diagnosis and prognosis. Diagnostic evaluation is different in these patients since stress testing is not possible or necessary to elicit an abnormality. Accordingly, both regional myocardial perfusion and regional left ventricular function would be expected to be abnormal. In the early hours (6 hours or less) of infarction, ^{201}Tl studies are positive in more than 90% of patients. As time passes after the acute event, the incidence of positive ^{201}Tl studies in patients with acute myocardial infarction decreases. For instance, after 24 hours, only 70%-80% of patients have positive ^{201}Tl studies. The stress and the ischemia associated with the acute event are partly responsible for the loss in sensitivity over time. Serial ^{201}Tl imaging is helpful in distinguishing between ischemic but viable and infarcted myocardium. However, there is no way to differentiate between acute infarct and myocardial scar using ^{201}Tl imaging.

The ejection fraction and degree of regional ventricular wall motion are helpful in assessing the degree of dysfunction. Wall motion abnormalities also occur with a high frequency in patients with acute ischemic events. Echocardiography demonstrates wall motion abnormalities in patients with myocardial infarction but is not as reliable as radionuclide cineangiography in assessing global ventricular function. Wall motion, however, is abnormal in patients with ischemia, acute infarction, and myocardial scar. Finally, ^{99m}Tc (stannous) pyrophosphate studies frequently demonstrate a "hot spot" in patients with acute myocardial infarction between 24–48 hours and one week after the acute event. This approach provides a means of differentiating between acute infarction and myocardial scar. It is useful when routine diagnostic methods fail to establish the diagnosis, especially in patients who present 24–72 hours after the onset of chest pain or in patients who have undergone cardiac surgery.

Recent data suggest that gamma-camera imaging after intravenous administration of radiolabeled cardiac myosin specific antibody allows earlier and more specific detection of clinical myocardial infarction than pyrophosphate does. FAb fragments of such antibody gain intracellular access with loss of membrane integrity.

Prognosis after acute myocardial infarction is related to the extent of myocardial infarct. The resting ejection fraction and the extent of persistent ^{201}Tl deficit have been shown to have prognostic power. Recent work has suggested that ECG, ^{201}Tl imaging, and radionuclide cineangiography during low-level stress may provide additional prognostic information when performed at the time of hospital discharge. In addition, a pyrophosphate study which demonstrates an annular appearance or remains positive for two weeks or more after the acute event has been shown to be associated with a worse prognosis.

EVALUATION OF THE COMPLICATIONS OF ISCHEMIC HEART DISEASE

The noninvasive imaging methods have been of considerable benefit in evaluating the complications of ischemic heart disease. These complications occur primarily following myocardial infarction and include left ventricular aneurysm, left ventricular pseudoaneurysm, rupture of the interventircular septum, papillary muscle dysfunction and rupture, and pericardial effusion. Generally, it is best to begin the diagnostic evaluation with echocardiography, since ultrasound can detect all the complications just listed. Radionuclide cineangiography is a good means of detecting ventricular aneurysm and pseudoaneurysm, and myocardial perfusion imaging is of help in evaluating the extent of infarction. With aneurysm, a discrete, moderate-sized defect is usually found, and the size of the ^{201} Tl defect is smaller than expected from the wall motion abnormality. This disparity is frequently even more marked with pseudoaneurysm, in which the akinetic zone may attain great size while the 201 Tl defect remains relatively small.

PART V

Acute Myocardial Ischemia

ECHOCARDIOGRAPHY

Daniel David, Chin C. Chen, and Joel Morganroth

THE CONTRACTILE PROPERTIES of the myocardial cell are closely linked to its metabolic state. Acute myocardial ischemia causes immediate and profound deterioration of myocardial contraction. The detection of acute change in myocardial contractility can, therefore, serve as a diagnostic marker for acute myocardial ischemia. This chapter reviews the role of echocardiography in the noninvasive detection of acute myocardial wall motion abnormalities as they relate to diagnostic considerations in the detection of spontaneous or exercise-induced myocardial ischemia and the acute phase of myocardial infarction.

ACUTE MYOCARDIAL ISCHEMIA

Animal Experiments

The experimental induction of acute myocardial ischemia results in almost instantaneous metabolic changes.[1] Within 30 to 60 seconds of myocardial ischemia, a marked decrease in the phosphocreatine level and a concomitant rise in inorganic orthophosphate and lactate levels can be detected. These changes reflect the instantaneous decrease in adenosine triphosphate synthesis and the accelerated process of anaerobic carbohydrate breakdown.[1, 2] The ischemia-induced hyperacute severe metabolic derangements result in profound mechanical changes which become apparent as global changes in the contractile pattern of the heart and as regional wall motion abnormalities. The changes in contractile patterns were first noted by Tennant and Wiggers[3] and were later confirmed in a number of experimental studies.[4–6] The hallmarks of acute ischemic changes in the affected myocardium are (1) hypocontractility, (2) paradoxic systolic motion, (3) loss of systolic thickening,[7, 8] and (4) an increase in ventricular internal dimensions. The normally perfused areas, however, may show a compensatory hypercontractile pattern (Table 9–1). These mechanical alterations precede the commonly accepted electric signs and criteria for myocardial ischemia, i.e., ST segment and T wave changes.[9, 10]

During the past ten years, ultrasonic methods have been used to study the effect of acute myocardial ischemia on wall motion properties.[11–16] Changes in wall motion patterns as well as a progressive increase in ventricular volume begin approximately 10 seconds after the initiation of experimental myocardial ischemia (Fig 9–1). The velocity of wall motion decreases, and soon a fragmentation of contraction pattern can be seen (Figs 9–2,B and C). This marks the transition into a pattern of paradoxic wall motion in which the ischemic segment moves away from the center of the ventricle during systole. The second clinically important feature of acute myocardial ischemia is the loss of systolic thickening of the myocardium (see Figs 9–2,B and C, and Fig 9–3). The extent of loss of systolic wall thickening is related to the ex-

TABLE 9–1.—REGIONAL WALL MOTION ABNORMALITIES DETECTED IN EXPERIMENTAL ANIMALS BY ULTRASONIC TECHNIQUES

ISCHEMIC OR INJURED AREA	
	Fragmentation of contraction
	Abnormal bulging during isovolumic systole
	Decreased amplitude of motion during systolic ejection
	Decreased velocity of motion during systolic ejection
	Impaired systolic wall thickening
NORMALLY PERFUSED AREA	
	Compensatory hyperactivity in healthy remote areas
	Transitional wall motion abnormalities in adjacent areas

tent of transmural involvement of the infarct.[17] Echocardiography has also demonstrated and confirmed that mechanical changes precede the commonly accepted electric signs of myocardial ischemia by at least 20–30 seconds (Fig 9–4).[18] Wall motion abnormalities detected by echocardiography may even be present in ischemic events that result only in minor ECG alterations. Thus, echocardiographic changes constitute a sensitive index for the presence of acute ischemia.

During the hyperacute phase of ischemia, the

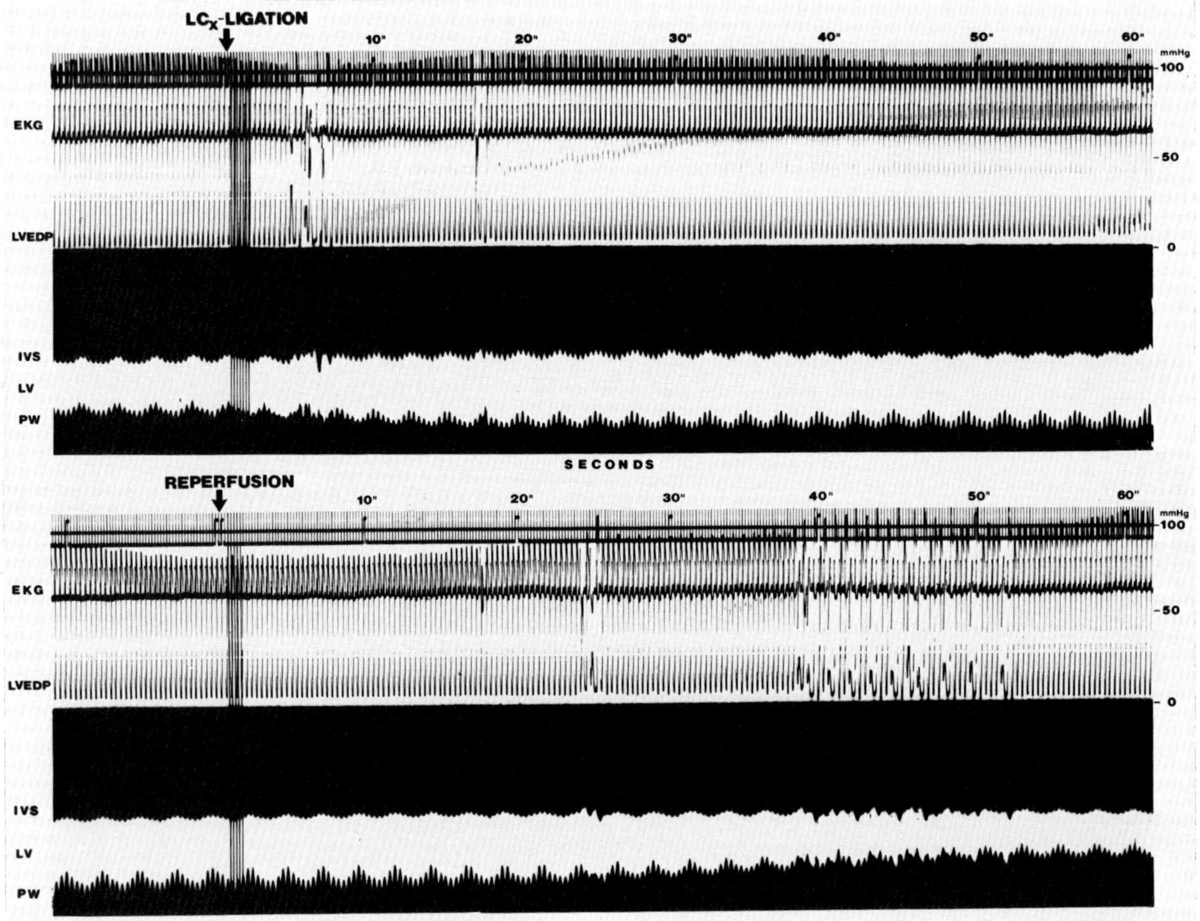

Fig 9–1.—*Top,* an M-mode echocardiographic trend recording of the left ventricle during the hyperacute experimental ligation period of the left circumflex coronary artery. *Bottom,* the immediate postreperfusion period. In both panels the electrocardiogram and left ventricular end-diastolic pressure *(LVEDP)* are recorded simultaneously with the echocardiogram that depicts the intraventricular septum *(IVS),* the left ventricular cavity *(LV),* and the left ventricular posterior wall *(PW).* Time from ligation and reperfusion is marked in 10-second intervals. Within 10 seconds after ligation *(top),* posterior wall motion pattern changes and the LV cavity size increases markedly and assumes its maximum expansion at 15–20 seconds. The LVEDP shows a concomitant gradual increase. Restitution of LV cavity size and LVEDP following reperfusion *(bottom)* is a much slower process.

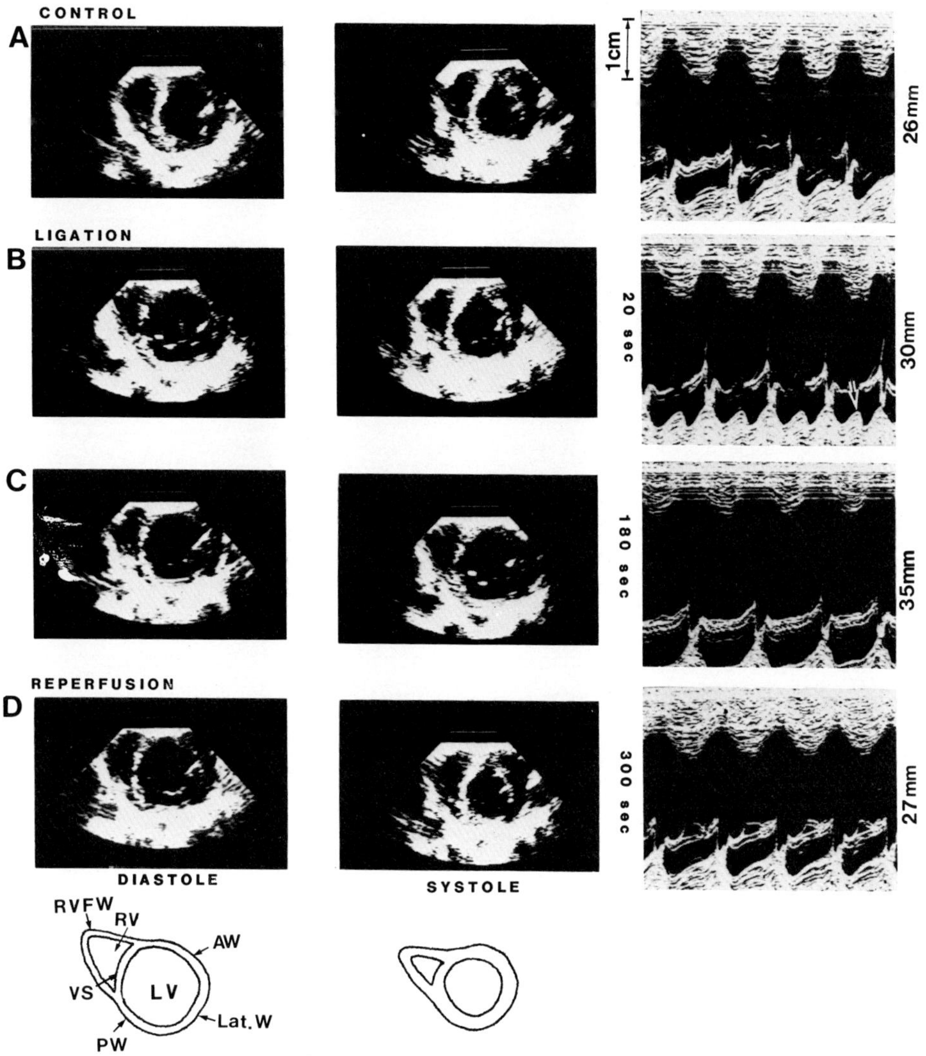

Fig 9–2.—The two-dimensional short-axis diastolic and systolic still frames as well as the corresponding M-mode recording of the left ventricular cavity demonstrate four stages of an experimental acute circumflex coronary artery ligation and reperfusion study. The short-axis views were taken at the level of the papillary muscles and depict the left and right ventricular *(LV, RV)* cavities. The anatomical location of the septum *(VS)* and the anterior *(AW)*, lateral *(Lat. W)*, and posterior walls *(PW)* as well as RV free wall *(RVFW)*, are depicted in the diagram below. As early as 20 seconds after coronary artery ligation, *(B)*, left ventricular cavity size both in the two-dimensional and M-mode has increased markedly (26 to 30 mm). The posterior wall on the M-mode echocardiogram shows a fragmentation of the contractile pattern which marks the transition into a paradoxic motion pattern and a further LV cavity increase *(C)*. Left ventricular cavity size and contractile pattern normalize 300 seconds after reperfusion *(D)*.

normal myocardium may show a compensatory hypercontractile pattern which gradually subsides and returns to the preischemic pattern after a short time. At that time the ischemic wall assumes a pattern of paradoxic hypocontractile motion.

Following reperfusion of the myocardium (after a short ischemic period), a reversal in the time sequence of normalization of electric and mechanical phenomena occurs.[18] The ECG ST-T segment changes return to control during the first minute after reinstitution of blood flow to the ischemic myocardium, whereas the depression of contrac-

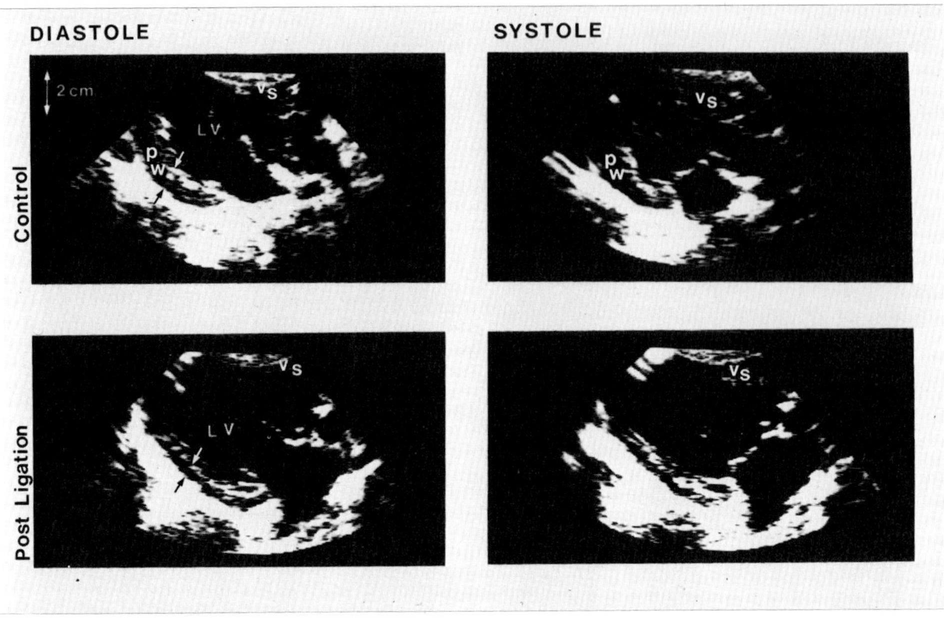

Fig 9–3.—Long-axis views of the left heart in diastole and systole during control and following experimental left circumflex coronary artery ligation. Note the diastolic thinning and inadequate systolic thickening of the posterior wall *(PW)* which are the echocardiographic hallmarks of acute myocardial ischemia *(arrows). VS,* ventricular spetum; *LV,* left ventricle.

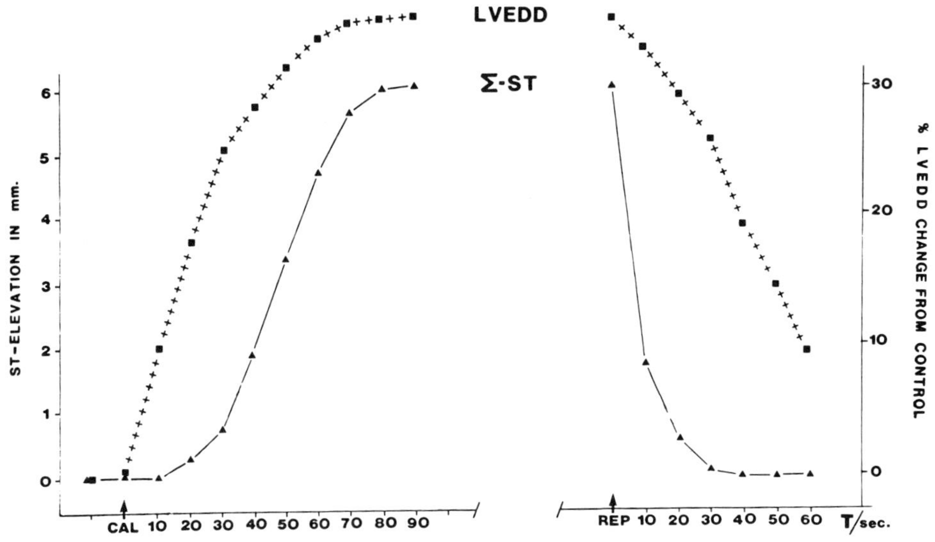

Fig 9–4.—Time course of electric and mechanical events immediately following an acute coronary artery ligation *(CAL)* and reperfusion *(REP)* in the canine model. Temporal left ventricular end-diastolic dimensional changes *(LVEDD)* in percent change from control are plotted against ST segment elevation in mm (Σ-*ST*). Whereas left ventricular volume increases almost immediately after CAL, an ST segment elevation of 1 mm or more is attained only 30–40 seconds after CAL. Following reperfusion, the reversal of electric and mechanical events can be seen. The ST segment returns to about normal range within 10–20 seconds after REP, whereas LVEDD shows a protracted course of normalization.

tility and the wall motion abnormalities undergo a protracted course of recovery that can last for minutes and even hours, depending on the duration of the ischemic process (Fig 9–2,D; Fig 9–4).[15, 18] Two-dimensional echocardiography (2DE) has also been used by Meltzer et al.[19] to estimate infarct size and the influence of various drugs such as phenylephrine and nitroglycerin on the extent of experimental myocardial damage.

These data suggest that: (1) Noninvasive echocardiographic visualization of wall motion abnormalities resulting from acute myocardial ischemia is possible. (2) Since mechanical changes are an early and sensitive index for ischemia, this method may be clinically suitable for detecting acute myocardial ischemia, coronary spasm, the acute phase of acute myocardial infarction, and ischemia induced by exercise stress testing. (3) Wall motion abnormalities as demonstrated by echocardiography may precede ECG changes of ischemia and may be the only sign of an ischemic process.

Clinical Observations

Spontaneously occurring transient myocardial ischemic attacks were observed by Widlansky et al.[20] using M-mode echocardiography in a patient with Prinzmetal's angina. The observed changes in myocardial contraction patterns showed a remarkable similarity to the results of the animal experiments cited above and underscore their validity. The patient had angiographically documented arterial spasm but no fixed obstruction in the distribution of the left anterior descending coronary artery. During ischemic episodes characterized by chest pain and associated with ST segment elevation and T wave peaking in the midprecordial leads, there was a marked loss of amplitude of systolic septal motion. The amplitude of septal motion returned to normal as the clinical episodes abated and ECG manifestations of the ischemic process resolved.

More common, and clinically more important, are transient myocardial ischemic episodes induced by exercise stress testing. This test constitutes a major step in the diagnostic evaluation of patients suffering from obstructive coronary artery disease. The sensitivity and specificity of the ECG changes in the diagnosis of exercise-induced ischemia are a subject of extensive research. Any noninvasive technique that has the ability to improve the predictive accuracy of exercise testing may enhance its power in the diagnosis of coronary patients. The previous section demonstrated the ability of echocardiography to detect acute episodes of myocardial ischemia. It follows, therefore, that exercise-induced wall motion abnormalities in the coronary patient can be diagnosed by echocardiography. New regional wall motion abnormalities have been demonstrated during exercise-induced ischemia by left ventricular cineangiography[21] and cardiac nuclear imaging techniques.[22]

The advantages of echocardiography over angiography or nuclear imaging are that it is the only technique in which dynamic changes in myocardial wall thickening in different regions of the heart can be evaluated. It is, of course, noninvasive, easily repeatable, and inexpensive. Echocardiography does not alter the function of the ventricle as angiographic contrast dye may, and a large number of cardiac cycles before, during, and after intervention can be studied. Compared to stress radionuclide angiography, echocardiography follows instantaneous events rather than combining several cardiac cycles. Moreover, it imposes no radiation exposure. Echocardiography can be used to evaluate changes in wall thickening as well as endocardial motion which cannot be assessed by gated blood pool scanning techniques.

M-Mode Echocardiography

Using M-mode echocardiography, Fogelman et al.[23] studied posterior wall motion in 30 normal subjects and 9 patients with coronary disease during 13 episodes of angina provoked by exercise. A significant increase in systolic and diastolic wall motion characteristics was observed in normal subjects during exercise; however, in the patients with coronary artery disease, resting overall wall motion characteristics were lower than in the normal subjects. During the initial phases of exercise these wall motion characteristics increased, but by the time the patients reached the angina level, wall motion in the ischemic region slowed markedly and fell below the resting values. These changes were reversible after the anginal attack had abated. (Table 9–2).

TABLE 9–2.—EXERCISE ECHOCARDIOGRAPHY

STUDY	NO. OF PATIENTS	FEASIBILITY	NEW RWMA† CORRELATED WITH: ANGINA	THALLIUM PERFUSION DEFECTS	ECG ST CHANGES
		M-Mode Echocardiography			
Fogelman et al.[23]*	39	Not stated	5/5	Not performed	39/39
Mason et al.[24]*	54	45%	13/13	Not performed	Not stated
		Two-Dimensional Echocardiography			
Wann et al.[25]	28	71%	10/10	6/6	4/10
Romijn et al.[26]	34	80%	14/15	13/15	Not stated
Morganroth et al.[27]	55	78%	19/20	Not performed	15/19

*Selected groups of patients.
†RWMA, regional wall motion abnormalities.

Mason et al.[24] examined 54 men during exercise testing. In only 13 (45%) patients and 11 normal volunteers could an analyzable echocardiographic recording during exercise be obtained (see Table 9–2). Changes in systolic wall thickening and left ventricular cavity dimensions during exercise were evaluated. Increased systolic wall thickening during exercise was seen in a significant number of myocardial segments recorded in the normal volunteers, whereas a reduction in systolic wall thickening during exercise was the hallmark in patients with coronary obstructive disease. A similar pattern was noted in regards to ventricular dimensional changes. During exercise in the normal volunteers, systolic percent change in ventricular diameter increased significantly as compared to the resting state. In the coronary patients, however, systolic percent change in ventricular diameter decreased significantly. These results emphasize the efficacy of M-mode echocardiography in the diagnosis of acute ischemia induced by exercise. The greatest limitation of exercise M-mode echocardiography is the difficulty of obtaining high-quality echocardiograms during exercise and the inherent problems of limited viewing areas.

Two-Dimensional Echocardiographic Studies

Recent endeavors in the use of 2DE in the detection of acute transient regional wall motion abnormalities have shown that 2DE provides better visual orientation than M-mode echocardiography. Wann et al.[25] studied 28 patients; analyzable echocardiographic data obtained during exercise in 20 (71%). In 10 patients with angiographically proved coronary stenosis, new areas of reversible segmental wall motion abnormalities during exercise echocardiography were found. Six of those 10 patients had reversible thallium 201 perfusion defects in areas corresponding to the regional wall motion abnormalities detected by echocardiography. It is important to note that of the 10 patients showing new regional wall motion abnormalities on exercise echocardiography, only 4 had exercise-induced ECG signs of ischemia (see Table 9–2). In a similar study by Romijn et al.,[26] 34 consecutive patients without previously known myocardial infarction were studied; 80% of the studies were analyzable. Fourteen of 15 patients with proved significant coronary artery disease and only 1 of 12 from the normal group had exercise-induced new wall motion abnormalities detected by 2DE. These results correlated well with radionuclide studies (see Table 9–2). Recently, we prospectively studied 55 patients undergoing diagnostic coronary angiography.[27] Analyzable exercise cross-sectional echocardiographic results were available in 43 (78%) (see Table 9–2). In 20 patients new regional wall motion abnormalities were detected during exercise (Fig 9–5), and in 19 of those 20, significant coronary artery disease was

TABLE 9–3.—ECHOCARDIOGRAPHIC FINDINGS DURING EXERCISE IN PATIENTS WITH CORONARY ARTERY DISEASE

Increase in contractility during ischemia-free exercise
Marked decrease in wall motion characteristics during exercise-induced ischemia
Increase in left ventricular internal dimensions during ischemia
Reversal of wall motion changes with subsequent rest

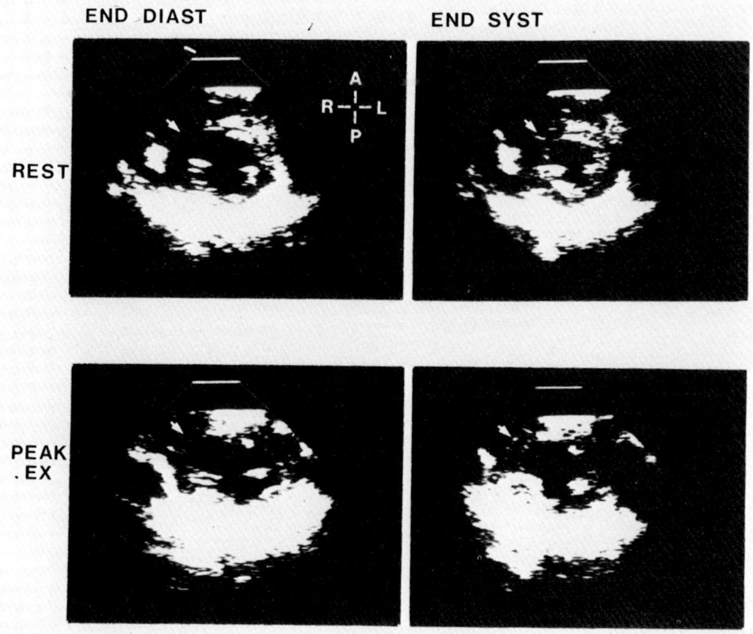

Fig 9–5.—Left ventricular short-axis end-systolic *(left)* and end-diastolic *(right)* views at the level of the papillary muscle in a patient with severe triple-vessel coronary artery disease and exercise-induced angina pectoris. *Small white arrow* points to the ventricular septum which, during rest *(top)* shows a normal systolic motion. However, during peak exercise *(bottom)*, the ventricular septum becomes markedly dyskinetic. Note also the marked increased in end-systolic volume during peak exercise, suggesting a decrease in regional ejection fraction. (From Morganroth J., et al.: *Am. J. Cardiol.* 47:20–26, 1981. Reproduced by permission of the *American Journal of Cardiology.*)

diagnosed angiographically. The 1 patient with new regional wall motion abnormality detected by normal angiography had cardiomyopathy. Of the 21 patients in whom no exercise-induced regional wall motion abnormalities were detected, 10 had normal coronary arteries on angiography, whereas 11 had significant coronary obstructive disease.

Thus, from the few studies available, it may be concluded that echocardiography is capable of detecting new regional wall motion abnormalities caused by acute myocardial ischemia occurring spontaneously or induced by exercise testing. These results suggest that exercise-induced regional wall motion abnormalities, as summarized in Table 9–3, are specific for the presence of ischemic heart disease; however, their absence does not exclude important coronary obstruction. The use of exercise 2DE improves the ability to obtain analyzable data, and the expected yield is in the range of 70%-80%. However, more data are necessary in order to evaluate the sensitivity and specificity of this method alone or in conjunction with ECG changes and other methods in the exercise evaluation of the coronary patient.

ACUTE MYOCARDIAL INFARCTION

M-Mode Echocardiography

Depression of the ischemic wall motion and an increase in ventricular volume during acute myocardial infarction were diagnosed on M-mode echocardiography as early as 1972 (Fig 9–6).[28, 29] Stud-

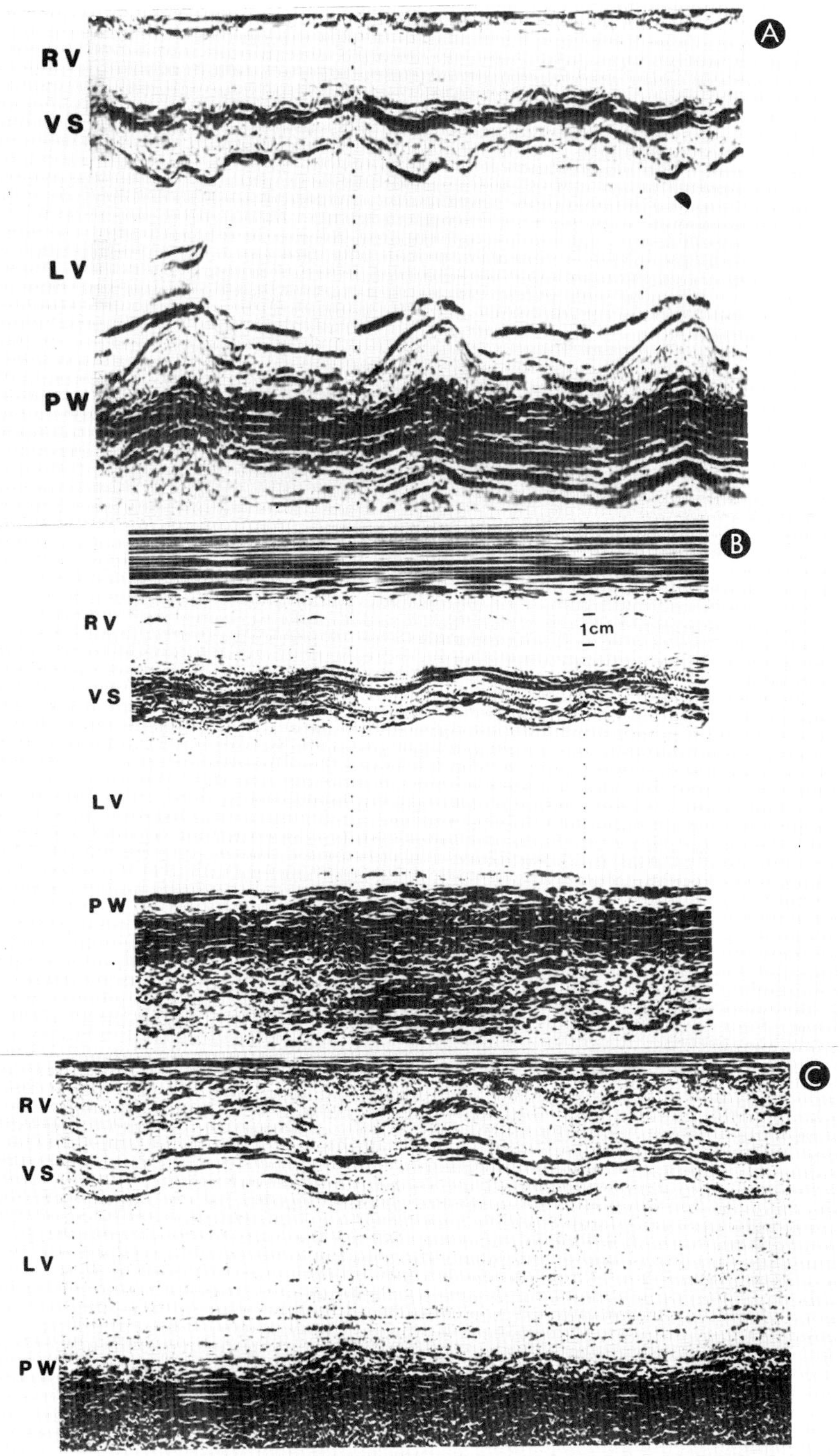
A
RV
VS
LV
PW
B
RV
1cm
VS
LV
PW
C
RV
VS
LV
PW

ies in patients admitted to coronary care units with the diagnosis of acute myocardial infarction have further confirmed that impaired amplitude of wall motion is highly associated with regional myocardial ischemia. In a series of 64 patients with acute transmural myocardial infarction, Corya et al.[30] reported abnormal echocardiographic wall motion that corresponded with the ECG site of infarction in 84% of cases (Table 9–4). In 30%, a hypercontractile motion pattern in the noninfarcted areas compatible with the results cited above in the animal experiments was seen. In another study by Heikkila and Nieminen,[31] a more lateral positioning of the M-mode echocardiographic transducer was used in order to detect wall motion abnormalities in the anterior wall and parts of the lateral wall. Using this approach, absent or paradoxic anterior left ventricular wall motion was a frequent finding in patients with anterior infarction, while anterior wall motion abnormalities were rarely seen in patients with inferior infarction (see Table 9–4).

Echocardiographically detected abnormal regional wall motion should not always be equated with coronary artery disease. Corya et al.[32] demonstrated that regional wall motion abnormalities on M-mode echocardiography may not be caused by coronary ischemia alone. Similar abnormalities can also be due to the motion of the entire heart within the chest, abnormal electric conduction patterns, and relative diastolic volume overload of the right and left ventricles such as seen in atrial septal defect. Ischemia induced by conditions other than coronary artery disease, such as idiopathic congestive cardiomyopathy, may also cause abnormal regional wall motion abnormalities. According to Corya et al.,[32] the loss of systolic thickening of the myocardium during the transition from diastole to systole seems to be the most important distinguishing feature of true acute myocardial ischemia. In their series of 40 patients with acute myocardial infarction (composed of equal numbers with anterior and inferior infarction), 18 of the 20 with anterior myocardial infarctions had abnormally decreased septal systolic thickening. Nineteen had abnormally decreased septal motion, and 18 had both decreased septal thickening and abnormal motion (see Table 9–4). Interestingly, 11 of these patients had systolic septal thinning. Of the 20 patients with inferior infarction, 13 had abnormally decreased posterior wall thickening, 18 had abnormally decreased posterior wall motion, and 13 had both thickening and wall motion abnormalities. Systolic thinning of the posterior wall was infrequently recorded. The authors concluded that abnormalities of wall motion and systolic thickening can be seen in cases other than acute ischemia—for instance, in patients with chronic coronary artery disease, especially those with antecedent myocardial infarction, and in some patients with cardiomyopathy. Systolic thinning, however, is highly suggestive of acute injury since it is an unusual finding outside the setting of acute myocardial ischemia. Nieminen and Heikkila[33] demonstrated abnormal wall motion patterns of the acutely infarcted left ventricular regions in all of 70 consecutively studied patients. Asynergy and paradoxic motion in the first 24 hours of infarct were typical for anterior wall infarction, whereas inferior wall infarcts showed hypokinesis or akinesis rather than paradoxic motion. From a prognostic point of view, it is interesting to note that in patients that subsequently died, no recovery of contractile patterns of the ischemic region and no compensatory hypercontractility of the normal segments were noticed (see Table 9–4).[33, 34] In another study from the same center, Heikkila and Nieminen[35] reported a good statistical correlation between the modifications in abnormal ST and T segment distribution caused by various drug interventions and wall motion abnormalities during acute myocardial ischemia (see Table 9–4). An in-

Fig 9–6.—M-mode echocardiographic changes during the course of an acute inferior wall myocardial infarction. **A,** a normally contracting posterior wall. Note the normal pattern of systolic thickening. **B,** during the acute phase of myocardial infarction, the posterior wall becomes akinetic and loses its ability for systolic thickening. However, the overall thickness of the posterior wall is not yet markedly reduced. **C,** the chronic state after the development of fibrosis in the posterior wall. Note loss of contractility, systolic thickening, and overall thinning of the posterior wall. *RV,* right ventricular cavity; *VS,* intraventricular septum; *LV,* left ventricular cavity; *PW,* left ventricular posterior wall.

TABLE 9–4.—ECHOCARDIOGRAPHY IN ACUTE MYOCARDIAL INFARCTION

		LOCATION AND EXTENT OF NEW RWMA* CORRELATED WITH	
STUDY	NO. OF PATIENTS	ECG SITE OF INFARCTION	OTHER PARAMETERS
		M-Mode Echocardiography	
Corya et al.[30]	64	84%	Rate of complications (CHF); mortality
Heikkila and Nieminen[31]	30	100%	Pathology (17 patients); rate of complications (CHF)
Corya et al.[32]	40	92%	. . .
Nieminen and Heikkila[33]	70	100%	Prognosis
Heikkila and Nieminen[35]	42	88%	Improvement in RWM in response to drug intervention
		Two-Dimensional Echocardiography	
Nixon et al.[39]	29	89%	Thallium 201 and Tc pyrophosphate radionuclide imaging
Heger et al.[40, 41]	37	97%	Pathology (4 patients); left ventricular function[50]
Horowitz et al.[42]	33	94%	Prognosis
Horowitz et al.[43]	60	87%	Cumulative CPK-MB curves; rate of complications (CHF, arrhythmias)

*RWMA, regional wall motion abnormalities.

crease in ischemia, as judged by the increase in ST segment shifts, was accompanied by deterioration of the contractile function of the ischemic region, and vice versa. The specific question of the prognostic value of M-mode echocardiography in patients with acute anteroseptal myocardial infarction was studied by Weiner et al.[36] In all 40 patients included in their study, the ECG presence of Q waves in the anterior wall indicated anterior wall infarction. Twenty-one patients had normal septal motion and systolic thickening, whereas 19 had abnormalities of one or both of these parameters. Only 5 patients of the 21 with normal septal motion developed congestive heart failure, but none of them died. Of the 19 patients with abnormal septal motion, 17 developed congestive heart failure and 6 died. These authors concluded, therefore, that although echocardiographic findings of septal motion were not diagnostic for anterior infarction, they were of marked prognostic value (see Table 9–4).

The use of M-mode recordings in the detection of regional wall motion abnormalities has important limitations that have been well defined.[37] The ice pick view of M-mode echocardiography does not allow for simultaneous evaluation of multiple regional wall motion changes or evaluation of many areas of the ventricle. For example, the left ventricular apex is rarely well examined by M-mode echocardiography. Because of these limitations, 2DE has a theoretical advantage of not only detecting multiple tomographic views of the left ventricle, but also in the determination of ventricle shape and function.

Two-Dimensional Echocardiography

Two-dimensional echocardiography offers the ability to evaluate regional abnormalities of myocardial motion with greater facility than M-mode echocardiography, since the field of the examination is not restricted to the narrow M-mode beam and the spatial orientation of the tomographic sections can be appreciated. Only a few studies on the specific role of 2DE in the diagnosis of acute myocardial infarction have been published. As early as 1977, Kisslo et al.[38] reported that 2DE studies lent themselves as readily to quantitative examination of regional wall motion abnormalities as did left ventricular cineangiograms. A good correlation between the radionuclide study and 2DE evaluation of the location and extent of the acute ischemic process have been reported by Nixon et al.,[39] thus confirming that 2DE is a reliable method to detect and localize regional contraction abnormalities during acute myocardial infarction and correlates well with the hemodynamic state of the patient (see Table 9–4).

In an attempt to use 2DE as a diagnostic tool for acute myocardial infarction, Heger et al.[40] studied 44 patients with acute myocardial infarction. These authors suggested a nine-segment subdivision of the left ventricle which included anterior, medial, posterior, and lateral quadrants at the mitral and papillary muscle levels and an apical segment recorded by placing the transducer directly over the apex and obtaining a long-axis scan. Complete studies allowing evaluation of these nine segments were achieved in 37 of 44 attempts. Nineteen of 20 patients with inferior infarction had asynergy in posterior segments; 14 patients with anterior infarction had asynergy in anterior segments; and in 3 patients with both anterior and inferior infarction, wall motion abnormalities were appropriately localized. In 4 patients, later pathologic localization of the infarction corresponded to the asynergic areas detected on 2DE (see Table 9–4). In a subsequent study by the same group and using the same criteria,[41] segmental asynergy was detected in all 44 patients with acute myocardial infarction. By wall motion criteria, patients could be separated into those having uneventful myocardial infarction, those having congestive heart failure, and those having other complications, such as acute ventricular septal defect ar acute mitral regurgitation. With a similar goal, we[42] studied a group of 80 patients admitted to the emergency room with acute chest pain syndrome. The echocardiographic short-axis view at the level of the papillary muscle and the mitral valve was obtained, as were the long-axis and the apical four-chamber views (Fig 9–7). Adequate 2DE studies were obtained in 65 patients (81%). Thirty-three patients had clinical evidence of acute myocardial infarction. Of those, 31 (94%) had regional wall motion abnormalities on the initial study. Thirty-two patients eventually did not develop myocardial infarction, and 27 of them (84%) did not show regional wall motion abnormalities on the first 2DE study (see Table 9–4). The group of patients showing initial regional wall motion abnormalities had an increased incidence of complications. In those patients without initial regional wall motion abnormalities, no complications were encountered. This study stresses the possible importance of 2DE in the diagnostic evaluation of the patient with acute chest pain syndrome and suggests some of the prognostic values of this noninvasive method. In a serial follow-up study of patients with acute myocardial infarction, we further studied 60 consecutive patients.[43] Dyskinetic and akinetic myocardial segments on serial 2DE studies were scored and related to the ECG localization and extent of the infarct, the rate of CPK-

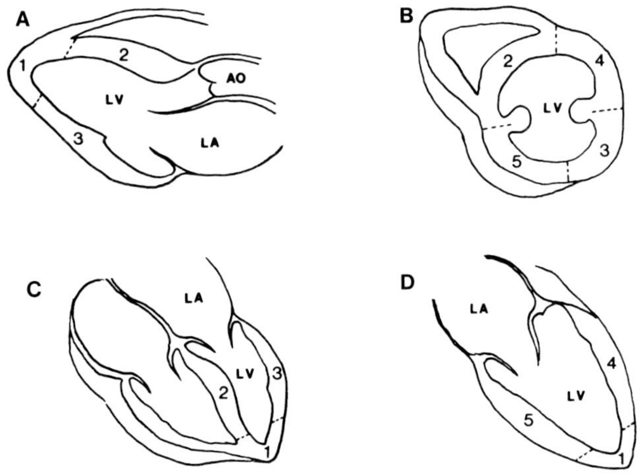

Fig 9–7.—Segmental delineation for the evaluation of segmental wall motion changes during acute myocardial infarction. The left ventricle was divided into 5 segments: apical *(1)*, septal *(2)*, lateral *(3)*, anterior *(4)*, and posterior *(5)*. Their relative location in the various two-dimensional views, long-axis *(A)*, short-axis *(B)*, apical four-chamber *(C)*, and apical two-chamber *(D)*, is shown. *LV*, left ventricle; *LA*, left atrium; *Ao*, aorta.

MB, and the clinical course. Analyzable data were obtained in 43 (71%) of the patients. In general, the segmental localization and scoring coincided with the ECG and enzymatic data. The mean abnormal segmental score for the whole group was 6.2 ± 3.8. This was significantly lower, 4.7 ± 3.4, in a subgroup of 26 patients with nontransmural infarction. Patients who developed complications had a significantly higher abnormal segmental score (8.4 ± 3.8) than the group with an uneventful course (4.3 ± 2.7). The prognostic value of 2DE in the course of acute myocardial infarction was also studied by Eaton et al.[44] Serial 2DE studies in 28 patients during the first two weeks after myocardial infarction were performed. Diastolic short-axis 2DEs at the level of the tips of the papillary muscles were evaluated serially in this study. The first echocardiogram was obtained within 60 hours of the acute event. Segment length and wall thickness were calculated by tracing endocardial and epicardial outlines using a computer-aided semiautomated contouring system. Eight patients showed evidence of infarct expansion with a proportional transmural thinning of the infarct zone and associated left ventricular dilation, while the remaining 20 patients failed to show these changes

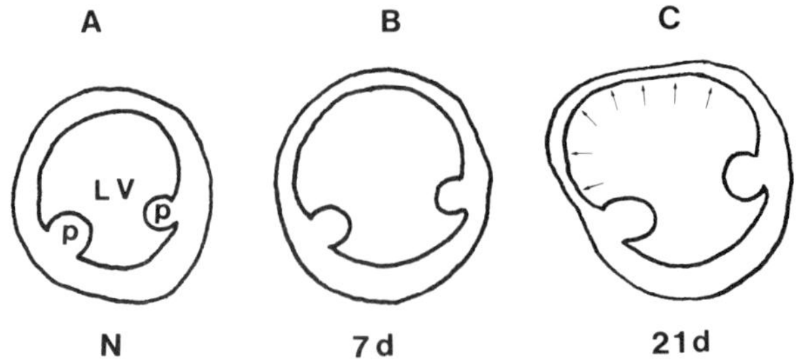

Fig 9–8.—Schematic delineation of short-axis views of the left ventricle *(LV)* at the level of the papillary muscles *(P)* in the normal patient *(A)*, 7 days after acute anterior wall myocardial infarction *(B)*, and 21 days later *(C)*. Note thinning of the wall and especially the expansion of the infarcted zone (adapted from Eaton et al.[44]).

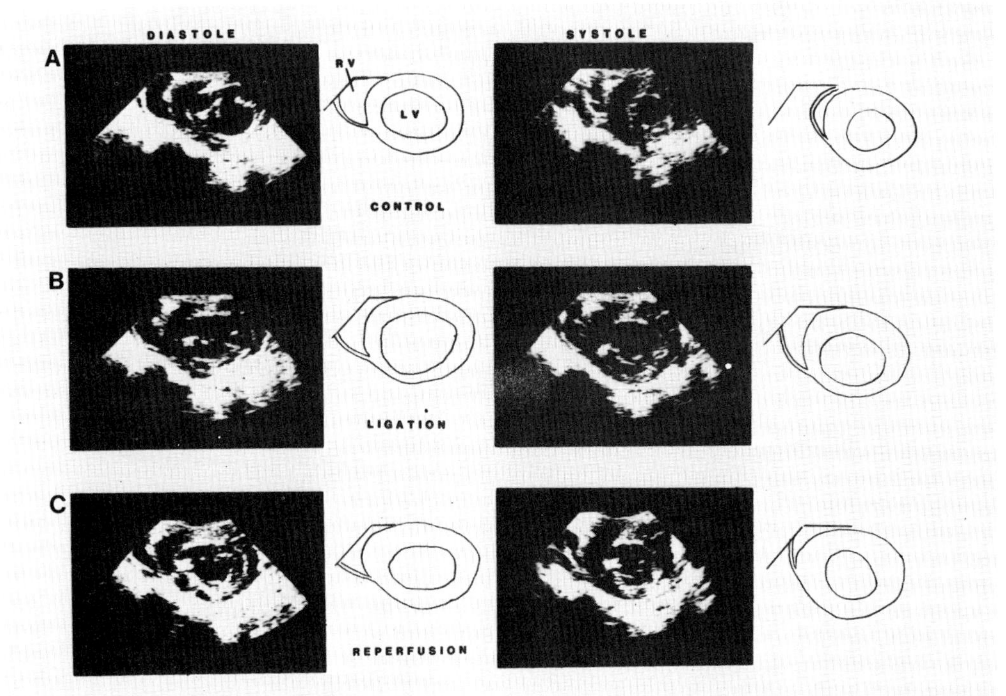

Fig 9–9.—Two-dimensional echocardiographic demonstration of right ventricular involvement in an acute ischemic process created by experimental ligation of the left circumflex coronary artery in a dog. The short-axis view of the left and right ventricles *(LV, RV)* at a level just below the mitral valve is shown. End-diastolic *(left panels)* and end-systolic *(right panels)* still frames during control *(A)*, ligation *(B)*, and postreperfusion *(C)* periods are depicted. Note marked thinning of the LV posterior wall, akinesis of the RV posterior and lateral wall, and marked increase in LV as well as RV internal dimensions during ischemia *(B)*.

(Fig 9–8). Patients with anterior and anteroseptal infarction seemed particularly prone to infarct expansion. By 8 weeks, 4 of the 8 patients who showed infarct expansion had died, while all 20 patients who did not show infarct expansion survived. Based on this study, these investigators contended that infarct expansion rather than further extension of the ischemic process with further necrosis of myocardial tissue may play a more important role than previously appreciated in patients surviving acute myocardial infarction. This study demonstrates that 2DE can be used to uncover topographic changes which occur in the evolution of an acute myocardial infarction and may have considerable clinical importance not only in assessing survival, but potentially in assessing interventions which may influence survival of such patients.

RIGHT VENTRICULAR INFARCTION

Another possible diagnostic use for echocardiography is the detection of right ventricular infarction. This clinical entity has lately gained increasing interest because of the high mortality in undiagnosed patients. It is characterized by a complex of clinical ECG and hemodynamic signs. The acute overload of the right ventricle in the presence of a posteroinferior wall infarction strongly suggests involvement of the right ventricle in the ischemic process.[45–47]

Acute echocardiographic changes in right ventricular performance can be seen in the canine model following ligation of the major artery supplying the posterior wall of the heart. Synchronous with the development of dyskinesia in the left ventricular wall, a marked dilation of the right ventricle takes place, with concomitant hypokinesis of the right ventricular posterior and lateral walls. The posterior septum is also largely involved in this process (Fig 9–9). In man, the acute overload of the right ventricle has been shown to significantly change the interventricular septal motion (Fig 9–10).[48]

Clinical echocardiographic studies of patients

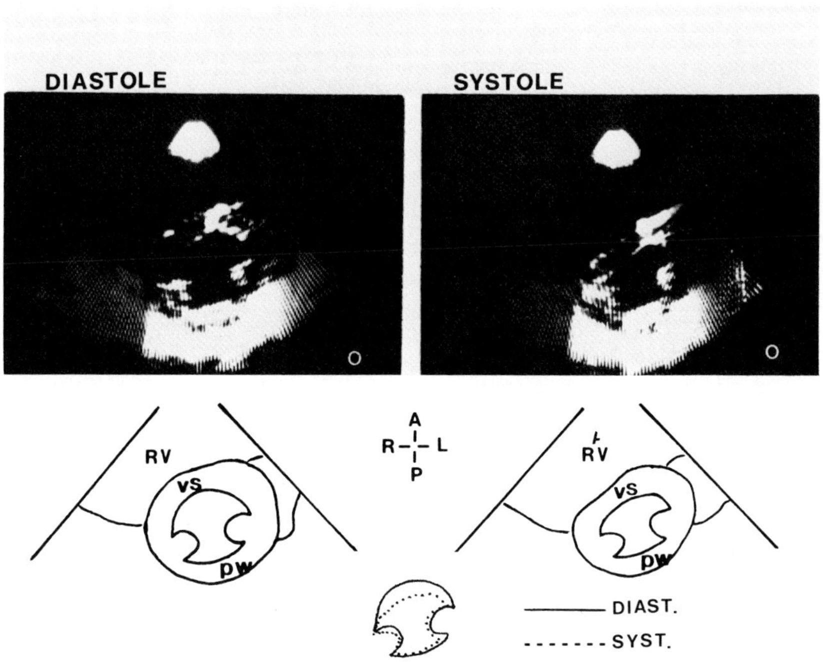

Fig 9–10.—Acute right ventricular infarction in a patient with an acute inferior wall myocardial infarction. The two-dimensional short-axis echocardiographic still frames during diastole and systole depict the left and right ventricular cavities *(LV, RV)*, the interventricular septum *(VS)*, and the left ventricular posterior wall. Note the enlarged RV cavity as well as the paradoxic septal motion during systole *(diagrams)*.

with acute right ventricular infarction are scant. Sharpe et al.,[49] examining noninvasive means of diagnosing right ventricular infarction, studied 26 consecutive patients with transmural myocardial infarction. In 6 of 15 patients with inferior myocardial infarction, involvement of the right ventricle was diagnosed by means of radionuclide studies. These findings correlated well with the echocardiographic finding of an enlarged and dyskinetic right ventricle in these patients. In a preliminary report on 5 patients, D'Arcy et al.[50] observed marked enlargement of the right ventricle, right ventricular anterolateral and apical segmental wall motion abnormalities, and paradoxic septal motion in 4. Contrast echocardiography in these patients revealed marked tricuspid valve insufficiency. Park et al.[51] studied 17 patients in whom right ventricular infarction was diagnosed by clinical, hemodynamic, and radioisotope studies, as well as on autopsy. Thirteen of these 17 patients showed right ventricular posterior wall and septal asynergy. In 10 patients, additional lateral and anterior segments of the right ventricle were involved. In 5 patients these changes persisted even after the normalization of hemodynamic parameters. Klein et al.,[52] in a yet unpublished echocardiographic study of 32 patients with suspected right ventricular infarction, found that in 26 patients the right ventricular cavity was enlarged (> 23 mm). In this group, 3 patients died, and pathologic studies confirmed the extensive involvement of the right ventricle in the necrotic process. These findings correlated well with radionuclide investigations performed in these patients.

From the studies reviewed above, it seems that echocardiography may serve as a simple noninvasive bedside method for detecting right ventricular infarction. Echocardiographically determined right ventricular enlargement and dyskinesia in the presence of an inferior wall myocardial infarction strongly suggest the involvement of the right ventricle in the ischemic process and warrant further investigative and therapeutic steps.

REFERENCES

1. Wollenberger A., Krause E.G.: Metabolic control characteristics of the acutely ischemic myocardium. *Am. J. Cardiol.* 22:349–359, 1968.
2. Krause E.G., Wollenberger A.: Über die Aktivierung der Phosphorylase und Glycolyserate im akut anoxischen Hundeherzen. *Biochem. Zeitschr.* 342:171, 1965.
3. Tennant R., Wiggers C.J.: Effective coronary occlusion on myocardial contraction. *Am. J. Physiol.* 112:351–361, 1935.
4. Tomoda H., et al.: Effects of ischemia and reoxygenation on regional myocardial performance of the dog. *Am. J. Physiol.* 221:1718–1721, 1971.
5. Heyndrickx G.R., et al.: Regional myocardial functional and electrophysiological alterations after brief coronary artery occlusion in conscious dogs. *J. Clin. Invest.* 56:978–985, 1975.
6. Theroux P., et al.: Regional myocardial functions during acute coronary artery occlusion and its modification by pharmacological agents in the dog. *Circ. Res.* 35:896–908, 1974.
7. Tyberg J.V., Parmley W.N.: Mechanics of myocardial ischemia. *Adv. Cardiol.* 23:40–51, 1978.
8. Heyndrickx G.R., et al.: Depression of regional blood flow and wall thickening after brief coronary occlusion. *Am. J. Physiol.* 234:H653–H659, 1978.
9. Schever J., Brachfelld N.: Coronary insufficiency: Relation between hemodynamic, electrical and biochemical parameters. *Circ. Res.* 18:178–189, 1966.
10. Chimovski J.E., et al.: Temporary coronary occlusion in conscious dogs: Collateral flow and electrocardiogram. *Am. J. Physiol.* 212:1025–1032, 1979.
11. Inoue K., et al.: Ultrasonic measurement of left ventricular wall motion in acute myocardial infarctions. *Circulation* 43:778–785, 1971.
12. Stefan G., Bing R.G.: Echocardiographic findings in experimental myocardial infarction of the posterior left ventricular wall. *Am. J. Cardiol.* 30:629–639, 1972.
13. Kerber R.E., Abboud F.M.: Echocardiographic detection of regional myocardial infarction. *Circulation* 47:997–1005, 1973.
14. Kerber R.E., et al.: Effects of inotropic agents on the localized dyskinesis of acutely ischemic myocardium: An experimental ultrasound study. *Circulation* 49:1038–1046, 1974.
15. Kerber R.E., et al.: Correlations between echocardiographically demonstrated segmental dyskinesis and regional myocardial perfusion. *Circulation* 52:1097–1104, 1975.
16. Kerber R.E., et al.: Effects of acute coronary occlusion on the motion and perfusion of the normal and ischemic interventricular septum: An experimental echocardiographic study. *Circulation* 54:928–935, 1976.
17. Weiss J.L., et al.: Relationship of systolic thickening to transmural extent of myocardial infarction in the dog. *Circulation* 62(suppl. III):328, 1980.
18. David D., et al.: Time sequence of mechanical and electrical alterations following coronary artery ligation and reperfusion. *Clin. Res.* 28:164A, 1980.
19. Meltzer R.S., et al.: Two-dimensional echocardiographic quantification of infarct size alteration by

pharmacologic agents. *Am. J. Cardiol.* 44:257–262, 1979.
20. Widlansky S., et al.: Coronary angiographic, echocardiographic, and electrocardiographic studies on a patient with variant angina due to coronary artery spasm. *Am. Heart J.* 90:631, 1975.
21. Sharma B., et al.: Left ventricular angiography on exercise: A new method of assessing left ventricular function and ischemic heart disease. *Br. Heart J.* 38:59–70, 1976.
22. Borer J.S., et al.: Real time radionuclide cineangiography in the non-invasive evaluation of global and regional left ventricular function at rest and during exercise in patients with coronary artery disease. *N. Engl. J. Med.* 296:839–844, 1977.
23. Fogelman A.M., et al.: Echocardiographic study of the abnormal motion of the posterior left ventricular wall during angina pectoris. *Circulation* 46:905–913, 1972.
24. Mason S.J., et al.: Exercise echocardiography detection of wall motion abnormalities during ischemia. *Circulation* 59:50–59, 1979.
25. Wann L.S., et al.: Exercise cross-sectional echocardiography in ischemic heart disease. *Circulation* 60:1300–1308, 1979.
26. Romijn K.H., et al.: Dynamic exercise cross-sectional echocardiography: Comparison to coronary arteriography and radionuclide angiography. *Circulation* 62(suppl. III):33, 1980.
27. Morganroth J., et al.: Exercise cross-sectional echocardiographic diagnosis of coronary artery disease. *Am. J.Cardiol.* 47:20–26, 1981.
28. Ratshin R.A., Rackley C.E., Russell R.O.: Serial evaluation of left ventricular volume and posterior wall movement in the acute phase of myocardial infarction using diagnostic ultrasound. *Am. J. Cardiol.* 29:286, 1972.
29. Smithen C., Wharton C., Sowton E.: Changes in left ventricular wall movement following exercise, atrial pacing, and acute myocardial infarction measured by reflected ultrasound. *Am. J. Cardiol.* 29:293, 1972.
30. Corya B.C., et al.: Echocardiography in acute myocardial infarction. *Am. J. Cardiol.* 36:1–10, 1975.
31. Heikkila J., Nieminen M.: Echoventriculographic detection, localization and quantification of left ventricular asynergy in acute myocardial infarction. *Br. Heart J.* 37:46, 1975.
32. Corya B.C., et al.: Systolic thickening and thinning of the septum and posterior wall in patients with coronary artery disease, congestive cardiomyopathy, and atrial septal defect. *Circulation* 55:109–114, 1977.
33. Nieminen M.S., Heikkila J.: Accuracy and usefulness of echoventriculography in acute myocardial infarction. *Acta Med. Scand. Suppl.* 627:152–163, 1978.
34. Nieminen N., Heikkila J.: Echoventriculography in acute myocardial infarction: III. Clinical correlations and implication of the non-infarcted myocardium. *Am. J. Cardiol.* 38:1–8, 1976.
35. Heikkila J., Nieminen M.S.: Rapid monitoring of regional myocardial ischemia with echocardiography and ST segment shift in man: Modification of "infarct size" and hemodynamics by dopamine and beta-blockade. *Acta Med. Scand. Suppl.* 623:71–95, 1978.
36. Weiner I., et al.: Prognostic value of echocardiographic evaluation of septal function in acute anteroseptal myocardial infarction. *Am. Heart J.* 97:726–732, 1979.
37. Feigenbaum H., et al.: Role of echocardiography in patients with coronary artery disease. *Am. J. Cardiol.* 37:775–786, 1976.
38. Kisslo J.A., et al.: A comparison of real time two-dimensional echocardiography and cineangiography in detecting left ventricular asynergy. *Circulation* 55:134–141, 1977.
39. Nixon J.V., Narahara K.A., Smitherman T.C.: Estimation of myocardial involvement in patients with acute myocardial infarction by two-dimensional echocardiography. *Circulation* 62:1248–1254, 1980.
40. Heger J.J., et al.: Cross-sectional echocardiography in an acute myocardial infarction: Detection localization of regional left ventricular asynergy. *Circulation* 60:531–538, 1979.
41. Heger J.J., et al.: Cross-sectional echocardiographic analysis of the extent of left ventricular asynergy in acute myocardial infarction. *Circulation* 61:1113–1118, 1980.
42. Horowitz R.S., et al.: Immediate diagnosis of acute myocardial infarction by two-dimensional echocardiography, unpublished.
43. Horowitz R.S., et al.: Immediate detection of a high-risk subset for in-hospital complication in patients with acute myocardial infarction using two-dimensional echocardiography, unpublished.
44. Eaton L.W., et al.: Regional cardiac dilatation after acute myocardial infarction. *N. Engl. J. Med.* 300:57, 1979.
45. Isner J.M., Roberts N.C.: Right ventricular infarction complicating left ventricular infarction secondary to coronary heart disease. *Am. J. Cardiol.* 42:885–895, 1978.
46. Lorell B., et al.: Right ventricular infarction: Clinical diagnosis and differentiation from cardiac tamponade and pericardial constriction. *Am. J. Cardiol.* 43:465–471, 1979.
47. Ratliff N.B., Hackel D.B.: Combined right and left ventricular infarction: Pathogenesis and clinicopathologic correlations. *Am. J. Cardiol.* 45:217–221, 1980.
48. Brinker J.A., et al.: Leftward septal displacement during right ventricular loading in man. *Circulation* 61:626–633, 1980.
49. Sharpe D.N., et al.: The non-invasive diagnosis of right ventricular infarction. *Circulation* 57:483–490, 1978.

50. D'Arcy B.J., et al.: Real time two-dimensional echocardiography in right ventricular infarction. *Am. J. Cardiol.* 45:436, 1980.
51. Park J.D., et al.: Assessment of asynergy in right ventricular infarction with real time two-dimensional echocardiography. *Circulation* 62(suppl. III):329, 1980.
52. Klein H.O., et al.: Echocardiography in right ventricular infarction, unpublished.

RADIONUCLIDE IMAGING

Jeffrey Leppo and Robert D. Okada

BECAUSE MYOCARDIAL INFARCTION is the leading cause of death in America,[1] efforts both to diagnose and to determine the severity of ischemic heart disease have been vigorously pursued. Radioisotope techniques in the coronary care unit have progressed from a research tool[2–5] to an important clinical modality in both university medical centers and community hospitals. Growth in this field is largely due to the use of portable imaging systems, improved computer technology, and the development of better imaging agents, as well as a refinement of existing techniques.

This chapter reviews the current status of radionuclide angiography, myocardial perfusion, and infarct-avid imaging in patients with myocardial infarction. The general principles behind the use of each radioisotope for myocardial radionuclide imaging can best be summarized by describing where the tracer is concentrated after an intravenous injection. Radionuclide angiography is performed with the radioisotope either attached to (equilibrium blood pool method) or mixed with (first-pass method) circulating red blood cells as they pass through the cardiac chambers during the study collection. Perfusion imaging depends on the direct relationship of the myocardial cell concentration of the tracer (thallium 201) to regional blood flow and to a rapid blood clearance of the isotope. Therefore, perfusion imaging demonstrates tracer uptake in normal tissue and diminished activity in abnormal tissue. In contrast, infarct-avid imaging reflects the concentration of radioisotope (technetium 99m pyrophosphate) activity in infarcted myocardium versus the lack of uptake in normal tissue. Therefore, infarct-avid tracers produce "hot spots" on myocardial scans during acute infarction.

This chapter discusses in turn the diagnosis and extent of infarction, the detection of associated ischemia, the assessment of physiologic parameters, and the derivation of prognostic information from myocardial scintigraphy. Table 10–1 presents much of this information in summary form.

DIAGNOSIS OF MYOCARDIAL INFARCTION

The clinical diagnosis of myocardial infarction relies on the triad of a typical history of prolonged chest pain, serial ECG changes,[6–10] and serum cardiac enzyme changes.[11–15] However, complicating factors such as recent open heart surgery, cardiopulmonary resuscitation, electric cardioversion, and intramuscular injections can impair the accuracy of enzyme changes as markers of infarction, while certain medications, ventricular hypertrophy, previous Q waves, and abnormal ECG conduction patterns can decrease the accuracy of an ECG diagnosis. Newer imaging techniques permit additional objective criteria for the diagnosis of infarction.

Radionuclide imaging techniques can suggest myocardial infarction by demonstrating a perfu-

TABLE 10–1.—Radionuclide Imaging in the Coronary Care Unit*

	Diagnosis of Myocardial Infarct <24 Hr	Diagnosis of Myocardial Infarct >24 Hr	Evaluate Extent of Infarct RV	Evaluate Extent of Infarct LV	Evaluate Ischemia	Assess Physiology	Prognosis In hosp.	Prognosis Long-term	Comments
Thallium 201	E	G	L	G-E	E	G	G	G-E	Best for early detection of infarct and ischemia; not always available in radiopharmacy; not able to assess RV infarct at rest; cannot differentiate old from acute infarction
Technetium 99m pyrophosphate	L-G	E	G	G	N	L	L-G	L-G	Best for detecting 2- to 4-day-old infarct; specificity problem of diffuse vs. focal uptake; need to get serial studies if initially negative
Radionuclide angiography	G	G	E	G-E	L	E	E	E	Best to assess early and late RV and LV function; may not detect small or subendocardial infarcts; cannot differentiate old from acute infarction

*E, excellent; G, good; L, limited; N, none; RV, right ventricle; LV, left ventricle.

sion defect or an accumulation of a tracer in damaged and necrotic tissue; cineangiography can demonstrate a severe segmental wall motion abnormality.

Thallium 201

Thallium 201 imaging done with the patient at rest within the first six hours of clinical presentation has been reported by Wackers and co-workers to be 100% sensitive for acute myocardial infarction.[16, 17] After an initial clinical study of patients with documented acute myocardial infarctions, Wackers et al. reported that ^{201}Tl imaging detected myocardial infarction in 44 of 44 patients studied within six hours, in 90 of 96 (94%) patients studied within 24 hours, and in 75 of 104 (72%) patients studied more than 24 hours after the chest pain episode. The majority of the false negative scan results occurred in patients with small or nontransmural infarcts, as determined by serial ECG and enzyme measurements.[17]

The potential value of ^{201}Tl imaging to select patients for admission to the coronary care unit was evaluated in 203 patients with an atypical history and ECG findings nondiagnostic for acute myocardial infarction who underwent imaging within 10 hours of chest pain symptoms. Subsequent enzyme determinations suggested acute myocardial infarction in 34 patients (17%); 30 had abnormal scans and the remaining four had questionable scan results. Of the remaining 169 patients, 14 had positive ^{201}Tl scans, which represents a specificity of 92%.[18] Other reports have supported a very high sensitivity of ^{201}Tl scans for infarction, apparently higher than either technetium 99m pyrophosphate imaging[19–21] or ECG Q waves.[22] The use of ^{201}Tl scans clinically to rule out a myocardial infarction appears to be a most sensitive early indicator (<24 hours) of underlying disease. As shown in Figure 10–1, the myocardial ^{201}Tl perfusion pattern can be used to localize the anatomical site of the infarction. Wackers et al. have noted good correlation (90% agreement) between the size of a myocardial scar as determined post mortem and as determined by quantitative analysis of ^{201}Tl scans performed shortly before death.[23] In this same report, ECG localization had only a 70% agreement with postmortem results and obviously could not reflect the size of necrotic

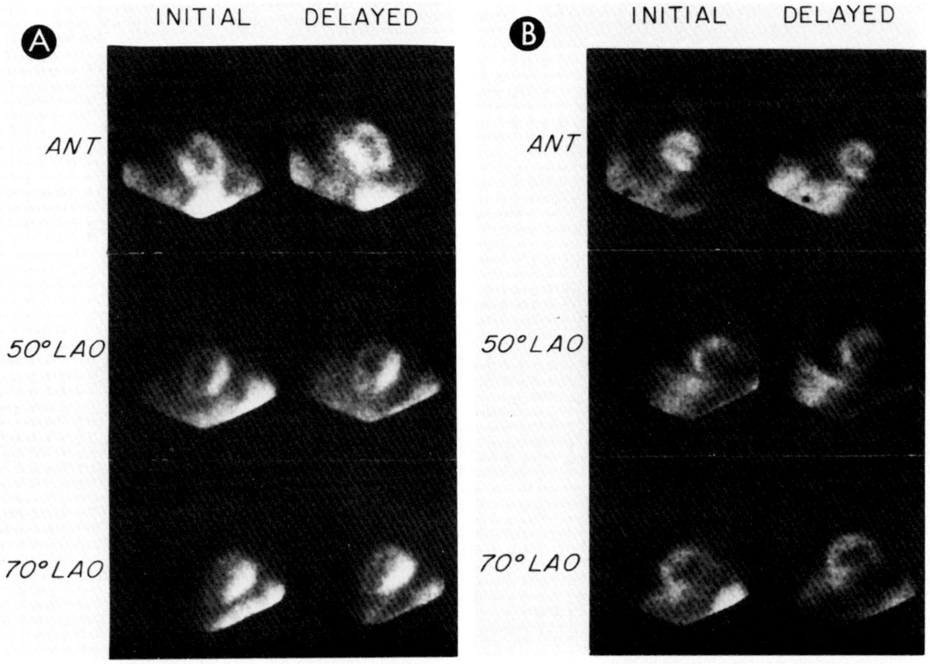

Fig 10–1.—Initial and delayed thallium 201 images in the anterior *(ANT)* and the 50-degree and the 70-degree left anterior oblique *(LAO)* views showing persistent defects. **A** is from a patient with an anterior septal and apical infarction; **B** is from a patient with an inferior-posterior infarction.

myocardium.[23] The ability of ^{201}Tl scanning to localize infarction has also been supported by studies which correlated scan defects to epicardial scars[24] at surgery and to akinesis as measured by analysis of contrast ventriculographic studies.[25]

A disadvantage to ^{201}Tl imaging in the detection of myocardial infarction is its inability to differentiate acute infarction from chronic scar tissue. Therefore, in patients who have had a previous infarction, an abnormal scan may not help in the diagnosis of acute damage unless a careful comparison with previous perfusion scans can be done. The presence of right ventricular infarction cannot be evaluated by ^{201}Tl studies performed in the resting state. The relatively short shelf life and high cost of the isotope also limits its availability to institutions that have a busy coronary care unit and must screen a large number of patients for potential infarction. However, if a dose is available, and if the diagnosis of infarction appears equivocal within 24 hours of presentation, a ^{201}Tl scan should provide useful information in the detection of coronary artery disease and infarction.

Technetium 99m Pyrophosphate

The use of infarct-avid tracers in the coronary care unit has mainly relied on technetium 99m pyrophosphate. The initial clinical experience as reported by Parkey and co-workers suggested that ^{99m}Tc-pyrophosphate imaging is extremely sensitive for detecting acute myocardial infarction.[26] These authors emphasize the need to prepare carefully the stannous pyrophosphate and technetium 99m, and they have demonstrated a good correlation between myocardial localization of the tracer and the presence of ECG Q waves. The highest sensitivity for acute infarction was noted to occur 24 to 72 hours after clinical presentation with acute chest pain.[26, 27] Other infarct-avid tracers such as technetium 99m (Sn) tetracycline[28] and glucoheptonate[29, 30] have not achieved widespread clinical usefulness. Although technetium 99m glucoheptonate has demonstrated positive results within six hours of acute infarction, the overall image appearance and target-to-background ratio are inferior to what can be obtained with pyrophosphate images.

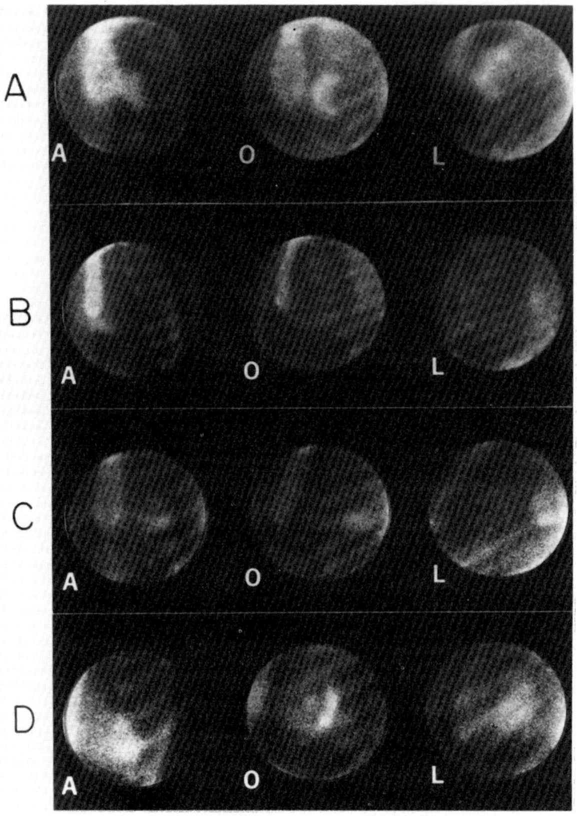

Fig 10–2.—Technetium 99m pyrophosphate scans in the anterior *(A)*, left anterior oblique *(O)*, and left lateral *(L)* views demonstrating focal myocardial tracer uptake after an acute infarction. *Panel A* shows an anterior-septal infarct; *panel B* shows an inferior infarct; *panel C* shows an apical infarct; *panel D* shows a posterior-lateral infarct.

Additional experimental and clinical studies have demonstrated that myocardial uptake of ^{99m}Tc-phosphorus radiopharmaceuticals is localized to necrotic tissue. There is a very good correlation between the size and site of tracer uptake and the size and site of acute infarction found on postmortem analysis. The exact mechanism of tracer uptake is still being studied, but present evidence suggests that calcium in the injured cell is able to form complexes with pyrophosphate.[31–33] Figure 10–2 shows the typical patterns of ^{99m}Tc-pyrophosphate uptake associated with different anatomical sites of infarction.

The overall method of ^{99m}Tc-pyrophosphate imaging and interpretation has been reviewed by Willerson et al.,[34] and their reported grading system for infarction is commonly followed. Images are graded from 0 to 4+ for activity: 0 = no activity, 1+ = minimal activity, 2+ = definite myocardial activity, 3+ = myocardial activity equal to bone activity, and 4+ = myocardial activity greater than bone activity. A score of 2+ or greater suggests acute myocardial infarction in this interpretation system and consistently results in a sensitivity of greater than 90% for a documented transmural infarction. The sensitivity of an intensity score of 2+ or greater in cases of subendocardial infarcts ranges from 51% to 100%. It is also important to note whether the myocardial tracer uptake is focal or diffuse (Fig 10–3), because the sensitivity for both transmural (>80%) and subendocardial (32%–44%) infarctions decreases when focal uptake is a criterion for positivity.[35–37] Specificity of myocardial ^{99m}Tc-pyrophosphate imaging is also quite dependent on the patient population and on whether focal uptake as well as intensity are considered as diagnostic criteria. It has been noted that abnormal pyrophosphate myocardial uptake occurs in only 2% of patients undergoing bone radionuclide imaging in the absence of clinical heart disease.[37] Table 10–2 lists some of the potential causes of an abnormal scan in the absence of acute infarction; all these causes may contribute to a decrease in specificity. Many false positive scans demonstrate diffuse or minimal (2+) uptake, but conditions such as previous infarction, aneurysm, myocardial and muscular skeletal trauma, and myocardial calcification may also be associated with intense focal uptake of ^{99m}Tc-pyrophosphate. In addition, several of these associated conditions may be present in a patient who is being evaluated for an acute myocardial infarct. Therefore, serial scans over ten days may be needed to establish a typical imaging pattern for acute infarction. Specifically, the intensity of tracer uptake should be maximal three to five days after the clinical event and should show no or only faint activity after ten days.[34] Although not all patients with an acute infarct will ultimately show normal patterns, and although certain conditions such as cardioversion may show a typical infarction pattern on serial scans, ^{99m}Tc-pyrophosphate imaging has limited usefulness if serial studies are needed to corroborate initially equivocal examinations. Therefore, the use of ^{99m}Tc-pyrophosphate imag-

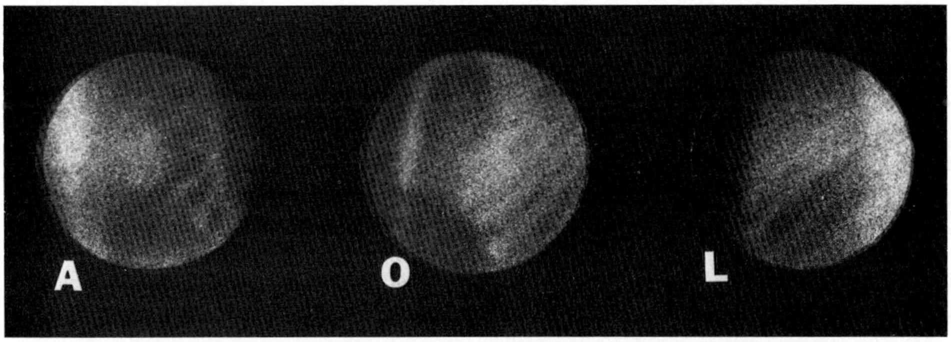

Fig 10–3.—Technetium 99m pyrophosphate scan in the anterior *(A)*, left anterior oblique *(O)*, and left lateral *(L)* views showing diffuse myocardial uptake in a patient with an acute subendocardial infarct.

ing is probably most useful in patients who do not have sufficient clinical or ECG evidence to establish a diagnosis of acute infarction three to four days after clinical symptoms.

There is another group of patients in whom ^{99m}Tc-pyrophosphate imaging appears to be extremely helpful. The diagnosis of acute myocardial infarction by traditional methods (history, ECG, enzymes) is difficult in patients who have recently had open heart surgery. Specifically, these patients cannot accurately report myocardial symptoms, the development of ECG Q waves is not sensitive, and cardiac enzyme levels are almost always elevated. Several reports[53, 64, 65] have demonstrated the ability of myocardial pyrophosphate uptake to reveal new postoperative infarction (Fig 10–4). In addition, postoperative ^{99m}Tc-pyrophosphate scans revert to normal following successful aneurysmectomy and valvular replacement in patients with preoperative uptake associated with aneurysm[64] or valvular calcification,[53] respectively.

TABLE 10–2.—Causes of Myocardial Uptake of ^{99m}Tc Pyrophosphate in the Absence of Acute Infarction

Previous myocardial infarction[38, 39]
Unstable angina[40–46]
Left ventricular wall motion abnormality[47, 48]
Left ventricular aneurysm[43, 47–49]
Cardiomyopathy[40]
Cardioversion[43, 50, 51]
Valvular calcification[31, 52, 53]
Myocardial trauma[54, 55]
Acute pericarditis[56]
Persistent blood pool activity[57, 58]
Breast tumors[26, 59]
Rib fracture[60, 61]
Calcified costal cartilage[62]
Skin lesions[63]

Other Infarct-Avid Agents

There have been recent reports of other infarct-avid radionuclide agents. Gamma camera studies using iodine-labeled myosin-specific antibody fragments have been reported by Khaw et al. in an experimental model of acute infarction.[66] The ^{131}I-labeled anticardiac myosin appears to bind only to myosin in necrotic myocytes, shows good localization of the site of infarction, and can be quickly concentrated to allow external imaging within a few hours after coronary occlusion.[66, 67] Positron transverse-sectional imaging with $Na^{18}F$ has also been reported in canine studies of an acute myocardial infarction. There is an inverse relationship between regional myocardial blood flow determined by radioactive microspheres and relative uptake of ^{18}F. Imaging comparisons of the site and extent of infarction appear to closely approximate findings on postmortem pathologic examinations.[68] Clinical application of these radionuclide compounds can be expected in the near future.

Radionuclide Angiography

The use of radionuclide techniques to assess noninvasively ventricular function in man has progressed from initial experiments with gated blood pool scans[69] and first-pass studies[70] to becoming an integral part of the clinical evaluation in cardiac patients. As reviewed by Berger et al.[71] and

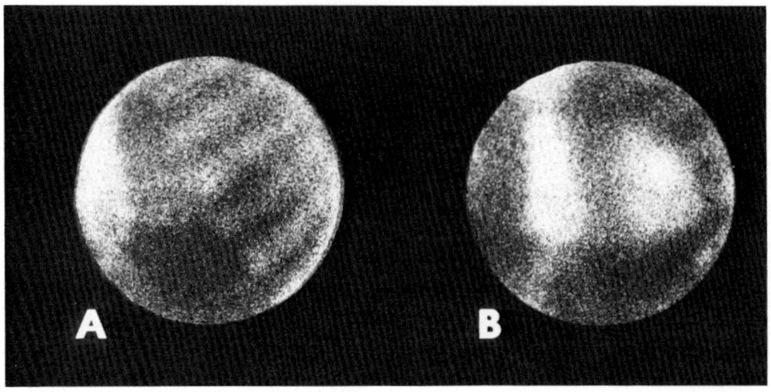

Fig 10–4.—Technetium 99m pyrophosphate scans in the left anterior oblique views before *(A)* and after *(B)* coronary artery bypass surgery. There is no focal uptake before surgery, but postoperatively the scan shows intense (4+) myocardial uptake consistent with an anterior-septal infarct.

Strauss et al.,[72] the technique of radionuclide angiography involves either (1) a nongated first-pass study of a tracer in transit through the cardiac chambers, in which several consecutive beats (four to seven) are summated to calculate ventricular indices, or (2) a gated collection of data from 200–250 cardiac cycles in which a single representative cycle is constructed to generate calculated indices and cineangiography. In this chapter, both first-pass and gated studies are included in the term, "radionuclide angiography" (RNA).

The correlation of RNA-determined left ventricular ejection fraction and regional wall motion with the findings at cardiac catheterization[73, 74] demonstrated that this technique could be used to study patients in the coronary care unit. Most reports of RNA in patients with acute myocardial infarction have not prospectively evaluated the diagnostic accuracy of this method for establishing a diagnosis in a group of patients admitted to rule out infarction. However, it is clear that measurements of both global left ventricular ejection fraction and regional wall motion and function are abnormal during the acute phase of infarction and

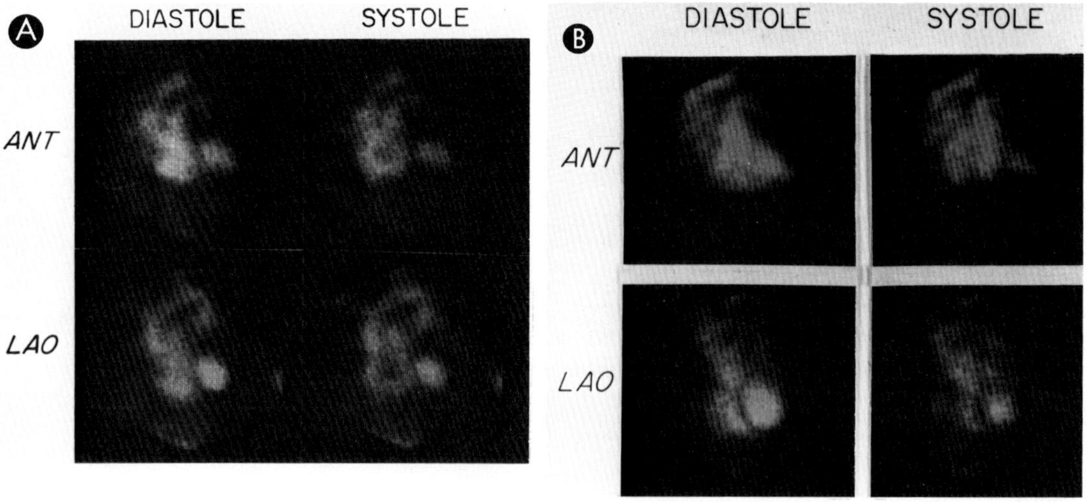

Fig 10–5.—Gated blood pool images in the anterior *(ANT)* and left anterior oblique *(LAO)* views showing abnormal regional contraction during an acute infarction. **A,** the anterior wall of the left ventricle shows diminished motion when the diastolic and systolic frames are compared in a patient with an acute anterior infarct. **B,** a regional contraction abnormality in the inferior-posterior wall in a patient with an acute infarction.

that these measurements can be used to detect the site and extent of damage.[75–79] Detection of acute infarction by RNA depends on the observation of abnormal regional wall motion, as shown in Figure 10–5. The highest specificity is associated with dyskinetic motion, but most reports define infarction as either akinetic or dyskinetic wall motion. The extent of infarction is usually expressed as a percentage of the left ventricular wall circumference. Unfortunately, it is difficult to distinguish acute from chronic infarction by evaluating regional wall motion.

EVALUATION OF THE EXTENT OF INFARCTION: INVOLVEMENT OF RIGHT AND LEFT VENTRICLE

The immediate prognosis for the patient with an acute infarction is based primarily on the extent of ventricular necrosis and severe ischemia, especially with respect to the development of cardiogenic shock.[80] Several reports have also demonstrated that after discharge, patients with larger infarctions have higher mortality,[81] more ventricular arrhythmia,[82] and poorer left ventricular pump function[83] than patients with smaller infarctions.

Dêmonstration of the site and extent of infarction by myocardial ^{201}Tl perfusion imaging correlates well with demonstration by postmortem analysis,[23] by epicardial scars at surgery,[24] and by akinesis on contrast ventriculography.[25] Experimental comparisons between the size of the defect on ^{201}Tl imaging and the weight of infarcted ventricular muscle demonstrate a linear correlation, but small (less than 5 gm) infarcts may not be detected.[85] Bulkley et al., using quantitative analysis of the circumferential profile of the ^{201}Tl scan, did not show a high correlation between defect size and the extent of necrosis as determined by postmortem evaluation in patients with fatal infarctions.[86] These investigators suggested that the discrepancy between necrosis size and defect size could be caused by peri-infarction ischemia, but serial images were not collected. However, patients with large defects on ^{201}Tl imaging had a significantly higher average percentage of myocardial necrosis (36%) than patients with smaller defects (13%).[86] An experimental report has shown that with careful attention to camera position, a quantitative analysis of ^{201}Tl scans in dogs correlates with infarct size with an *r* value of 0.88.[87]

The ability of serial ^{201}Tl myocardial scans to detect ischemia versus infarction has been well documented[88–90] and will be more fully discussed in later sections. It is evident tht defects identified on resting ^{201}Tl myocardial perfusion studies do correlate with either scar tissue or severe coronary artery disease in patients who may experience chest pain at rest.[91–93] The observation that some of these resting defects disappear after coronary bypass surgery attests to both reversibility of the flow disparity and viability of the myocardium, as well as to the severity of the coronary arterial lesion.[94]

The right ventricle is not usually visualized on a resting ^{201}Tl myocardial study[21] except in cases of pressure or volume overload.[95] Therefore, ^{201}Tl radionuclide imaging is of limited value in the evaluation of right ventricular infarction.

Results obtained from ^{99m}Tc-pyrophosphate imaging to assess the site and extent of a myocardial infarction appear to be somewhat less accurate than results obtained in the same patients with ^{201}Tl myocardial studies.[19–21, 96, 97] Comparisons between infarct size by enzyme determination and extent of myocardial uptake of ^{99m}Tc-pyrophosphate do not show a good correlation, while left ventricular ejection fraction and size of a defect on ^{201}Tl scans correlate well.[97] One reason for the poor results of ^{99m}Tc-pyrophosphate infarct sizing is that pyrophosphate uptake depends on some residual flow to the infarcted myocardium. In addition, Berger et al. noted that ^{99m}Tc-pyrophosphate myocardial imaging tends to overestimate the extent of the perfusion abnormality noted on ^{201}Tl imaging. This disparity between thallium and pyrophosphate scans has been partly attributed to the image produced: a hot spot of myocardial pyrophosphate uptake depicts an edge-to-edge image while a thallium cold spot is produced by a central myocardial region of diminished activity. Quantitation of the extent of myocardial uptake of pyrophosphate is difficult using planar imaging, and

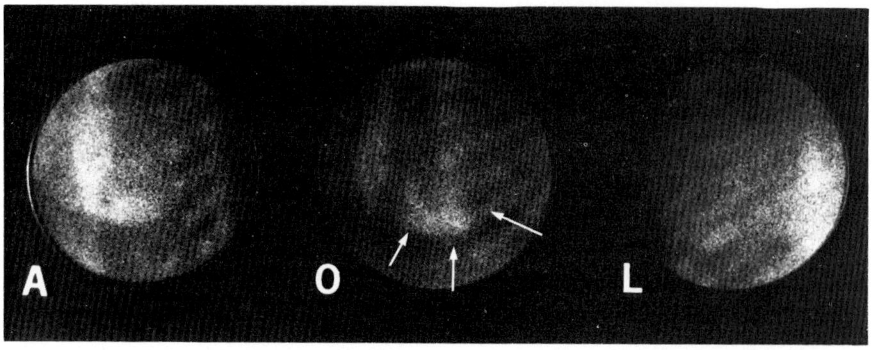

Fig 10–6.—Technetium 99m pyrophosphate scan in the anterior *(A),* left anterior oblique *(O),* and left lateral *(L)* views showing right ventricular uptake of the tracer. In the oblique view, the *center arrow* points to the septum and the *left arrow* points to the right ventricle. *Right arrow* points to tracer uptake in the inferior wall of the left ventricle.

techniques that employ tomography may prove helpful. In addition, hot spot scans and ^{201}Tl scans are not ordinarily done simultaneously. The difference in imaging time could lead to systematic errors when the two techniques are compared.

It does seem clear that myocardial uptake of ^{99m}Tc-pyrophosphate is related to actual necrosis of tissue in the setting of an infarction.[31–32] Other workers have employed precise measurements of serial serum enzyme levels to demonstrate that myocardial ^{99m}Tc-pyrophosphate uptake correlates with extent of infarction in 90% of studies. The problem of timing the imaging with both the peak of myocardial uptake and the clinical course of infarction is a problem when evaluating the size of ventricular injury.

The ability of infarcted right ventricular tissue to concentrate ^{99m}Tc-pyrophosphate has been documented and can be an important clinical evaluation.[21, 98] A hot spot scan positive for right ventricular infarction is shown in Figure 10–6. Clinical detection of right ventricular infarction and subsequent dilation is difficult when done by ECG and enzyme determinations alone. The associated clinical syndrome of shock, elevated right heart pressure, and normal pulmonary capillary wedge pressure requires therapy different from therapy for left ventricular muscle failure. A pathologic study reports that 14% of all infarctions have right ventricular involvement. However, all of the observed cases of right ventricular necrosis occurred in patients with transmural posteroseptal left ventricular infarcts. Furthermore, 50% of the patients with posteroseptal transmural left ventricular infarction had evidence of right ventricular necrosis.[99] The clinical observation of positive right ventricular uptake of ^{99m}Tc-pyrophosphate in approximately 40% of inferior wall infarcts[21, 98] appears to correlate with these postmortem studies.

The site and extent of left ventricular necrosis can be evaluated by RNA techniques. Several reports have demonstrated that quantitative measurements of left ventricular ejection fraction and the percentage of ventricular circumference with akinetic or dyskinetic wall motion correlate with infarct size as determined by serum enzyme determinations and mortality after infarction.[75–77, 100] Radionuclide angiography appears to be especially helpful in evaluating the site and extent of a left ventricular aneurysm. The accuracy of site determination is reported to be 96% when compared with contrast angiography.[101] It is important to note that RNA studies should include posterior oblique views to adequately assess the extent of the aneurysm and viable myocardium.

The relative ease of obtaining a computer-automated left ventricular ejection fraction determination and its high correlation with the extent of necrosis make RNA studies important in evaluating patients in the coronary care unit. The pumping function of the left ventricle is inherently limited by the amount of functioning myocardium, and it is not surprising to find that global ejection fraction is one of the single best measurements of the extent of myocardial damage.

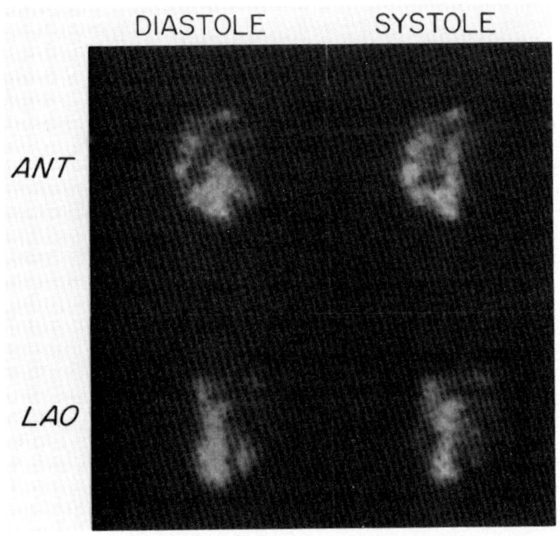

Fig 10–7.—Gated blood pool images showing an acute right ventricular infarction. Note the enlarged right ventricle in diastole which does not contract normally in systole; the left ventricle appears normal in size and contractions.

Radionuclide angiography has demonstrated right ventricular dysfunction in association with inferior and posterior myocardial infarctions. These reports,[102, 103] using criteria that included chamber enlargement, segmental wall akinesis, and reduced ejection fraction, were among the first reports of a noninvasive method that clearly offered significant diagnostic accuracy in this difficult clinical syndrome. An example is shown in Figure 10–7. Pathologic studies confirm the association between right ventricular infarction and regional wall fibrosis as well as between right ventricular infarction and cavity enlargements.[99] Radionuclide angiography appears to be the best means of evaluating the site and extent of right ventricular infarction. It is especially helpful in differentiating cardiogenic shock caused by right-sided dysfunction from acute left ventricular pump failure.[102]

EVALUATION OF ISCHEMIA

The continuation of chest pain and other markers of ischemia in the presence of a myocardial infarction is generally considered to require more vigorous therapy aimed at preventing infarct extension. Therefore, it is important to employ objective methods in the detecton of ischemic but viable myocardium in the coronary care unit.

Serial ^{201}Tl myocardial imaging performed at rest (Fig 10–8) can detect the presence of ischemia as manifested by chest pain at rest,[91, 92] reversible wall motion abnormalities,[94] and severe multivessel coronary artery disease.[93] The observation that ^{201}Tl redistribution occurs in all viable tissue regardless of the regional myocardial blood flow during the administration of the tracer has been used to detect ischemic or flow-restricted myocardium with ^{201}Tl imaging. Thallium 201 redistribution can be documented with serial gamma camera imaging by observing a complete or partial disappearance of an initial defect on subsequent myocardial scans.[88, 104] The initial experience with ^{201}Tl redistribution involved serial imaging after a standard exercise stress test. At the same time, Maseri and co-workers were performing sequential ^{201}Tl myocardial scans in patients who were experiencing variant angina or impending infarctions.[91, 92] The patients who had angina at rest clearly demonstrated the utility of ^{201}Tl imaging to detect a reduction in regional blood flow to viable myocardium. The use of careful ECG monitoring and coronary catheterization studies along with the radionuclide imaging findings helped to document coronary spasm as an important mechanism in the clinical setting of angina at rest.[91–92] Subsequent ^{201}Tl imaging studies have also documented a resting flow disparity in patients with unstable angina pectoris. Defects in these patients are probably associated with a reduction of myocardial blood flow at rest, which produces the clinical picture of unstable angina.[94, 105] Serial imaging in patients with myocardial infarction has demonstrated ^{201}Tl redistribution in patients considered by the investigators to have ischemic myocardium surrounding their infarctions.[106] A similar proposed mechanism of a zone of ischemia surrounding a zone of infarction was used to explain the discrepancy between large defects on ^{201}Tl myocardial scans and the extent of ventricular necrosis at autopsy.[86] Presently, prospective studies are needed to better define the

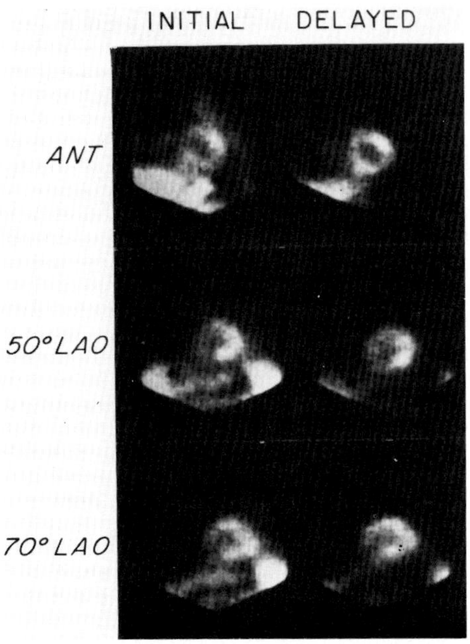

Fig 10–8.—Thallium 201 scan in a patient with an acute infarction shows a persistent defect in the apical region. There is also a transient defect in the inferior (*ANT* view) and septal *(50° LAO)* walls, suggesting ischemia at rest.

therapeutic and prognostic significance of ^{201}Tl redistribution in the acute phase of myocardial infarction.

Myocardial uptake of ^{99m}Tc-pyrophosphate has been reported in some patients with unstable angina,[40–46] although the possibility of subclinical myocardial damage in these patients is an alternative explanation. It does appear that ^{99m}Tc-pyrophosphate imaging has little application in the clinical setting of ongoing ischemia other than to establish the presence of new infarction[45] and to give prognostic information.

Radionuclide angiography studies performed at rest usually cannot be used to detect potentially ischemic myocardium unless an intervention study is compared with a resting examination. The intervention typically performed is exercise stress testing, which is not appropriate in the setting of ischemia during an acute myocardial infarction. Ramanathan et al. have reported that RNA studies done 6 to 24 hours post infarction can show regional wall motion improvement after nitroglycerin administration.[107] This observation may suggest resting ischemia in addition to the myocardial infarction and is based on previous work by Banka et al. using contrast ventriculography.[108] The potential to intervene and salvage these myocardial regions which respond to nitroglycerin has not been critically evaluated. In addition, Shah et al. have reported that anterior wall motion abnormalities were more frequent and severe in patients who had more than 1 mm of ST segment depression in ECG leads V_1–V_6 in conjunction with a new inferior wall infarction.[109] These observations may help answer clinically important questions on primary ECG changes versus reciprocal alterations.

ASSESSMENT OF PHYSIOLOGIC PARAMETERS

One important advantage of noninvasive radionuclide imaging of patients with myocardial infarction is that data on myocardial perfusion, amount of necrosis, and cardiac function can be easily collected in a serial fashion during the course of admission to the coronary care unit. For example, physiologic parameters such as global and regional wall motion of the left and right ventricle can be assessed in conjunction with regional blood flow, viability, and extent of necrosis. Radionuclide studies can help physicians gain a better understanding of the pathophysiology of myocardial infarction starting with the initial period of injury, through the development of necrosis and impaired cardiac function, to healing and recovery.

Experimental and clinical research on myocardial infarction using radioisotope methods is progressing quickly, especially in the field of positron emission transaxial tomography. Sobel et al.[110] and Ter-Pogossian et al.[111] have reported myocardial imaging of ^{11}C-labeled palmitate using a specially designed radiation detector device. This technique of imaging takes advantage of the high avidity for fatty acids (palmitate) in normal myocardial cells. Normal heart cells rapidly extract and metabolize fatty acids for energy production. However, during ischemic or hypoxic periods, the uptake and metabolism of fatty acids are greatly impaired. Initial reports suggest that ^{11}C-palmitate can be used to detect alterations in myocardial metabolism induced by ischemia and accurately to quantify the size of infarcted or ischemic tissue using tomographic reconstruction.[110, 111] Recently, investigators have described the regional kinetics of ^{201}Tl in canine models with transient[112] or fixed stenoses.[113] These experimental reports suggest that quantitative analysis of regional myocardial ^{201}Tl activity over time may be able to evaluate the absolute level of flow disparity associated with angina pectoris at rest. In addition, the amount and time course of ^{201}Tl redistribution around an area of infarction may be related to collateral supply[114] and the extent of viable myocardium. Repeated ^{201}Tl scans can also be done during the hospital course to document the extension of an infarct.

The use of ^{99m}Tc-pyrophosphate imaging to assess parameters other than myocardial infarction is limited. Recent experimental studies have evaluated the ability of infarct-avid imaging to detect the extension of myocardial injury. Technetium 99m pyrophosphate myocardial images were obtained on three consecutive days after a coronary occlusion in a dog. Between day 2 and 3, an additional coronary occlusion was performed. Although serial imaging did not detect new pyrophosphate uptake in the myocardial region infarcted between day 2 and 3, quantification of the infarct size on the final scan correlated with infarct weight.[115] Another experimental imaging study in dogs demonstrated faster myocardial uptake of technetium 99m pyrophosphate after reperfusion of an infarct than during occlusion necrosis.[116]

Radionuclide angiography in patients with routine and complicated myocardial infarcts yields important information on cardiac function, thus allowing a better understanding of the basic pathophysiology of this disease process. Several reports of sequential RNA studies have shown that global left ventricular ejection fraction is an extremely sensitive indicator of the extent of ventricular damage.[75, 77, 79, 103, 107, 117] The utility of RNA to assess congestive heart failure has been demonstrated by Nichols et al.[118] Radionuclide angiography can be used to evaluate ventricular size and function, to screen patients prior to cardiac catheterization, and to determine specific patterns of ventricular dysfunction, all of which facilitate the choice of surgical or medical intervention and provide important prognostic information. Radionuclide angiography can also detect left ventricular volume overload by detecting an elevated stroke volume ratio (left ventricular stroke counts/right ventricular stroke counts). Specifically, this stroke volume ratio is abnormal with mitral regurgitation secondary to papillary muscle rupture.[119] Left-to-right cardiac shunts secondary to acute ventricular septal rupture can be evaluated by RNA techniques which evaluate the transit of the tracer through the pulmonary circulation, from which is derived a pulmonic to systemic flow ratio.[120] It is possible to assess the effect of acute drug interventions during an infarct using RNA. Currently, a large cooperative study to limit infarct size with medical therapy is being evaluated with cardiac radionuclide imaging studies.

PROGNOSIS POST INFARCTION: IN HOSPITAL

The growth of coronary care units over the past two decades has had a major impact on preventing sudden electric deaths during the course of an acute myocardial infarction. It now appears that the extent of ventricular damage and the limitation of injury are factors which also need to be evaluated. Early mortality during an acute infarction is related to infarct size.[121, 122] The development of cardiogenic shock and pump failure is also related to the percentage of ventricular necrosis.[80] As reviewed in this section, radionuclide imaging studies have been useful in identifying patients who are at higher risk during their stay in the coronary care unit. However, a great deal of experience still needs to be accumulated before these noninvasive methods can be recommended as part of a routine evaluation of infarct patients.

Thallium 201 myocardial scans performed at rest early in the course of an infarction have been shown to predict mortality. The size of the perfusion defect even in the absence of congestive heart failure or shock was noted to correlate with in-hospital mortality.[86, 123] Other investigators have reported that an increase in defect size on subsequent ^{201}Tl scans was also associated with a poor clinical course,[17] probably due to infarct exten-

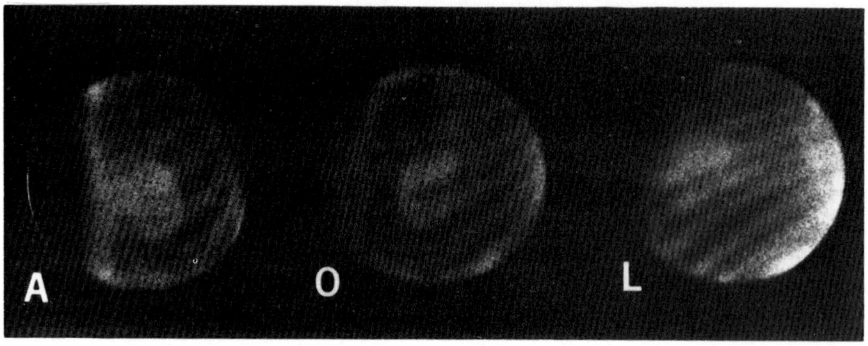

Fig 10–9.—Technetium 99m pyrophosphate scan in a patient with an acute anterior infarct. The myocardial uptake of the tracer demonstrates a doughnut pattern, seen best in the anterior and oblique views.

sion. It should be noted that ^{201}Tl redistribution was not evaluated by serial imaging in these reports of prognosis based on defect size. Further clinical experience and the evaluation of ischemic yet viable as compared with infarcted myocardium needs to be done to better appreciate the optimal use of ^{201}Tl imaging to predict a clinical course in the early phase of infarction.

Rude et al. observed that myocardial uptake of ^{99m}Tc-pyrophosphate in a "doughnut" pattern (Fig 10–9) has significant clinical implications.[124] Infarct size determined by serum enzyme measurements in patients with a doughnut pattern on a ^{99m}Tc-pyrophosphate scan is usually larger than in patients who do not have such a pattern. The increased risk of complications such as conduction abnormalities and congestive heart failure and a higher mortality in patients with a doughnut pattern is probably explained by a larger amount of ventricular damage. The explanation for this particular pattern appears to be a large myocardial infarct with a central core of ischemic necrosis associated with such a marked reduction in perfusion that the tracer cannot really accumulate. Therefore, a rim of intense ^{99m}Tc-pyrophosphate surrounds a region with myocardial uptake that is essentially the same as the normal myocardium, even though it is completely necrotic.[124] This pattern of myocardial tracer uptake is usually associated with anterior wall infarctions. There is no reported experience of altering the clinical course of patients with this type of scan pattern.

Radionuclide angiography in the acute stage of myocardial infarction provides excellent prognostic data. The size of myocardial infarction can be assessed by evaluation of regional wall motion abnormalities[100] and measurement of global ejection fraction.[75] The association between higher mortality and lower ejection fraction and/or percentage of akinetic wall motion is expected. Several reports have shown that early mortality is associated with a decreased ejection fraction by RNA.[75–77, 79, 125] The mean left ventricular ejection fraction in the high-risk group varied from 25% to 35%, while the lower risk group typically had an ejection fraction of more than 35% to 40%. Wynne et al.[79] also found a higher mortality in infarct patients with a decrease in regional ejection fraction in the noninfarcted regions as well as in the infarcted regions. This observation supports the concept of "ischemia at a distance," which implies that early mortality postinfarction is related to the extent of coronary artery disease not only in the infarcted regions but also in the noninfarcted but jeopardized segments.[126] The consistent association of reduced cardiac function and high mortality demonstrates that a high-risk subpopulation of infarct patients can be easily detected by RNA. In addition, serial measurements during the hospital course can be compared to the initial study to determine the progression of disease during hospitalization or the effect of therapeutic interventions. Unfortunately, it is not yet known whether available interventions can alter the poor prognosis associated with decreased left ventricular function. However, demonstration of a fall in or a persistently low level of ventricular performance should suggest the need for close observation and possibly more aggressive therapy.

LONG-TERM PROGNOSIS POST INFARCTION

In a patient with known coronary artery disease, the long-term prognosis is related to the number of major coronary vessels involved and to the level of left ventricular function.[127–130] In patients who have had a myocardial infarction, the presence of postinfarction angina also is associated with a higher mortality and morbidity.[130, 131] The observation of an ischemic response (ST segment depression) on submaximal treadmill testing before discharge is associated with higher mortality even in the absence of chest pain in postinfarction patients.[132–133] Therefore, the noninvasive evaluation of a patient to determine prognosis following myocardial infarction should concentrate on the assessment of overall cardiac impairment and on the number of stenosed coronary arteries.

Thallium 201 imaging can adequately assess the extent of scar tissue, as noted previously.[23, 100] Patients with relatively large defects have been shown to have an increased mortality.[123] Although little improvement in the clinical course of a patient with a large amount of myocardial necrosis may be expected, it is reasonable to expect that patients with ischemic or potentially ischemic regions should benefit from therapeutic interventions.

Gibson et al. reported that 13 of 25 patients with new inferior wall infarcts had anterior as well as inferior wall defects on resting ^{201}Tl scans.[134] The defect in the anterior wall was transient in 10 patients and was assumed to represent a significant left anterior descending artery stenosis. The group with associated anterior wall defects had a greater complication rate, including angina, recurrent infarction, congestive heart failure, and death.[134] Turner et al. used submaximal treadmill testing with ^{201}Tl three weeks post infarction to evaluate residual jeopardized myocardium.[135] All patients in this series had cardiac catheterization, and an exercise-induced ^{201}Tl defect or ST segment depression had a predictive value of 95% for multivessel coronary artery disease. The ^{201}Tl scan was more sensitive than ECG alone and correctly identified most myocardial segments that were supplied by arteries with a stenosis of greater than 70%.[135] Dunn et al. noted that a stress-induced ^{201}Tl defect involving two vascular regions (Fig 10–10) correlated with multivessel disease after myocardial infarction.[136] In this study, the incidence of exercise-induced ST segment depression was not significantly different for single-vessel versus mul-

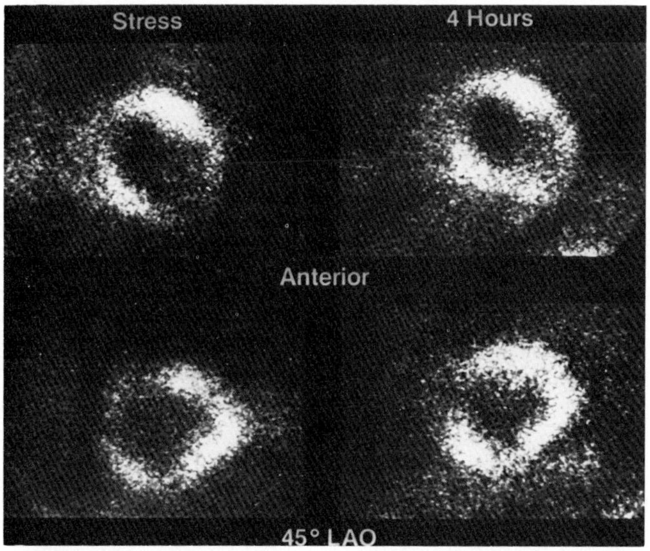

Fig 10–10.—Exercise thallium 201 scan from a patient after anterior wall infarction. The stress anterior and 45-degree LAO views show defects in the anterior, apical, and septal walls that decrease in size on the 4-hour images. This suggests infarction with surrounding ischemia in a patient who had triple-vessel coronary disease.

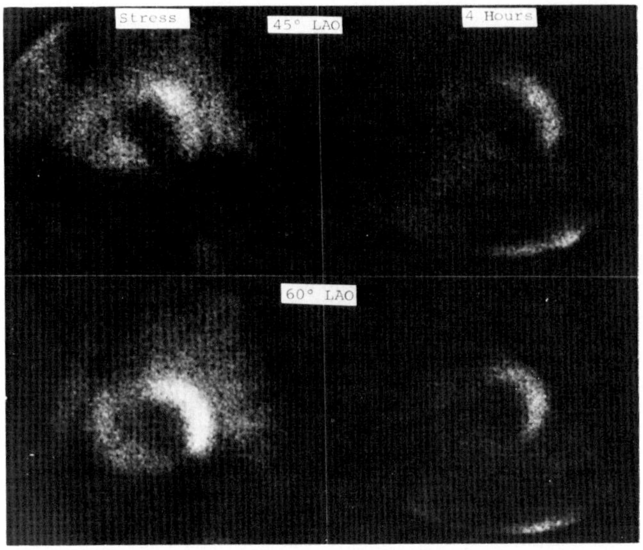

Fig 10–11.—Exercise thallium 201 scan in a patient after anterior septal infarct demonstrates persistent anterior, apical, and septal wall defects. The stress images show increased lung uptake that disappears on the 4-hour images, suggesting left ventricular dysfunction during stress.

tivessel coronary artery disease, while multiple ^{201}Tl scan defects were noted in 12% of patients with single-vessel disease and in 85% of those with multivessel disease.[136]

The observation of increased lung uptake on stress ^{201}Tl studies in postinfarction patients (Fig 10–11) suggests exercise-induced left ventricular dysfunction.[137, 138] In postinfarction patients, exercise test and ^{201}Tl imaging are done to detect remote infarctions[139] and to correlate segmental defects with additional coronary stenoses. Investigators have compared regional myocardial ^{201}Tl distribution with coronary anatomy and have demonstrated a good sensitivity of ^{201}Tl imaging for detecting left anterior descending and right coronary artery disease. However, sensitivity for circumflex coronary artery disease may be as low as 75%.[140, 141] Finally, the use of ^{201}Tl redistribution to distinguish viable myocardium from scar can be used to guide surgical revascularization even in the presence of regional wall motion abnormalities.[142]

Technetium 99m pyrophosphate imaging can also be of value in the evaluation of the postinfarction patient. Olson et al. have reported that persistently positive myocardial uptake (three to six months after infarct) (Fig 10–12) is associated with a higher incidence of complications (42%) than scans which show a return to normal.[143] Myocardial uptake of pyrophosphate in patients after infarction or with angina has been noted to revert to normal after coronary artery bypass surgery,[144] which suggests that the myocardial abnormality causing the uptake is not permanent. As noted above, patients having a doughnut pattern on the scan during the acute phase of their infarction have a poorer in-hospital prognosis.[124] After hospital discharge, these patients have a high incidence of complications during the first year post infarction.[145]

Several reports have demonstrated that RNA

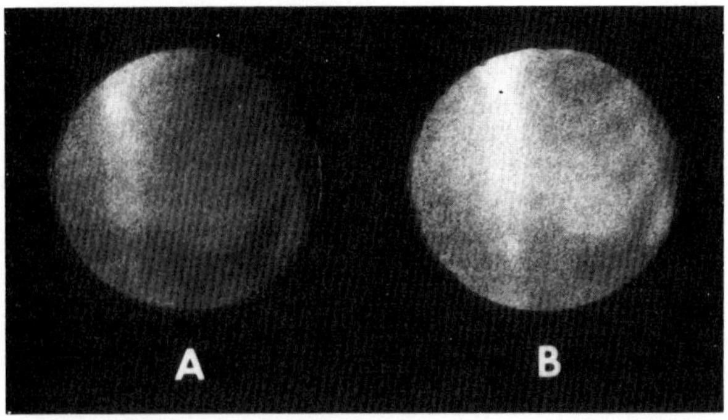

Fig 10–12.—Technetium 99m pyrophosphate scans (anterior view) in a patient during *(A)* and three months after *(B)* an anterior infarct. Myocardial uptake of the tracer persisted, and the patient died suddenly one week after the follow-up scan.

studies prior to discharge can provide useful prognostic information after an infarction. Initial reports related resting left ventricular ejection fraction measurements to mortality, especially if the ejection fraction was reduced.[77, 146] In addition, ventricular ectopy was predictive of sudden death only when associated with an ejection fraction of less than 40%.[146] The combination of exercise stress with RNA studies has also produced important prognostic information. Pulido et al.[147] noted that patients with anterior infarcts have lower resting ejection fractions than patients with inferior or subendocardial infarcts. In response to exercise, patients with anterior infarcts have a significant fall in ejection fraction, while no change or a slight increase is noted in patients with inferior and subendocardial infarction, respectively.[147] Paine et al.[148] studied 100 patients four months after infarction and reported a good correlation between multivessel coronary artery disease and a fall in ejection fraction during exercise. The combination of ST segment elevation and a relatively large fall in ejection fraction accurately predicted large akinetic segments on contrast ventriculography.[148] These RNA results are supported by a cardiac catheterization study of 106 post–myocardial infarction patients in whom the amount of akinesis (extent of infarction) and an ejection fraction of less than 40% were the best predictors of mortality.[149] It is also important to note that the ejection fraction response to submaximal exercise improves during cardiac rehabilitation.[150]

Another important aspect of follow-up after an infarction is the detection of a ventricular aneurysm. Radionuclide angiography has been reported to accurately detect an aneurysm and can be used to assess medical or surgical intervention.[151–153] Radionuclide angiography can be used to evaluate the nonaneurysmal myocardium during rest and exercise, which provides valuable information about the functional cardiac reserve of a patient prior to selecting a therapeutic intervention.

In summary, the value of different radionuclide studies during the clinical course of a myocardial infarction is variable. Myocardial perfusion imaging with ^{201}Tl is the most sensitive test for detecting an acute infarct soon after initial symptomatic presentation and is also the best technique for evaluating the presence of associated ischemia. Thallium 201 imaging is limited by its inability to detect right ventricular infarction and to differentiate between new and old scar tissue. Although new infarct-avid imaging agents are being evaluated, ^{99m}Tc-pyrophosphate is presently the best hot spot scanning agent, especially in detecting three- to five-day old infarcts. In addition, right ventricular involvement can also be detected. The limitations of this tracer include the observation of myocardial uptake without acute necrosis, especially when a diffuse pattern of tracer uptake is interpreted as positive, and the need to get serial scans if the initial (day 1 to 2) images are negative. Radionuclide angiography is the best available technique for evaluating right and left ventricular function and for assessing the patient's prognosis; it is the imaging technique that best utilizes computer quantitation. Therefore, RNA studies are highly reproducible and serial measurements can easily be obtained. It is limited in its ability to evaluate ischemia at rest and cannot differentiate old from acute regional wall motion abnormalities.

RADIATION SAFETY IN THE CORONARY CARE UNIT

Prior to all myocardial scanning studies a radioactive drug (radiopharmaceutical) is administered intravenously. The patient then becomes a source of radiation exposure, the extent of which depends on the species of radionuclide, the class of radiopharmaceutical, and the time after the administration.

Specific precautions can be formulated for each radiopharmaceutical agent so that patient care can be delivered with the least radiation exposure to medical personnel. Precautions generally correlate with the type of exposure, as listed below.

External exposure.—Exposure to radiation emitted from within the patient or from the patient's radioactive excreta (urine, feces, blood). The radiation must then penetrate into deeper tissue to do damage.

Contamination.—Deposition of radioactive material in any place where it is not desired and particularly where its presence may be harmful to personnel.

Internal exposure.—Exposure to radiation from a source within the body as a result of accidental deposition, usually from a contaminated hand which transfers the radioactivity to the mouth during eating or drinking.

A radiation safety profile can be outlined for agents used in myocardial scanning procedures. Important points to consider include the scan name, agent, physical half-life of radionuclide, the purpose of the scan, patient preparation, scan procedure, and nursing precautions.

The two radiopharmaceuticals most widely used in the coronary care unit are thallium 201 and technetium 99m, which are used in myocardial perfusion imaging and hot spot and radionuclide angiography scans, respectively. The purpose of the scans has been outlined in this chapter. There is no special patient preparation to be done prior to the study. Imaging may be done up to three to six hours after ^{201}Tl injection and up to three hours after technetium administration.

The physical properties of these isotopes include the following:

Physical half-life.—The time required for a radioactive substance to lose 50% of its activity by radioactive decay. (Thallium 201 = 73 hours, technetium 99m = 6.06 hours.)

Type of radioactive emission.—Both agents emit photons (γ-rays or x-rays) which have the ability to penetrate tissue with a minimum of interaction. However, these same photons are stopped and detected with gamma camera crystals during a scanning procedure.

Quantity of radioactivity administered.—This measurement of activity is expressed in millicuries. One millicurie is equal to 3.7×10^7 atoms decaying per second, or 2.2×10^9 atoms decaying per minute. After each decay radiations are emitted (photons) unique to a particular radionuclide. (Thallium 201 = 1.5–2.0 mCi, technetium 99m = 20 mCi.)

There are no nursing precautions recommended for ^{201}Tl studies, but there is slight urine activity for up to six hours after technetium studies. Gloves should be worn when handling urine collections during this early postscan stage. In addition, blood pool studies with technetium-labeled red blood cells will have blood activity for up to 24 hours and gloves should be worn during postscan blood sampling.

No studies have documented a significant radiation exposure to personnel in a coronary care unit environment. A radiation safety plan should be outlined for individual units based on the number and type of nuclear studies performed. It is essential that coronary care unit personnel have an opportunity to discuss this plan with the radiation safety officer and with nuclear medicine and cardiology specialists and that an ongoing communication and monitoring system be implemented. Cardiovascular nuclear medicine studies pose no health problems in a properly organized department.

REFERENCES

1. The American Heart Association: *Heart Facts 1981;* 1980.
2. Carr E.A. Jr., Beierwaltes W.H., Patno M.E., et al.: The detection of experimental infarcts by photoscanning. *Am. Heart J.* 64:650–660, 1962.
3. Donato L., Bartolomei G., Giordani R.: Evaluation of myocardial blood perfusion in man with radioactive potassium or rubidium and precordial counting. *Circulation* 29:195–203, 1964.
4. Carr E.A. Jr., Gleason G., Shaw J., et al.: The direct diagnosis of myocardial infarction by photoscanning after the administration of cesium-131. *Am. Heart J.* 68:627–636, 1964.
5. Romhilt D.W., Adolph A.J., Sodd V.J., et al.: Cesium-129 myocardial scintigraphy to detect myocardial infarction. *Circulation* 48:1242–1251, 1973.
6. Samson W.E., Scher A.M.: Mechanism of S-T segment alteration during acute myocardial injury. *Circ. Res.* 8:780, 1960.
7. Horan L.G., Flowers N.C., Johnson J.C.: Significance of the diagnostic Q wave in myocardial infarction. *Circulation* 43:428, 1971.
8. Nelson C.V., Rand P.W., Angelakos E.T., et al.: Effects of intracardiac blood on the spatial vectorcardiogram: I. Results in the dog. *Circ. Res.* 31:95, 1972.
9. Braunwald E., Maroko P.R.: ST-segment potentials and mappings: Theory and experiments. *Circulation* 54:529, 1976.
10. Vincent G.M., Abildskov J.A., Burgess M.J.: Mechanisms of ischemic ST-segment displacement: Evaluation by direct current recordings. *Circulation* 56:599, 1977.
11. Jennings R.B., Kaltenbach J.P., Smetters G.W.: Enzymatic changes in acute myocardial ischemic injury. *Arch. Pathol.* 64:10, 1957.

12. Agress C.M., Kin J.H.C.: Evaluation of enzyme tests in the diagnosis of heart disease. *Am. J. Cardiol.* 6:641, 1960.
13. Shell W.E., Kjekshus J.K., Sobel B.E.: Quantitative assessment of the extent of myocardial infarction in the conscious dog by means of analysis of serial changes in serum creatine phosphokinase activity. *J. Clin. Invest.* 50:2614, 1971.
14. Sobel B.E., Shell W.E.: Serum enzyme determinations in the diagnosis and assessment of myocardial infarction. *Circulation* 45:471, 1972.
15. Hearse D.J.: Myocardial enzyme leakage. *J. Mol. Med.* 2:185, 1977.
16. Wackers F.J.T., Schoot J.B., Sokole E.B., et al.: Noninvasive visualization of acute myocardial infarction in man with thallium-201. *Br. Heart J.* 37:741–744, 1975.
17. Wackers F.J.T., Sokole E.B., Samson G., et al.: Value and limitations of thallium-201 scintigraphy in the acute phase of myocardial infarction. *N. Engl. J. Med.* 295:1–5, 1976.
18. Wackers F.J.T., Lie K.I., Liem K.L., et al.: Potential value of thallium-201 scintigraphy as a means of selecting patients for the coronary care unit. *Br. Heart J.* 41:111–117, 1979.
19. Henning H., Schelbert H., Righetti A., et al.: Dual myocardial imaging with technetium-99m pyrophosphate and thallium-201 for detecting, localizing, and sizing acute myocardial infarction. *Am. J. Cardiol.* 40:147–155, 1977.
20. Berger H.J., Gottschalk A., Zaret B.L.: Dual radionuclide study of acute myocardial infarction: Comparison of thallium-201 and technetium-99m stannous pyrophosphate imaging in man. *Ann. Intern. Med.* 88:145–154, 1978.
21. Wackers F.J.T., Lie K.I., Busemann E., et al.: Prevalence of right ventricular involvement in inferior wall infarction assessed with myocardial imaging with thallium-201 and technetium-99m pyrophosphate. *Am. J. Cardiol.* 42:358–362, 1978.
22. Ritchie J.L., Zaret B.L., Strauss H.W., et al.: Myocardial imaging with thallium-201: A multicenter study in patients with angina pectoris or acute myocardial infarction. *Am. J. Cardiol.* 42:345–350, 1978.
23. Wackers F.J.T., Becker A.E., Samson G., et al.: Location and size of acute transmural myocardial infarction estimated from thallium-201 scintiscans: A clinical study. *Circulation* 56:72–78, 1977.
24. Leppo J., Yipintsoi T., Blankstein R., et al.: Thallium-201 myocardial scintigraphy in patients with triple-vessel disease and ischemic exercise stress tests. *Circulation* 59:714–721, 1979.
25. Niess G.S., Logic J.R., Russell R.O. Jr., et al.: Usefulness and limitations of thallium-201 myocardial scintigraphy in delineating location and size of prior myocardial infarction. *Circulation* 59:1010, 1979.
26. Parkey R.W., Bonte F.J., Meyer S.L., et al.: A new method for radionuclide imaging of acute myocardial infarction in humans. *Circulation* 50:540–546, 1974.
27. Willerson J.T., Parkey R.W., Bonte F.J., et al.: Technetium stannous pyrophosphate myocardial scintigrams in patients with chest pain of varying etiology. *Circulation* 51:1046, 1975.
28. Holman B.L., Lesch M., Zweiman F.G.: Detection and sizing of acute myocardial infarcts with ^{99}Tc (Sn) tetracycline. *N. Engl. J. Med.* 291:159, 1974.
29. Rossman D.J., Strauss H.W., Siegel M.E., et al.: Accumulation of 99m Tc-glucoheptonate in acutely infarcted myocardium. *J. Nucl. Med.* 16:875, 1975.
30. Alonso D.R., Jacobstein J.G., Cipriano P.R., et al.: Early quantification of experimental myocardial infarction with technetium-99m glucoheptonate: Scintigraphic and anatomic studies. *Am. J. Cardiol.* 42:251, 1978.
31. Buja L.M., Parkey R.W., Stokely E.M., et al.: Pathophysiology of technetium-99m stannous pyrophosphate and thallium-201 scintigraphy of acute anterior myocardial infarcts in dogs. *J. Clin. Invest.* 57:1508, 1976.
32. Buja L.M., Tofe A.J., Kulkarni P.V., et al.: Sites and mechanisms of localization of technetium-99m phosphorus radiopharmaceuticals in acute myocardial infarcts and other tissues. *J. Clin. Invest.* 60:724, 1977.
33. Poliner L.R., Buja L.M., Parkey R.W., et al.: Clinicopathologic findings in 52 patients studied by technetium-99m stannous pyrophosphate myocardial scintigraphy. *Circulation* 59:257, 1979.
34. Willerson J.T., Parkey R.W., Buja L.M., et al.: Detection of acute myocardial infarcts using myocardial scintigraphic techniques, in Parkey R.W., Bonte F.J., Buja L.M., et al. (eds.): *Clinical Nuclear Cardiology*. New York, Appleton-Century-Crofts, 1979, p. 141.
35. Willerson J.T., Parkey R.W., Bonte F.J., et al.: Acute subendocardial infarction in patients: Its detection by technetium-99m stannous pyrophosphate scintigrams. *Circulation* 51:436, 1975.
36. Massie B.M., Botvinick E.H., Werner J.A., et al.: Myocardial scintigraphy with technetium-99m stannous pyrophosphate: An insensitive test for nontransmural myocardial infarction. *Am. J. Cardiol.* 43:186, 1979.
37. Lyons K.P., Olson H.G., Aronow W.S.: Pyrophosphate myocardial imaging. *Semin. Nucl. Med.* 10:168, 1980.
38. Olson H.G., Lyons K.P., Aronow W.S., et al.: Follow-up technetium-99m stannous pyrophosphate myocardial scintigrams after acute myocardial infarction. *Circulation* 56:181, 1977.
39. Malin F.R., Rollow F.D., Gertz E.W.: Sequential myocardial scintigraphy with technetium-99m stannous pyrophosphate following myocardial infarction. *J. Nucl. Med.* 19:1111, 1978.

40. Perez L.A., Hayt D.B., Freeman L.M.: Localization of myocardial disorders other than infarction with 99m-Tc-labelled phosphate agents. *J. Nucl. Med.* 17:241, 1976.
41. Donsky M.S., Curry G.C., Parkey R.W., et al.: Unstable angina pectoris: Clinical, angiographic, and myocardial scintigraphic observations. *Br. Heart J.* 38:257, 1976.
42. Abdulla A.M., Canedo M.I., Cortez B.C., et al.: Detection of unstable angina by ^{99m}technetium pyrophosphate myocardial scintigraphy. *Chest* 69:168, 1976.
43. Prasquier R., Taradash M.R., Botvinick E.H., et al.: The specificity of the diffuse pattern of cardiac uptake in myocardial infarction imaging with technetium-99m stannous pyrophosphate. *Circulation* 55:61, 1977.
44. Ahmad M., Dubiel J.P., Logan K.W., et al.: Limited clinical diagnostic specificity of technetium-99m stannous pyrophosphate myocardial imaging in acute myocardial infarction. *Am. J. Cardiol.* 39:50, 1977.
45. Jaffe A.S., Klein M.S., Patel B.R., et al.: Abnormal technetium-99m pyrophosphate images in unstable angina: Ischemia versus infarction? *Am. J. Cardiol.* 44:1035, 1979.
46. Holman B.L., Lesch M., Alpert J.S.: Myocardial scintigraphy with technetium-99m pyrophosphate during the early phase of acute infarction. *Am. J. Cardiol.* 41:39, 1978.
47. Ahmad M., Dubid J.P., Verdon T.A. Jr., et al.: Technetium-99m stannous pyrophosphate myocardial imaging in patients with and without left ventricular aneurysm. *Circulation* 53:833, 1976.
48. Crowley M.J., Mantle J.A., Rogers W.J., et al.: Technetium-99m stannous pyrophosphate myocardial scintigraphy: Reliability and limitations in assessment of acute myocardial infarction. *Circulation* 56:192, 1977.
49. Curry R.C., Jackmon W.M.: Persistently positive Tc-pyrophosphate myocardial scintigram in patients with a left ventricular aneurysm. *Clin. Nucl. Med.* 1:91, 1976.
50. Pugh B.R., Buja L.M., Parkey R.W., et al.: Cardioversion and "false positive" technetium-99m stannous pyrophosphate myocardial scintigraphy. *Circulation* 54:399, 1976.
51. Davidson R., Spies S.M., Przybylek J., et al.: Technetium-99m stannous pyrophosphate myocardial scintigraphy after cardiopulmonary resuscitation with cardioversion. *Circulation* 60:292, 1979.
52. Epstein D.A., Solar M., Levin E.J.: Demonstration of long-standing metastatic soft tissue calcification by 99m Tc-diphosphate. *A.J.R.* 128:145, 1977.
53. Righetti A., O'Rourke R.A., Schelbert H., et al.: Usefulness of preoperative and postoperative Tc-99m (Sn) pyroscans in patients with ischemic and valvular heart disease. *Am. J. Cardiol.* 39:43, 1977.
54. Chiu C.L., Roelofs J.D., Go R.T., et al.: Coronary angiographic and scintigraphic findings in experimental cardiac contusion. *Radiology* 116:679, 1975.
55. Go R.T., Doty D.B., Chiu C.L.: A new method of diagnosing myocardial contusion in man by radionuclide imaging. *Radiology* 116:107, 1975.
56. Lyons K.P., Olson H.G., Brown W.T., et al.: Persistence of an abnormal pattern on Tc-99m pyrophosphate myocardial scintigraphy of acute myocardial infarction. *Clin. Nucl. Med.* 1:253, 1976.
57. Klein M.S., Coleman E., Roberts R., et al.: False positive Tc(Sn) pyrophosphate myocardial infarct images related to delayed blood pool clearance. *Clin. Nucl. Med.* 1:45, 1976.
58. Stokely E.M., Parkey R.W., Bonte F.J., et al.: Gated blood pool imaging following 99m Tc stannous pyrophosphate imaging. *Radiology* 120:433, 1976.
59. Serafini A.N., Raskin M.M., Zand L.C., et al.: Radionuclide breast scanning in carcinoma of the breast. *J. Nucl. Med.* 15:1149, 1974.
60. Hisada K., Suzuki Y., Iimori M.: Technetium 99m pyrophosphate bone imaging in the evaluation of trauma. *Clin. Nucl. Med.* 1:18, 1976.
61. Rosenthall L., Hill R.O., Chuang S.: Observation on the use of 99m Tc-phosphate imaging in peripheral bone trauma. *Radiology* 119:637, 1976.
62. Kim E.: Calcified costal cartilage as a cause of false interpretation on myocardial imaging. *Clin. Nucl. Med.* 1:159, 1976.
63. Bossuyt A., Verbeelen D.: Accumulation of ^{99m}Tc pyrophosphate in the skin lesions of pseudoxanthoma elasticum. *Clin. Nucl. Med.* 1:245, 1976.
64. Platt M.R., Mills L.J., Parkey R.W., et al.: Perioperative myocardial infarction diagnosed by technetium 99m stannous pyrophosphate myocardial scintigrams. *Circulation* 54(suppl. 3):24–27, 1976.
65. Raabe D.S. Jr., Morise A., Sbarbaro J.A., et al.: Diagnostic criteria for acute myocardial infarction in patients undergoing coronary artery bypass surgery. *Circulation* 62:869, 1980.
66. Khaw B.A., Gold H.K., Leinbach R.C., et al.: Early imaging of experimental myocardial infarction by intracoronary administration of ^{131}I-labeled anticardiac myosin $(Fab_1)_2$ fragments. *Circulation* 58:1137, 1978.
67. Khaw B.A., Fallon J.T., Beller G.A., et al.: Specificity of localization of myosin specific antibody fragments in experimental myocardial infarction: Histologic, histochemical, autoradiographic and scintigraphic studies. *Circulation* 60:1527, 1979.
68. Cochavi S., Pohost G.M., Elmaleh D.R., et al.: Transverse-sectional imaging with $Na^{18}F$ in myocardial infarction. *J. Nucl. Med.* 20:1013, 1979.
69. Mullins C.B., Mason D.T., Ashburn W.L., et al.: Determination of ventricular volume by radioisotope angiography. *Am. J. Cardiol.* 24:72, 1969.

70. Mason D.T., Ashburn W.L., Harbert J.C., et al.: Rapid sequential visualization of the heart and great vessels in man using the wide field Anger scintillation camera. *Circulation* 39:19, 1969.
71. Berger H.J., Matthay R.A., Pytlik L.M., et al.: First-pass radionuclide assessment of right and left ventricular performance in patients with cardiac and pulmonary disease. *Semin. Nucl. Med.* 9:275, 1979.
72. Strauss H.W., McKusick K.A., Boucher C.A., et al.: Of lines and laces: The eighth anniversary of the gated blood pool scan. *Semin. Nucl. Med.* 9:296, 1979.
73. Strauss H.W., Zaret B.L., Hurley P.J., et al.: Scintiphotographic method for measuring left ventricular ejection fraction in man without cardiac catheterization. *Am. J. Cardiol.* 28:575, 1971.
74. Zaret B.L., Strauss H.W., Hurley P.J., et al.: A noninvasive scintiphotographic method for detecting regional ventricular dysfunction in man. *N. Engl. J. Med.* 284:1165, 1971.
75. Kostuk W.J., Ehsani A.A., Karliner J.S., et al.: Left ventricular performance after myocardial infarction assessed by radioisotope angiocardiography. *Circulation* 47:242, 1973.
76. Rigo P., Murray M., Strauss H.W., et al.: Left ventricular function in acute myocardial infarction evaluated by gated scintiphotography. *Circulation* 50:678, 1974.
77. Schelbert H.R., Henning H., Ashburn W.L., et al.: Serial measurements of left ventricular ejection fraction by radionuclide angiography early and late after myocardial infarction. *Am. J. Cardiol.* 38:407, 1976.
78. Schad N.: Nontraumatic assessment of left ventricular wall motion and regional stroke volume after myocardial infarction. *J. Nucl. Med.* 18:333, 1977.
79. Wynne J., Sayres M., Maddox D.E., et al.: Regional left ventricular function in acute myocardial infarction: Evaluation with quantitative radionuclide ventriculography. *Am. J. Cardiol.* 45:203–209, 1980.
80. Page D.L., Caulfield J.B., Kastor J.A., et al.: Myocardial changes associated with cardiogenic shock. *N. Engl. J. Med.* 285:134–137, 1971.
81. Davis H.T., DeCamilla J., Bayer L.W., et al.: Survivorship patterns in the posthospital phase of myocardial infarction. *Circulation* 60:1252–1258, 1979.
82. Roberts R., Husain A., Ambros D., et al.: Relation between infarct size and ventricular arrhythmia. *Br. Heart J.* 37:1169–1175, 1975.
83. Miller R.R., Olson H.G., Vismara L.A., et al.: Pump dysfunction after myocardial infarction: Importance of location, extent, and pattern of abnormal left ventricular segmental contraction. *Am. J. Cardiol.* 37:340–344, 1976.
84. Sullivan W., Vlodaver Z., Tuna B., et al.: Correlation of electrocardiographic and pathologic findings in healed myocardial infarction. *Am. J. Cardiol.* 42:724–732, 1978.
85. Mueller T.M., Marcus M.L., Ehrhardt J.C., et al.: Limitations of thallium-201 myocardial perfusion scintigrams. *Circulation* 54:640, 1976.
86. Bulkley B.H., Silverman K., Weisfeldt M.L., et al.: Pathologic basis of thallium-201 scintigraphic defects in patients with fatal myocardial injury. *Circulation* 60:785–791, 1979.
87. Nelson A.D., Khullar S., Leighton R.F., et al.: Quantification of thallium-201 scintigrams in acute myocardial infarction. *Am. J. Cardiol.* 44:664, 1979.
88. Pohost G.M., Zir L.M., Moore R.H., et al.: Differentiation of transiently ischemic from infarcted myocardium by serial imaging after a single dose of thallium-201. *Circulation* 55:294, 1977.
89. Massie B.M., Botvinick E.H., Brundage B.H., et al.: Relationship of regional myocardial perfusion to sequential wall motion. *Circulation* 58:1154, 1978.
90. Bodenheimer M.M., Banka V.S., Fooshee C., et al.: Relationship between regional myocardial perfusion and the presence, severity and reversibility of asynergy in patients with coronary heart disease. *Circulation* 58:789, 1978.
91. Maseri A., Parodi O., Severi S., et al.: Transient transmural reduction of myocardial blood flow demonstrated by thallium-201 scintigraphy as a cause of variant angina pectoris. *Circulation* 54:280, 1976.
92. Maseri A., Severi S., Nes M.D., et al.: "Variant" angina: One aspect of a continuous spectrum of vasospastic myocardial ischemia. *Am. J. Cardiol.* 42:1019, 1978.
93. Gewirtz H., Beller G., Strauss H.W., et al.: Transient defects of resting thallium scans in patients with coronary artery disease. *Circulation* 59:707, 1979.
94. Berger B.C., Watson D.D., Burwell L.R., et al.: Redistribution of thallium at rest in patients with stable and unstable angina and the effect of coronary artery bypass surgery. *Circulation* 60:1114, 1979.
95. Ohsuzu F., Handa S., Kondo M., et al.: Thallium-201 myocardial imaging to evaluate right ventricular overloading. *Circulation* 61:610, 1980.
96. Parkey R.W., Bonte F.J., Stokely E.M., et al.: Acute myocardial infarction imaged with ^{99m}Tc-stannous pyrophosphate and ^{201}Tl: A clinical evaluation. *J. Nucl. Med.* 17:771, 1976.
97. Sharpe D.N., Botvinick E.H., Shames D.M., et al.: The clinical estimation of acute myocardial infarct size with ^{99m} technetium pyrophosphate scintigraphy. *Circulation* 57:307, 1978.
98. Sharpe D.N., Botvinick E.H., Shames D.M., et al.: The noninvasive diagnosis of right ventricular infarction. *Circulation* 57:483, 1978.
99. Inser J.M., Roberts W.L.: Right ventricular in-

farction complicating left ventricular infarction secondary to coronary heart disease. *Am. J. Cardiol.* 42:885, 1978.
100. Morrison J., Coromilas J., Munsey D., et al.: Correlation of radionuclide estimates of myocardial infarction size and release of creatine kinase MB in man. *Circulation* 62:277–287, 1980.
101. Winzelberg G.G., Strauss H.W., Bingham J.B., et al.: Scintigraphic evaluation of left ventricular aneurysm. *Am. J. Cardiol.* 46:1138–1143, 1980.
102. Rigo P., Murray M., Taylor D.R., et al.: Right ventricular dysfunction detected by gated scintiphotography in patients with acute myocardial infarction. *Circulation* 52:268–274, 1975.
103. Reduto L.A., Berger H.J., Cohen L.S., et al.: Sequential radionuclide assessment of left and right ventricular performance after acute transmural myocardial infarction. *Ann. Intern. Med.* 89:441–447, 1978.
104. Pohost G.M., Alpert N.M., Ingwall J.S., et al.: Thallium redistribution: Mechanisms and clinical utility. *Semin. Nucl. Med.* 10:70–93, 1980.
105. Wackers F.J.T., Lie K.I., Liem K.L., et al.: Thallium-201 scintigraphy in unstable angina pectoris. *Circulation* 57:738–742, 1978.
106. Smitherman T.C., Osborn R.C., Narahara K.A.: Serial myocardial scintigraphy after a single dose of thallium-201 in men after acute myocardial infarction. *Am. J. Cardiol.* 42:177–182, 1978.
107. Ramanathan K.B., Bodenheimer M.M., Banka V.S., et al.: Severity of contraction abnormalities following acute myocardial infarction in man: Response to nitroglycerin. *Circulation* 60:1230–1237, 1979.
108. Banka V.S., Bodenheimer M.M., Shah R., et al.: Intervention ventriculography: Comparative value of nitroglycerin, postextrasystolic potentiation, and nitroglycerin and postextrasystolic potentiation. *Circulation* 53:632–636, 1976
109. Shah P.K., Pichler M., Berman D.S., et al.: Noninvasive identification of a high risk subset of patients with acute inferior myocardial infarction. *Am. J. Cardiol.* 46:915–921, 1980.
110. Sobel B.E., Weiss E.S., Welch M.J., et al.: Detection of remote myocardial infarction in patients with positron emission transaxial tomography and intravenous ^{11}C-palmitate. *Circulation* 55:853–857, 1977.
111. Ter-Pogossian M.M., Klein M.S., Markham J., et al.: Regional assessment of myocardial metabolic integrity in vivo by positron emission tomography with ^{11}C-labeled palmitate. *Circulation* 61:242–255, 1980.
112. Beller G.A., Watson D.D., Ackell P., et al.: Time course of thallium-201 redistribution after transient myocardial ischemia. *Circulation* 61:791–797, 1980.
113. Pohost G.M., Okada R.D., O'Keefe D.D., et al.: Thallium redistribution in dogs with severe coronary artery stenosis of fixed caliber. *Circ. Res.* 48:439–446, 1981.
114. Verani M.S., Jhingran S., Attar M., et al.: Poststress redistribution of thallium-201 in patients with coronary artery disease, and with and without prior myocardial infarction. *Am. J. Cardiol.* 43:1114–1122, 1979.
115. Kronenberg M.W., Wooten N.E., Friesinger G.C., et al.: Scintigraphic characteristics of experimental myocardial infarct extension. *Circulation* 60:1130–1140, 1979.
116. Long R., Symes J., Allard J., et al.: Differentiation between reperfusion and occlusion myocardial necrosis with technetium-99m pyrophosphate scans. *Am. J. Cardiol.* 46:413–418, 1980.
117. Borer J.S., Rosing D.R., Miller R.H., et al.: Natural history of left ventricular function during 1 year after acute myocardial infarction: Comparison with clinical, electrocardiographic and biochemical determinations. *Am. J. Cardiol.* 46:1–12, 1980.
118. Nichols A.B., McKusick K.A., Strauss H.W., et al.: Clinical utility of gated cardiac blood pool imaging in congestive left heart failure. *Am. J. Med.* 65:785–793, 1978.
119. Rigo P., Alderson P.O., Robertson R.M., et al.: Measurement of aortic and mitral regurgitation by gated cardiac blood pool scans. *Circulation* 60:306–312, 1979.
120. Askenasi J., Ahnberg D.S., Korngold E., et al.: Quantitative radionuclide angiocardiography: Detection and quantitation of left to right shunts. *Am. J. Cardiol.* 37:382–387, 1976.
121. Sobel B.E., Bresnahan G.F., Shell W.E., et al.: Estimation of infarct size in man and its relation to prognosis. *Circulation* 46:640, 1972.
122. Norris R.M., Whitlock R.M.L., Barratt-Boyes C., et al.: Clinical measurement of myocardial infarct size: Modification of a method for the estimation of total creatine phosphokinase release after myocardial infarction. *Circulation* 51:614, 1975.
123. Silverman K.J., Becker L.C., Bulkley B.H., et al.: Value of early thallium-201 scintigraphy for predicting mortality in patients with acute myocardial infarction. *Circulation* 61:996–1003, 1980.
124. Rude R.E., Parkey R.W., Bonte F.J., et al.: Clinical implications of the technetium-99m stannous pyrophosphate myocardial scintigraphic "doughnut" pattern in patients with acute myocardial infarcts. *Circulation* 59:721–729, 1979.
125. Schulze R.A., Rouleau J., Rigo P., et al.: Left ventricular function and ventricular arrhythmias in the late hospital phase of acute myocardial infarction. *Circulation* 52:1006–1011, 1975.
126. Schuster E.H., Bulkley B.H.: Ischemia at a distance after acute myocardial infarction: A cause of early postinfarction angina. *Circulation* 62:509–515, 1980.
127. Freisinger G.C., Page E.E., Ross R.S.: Prognos-

tic significance of coronary arteriography. *Trans. Assoc. Am. Phys.* 93:78–92, 1970.
128. Operman A., Jones W.B., Riley C.P., et al.: Natural history of coronary artery disease. *Bull. N.Y. Acad. Med.* 48:1109–1125, 1972.
129. Bruschke A.V.G., Proudfit W.L., Sones F.M. Jr.: Progress study of 590 consecutive nonsurgical cases of coronary disease followed 5–9 years: I. Arteriographic correlations. *Circulation* 47:1147–1153, 1973.
130. Harris P.J., Harrell F.E., Lee K.L., et al.: Survival in medically treated coronary artery disease. *Circulation* 60:1259–1269, 1979.
131. Kannel W.B., Sorlie P., McNamara P.M.: Prognosis after initial myocardial infarction: The Framingham study. *Am. J. Cardiol.* 44:53–59, 1979.
132. Ellestad M.H., Wan M.K.C.: Predictive implications of stress testing followup of 2700 subjects after maximum treadmill stress testing. *Circulation* 51:363–369, 1975.
133. Theroux P., Waters D.D., Halphen C., et al.: Prognostic value of exercise testing soon after myocardial infarction. *N. Engl. J. Med.* 301:341–345, 1979.
134. Gibson R.S., Taylor G.J., Watson D.D., et al.: Prognostic significance of resting anterior thallium-201 defects in patients with inferior myocardial infarction. *J. Nucl. Med.* 21:1015–1021, 1980.
135. Turner J.D., Schwartz K.M., Logic J.R., et al.: Detection of residual jeopardized myocardium 3 weeks after myocardial infarction by exercise testing with thallium-201 myocardial scintigraphy. *Circulation* 61:729–737, 1980.
136. Dunn R.F., Freedman B., Bailey I.K., et al.: Noninvasive prediction of multivessel disease after myocardial infarction. *Circulation* 62:726–734, 1980.
137. Boucher C.A., Zir L.M., Beller G.A., et al.: Increased lung uptake of thallium-201 during exercise myocardial imaging: Clinical, hemodynamic and angiographic implications in patients with coronary artery disease. *Am. J. Cardiol.* 46:189–196, 1980.
138. Bingham J.B., McKusick K.A., Strauss H.W., et al.: Influence of coronary artery disease on pulmonary uptake of thallium-201. *Am. J. Cardiol.* 46:821–826, 1980.
139. Blood D.K., McCarthy D.M., Sciacca R.R., et al.: Comparison of single-dose and double-dose thallium-201 myocardial perfusion scintigraphy for the detection of coronary artery disease and prior myocardial infarction. *Circulation* 58:777–788, 1978.
140. Massie B.M., Botvinick E.H., Brundage B.H.: Correlation of thallium-201 scintigrams with coronary anatomy: Factors affecting region by region sensitivity. *Am. J. Cardiol.* 44:616–622, 1979.
141. Rigo P., Bailey I.K., Griffith L.S.C., et al.: Value and limitations of segmental analysis of stress thallium myocardial imaging for localization of coronary artery disease. *Circulation* 61:973–981, 1980.
142. Akins C.W., Pohost G.M., DeSanctis R.W., et al.: Selection of angina-free patients with severe left ventricular dysfunction for myocardial revascularization. *Am. J. Cardiol.* 46:695–700, 1980.
143. Olson H.G., Lyons K.P., Aronow W.S., et al.: Prognostic value of a persistently positive technetium-99m stannous pyrophosphate myocardial scintigram after myocardial infarction. *Am. J. Cardiol.* 43:889–898, 1979.
144. Lyons K.P., Olson H.G., Kuperus J., et al.: Correlations of Tc-99m pyrophosphate myocardial scintigraphy and the results of coronary-artery bypass surgery. *J. Nucl. Med.* 19:1116–1120, 1978.
145. Ahmad M., Logan K.W., Martin R.H.: Doughnut pattern of technetium-99m pyrophosphate myocardial uptake in patients with acute myocardial infarction: A sign of poor long-term prognosis. *Am. J. Cardiol.* 44:13–17, 1979.
146. Schulze R.A., Strauss H.W., Pitt B.: Sudden death in the year following myocardial infarction: Relation to ventricular premature contractions in the late hospital phase and left ventricular ejection fraction. *Am. J. Med.* 62:192–199, 1977.
147. Pulido J.I., Doss J., Tweig D., et al.: Submaximal exercise testing in patients after acute myocardial infarction: Myocardial scintigraphic and electrocardiographic observations. *Am. J. Cardiol.* 42:19–28, 1978.
148. Paine T.D., Dye L.E., Roitman D.I., et al.: Relation of graded exercise test findings after myocardial infarction to extent of coronary artery disease and left ventricular dysfunction. *Am. J. Cardiol.* 42:716–723, 1978.
149. Taylor G.J., Humphries J.O., Mellits E.D., et al.: Predictors of clinical course, coronary anatomy and left ventricular function after recovery from acute myocardial infarction. *Circulation* 62:960–969, 1980.
150. Jensen D., Atwood J.E., Froelicher V., et al.: Improvement in ventricular function during exercise studied with radionuclide ventriculography after cardiac rehabilitation. *Am. J. Cardiol.* 96:770–777, 1980.
151. Froehlich R.T., Falsetti H.L., Doty D.B., et al.: Prospective study of surgery for left ventricular aneurysm. *Am. J. Cardiol.* 45:923–931, 1980.
152. Stephens J.D., Dymond D.S., Stone D.L., et al.: Left ventricular aneurysm and congestive heart failure: Value of exercise stress and isosorbide dinitrate in predicting hemodynamic results of aneurysmectomy. *Am. J. Cardiol.* 45:932–939, 1980.
153. Borer J.S., Jacobstein J.G., Bacharach S.L., et al.: Detection of left ventricular aneurysm and evaluation of effects of surgical repair: the role of radionuclide cineangiography. *Am. J. Cardiol.* 45:1103–1106, 1980.

PART VI

Complications of Myocardial Infarction

ECHOCARDIOGRAPHY

William E. Strauss and Alfred F. Parisi

ECHOCARDIOGRAPHY is particularly well suited to identifying a number of complications of myocardial infarction because of the effects of such complications on cardiac anatomy and function. In general, these effects can be imaged because (1) a substantial amount of myocardium has been damaged, (2) specific regions of the myocardium have been damaged, with additional consequences (e.g., papillary muscle rupture, ventricular septal defect), and (3) there is further pathologic interplay between blood elements and the region of myocardial damage (e.g., thrombus formation). A list of complications of acute myocardial infarction is given in Table 11–1; those in which echocardiography has made an important contribution or has a potentially important role are discussed herein.

VENTRICULAR ANEURYSMS

Ventricular aneurysms, which are circumscribed, noncontractile areas of infarcted left ventricle, develop in approximately 12%–15% of patients who survive myocardial infarction. This complication can cause congestive heart failure, precipitate ventricular tachyarrhythmias, or predispose to systemic embolization. In carefully selected cases surgical intervention has proved effective in improving symptoms and hemodynamics. Although clinical, ECG, and conventional radiographic techniques can suggest the presence of a ventricular aneurysm, these methods are nonspecific and insensitive: 40%–50% of discrete aneurysms remain undiagnosed prior to angiography or postmortem examination if only ECG and chest roentgenography are used as screening techniques prior to more definitive study by contrast ventriculography. However, x-ray contrast studies are not without risks, especially if mural thrombi within the wall of the aneurysm are dislodged during ventriculography, producing systemic embolization.

M-mode echocardiography has long been recognized as capable of detecting ventricular aneurysms.[1, 2] In a typical examination with the transducer in a standard location, a scan of the left ventricle from base to apex shows that the cavity expands or fails to taper as the region of the papillary muscles is approached. This finding is often associated with the presence of a left ventricular aneurysm.[3] Another observation associated with left ventricular aneurysm is localized displacement of the posterior left ventricular wall.[1, 2] Many, but not all, left ventricular aneurysms fall within the path of a standard M-mode examination procedure. Weyman and co-workers[4] noted that in a series of 31 patients with angiographically proved left ventricular aneurysms, two-dimensional echocardiography (2DE) detected 100% of these defects, while M-mode studies were successful in detecting the abnormality 47% of the time. The 2DE studies clearly defined localized interruption in the diastolic configuration of the left ventricular wall that corresponded in each case to a similar location on the angiogram. Others have noted paradoxic movement of the wall of the aneurysm

TABLE 11–1.—Complications of Acute Myocardial Infarction

Complication	Echocardiographic Manifestations
Early	
Arrhythmias	Not applicable
Heart block and/or marked bradycardia	Not applicable
Shock	Large areas of noncontractile LV myocardium. Right ventricular infarction: impaired RV wall motion, increased RV size with or without abnormal septal motion; absence of pericardial fluid
Pulmonary edema (congestive heart failure)	Large areas of noncontractile LV myocardium and/or anatomical complications (e.g., ventricular septal defect)
Subacute	
Infarct extension/expansion	Expansion demonstrated by disproportionate transmural diastolic thinning and associated regional ventricular dilation on 2DE
Severe mitral regurgitation secondary to papillary muscle dysfunction or rupture	Rupture demonstrated by visualization of untethered mitral valve leaflet on 2DE
Acute ventricular septal defect	2DE visualization of septal rent; negative contrast effect after IV fluid injection
Subacute to late	
Ventricular aneurysm	Localized interruption in the diastolic configuration of LV wall; orifice to aneurysm is wide
Ventricular pseudoaneurysm	Demonstration of narrow neck leading into the false aneurysm cavity
Thromboembolism	Visualization of LV thrombus

compared to the remaining noninfarcted ventricular wall.[5] Typical examples of left ventricular aneurysms detected by 2DE are shown in Figure 11–1. Since it is highly specific and has no associated morbidity, 2DE should be considered the initial noninvasive screening procedure for detecting ventricular aneurysm. Positive findings on an adequately performed examination should be considered diagnostic; further action will depend on an individual patient's needs. If a technically adequate 2DE study is negative it is reasonable to proceed no further: if the 2DE examination is not definitive, alternative procedures may be entertained.

VENTRICULAR PSEUDOANEURYSMS

Rupture of the left ventricular myocardium usually results in sudden and fatal hemopericardium. However, if adhesions are present, the hemorrhage may be locally contained by the pericardium. Subsequent organization of this self-limiting myocardial rupture produces a thrombus-lined pericardial sac devoid of myocardial tissue. In contrast, true left ventricular aneurysms are abnormal outpouchings of infarcted left ventricular myocardium.

In the patient who has not had antecedent cardiac trauma or surgery, myocardial infarction is the leading cause of pseudoaneurysm formation.[6] Unlike the orifice to a true aneurysm, which is very wide, the orifice to a false aneurysm tends to be narrow. By virtue of this anatomical feature, false ventricular aneurysms are often detectable by echocardiography. M-mode echocardiography has been reported to detect both posterior pseudoaneurysms[7, 8] (Fig 11–2) and septal pseudoaneurysms[6] (Fig 11–3), in each instance demonstrating discontinuity between an ectopic cavity and the true confines of the ventricle. However, M-mode echocardiography does not provide reliable visualization of the orifice to the pseudoaneurysm. Two-dimensional echocardiography greatly facilitates recognition of the narrow orifice leading into the false aneurysm cavity (Fig 11–4).[9–12] Successful differentiation of pseudoaneurysms from true left ventricular aneurysms was made in two series of cases angiographically or pathologically documented[11, 12] by comparison of the width of the orifice to the internal diameter of aneurysmal dilation. The maximal internal width of the pseudo-

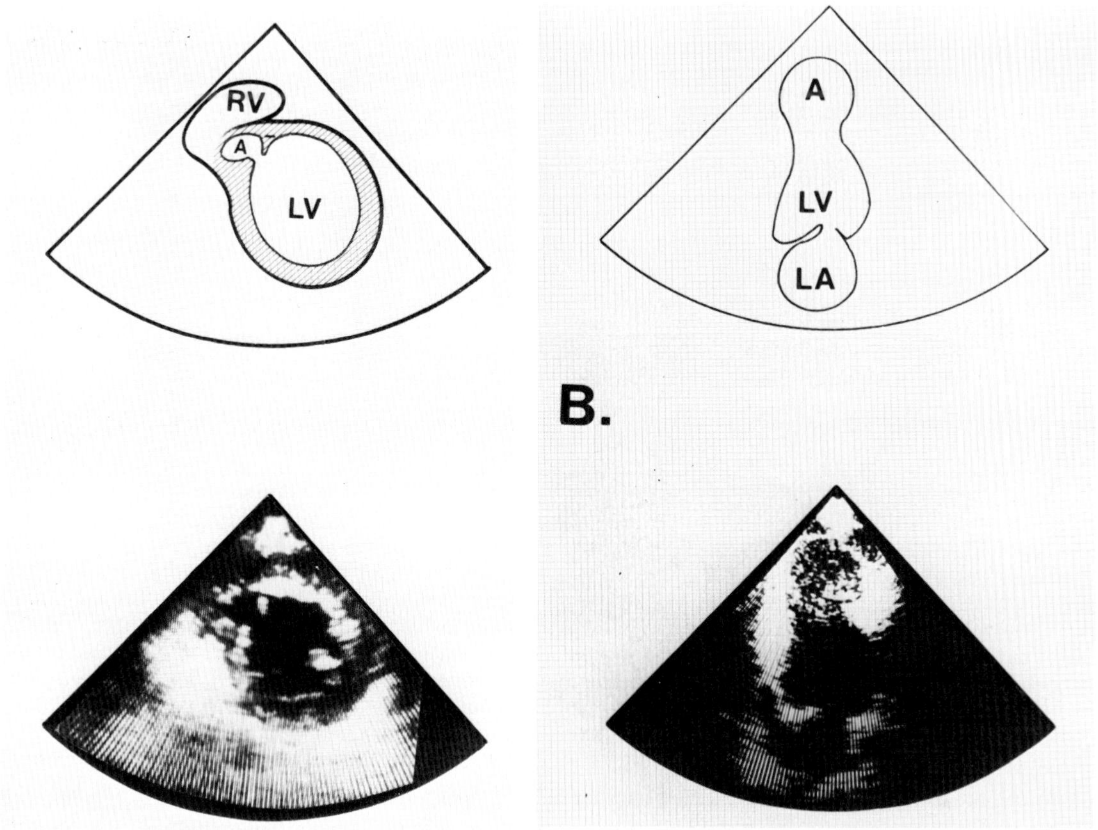

Fig 11–1.—Left ventricular aneurysm. *Left,* aneurysm of the interventricular septum in a patient with remote anterior myocardial infarction. This type of aneurysm is more likely to be missed on M-mode scanning than is an apical aneurysm. *Right,* apical left ventricular aneurysm seen with an apical view on two-dimensional echocardiography. The cloud of echoes within the aneurysmal chamber suggests a left ventricular thrombus. *A,* aneurysm; *LA,* left atrium; *LV,* left ventricle; *MV,* mitral valve; *RV,* right ventricle.

aneurysm orifice (Omax) was smaller than the maximal parallel internal diameter (Dmax) of the aneurysmal sac, with the ratio Omax/Dmax never exceeding 0.5 (Fig 11–5).[12] In contrast, true aneurysms resulted in local dilation of the ventricular wall so that the maximal internal width of the aneurysm mouth was nearly equal to the maximal internal diameter of the aneurysm, producing a ratio Omax/Dmax of 0.9–1.0.

Detection of false aneurysms is more than academic, since false aneurysms are prone to fatal rupture, a complication very rarely encountered with a true left ventricular aneurysm. Moreover, the false aneurysm is readily amenable to surgery, which is the treatment of choice. Thus, echocardiography, particularly 2DE, is a key examination in the patient with an abnormally bulging radiographic cardiac silhouette after myocardial infarction. Since the primary clue to distinguishing between true and false aneurysm is a narrowed orifice to the aneurysm cavity, false aneurysms will *not* be detected on standard chest roentgenograms.

PAPILLARY MUSCLE DYSFUNCTION AND RUPTURE

Mitral valve regurgitation may arise from anatomical or functional derangements of the papillary muscles. Papillary muscle dysfunction can be caused by ischemia or infarction that leads to asyn-

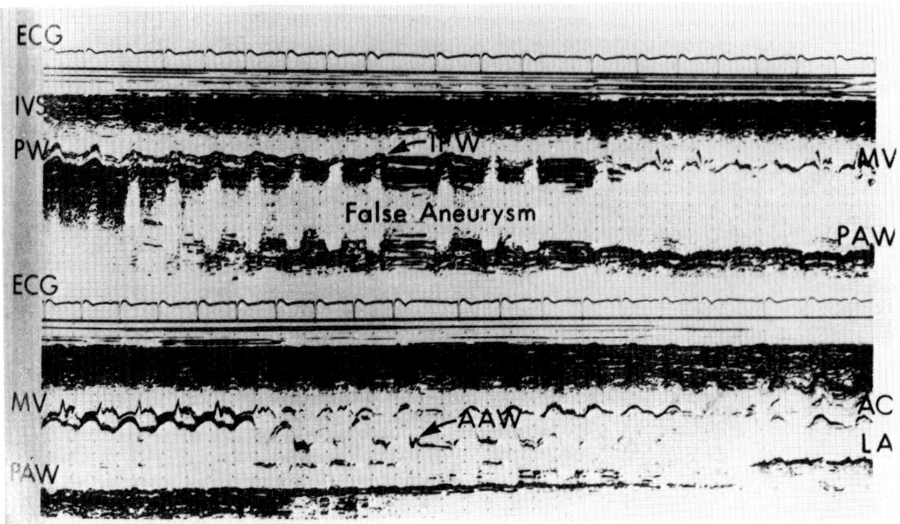

Fig 11–2.—Continuous sweep of M-mode echocardiography recorded through fifth intercostal space. Note excellent motion of both septum and left ventricular posterior wall *(PW)* at apex *(top strip, left).* False aneurysm is recorded behind left ventricle and occupies almost entire lower portion of both strips. Both borders of its orifice are formed at the discontinuity of infarcted left ventricular PW in top strip and at junction of posterior mitral valve leaflet and anterior aneurysmal wall in lower strip. Aorta and left atrium appear in *bottom strip, right. AAW,* anterior aneurysmal wall; *IVS,* interventricular septum; *MV,* mitral valve; *PAW,* posterior aneurysmal wall. (From Thanovaro et al.[8] Reproduced by permission of the *Southern Medical Journal.*)

ergic contraction of the muscles, or by ventricular dilation or aneurysms that produce sufficient malalignment of the papillary muscle tethering mechanisms to result in mitral regurgitation. Although these two mechanisms were initially proposed by Burch in 1963, M-mode echocardiography has been unable to show the anatomical basis for these two possible explanations. Since 2DE permits real-time evaluation of the anatomical and functional relationships of intracardiac structures, differentiation between these functional mechanisms has been reported. In a series of 14 patients with papillary muscle dysfunction, two abnormal patterns of mitral valve closure have been identified by 2DE: 3 patients had *mitral valve prolapse* associated with inferoposterior wall akinesis and increased tissue echo density consistent with papillary muscle fibrosis, 9 patients with ventricular enlargement or aneurysm had *apically displaced mitral leaflet coaptation,* and the remaining 2 patients had both patterns.[13]

Papillary muscle rupture is a devastating complication of acute myocardial infarction. It produces mitral regurgitation, which acutely imposes a large volume overload on the left heart. The precise magnitude of the volume load depends on the exact anatomical site of papillary muscle rupture. Papillary muscle rupture is usually suspected from the sudden appearance of a loud systolic murmur, which may be impossible to distinguish at the bedside from the murmur of a ruptured interventricular septum. If a head of a papillary muscle rather than an entire papillary muscle ruptures, it is possible that the patient can survive and undergo diagnostic evaluation that will allow its confirmation and the possibility for surgical repair. Rupture of an entire papillary muscle generally produces such a catastrophic deterioration that effective intervention is extremely difficult or impossible.

Ventricular angiography is a definitive procedure which can detect papillary muscle rupture but which carries a significant risk in a patient who is sufficiently decompensated. Right heart catheterization by means of a Swan-Ganz catheter has proved very helpful but has limitations: in the context of tachycardia or atrial fibrillation, differentiation of elevated pulmonary artery pressure

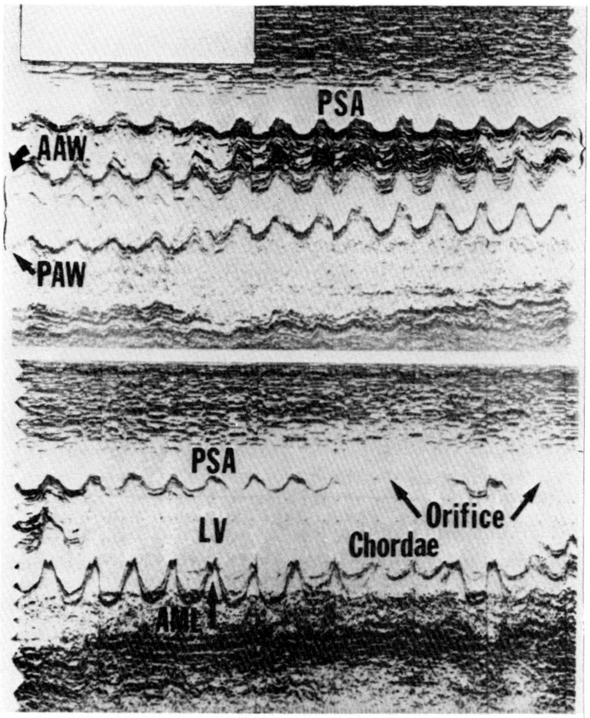

Fig 11–3.—Continuous M-mode scan from the aorta *(top left)* to the apex of the left ventricle *(bottom right).* The strip chart record has been divided at the serrated edges for illustrative purposes. *AO,* aortic root; *AAW,* anterior aortic wall; *PAW,* posterior aortic wall; *S,* interventricular septum; *AML,* anterior mitral leaflet; *LV,* left ventricle. The thin posterior wall of the pseudoaneurysm *(PSA)* abuts the septum; at the level of the chordae tendineae there is open communication between the *LV* and *PSA.*

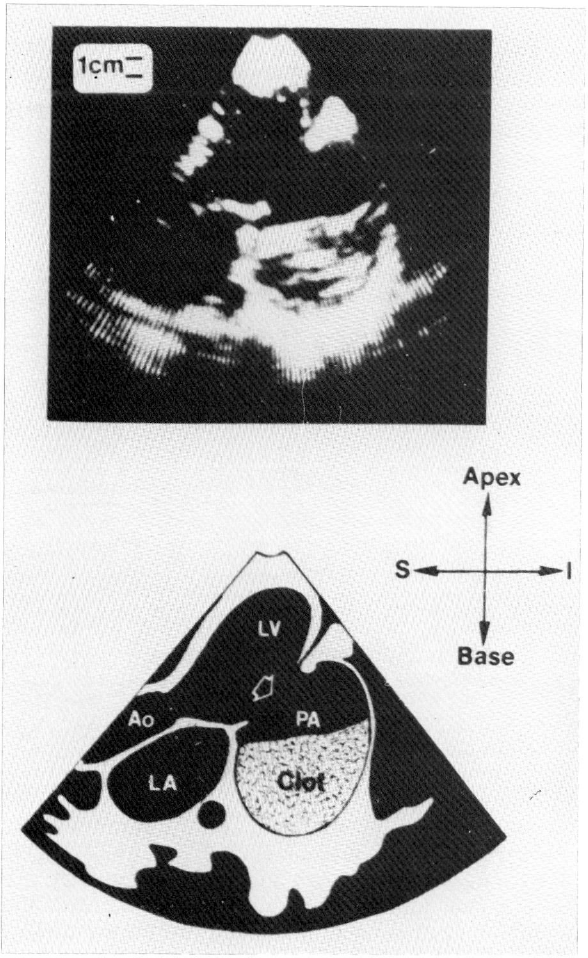

Fig 11–4.—*Top,* 2DE in apical two-chamber projection of a patient with a pseudoaneurysm of the left ventricle. *Bottom,* schematic drawing of the orientation of the cardiac chambers and the pseudoaneurysm *(PA). Ao,* aorta, *I,* inferior, *LA,* left atrium, *LV,* left ventricle, *S,* superior. (From Catherwood et al.[11] Reproduced by permission of the American Heart Association.)

waveforms from elevated V waves secondary to mitral regurgitation is often difficult. The latter finding of mitral regurgitation also does not distinguish between papillary muscle rupture and dysfunction. M-mode echocardiography has documented features of papillary muscle ruptures, including bizarre diastolic fluttering of the posterior leaflet of the mitral valve suggesting an unhinging of the mitral valve apparatus (Fig 11–6).[14] As with ruptured chordae tendineae, papillary muscle rupture will lead to flail anterior or posterior mitral leaflets; a flail valve can be readily appreciated on 2DE as one of the mitral leaflets swings freely beyond the anticipated line of valve closure at the atrioventricular ring into the left atrial cavity during systole.[15] Also noted is loss of normal systolic coaptation of the two mitral valve leaflets (Fig 11–7).[16] The diagnosis of flail leaflet, whether secondary to ruptured chordae or papillary muscle, is usually made by inference with M-mode echocardiography, since the full excursion of the flail leaflet in a superior direction into the left atrium is difficult to appreciate. In contrast, direct visualization of the untethered mitral valve leaflet into the left atrium is more readily imaged by 2DE.

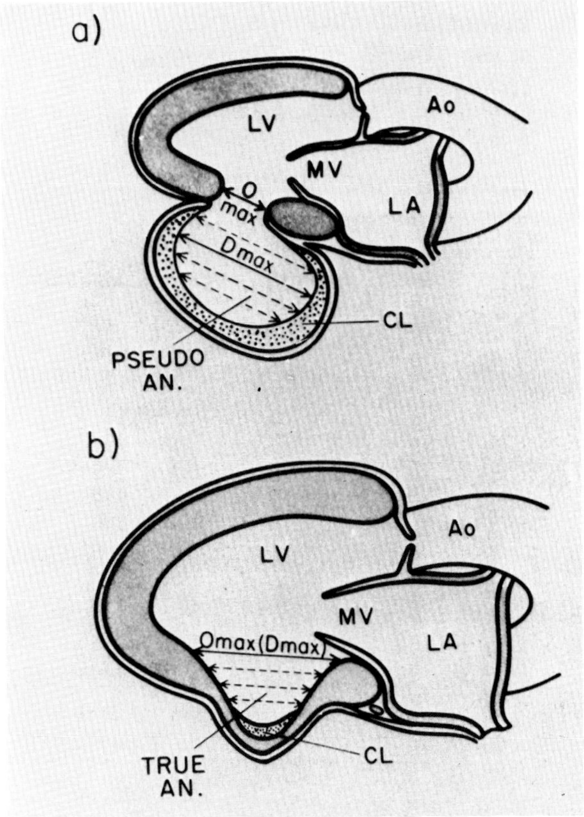

Fig 11–5.—Schematic illustrations of the two types of left ventricular aneurysm. In a pseudoaneurysm *(a)*, the maximal internal width of its neck or opening *(Omax)* is much smaller than the maximal parallel internal diameter *(Dmax)* of the aneurysmal sac. In a true aneurysm *(b)*, the maximal internal width of the mouth or opening *(Omax)* is usually equal to, or wider than, any other parallel internal diameter *(dashed lines)* in the aneurysmal cavity. Therefore, in this example Omax represents the maximal parallel internal diameter *(Dmax)*. *Ao,* aorta, *Cl,* clot, *LA,* left atrium, *LV,* left ventricle, *MV,* mitral valve. (From Gatewood et al.[12] Reproduced by permission of the *American Journal of Cardiology.*)

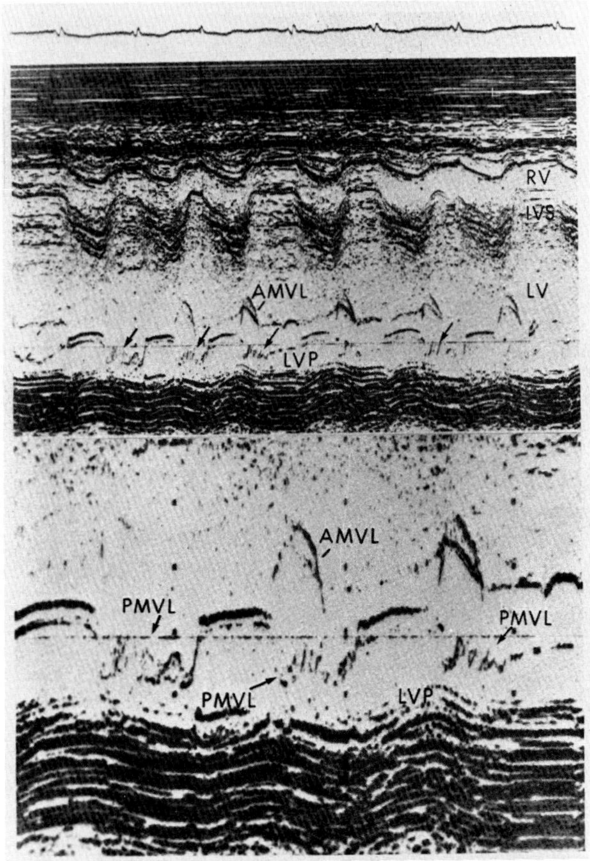

Fig 11–6.—*Top,* echocardiogram showing hyperdynamic motion of interventricular septum *(IVS),* poorly moving left ventricular posterior wall *(LVP),* enlarged left ventricle *(LV),* and bizarre fluttering motion of posterior leaflet of mitral valve in diastole, as shown by *arrows. Bottom,* enlarged view, highlighting fluttering motion of posterior mitral valvular leaflet *(PMVL),* as indicated by *arrows.* Left ventricular posterior wall *(LVP)* is hypokinetic. *RV,* right ventricle, *AMVL,* anterior mitral valvular leaflet. (From Ahmad et al.[14] Reproduced by permission of *Chest.*)

VENTRICULAR SEPTAL RUPTURE

Rupture of the interventricular septum is an infrequent but grave complication of myocardial infarction. Estimated to occur in approximately 1% of all myocardial infarctions, it is more common with anterior than with inferior infarcts and is usually seen within the first two weeks of the insult. Twenty-four percent of patients with this complication die within the first 24 hours, 65% are dead within two weeks, and only 17% live beyond one year.[17] However, prompt diagnosis and surgical correction can improve survival. Differentiation from acute mitral insufficiency is often impossible by clinical features and generally is accomplished by a right heart catheterization. Re-

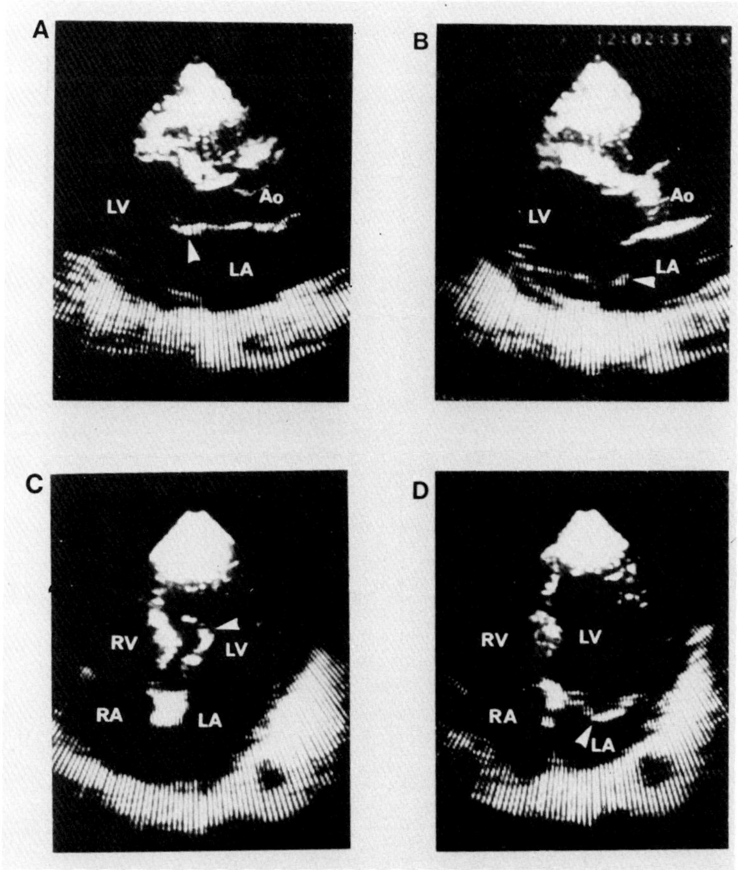

Fig 11–7.—Example of flail mitral valve imaged with 2DE. *Upper two panels* demonstrate precordial long-axis views of the left ventricle during diastole **(A)** and systole **(B),** showing the anterior mitral leaflet *(arrowhead)* swinging back into the left atrium *(LA)* during systole. *Lower two panels* are apical four-chamber views that further demonstrate the abnormal motion of the anterior mitral leaflet *(arrowhead),* freely flailing into the left ventricle *(LV)* during diastole **(C)** and into the left atrium during systole **(D).** In addition, the apical views show a thickened echo-dense area of the high septum, a finding often associated with a flail anterior mitral leaflet. *Ao,* aorta, *RA,* right àtrium, *RV,* right ventricle.

cently it has become apparent not only that can this diagnosis be made noninvasively by echocardiography but also that information concerning size and location of the defect can be ascertained as well. M-mode echocardiography is limited by the relative narrowness of the ultrasound beam. Certain features, although nonspecific, are of value in the diagnosis of septal rupture. Right ventricular enlargement without abnormal septal motion[18] has generally been reported. Abnormal mitral valve motion with transient complete closure during diastole[18] and abrupt posterior motion of a hyperdynamic septum early in diastole have also been noted.[19] Direct visualization of loss of septal continuity is unlikely to be detected by M-mode. echocardiography because the septal rent may be irregular and obliquely located relative to the echo beam direction from a parasternal or precordial transducer location. Nevertheless, one case has been reported that showed discontinuity of the interventricular septum below the AV junction.[20] The infrequency of the finding attests to the difficulty of detecting ventricular septal defect on M-mode echocardiography.

Two-dimensional echocardiography allows more complete inspection of the interventricular septum with direct visualization of septal defects. Using an apical four-chamber view in which the length

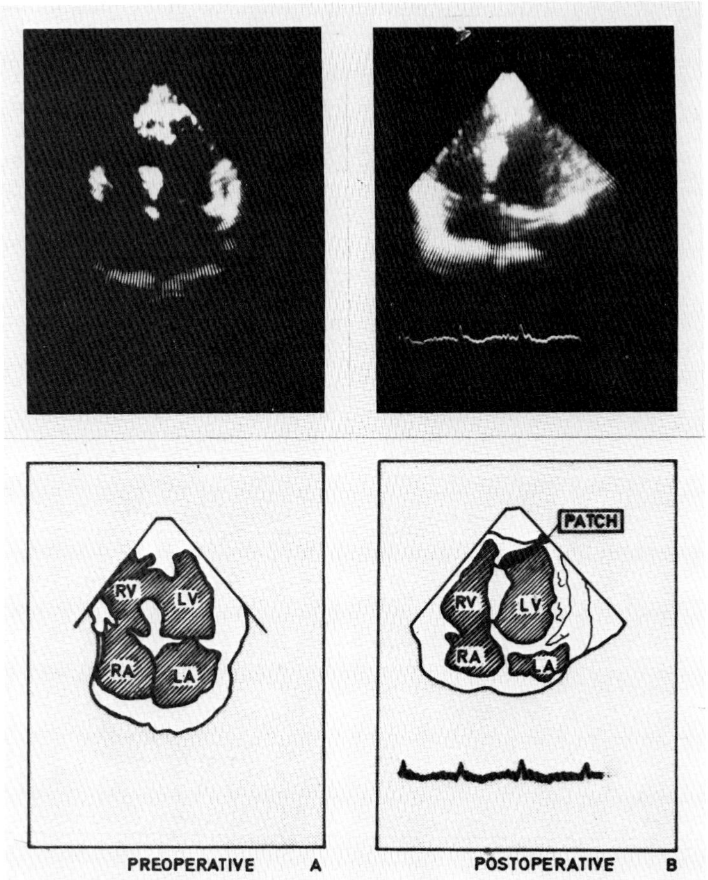

Fig 11–8.—Preoperative and postoperative Polaroid frames of two-dimensional echocardiograms. *Left,* a large defect is evident in the lower interventricular septum. *Right,* postoperative study showing successful repair as indicated by the bright echoes from the patch closing the defect. (From Farcot et al.[21] Reproduced by permission of the *American Journal of Cardiology.*)

of the septum was delineated, Farcot et al. identified three consecutive patients with ventricular septal rupture in the course of acute anterior infarction.[21] In two of the three, the defect was imaged as an oblique rent from the distal left ventricle to the proximal right ventricle, while in the third patient a large orifice was evident in the distal septum (Fig 11–8). Short-axis, parasternal views have also been employed to diagnose a septal defect complicating inferior infarction.[22]

A specific, though insensitive, means of documenting flow through a septal defect may be the peripheral injection of echo-producing contrast material (dextran, indocyanine green, or saline). In acute ventricular septal defects there is shunting of blood from the high-pressure left ventricle to the lower-pressure right ventricle and consequent washout of the injected microbubbles (negative contrast effect).[21] Occasionally, especially after a premature beat, there is a small amount of right-to-left shunting, and the microbubbles can be detected traversing the septal defect into the left ventricle.[22]

Right heart catheterization can document the step-up in oxygen saturation compatible with the septal defect. However, 2DE additionally offers an appreciation of the spatial relationships of intracardiac structures, the distribution and extent of myocardial damage, and the size and exact location of the septal defect.

LEFT VENTRICULAR THROMBI

Left ventricular thrombi are important and potentially catastrophic sequelae to myocardial infarction. Although commonly detected at postmortem examination,[23] prior to the advent of 2DE they were found only if ventriculography were performed, or they might be suspected if an embolic event occurred. The presumed mechanism for embolic events after myocardial infarction is formation of a mural thrombus with secondary embolization. Although studies of the efficacy of anticoagulation after infarction have failed to show a significant decrease in mortality with therapy, reduction in the occurrence of peripheral embolization has been noted.[24] A sensitive noninvasive technique may enable physicians to detect patients at risk for embolization and to institute appropriate therapy.

Although well recognized for its ability to detect nonthrombotic tumors and masses in the left atrium and ventricle, M-mode echocardiography is insensitive for detecting thrombi within the left ventricle.[25, 26] Although occasional positive studies have been reported (Fig. 11–9),[27, 28] the technique is hindered by its intrinsic lack of spatial sampling, which often precludes full visualization of the cardiac apex.

Two-dimensional echocardiography enables full visualization of the entire left ventricle with multiple views, making available a number of sector images of any suspicious areas.[25, 26, 29, 30] Although standard parasternal windows have been used, the apical four-chamber[29] and the subxiphoid transducer locations[30] appear especially effective for thrombus detection. Multiple gain and reject adjustments are required to ensure adequate definition of the pericardium, epicardium, endocardium, and thrombus margin. In the largest series to date, Asinger and co-workers reported 25 patients with 2DE findings characteristic of thrombus: in 20, the findings were confirmed by surgery, angiography, or postmortem examination, while in the remaining 5 the findings were felt to be unequivocal for thrombus[29] but independent confirmation was lacking. Clear delineation of the thrombus margin adjacent to but distinct from the endocardial echoes was considered essential to the correct diagnosis of thrombus (Fig 11–10). All of the patients in this series had wall motion abnor-

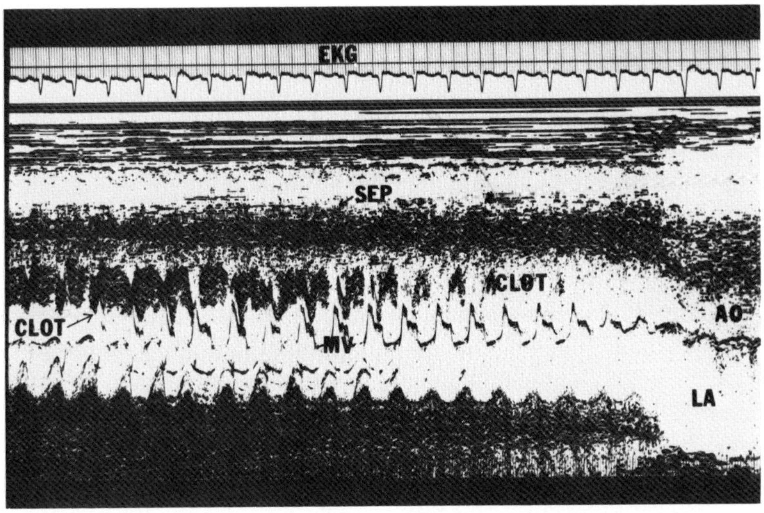

Fig 11–9.—Preoperative M-mode echocardiographic scan from the left ventricle to the aortic root *(AO)* and left atrium *(LA)*. A dense mass of echoes, representing left ventricular clot subsequently confirmed at surgery, is visualized between the septum *(SEP)* and the mitral valve leaflets *(MV)*. The left atrium and left ventricle are enlarged. Septal movement is hypokinetic. (From Come et al.[27] Reproduced by permission of the *American Heart Journal.*)

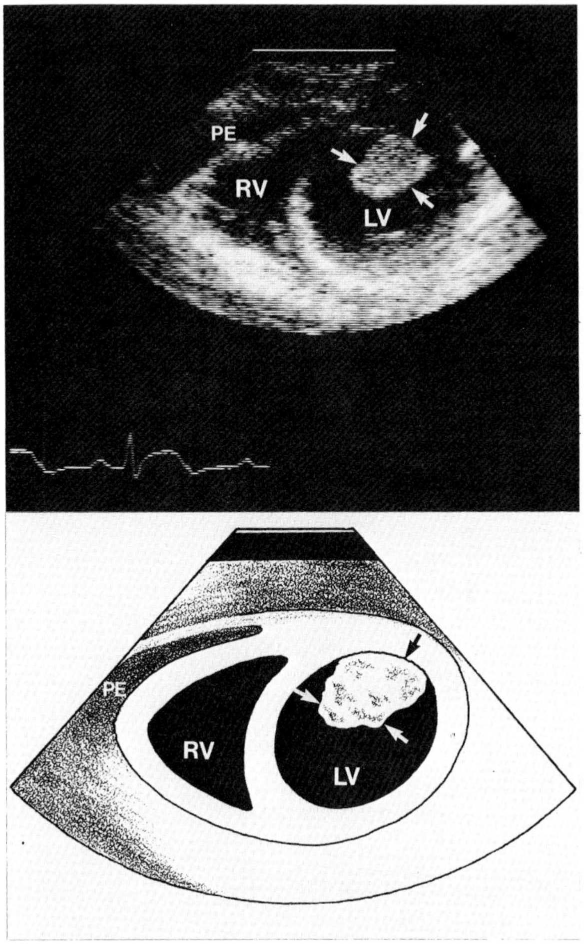

Fig 11–10.—Apical short-axis view of echocardiogram *(top)* obtained 7 days after acute anterior myocardial infarction. *Bottom,* artist's drawing. A large protruding apical thrombus *(arrows)* is present and demonstrates increased echo density compared with that of surrounding myocardium. A small pericardial effusion *(PE)* is also present. *LV,* left ventricular cavity, *RV,* right ventricular cavity. (From Asinger et al.[29] Reproduced by permission of the *American Journal of Cardiology.*)

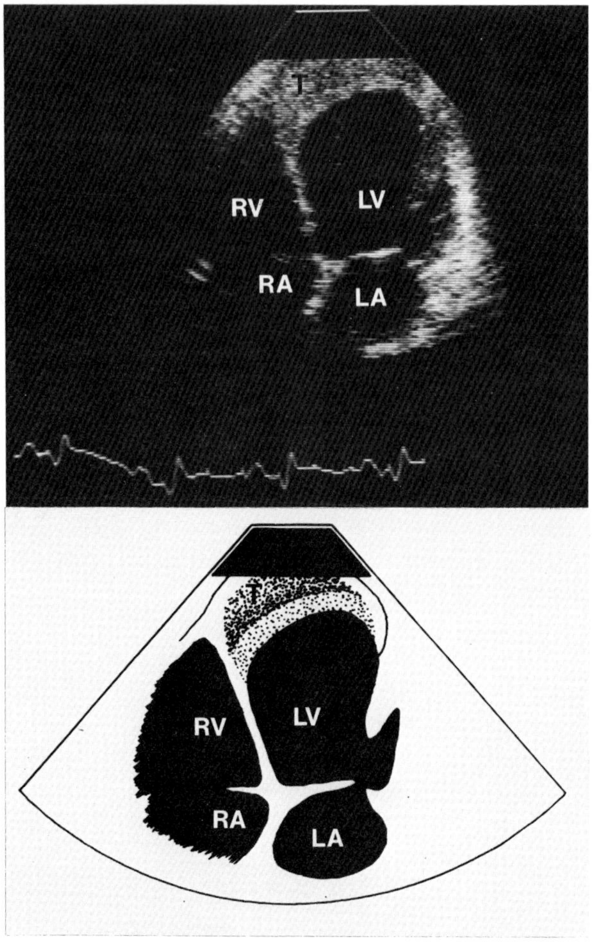

Fig 11–11.—Apical four-chamber view demonstrating a mural thrombus *(T)* with layering. A layer approximately 5 mm thick adjacent to the left ventricular *(LV)* cavity is present and is of increased echo density when compared with the remainder of the thrombus. (From Asinger et al.[29] Reproduced by permission of the *American Journal of Cardiology.*)

malities—dyskinesis, hypokinesis, or akinesis—adjacent to the mass. This study and others[26, 30] confirm that the overwhelming majority of left ventricular thrombi are apical in location and best diagnosed by apical or subcostal views. Free motion of the thrombus margin into the ventricular lumen was infrequently noted but was helpful in making the correct diagnosis, as was a layering effect of different acoustical density or a texture distinct from the adjacent myocardium (Fig 11–11). A shaggy, irregular border of the thrombus in coronary patients with recent embolization suggested fresh thrombi and differed from the circumscribed, smooth appearance of thrombi in patients with chronic cardiomyopathies.[26] Serial examinations showing the disappearance of a mass in a patient with subsequent embolization or on anticoagulant therapy supports the diagnosis of left ventricular thrombus, as does the new appearance of an echo-dense mass in the early postinfarct period.[29]

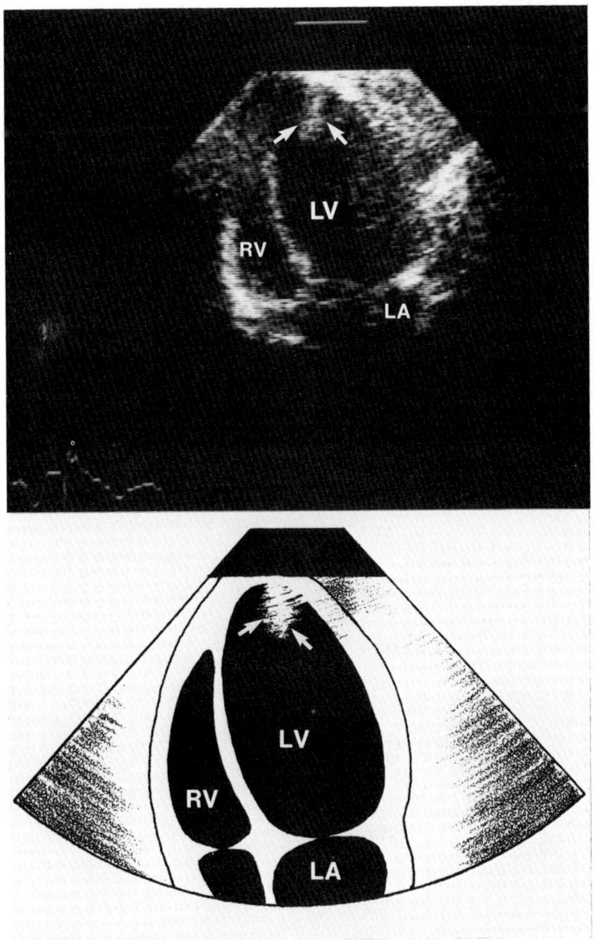

Fig 11–12.—Apical four-chamber view of a heart with previous infarction. Reverberation artifact from the apex is present *(arrows)* and simulates a protruding intracavitary thrombus. *Arrows* indicate this reverberation artifact. (From Asinger et al.[29] Reproduced by permission of the *American Journal of Cardiology.*)

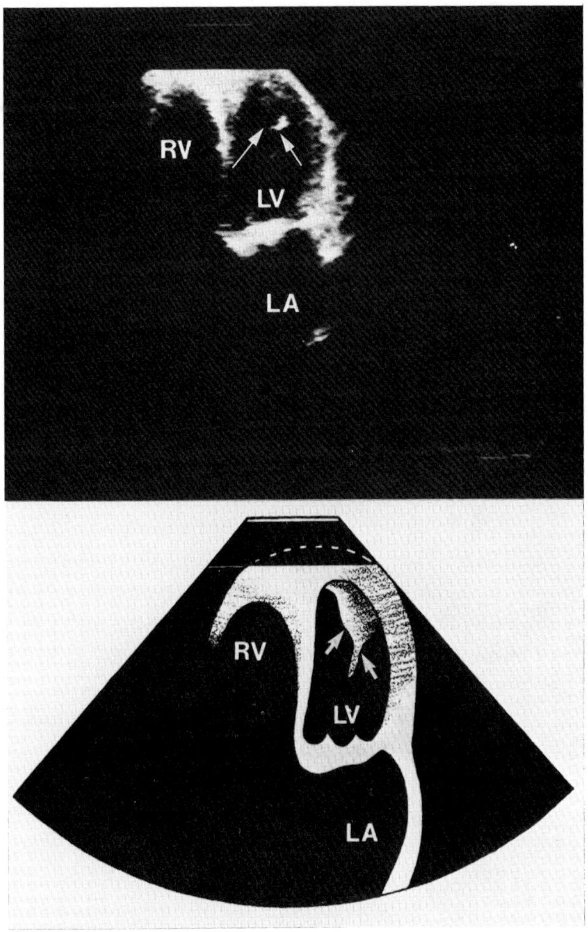

Fig 11–13.—Apical two-chamber view of a heart after mitral valve replacement. A partially amputated papillary muscle with chordal remnants is present *(arrows)* and simulates a thrombus. However, it is in the position of the papillary muscle, and no wall motion abnormalities were present. (From Asinger et al.[29] Reproduced by permission of the *American Journal of Cardiology.*)

It is increasingly evident that 2DE is a very useful method for detecting left ventricular thrombi. Catheterization of the left ventricle and contrast ventriculography are potentially hazardous since they may dislodge the clot. Although reasonably specific, ventriculography is also relatively insensitive: only 41% of left ventricular clots are detected by this technique in patients in whom thrombi were subsequently identified at surgery.[31] Since the ability to detect and follow the course of thrombi has therapeutic implications, great emphasis has to be placed on accurate diagnosis and the avoidance of false positive studies. Falsely positive diagnoses may result from the problems inherent in the technique itself or from inaccurate identification of normal or pathologic intracardiac structures.[29] Problems such as near field artifact or intense side lobes from areas of myocardial scars can be minimized by obtaining multiple sector orientations (Fig 11–12). Spurious echoes disappear with changes in transducer location and orientation, whereas the margin of a true thrombus should be reproducibly imaged in the same position in the left ventricle. Structures such as papillary muscles, muscular trabeculae, chordae tendineae, and tangential left ventricular wall can be distinguished from true thrombi by their location and appearance as well as with the use of multiple views and orientations (Fig 11–13). Thus 2DE offers a means for the accurate and safe diagnosis of left ventricular thrombi. Additionally, it may offer a way to screen patients at high risk—e.g., in the first week after large anterior or apical infarction or soon after the development of thrombi—and to make serial evaluation of responses to anticoagulant therapy.

RIGHT VENTRICULAR INFARCTION

Acute myocardial infarction is usually associated with dysfunction of the left ventricle. The early belief that elevation of the central venous pressure in patients with acute myocardial infarction was always secondary to left ventricular dysfunction was proved incorrect once hemodynamic monitoring of the pressures of both ventricles was undertaken. The increase in central venous pressure in myocardial infarction may depend not only on the severity of the involvement of the left ventricle, but also on involvement of the right ventricle.[32, 33] The clinical syndrome of right ventricular infarction in patients with inferior or inferoposterior infarction, in whom there is the triad of elevated systemic venous pressure, hypotension, and clear lungs, has been well described.[32, 34] These patients have a characteristic hemodynamic pattern: right ventricular filling pressures are elevated, being equal to or greater than those of the left ventricle.[32, 34, 35] This clinical and hemodynamic picture can also be mimicked by acute massive pulmonary embolism or acute cardiac tamponade.

Right ventricular infarction frequently goes unrecognized or misdiagnosed even when hemodynamic monitoring has been used. Echocardiography can help to arrive at the correct diagnosis. Lorell at el.[34] reported a series of 12 patients with right ventricular infarction. All were hypotensive, and 11 had pericardial friction rubs. Seven had equilibration of the right atrial, pulmonary artery diastolic, and pulmonary capillary wedge pressures; of these 7, 5 had pulsus paradoxus, 5 had a "dip and plateau" pattern on the right ventricular pressure tracings, and 2 had a positive Kussmaul's sign. This constellation of findings—all secondary to right ventricular dysfunction—can easily be mistaken for cardiac tamponade. Indeed, the latter diagnosis was made in 4 of the 12 patients, and 3 underwent pericardiocentesis or pericardial exploration under cardiopulmonary bypass. However, 4 patients also had echocardiograms disclosing *absence of pericardial effusion* and evidence of right ventricular enlargement. The features of right ventricular infarction on M-mode echocardiography have been quite consistent:[34, 36] an increase in right ventricular size with an increased RV/LV minor-axis ratio. Paradoxic motion of the

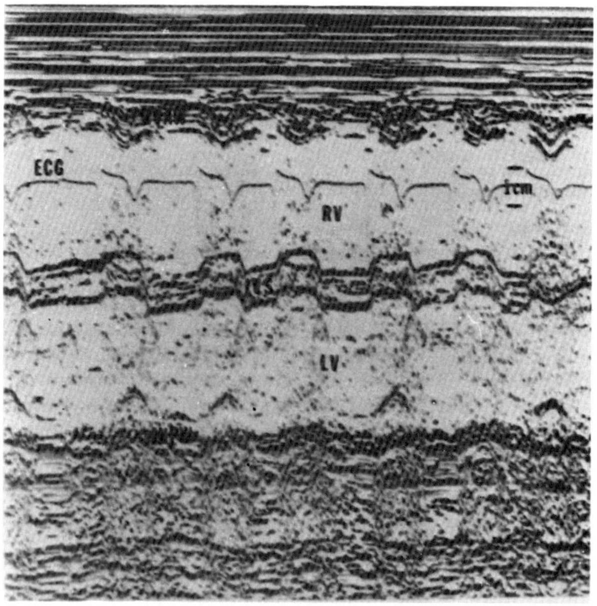

Fig 11–14.—Echocardiogram showing enlarged right ventricular *(RV)* cavity (3.7 cm), small left ventricle *(LV)* (2.9 cm), preserved motion of the right ventricular anterior wall *(RVAW),* and left ventricular posterior wall *(LVPW).* In addition, the interventricular septum *(IVS)* shows abnormal motion and diminished thickening during systole. *CW,* chest wall. (From Elkyam et al.[36] Reproduced by permission of *Catheterization and Cardiovascular Diagnosis.*)

interventricular septum has also been noted. These findings suggest right ventricular volume overload secondary to poor right ventricular contraction (Fig 11–14). In addition, ischemia of the septum may also play a role.

Findings on 2DE parallel those of M-mode echocardiography: right ventricular enlargement in both long- and short-axis planes and paradoxic movement of the septum.[37] Furthermore, regional right ventricular contraction abnormalities appear to be a critical element in establishing this diagnosis. Since 2DE allows a more systematic exploration of regional RV function, it is not surprising that it will offer advantages over M-mode in this regard. Thus, in a series of 10 patients with right ventricular infarction, each patient had some degree of right ventricular wall motion abnormality; all 10 had akinesis of the diaphragmatic wall, 7 of these 10 had akinesis of the right ventricular free wall, and an equal number had abnormal septal motion. Interestingly, evidence of tricuspid regurgitation was noted in 8 of 9 patients after contrast ("bubble") injections.[37]

Thus, not all patients who develop a pericardial friction rub in the course of myocardial infarction have significant pericardial effusions. In the absence of echocardiographically detectable effusion, cardiac tamponade is a very unlikely complication of acute myocardial infarction. Patients with tamponade not only show signs of effusion, but are very likely to show signs of right ventricular compression. In patients with inferior myocardial infarction who develop a pericardial friction rub and elevated neck veins, the distinction between right ventricular infarction and postinfarction pericarditis with cardiac tamponade accounting for impaired ventricular filling can be considerably facilitated by the use of echocardiography.

ADVANTAGES AND LIMITATIONS OF 2DE IN MYOCARDIAL INFARCTION

Two-dimensional echocardiography offers distinct advantages for evaluating myocardial structure and function in myocardial infarction not currently available by other methods. First and foremost, it makes available the most comprehensive information of any noninvasive imaging technique. From a single bedside examination, one can appreciate not only myocardial structure and function, but also the area around the heart and the function of the cardiac valves. In addition, the resolution obtainable with echocardiography is superior to that of any other widely used noninvasive imaging modality. The relatively high degree of resolution obtainable is particularly useful in detecting special complications of infarction that can affect small and highly localized anatomical regions of the ventricle, such as papillary muscle dysfunction and formation of mural thrombi. Another advantage of echocardiography in this setting is that it can be repeated, if necessary, multiple times on a daily basis without the concern of exposing the patient to ionizing radiation.

The principal limitation of echocardiography lies in the fact that high-quality diagnostic images can be obtained only 70% to 80% of the time, depending on the investigator and the patient population. Since acute myocardial infarction is so prevalent, this still represents an impressive number of patients in whom the technique may be diagnostically useful. Difficulties with image quality are being overcome in part through improved techniques of examination using different approaches to viewing endocardial and myocardial targets; further development of instrumentation will be necessary to achieve a success rate with ultrasound comparable to that of radionuclide imaging techniques. Recent development of lighter, more portable units should result in an even more widespread application of 2DE in the coronary care unit setting, while emphasis on quantification heralds a new era of application of echocardiography to acute myocardial infarction.

REFERENCES

1. Peterson J.L., Johnson W., Hessel E.A., et al.: Echocardiographic recognition of left ventricular aneurysm. *Am. Heart J.* 83:244, 1972.
2. Kreamer R., Kerber R.E., Abboud F.R.: Ventricular aneurysm: Use of echocardiography. *J. Clin. Ultrasound* 1:60, 1973.
3. Dillon J.C., Feigenbaum H., Weyman A.E., et al.: Echocardiography in the evaluation of patients for aneurysmectomy. *Circulation* 53:657, 1976.

4. Weyman A.E., Peskoe S.M., Williams E.S., et al.: Detection of left ventricular aneurysms by cross-sectional echocardiography. *Circulation* 54:936, 1976.
5. Kambe T., Nishimura K., Hibi N., et al.: Real time observation of left ventricular aneurysm by B mode echocardiography. *J. Clin. Ultrasound* 6:405, 1978.
6. Davidson K.H., Parisi A.F., Harrington J.J., et al.: Pseudoaneurysms of the left ventricle: An unusual echocardiographic presentation. *Ann. Intern. Med.* 86:430, 1977.
7. Morcerf F.P., Duart E.P., Salcedo E.E., et al.: Echocardiographic findings in false aneurysm of the left ventricle. *Cleveland Clin. Q.* 43:71, 1976.
8. Thanavaro S., Biggs F.D., Kleiger R.E., et al.: Posterior pseudoaneurysm of the left ventricle: A prospective echocardiographic diagnosis. *South. Med. J.* 72:52b, 1979.
9. Sears T.D., Yee S.O., Starke H., et al.: Left ventricular pseudoaneurysm identified by cross-sectional echocardiography. *Ann. Intern. Med.* 90:935, 1979.
10. Katz R.J., Simpson A., DiBianco R., et al.: Noninvasive diagnosis of left ventricular pseudoaneurysm: Role of two-dimensional echocardiography and radionuclide gated pool imaging. *Am. J. Cardiol.* 44:372, 1979.
11. Catherwood E., Mintz G.S., Kotler M.N., et al.: Two-dimensional echocardiographic recognition of left ventricular pseudoaneurysm. *Circulation* 62:294, 1980.
12. Gatewood R.P., Nanda N.C.: Differentiation of left ventricular pseudoaneurysm from true aneurysm with two-dimensional echocardiography. *Am. J. Cardiol.* 46:869, 1980.
13. Ogawa S., Hubbard F.E., Mardelli T.J., et al.: Cross-sectional echocardiographic spectrum of papillary muscle dysfunction. *Am. Heart J.* 97:312, 1979.
14. Ahmad S., Kleiger R.E., Connors J., et al.: Echocardiographic diagnosis of rupture of a papillary muscle. *Chest* 73:232, 1978.
15. Mintz G.S., Kotler N.N., Segal B.L., et al.: Two-dimensional echocardiographic recognition of ruptured chordae tendineae. *Circulation* 57:255, 1978.
16. Child J.S., Skorton D.J., Taylor R.D., et al.: Cross-sectional and M-mode echocardiographic features of flail mitral leaflets, abstracted. *Am. J. Cardiol.* 43:411, 1979.
17. Sanders R.J., Kern W.H., Blount S.G. Jr.: Perforation of the interventricular septum complicating myocardial infarction: A report of eight cases, one with cardiac catheterization. *Am. Heart J.* 51:736, 1956.
18. Chandraratna P.A.N., Balachandran P.K., Shah P.H., et al.: Echocardiographic observations on ventricular septal rupture complicating acute myocardial infarction. *Circulation* 51:506, 1975.
19. DeJoseph R.L., Seides S.F., Lindner A., et al.: Echocardiographic findings of ventricular septal rupture in acute myocardial infarction. *Am. J. Cardiol.* 36:346, 1975.
20. Kerin N.Z., Edelstein J., DeRue R.G.: Ventricular septal defect complicating acute myocardial infarction. *Chest* 70:560, 1976.
21. Farcot J.C., Boisanti L., Rigand M., et al.: Two-dimensional echocardiographic visualization of ventricular septal rupture after acute myocardial infarction. *Am. J. Cardiol.* 45:370, 1980.
22. Scanlon J.G., Seward J.B., Tajik A.J.: Visualization of ventricular septal rupture utilizing wide-angle two-dimensional echocardiography. *Mayo Clin. Proc.* 54:381, 1979.
23. Jordan R.A., Miller D., Edwards J.E., et al.: Thromboembolism in acute and in healed myocardial infarction: I. Intracardiac mural thrombosis. *Circulation* 6:1, 1952.
24. Ebert R.V.: Anticoagulants in acute myocardial infarction: Results of a cooperative clinical trial. *J.A.M.A.* 225:724, 1973.
25. Ports T.A., Cogan J., Schiller N.B., et al.: Echocardiography of left ventricular masses. *Circulation* 58:528, 1978.
26. DeMaria A.N., Bommer W., Neuman A., et al.: Left ventricular thrombi identified by cross-sectional echocardiography. *Ann. Intern. Med.* 90:14, 1979.
27. Come P.C., Markis J.E., Vine A.S., et al.: Echocardiographic diagnosis of left ventricular thrombi. *Am. Heart J.* 100:523, 1980.
28. DeJoseph R.L., Shiroff R.A., Levinson L.W., et al.: Echocardiographic diagnosis of intraventricular clot. *Chest* 71:417, 1977.
29. Asinger R.W., Mikell F.L., Sharma B., et al.: Observations on detecting left ventricular thrombosis with two-dimensional echocardiography: Emphasis on avoidance of false positive diagnoses. *Am. J. Cardiol.* 47:145, 1981.
30. Meltzer R.S., Guthaner D., Rakowski H., et al.: Diagnosis of left ventricular thrombi by two-dimensional echocardiography. *Br. Heart J.* 42:261, 1979.
31. Swan H.J.C., Magnusson P.T., Buchbinder N.A., et al.: Aneurysm of the cardiac ventricle: Its management by medical and surgical intervention. *West. J. Med.* 129:26, 1978.
32. Cohn J.N., Guiha N.H., Broder M.I., et al.: Right ventricular infarction: Clinical and hemodynamic features. *Am. J. Cardiol.* 33:209, 1974.
33. Rackley C.E., Russel R.O.: Right ventricular function in acute myocardial infarction. *Am. J. Cardiol.* 33:927, 1974.
34. Lorell B., Leinbach R.C., Pohost G.M., et al.: Right ventricular infarction: Clinical diagnosis and differentiation from cardiac tamponade and pericardial constriction. *Am. J. Cardiol.* 43:465, 1979.
35. Rotman M., Ratliff N.B., Hawley J.: Right ventric-

ular infarction: A haemodynamic diagnosis. *Br. Heart J.* 36:941, 1974.

36. Elkayam U., Halprin S.L., Frishman W., et al.: Echocardiographic findings in cardiogenic shock due to right ventricular myocardial infarction. Catheterization and Cardiovascular Diagnosis 5:289, 1979.
37. D'Arcy B.J., Nanda N.C.: Two-dimensional echocardiographic features of right ventricular infarction. *Circulation* 65:167,1982.

RADIONUCLIDE IMAGING

Mary D. Osbakken and Robert D. Okada

SEVERAL ANATOMICAL and pathophysiologic complications can result from myocardial infarction. Acute obstruction of coronary blood flow causes anoxia, which results in a process of cellular necrosis in the area supplied by the respective coronary artery. Obstruction of the coronary artery initiates a host of pathophysiologic responses, including (1) muscle cell membrane damage, with resultant release of cellular contents (creatine phosphokinase), (2) an inflammatory response consisting of lymphocyte migration to the damaged area to begin the healing process after infarction, (3) wall motion abnormalities and sometimes papillary muscle dysfunction due to mechanical dysfunction of the damaged muscle, (4) depression of global ventricular function as evidenced by decreased right and/or left ventricular ejection fraction, decreased cardiac output, increased end-diastolic pressure and volume, increased end-systolic volume, and increased pulmonary blood volume, and (5) rupture of necrotic muscle, with resultant production of ventricular septal defect, ventricular free wall rupture, pseudoaneurysm (due to contained rupture of the ventricular free wall), and severe mitral regurgitation (due to papillary muscle rupture).

Recent advances in noninvasive nuclear cardiology techniques allow evaluation of each of the cited pathophysiologic processes that result from myocardial infarction. This chapter examines appropriate modalities for delineating each complication (Table 12–1).

OBSTRUCTION OF CORONARY ARTERY PERFUSION IN MYOCARDIAL INFARCTION: EVALUATION WITH THALLIUM SCANS

Acute Infarct

Thallium radionuclide imaging has been used to evaluate the extent of myocardial damage during an acute myocardial infarction[1–6] and to predict subsequent mortality,[4] based on the percentage of infarcted myocardium. Chapter 10 discusses the use of ^{201}Tl imaging during an acute myocardial infarction. Semiquantitative ^{201}Tl scan analyses performed later in the postinfarction period have proved helpful in predicting the extent and location of stenosis.[7]

Chronic Effects of Myocardial Infarction

Thallium imaging is useful for determining the existence of remote myocardial infarction in patients without a historically or ECG-documented previous infarction and who present with congestive heart failure or arrhythmias.[8] Defects on exercise-redistribution ^{201}Tl scans support the diagnosis either of coronary artery disease or of arrhythmias as a cause of heart failure. Patients with persistent ^{201}Tl scan defects often have decreased ventricular reserve function on gated blood pool

TABLE 12–1.—Consequences of Myocardial Infarction and Nuclear Cardiology Studies Used in Their Evaluation

PATHOPHYSIOLOGIC EVENT	NUCLEAR CARDIOLOGY STUDY
Obstruction of coronary artery perfusion	Thallium scan
Myocardial cell damage and inflammatory changes	Antimyosin Ab imaging, indium-labeled WBC imaging
Intraventricular thrombosis	Indium 111 platelets
Ca++ metabolism derangement	Technetium pyrophosphate
Myocardial function abnormalities	Multigated blood pool and first-pass scan
Wall motion abnormalities	
Hypokinesis	
Akinesis	
Dyskinesis, aneurysm formation	
Papillary muscle dysfunction with mitral regurgitation	(Regurgitant fraction via multigated blood pool scan)
Depression of global function: right and left ventricle	
Ejection fraction	
End-systolic volume	
Cardiac output	
Pulmonary blood volume	
Gross anatomical changes of the myocardium	Multigated blood pool and first-pass scan
Ventricular septal defect	(Shunt study)
False aneurysm	
Papillary muscle rupture	
Pericardial effusion	Multigated blood pool scan

scans (no change or a decrease in exercise ejection fraction from the resting value).[9] Most of these patients have clinical or angiographic evidence of prior myocardial infarction. The size of defects on ^{201}Tl scans frequently corresponds to the proportion of hypokinetic, akinetic, or dyskinetic areas as seen on contrast[10] or radionuclide ventriculograms.[7] Thus, information obtained on a ^{201}Tl scan alone can indicate potential ventricular dysfunction. Exercise-redistribution ^{201}Tl scanning several weeks to months after an acute myocardial infarction has been found to be more useful than clinical findings in detecting jeopardized myocardium.[11]

DAMAGE TO MYOCARDIAL CELLS AND INFLAMMATORY RESPONSE TO ACUTE ISCHEMIC DAMAGE

Acute ischemic processes associated with myocardial infarction cause anoxic damage to the individual myocardial cells, resulting in membrane disruption in some of these cells. Recently, several investigators have devised a new method of infarct imaging based on this pathologic process of membrane leakiness.[12–14] Antimyosin antibodies tagged with iodine were synthesized that were specific to the contents of the myocardial cells. Infarcted myocardium was found to accumulate radioactivity which was assumed to be due to ^{31}I-Ab or ^{125}I-Ab crossing the leaky cell membrane and binding to its respective antigen, cardiac myosin. This type of imaging based on pathophysiologic processes has been extensively investigated in dog models, and it has recently been used in patients.

Accumulation of white blood cells in the damaged edematous area surrounding an acute myocardial infarction has been characterized histologically.[15–17] Recently, radionuclide imaging characterization of this process in dogs with experimental infarctions was performed using ^{111}In-labeled autologous leukocytes.[18] Both epicardial and endocardial accumulation depended on the extent of blood flow to each area, with the greatest uptake occurring in the zones of lowest flow. However, the time patterns of infiltration were different: maximum infiltration in epicardial areas occurred within 24 hours, while maximal uptake in endocardial areas occurred within 72 hours after

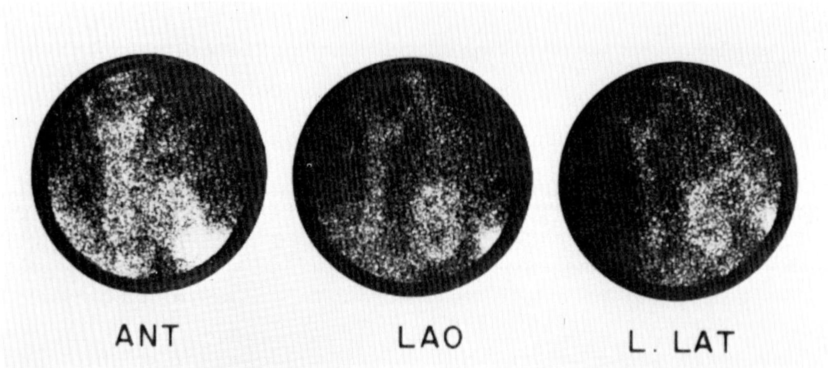

Fig 12–1.—Cardiac images from a patient with acute anterior wall myocardial infarction imaged 24 hours after the injection of ^{111}In-labeled leukocytes. Intense focal cardiac uptake is seen in all three views in a "doughnut" pattern. (From Davis R.A., et al.: *Circulation* 63:829, 1981. Reproduced by permission of the American Heart Association.)

infarction. If the ^{111}In-labeled leukocytes were injected 120 hours after infarction, no uptake occurred. Thus, the inflammatory process that results from myocardial insult (necrosis) can be used to evaluate the occurrence time and extent of the damage. The potential use of this diagnostic tool has been investigated preliminarily in limited clinical situations and appears to have potential in determining the presence and age of infarction in patients (Fig 12–1).[19]

INTRAVENTRICULAR THROMBOSIS

Indium-111 platelet imaging has been used recently to detect left ventricular thrombi in patients with remote myocardial infarction.[20, 21] Preliminary data show that platelet imaging is accurate in detecting thrombus in the ventricular cavity and probably most precisely detects dynamically active thrombi. Platelet imaging in 44 patients with either previous myocardial infarction or cardiomyopathy resulted in 10 positive studies.[20] In this series, the positive studies were found only in patients who had left ventricular aneurysms secondary to previous myocardial infarction. The time

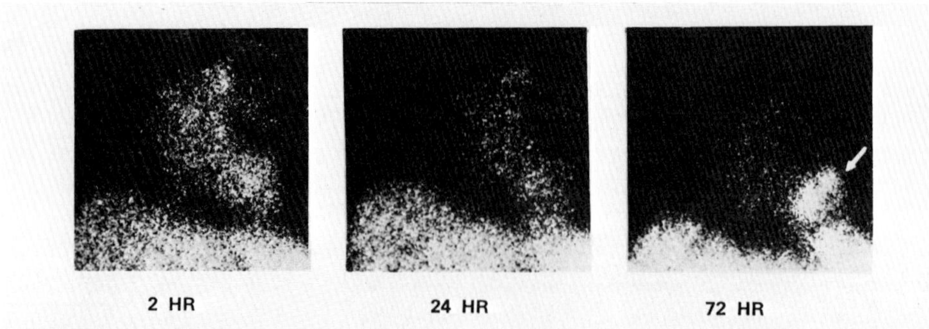

Fig 12–2.—Anterior views of indium-111-platelet localization to intramural thrombus found in a ventricular aneurysm. On serial images obtained 2 and 24 hours after injection of ^{111}In-labeled platelets, no discrete area of activity greater than the cardiac blood pool could be distinguished. On images obtained at 72 hours, intense ^{111}In-labeled platelet activity at the cardiac apex was apparent, while background blood pool activity had decreased. (From Stratton J.R., et al.: *Am. J. Cardiol.* 47:874–881, 1981. Reproduced by permission.)

course of positivity varied: no study was positive 2 hours after injection, 5 were positive 24 hours after injection, and all were positive 72 hours after injection of ^{111}In-labeled platelets (Fig 12–2). This time course indicates that platelet migration to these thrombi is an active process that continues throughout the period of thrombus formation and dissolution.

MYOCARDIAL NECROSIS WITH DERANGED CALCIUM METABOLISM: EVALUATION WITH TECHNETIUM PYROPHOSPHATE IMAGING

Ischemic damage to the heart can cause deranged calcium metabolism; i.e., myocardial necrosis is associated with increased calcium accumulation with resultant calcification of the mitochondria.[22] This pathophysiologic mechanism has been employed to effectively image the damaged myocardium in the following manner. (1) Pyrophosphate is known to complex with calcium. (2) When pyrophosphate is labeled with a radioactive substance, such as technetium, subsequent complexes with calcium pyrophosphate are radioactive and can be imaged. Thus, the deranged cardiac calcium metabolism can be used to evaluate the existence, extent, and sites of myocardial necrosis. This principle has been used extensively to diagnose patients with acute myocardial infarction.

Prognostic implications based on pattern and extent of uptake of technetium pyrophosphate have been made.[23–25] Diffuse intense uptake has been associated with a much higher complication rate than focal uptake.[23] These complications consist of infarct extension, congestive heart failure, refractory arrhythmias, and sudden death. Patients with a "doughnut" pattern (intense peripheral uptake and relatively less central uptake) localized to the anterior or lateral wall had a higher complication rate than clinically similar patients without this pattern of uptake (Fig 12–3).[24, 25] Thirty of 45 patients (67%) with anterolateral doughnut patterns

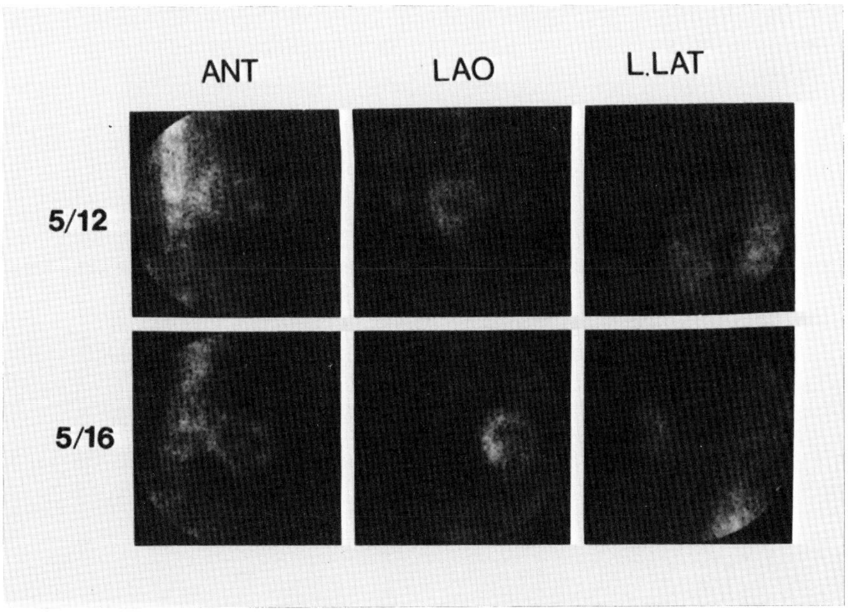

Fig 12–3.—Technetium 99m pyrophosphate myocardial images in the anterior *(ANT)*, left anterior oblique *(LAO)*, and left lateral *(L. LAT)* views demonstrating a doughnut pattern *(top)*. *Bottom*, a ^{99m}Tc-pyrophosphate myocardial scan obtained 4 days later in the same projection. The doughnut pattern is frequently associated with complications of heart failure and early death after a myocardial infarction. (From Rude R.E., et al.: *Circulation* 59:721–730, 1979. Reproduced by permission of the American Heart Association.)

developed left ventricular failure.[24] In another study, five of six patients with anterior doughnut patterns died within one year of infarction.[25] Patients with persistently positive scans several weeks to months after acute infarction have also been found to have a higher complication rate.[26] The continuation of positivity was thought to be due to continued derangement of calcium metabolism as in aneurysmal tissue or in tissue which continually has relative ischemia. Patients with this type of pathology could, indeed, be expected to have complications such as unstable angina, ventricular dyssynergy, and electric irritability.

MYOCARDIAL FUNCTIONAL ABNORMALITIES AFTER ACUTE INFARCT: EVALUATION WITH FIRST-PASS OR MULTIGATED BLOOD POOL IMAGING

Ischemic damage to cardiac muscle can cause production of acute or chronic hypokinetic, akinetic, and dyskinetic muscle segments. In addition, ventricular aneurysm formation and papillary muscle dysfunction and ventricular muscle rupture can result. Regional wall motion abnormalities of both the right and left ventricle, the effects of papillary muscle dysfunction, and the effects of muscle rupture can be evaluated with first-pass or multigated blood pool imaging, or both.

Wall Motion Abnormalities

Asynergy in the zone of acute infarction has been demonstrated and some investigators have found improvement of asynergy after sublingual administration of nitroglycerin.[27] This improvement in function is thought to be due to alleviation of ischemia in peri-infarction areas. Wall motion abnormalities due to remote infarctions have also been evaluated with rest and intervention radionuclide imaging ventriculography.[27–29] Exercise multigated blood pool scanning may reveal wall motion abnormalities not seen at rest which are associated with decreased left ventricular reserve function (decrease in ejection fraction with progressive exercise). This type of evaluation is helpful in determining a patient's functional capacity.[28, 30]

True Aneurysm Formation

It is difficult to determine how frequently left ventricular aneurysm formation occurs after myocardial infarction because few patients undergo in-

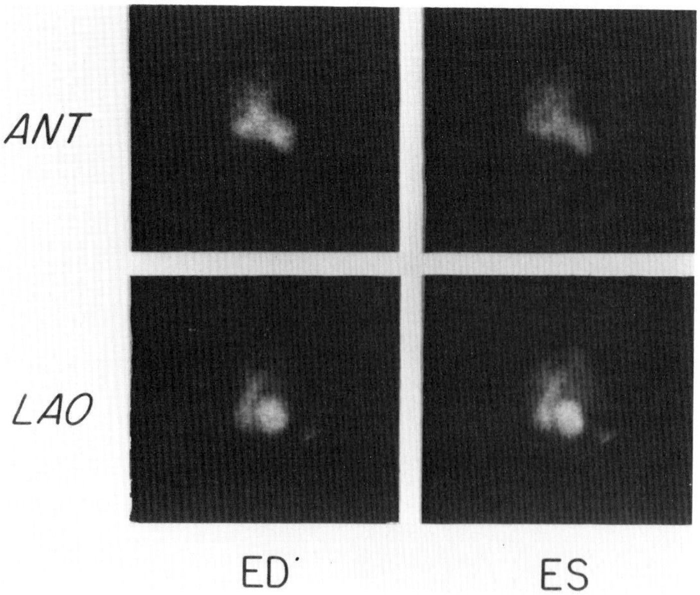

Fig 12–4.—End-diastolic *(ED)* and end-systolic *(ES)* blood pool images from a patient with an anterior-apical aneurysm. The left ventricular ejection fraction was 15%.

vasive or noninvasive studies to delineate cardiac anatomy after the acute event. However, aneurysm formation is a sufficiently frequent problem that clinical investigators have looked at various methods to diagnose this complication, especially in patients with resultant congestive heart failure, arrhythmias, and embolic events. Recently, radionuclide imaging has been used in an attempt to better define this anatomical defect.[28, 31–35]

Gated blood pool scans have been used to differentiate patients with localized ventricular aneurysms from those with diffuse left ventricular hypokinesis (Fig 12–4).[31, 35] Excellent correlation has been found between gated scan data and contrast angiographic data. In one study, gated radionuclide imaging detected 61 of 64 aneurysms demonstrated by contrast angiography.[35] Anterior and anterior-apical aneurysms were most frequently demonstrated, while posterior basal aneurysms were more difficult to diagnose. In this same study, radionuclide imaging was negative for aneurysm in 100% of 74 patients who had normal contrast angiograms. Thus, the overall accuracy of gated scans in detecting aneurysms was 96%. First-pass radionuclide imaging can also be used to accurately detect left ventricular aneurysms.[32, 33] Again, the extent of akinesis detected via scan has closely correlated with that found by contrast angiography.[33]

Technetium pyrophosphate (infarction "hot spot" imaging) has also been found to accumulate in aneurysms and in dyskinetic segments of myocardium, most likely due to deranged calcium metabolism.[36–38] However, this finding is not consistently associated with ventricular aneurysms (accuracy less than 50%) and therefore technetium pyrophosphate imaging is not a reliable study for diagnosing aneurysms.

Papillary Muscle Dysfunction

Papillary muscle dysfunction resulting from infarction can cause acute or chronic mitral regurgitation. Evaluation of this consequence of myocardial damage can be done with gated or first-pass scans which can be used to gather anatomical data on left atrial and ventricular size and thereby determine the likelihood of a volume overload. In acute mitral regurgitation, the left atrium and left ventricle are not dilated or are only minimally dilated, whereas in chronic mitral regurgitation both the left atrium and ventricle are dilated (Fig 12–

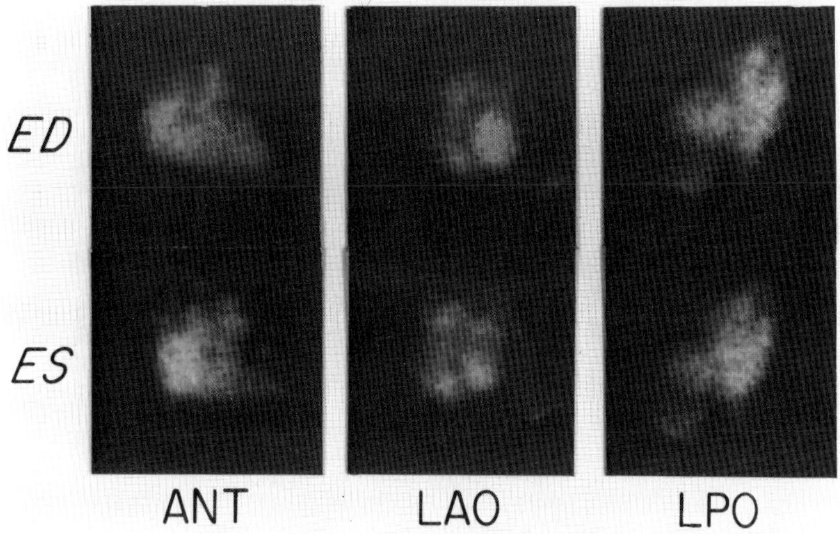

Fig 12–5.—End-diastolic *(ED)* and end-systolic *(ES)* blood pool images from a patient with an inferior myocardial infarction and mitral regurgitation secondary to papillary muscle dysfunction. The anterior *(ANT)* and left posterior oblique *(LPO)* projections demonstrate inferior wall hypokinesis and an increase in end-diastolic and stroke volumes. The left anterior oblique *(LAO)* projection demonstrates apical inferior hypokinesis.

5). In addition to anatomical data, regurgitant fraction can be estimated with gated equilibrium scans by measuring stroke volume (using counts) of both the right and left ventricle. The regurgitant fraction is[39–42]:

$$100 \times \frac{\text{left ventricular stroke volume} - \text{right ventricular stroke volume)}}{\text{left ventricular stroke volume}}$$

Regurgitation of blood from the left ventricle to the left atrium can cause increasing pressures in both chambers, which can be transmitted into the pulmonary venous system. The increase in pulmonary venous pressure increases the relative pulmonary blood volume in the lung apices compared to the bases. The increased apex to base volume or counts ratio can be determined from multigated blood pool scans (Fig 12–6). Any apex to base ratio greater than unity has been found to correlate with an increase in pulmonary venous pressure.[43]

Depression of Pump Function

Rest Studies

Myocardial function is generally acutely depressed during myocardial infarction and may continue to be depressed chronically. Measurement of ventricular function parameters such as ejection fraction, cardiac output, end-diastolic and end-systolic volume changes, and pulmonary blood volume distribution with first-pass or gated scans yields important information on ventricular decompensation.[27–35, 44–48] Schelbert et al.[44] performed serial measurements of left ventricular ejection fraction during the first five days after infarction in 50 patients. Ejection fraction was depressed to varying degrees in the majority of patients. It improved over the five-day period in 27 of 50 patients and was unchanged or decreased in 23. Patients with lower initial ejection fractions had more severe and more frequent complications (congestive heart failure, angina, arrhythmias). Late follow-up (two to three months later) in 43 of the 50 patients showed improvement of function in 61%, deterioration in 23%, and no change in 16%. It was suggested by these authors that early serial measurements of ejection fraction may be helpful in predicting morbidity and mortality. Patients with either a low initial ejection fraction or decreased ejection fraction on serial measurement had a greater early mortality and a higher incidence of long-term ventricular dysfunction. Shah et al.[45] reported that left ventricular ejection fraction was significantly reduced in patients with acute anterior infarction but not with inferior infarction. In addition, an ejection fraction less than 30% was of prognostic value in predicting a group of patients with a higher hospital morbidity and mortality.

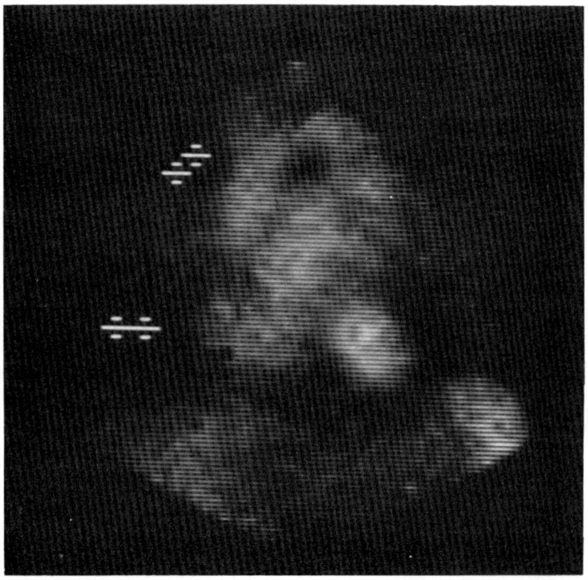

Fig 12–6.—Regions of interest have been located over the right lung apex and base on the end-systolic frame of a blood pool study. An apex-to-base ratio greater than unity was found to correlate with an increased pulmonary capillary wedge pressure.

Right Ventricular Function

Right ventricular function in patients after acute infarction can be evaluated in a manner similar to that used to evaluate left ventricular function.[46, 47, 49, 50] Algorithms have been developed that are fairly reliable for the determination of right ventricular ejection fraction. Depression of right ventricular ejection fraction at rest has been found in patients with right ventricular infarction. Exercise intervention ventriculography has been studied for the right ventricle as well as for the left ventricle. Right ventricular reserve function as determined by exercise ejection fraction response is depressed in some patients with clinical evidence of isolated left ventricular dysfunction, as well as in those with isolated right or combined right and left ventricular infarction.

GROSS ANATOMICAL CHANGES OF THE MYOCARDIUM (MUSCLE RUPTURE)

Ventricular Septal Defect

Infarction of the interventricular septum may cause septal rupture with resultant left-to-right shunt formation. The resultant acute volume overloads of both the right and left ventricle may be evidenced as chamber dilation with supernormal ejection fractions. Sequential first-pass studies can be performed to evaluate the site and extent of left-to-right shunt[51, 52] from ventricular septal defects. Regions of interest are located over the superior vena cava, right and left lungs, right atrium, right ventricle, pulmonary outflow tract, and left ventricle, and time-activity curves are generated. The superior vena cava curve is used to generate a bolus score (first transit of 2–6 seconds is a good bolus score). Then, first circulation *(A)* and recirculation curves *(B)* are generated for the other structures. Areas are determined for each first circulation and recirculation curve. Pulmonary to systemic flow ratios are determined by the equation, $A-B/A$. A ratio of 1.5:1 or greater for any vascular structure is evidence of a left-to-right

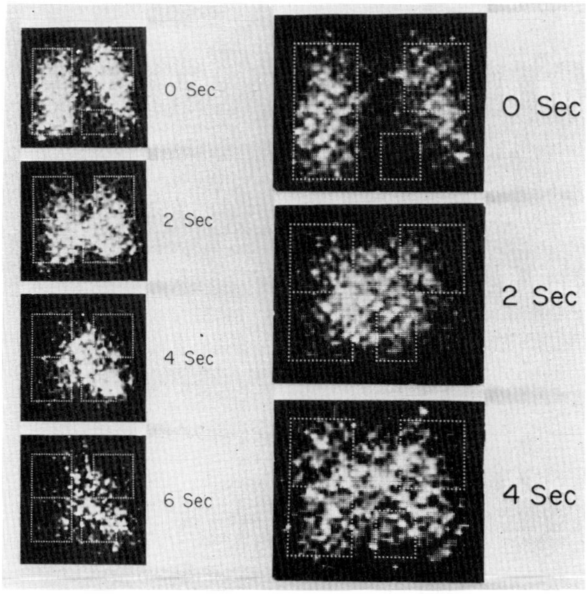

Fig 12–7.—*Left,* serial 0.5-second positron camera images of $C^{15}O_2$ activity in a normal patient taken 2, 4, and 6 seconds after peak inhalation (0 seconds). Various regions of interest, delineated by *dotted squares,* are located over the lung fields and heart area. These images show normal washout of tracer from the lungs and accumulation of activity in the heart region. Lung activity is almost entirely cleared by 6 seconds. *Right,* serial 0.5-second positron camera images of $C^{15}O_2$ activity obtained 2 and 4 seconds after peak inhalation (0 seconds) in a patient with an atrial septal defect. In this patient, normal pulmonary washout of tracer is observed at 2 seconds, but 4 seconds after inhalation there is early reappearance of activity in the lungs, reflecting left-to-right shunt flow. (From Boucher C.A., et al.: *Circulation* 56:632–640, 1977. Reproduced by permission of the American Heart Association.)

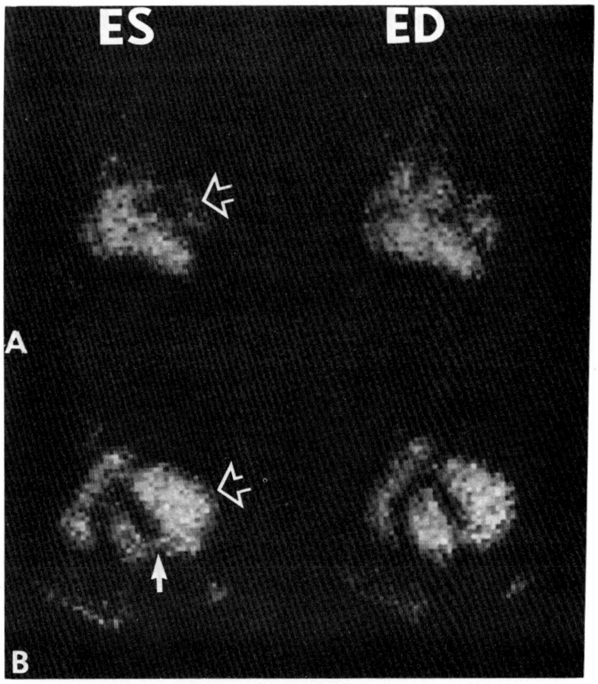

Fig 12–8.—Anterior *(A)* and left anterior oblique *(B)* end-systolic *(ES)* and end-diastolic *(ED)* gated cardiac blood pool scintiscans. Note large false aneurysm *(open arrows)* with narrow-necked connection to left ventricle *(solid arrow).*

shunt. The origin of the shunt can be determined by locating the first site of early recirculation.

Left-to-right shunts can also be determined by evaluation of pulmonary clearance of inhaled radioactive substances such as oxygen 15.[53, 54] Patients are imaged sequentially with a gamma camera after inhalation of radioactive gas (Fig 12–7). Regions of interest are located over the lungs, and time-activity curves are generated. In normal subjects the radioactivity clears exponentially. In patients with a left-to-right shunt, pulmonary clearance has an abnormal upward deviation in the exponential pulmonary clearance pattern.

Rupture of Ventricular Free Wall: False Aneurysm Formation

Infarction in the ventricular free wall can cause extensive necrosis which on occasion can result in muscle rupture. If the patient survives this event, a false aneurysm is formed. Radionuclide studies have contributed much to the understanding and diagnosis of this disastrous event.[55–61] Sequential first-pass studies demonstrate differential filling, with the true ventricular cavity filling first and the false aneurysm filling somewhat later.[55] Two chambers can also be identified on gated equilibrium scans. The typical appearance is of two chambers, separated by a neck of radiolucency. One chamber (left ventricle) is contractile and the second (the false aneurysm) is noncontractile (Figs 12–8, 12–9, and 12–10).[60] Thallium scans done in patients with false aneurysms show absence of perfusion (persistent defect) in the area of the pseudoaneurysm (see Fig 12–9).[60]

Pseudoaneurysm should be suspected in patients who have refractory congestive heart failure, arrhythmias, and embolic events. Radionu-

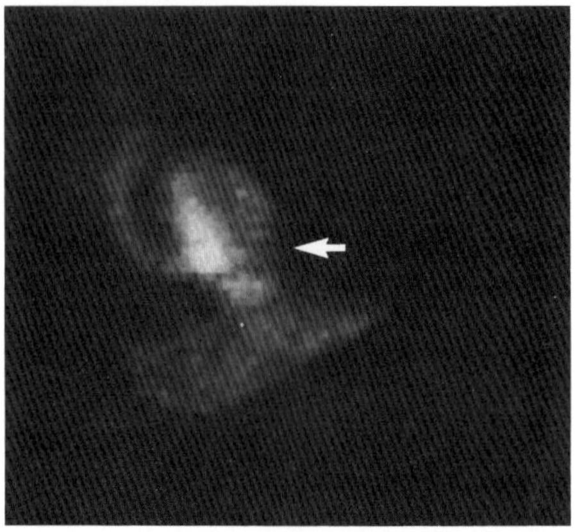

Fig 12–9.—Fifty-degree left anterior oblique ^{201}Tl myocardial perfusion scintiscan from same patient as in Figure 12–8. Note focal thallium defect in posterior left ventricular wall *(arrow)* in area of narrow-necked connection to false aneurysm.

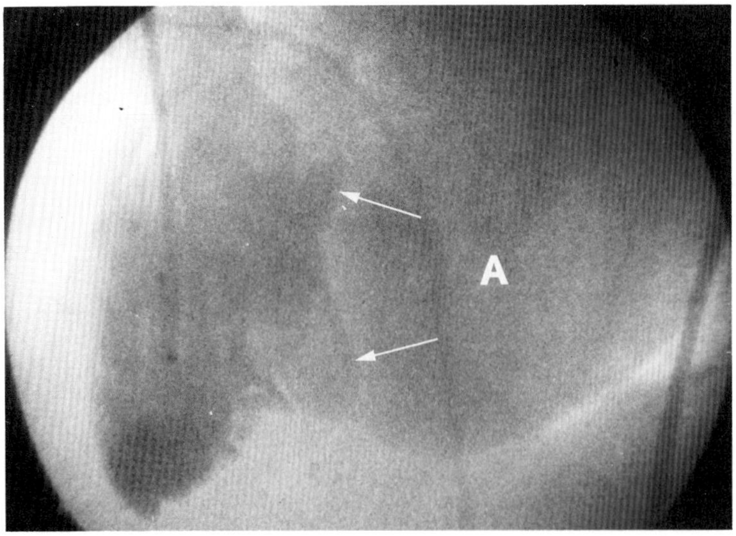

Fig 12–10.—Left anterior oblique contrast left ventriculogram from same patient as in Figure 12–8 and 12–9. Note false left ventricular aneurysm *(A)* with narrow-necked connection *(arrows)* to true ventricular cavity.

clide studies can be helpful in the early diagnosis of this frequently fatal complication of myocardial infarction.

Rupture of Papillary Muscle

Rupture of a papillary muscle body is usually fatal. However, patients can survive rupture of a papillary muscle head. The radionuclide imaging findings are similar to, although more extensive than, those described previously for papillary muscle dysfunction.

PERICARDIAL EFFUSION

Fluid can accumulate in the pericardial space for a number of reasons after a myocardial infarction and thus potentially cause cardiac tamponade, depending on the speed and amount of accumulation. The inflammatory process resulting after transmural myocardial infarction can cause fluid accumulation. Rupture of a ventricular free wall can also cause pericardial fluid accumulation. Pericardial fluid can be detected as a photon-deficient area surrounding the heart on a gated blood pool scan.

REFERENCES

1. Smitherman T.C., Osborn R.C., Narakara K.A.: Serial myocardial scintigraphy after a single dose of thallium-201 in men after acute myocardial infarction. *Am. J. Cardiol.* 42:177-182, 1978.
2. Fletcher J.W., Mueller H.S., Rao P.S.: Sequential thallium-201 myocardial scintigraphy after acute infarction in man. *Radiology* 136:191-195, 1980.
3. Nelson A.D., Khullar S., Leighton R.F., et al.: Quantitation of thallium-201 scintigrams in acute myocardial infarction. *Am. J. Cardiol.* 44:664-670, 1979.
4. Silverman K.J., Becker L.C., Bulkley B.H., et al.: Value of early thallium-201 scintigraphy for predicting mortality in patients with acute myocardial infarction. *Circulation* 60:996-1003, 1979.
5. Pohost G.M., Zir L.M., Moore R.H., et al.: Differentiation of transiently ischemic from infarcted myocardium by serial imaging after a single dose of thallium-201. *Circulation* 55:294-302, 1976.
6. Wackers F.J.: Thallium-201 myocardial scintigraphy in acute myocardial infarction and ischemia. *Semin. Nucl. Med.* 10:127-145, 1980.
7. Gibson R.S., Taylor G.J., Watson D.D., et al.: Predicting the extent and location of coronary artery disease during the early postinfarction period by quantitative thallium-201 scintigraphy. *Am. J. Cardiol.* 47:1010–1019, 1981.
8. Tiefenbrynn A.J., Biello D.R., Geltman E.M., et al.: Gated cardiac blood pool imaging and thallium-201 myocardial scintigraphy for detection of remote myocardial infarction. *Am. J. Cardiol.* 47:1–9, 1981.
9. Kirshenbaum H.D., Okada R.D., Boucher C.A., et al.: Relationship of thallium-201 myocardial perfusion to regional and global ventricular function. *Am. Heart J.* 101:734–739, 1981.
10. Niess G.S., Logic J.R., Russell R.O., et al.: Usefulness and limitations of thallium-201 myocardial scintigraphy in delineating location and size of prior myocardial infarction. *Circulation* 59:1010–1019, 1979.
11. Turner J.D., Schwartz K.M., Logic J.R., et al.: Detection of residual jeopardized myocardium three weeks after myocardial infarction by exercise testing with thallium-201 myocardial scintigraphy. *Circulation* 61:729–737, 1980.
12. Khaw B.V., Gold H.K., Leinbach R.C., et al.: Early imaging of experimental myocardial infarction by intracoronary administration of I131-labeled anticardiac myosin $(Fabl)_2$ fragments. *Circulation* 58:1137–1142, 1978.
13. Khaw B.A., Beller G.A., Haber E.: Experimental infarct imaging following intravenous administration of Iodine-131 labeled antibody $(Fabl)_2$ fragments specific for cardiac myosin. *Circulation* 57:743–750, 1977.
14. Khaw B.A., Fallon J.T., Beller G.A., et al.: Specificity of localization of myosin-specific antibody fragments in experimental myocardial infarction: Histologic, histochemical, autoradiographic, and scintigraphic studies. *Circulation* 60:1527–1531, 1979.
15. Mallory G.K., White P.D., Salcedo-Salgar J.: The speed of healing of myocardial infarction. *Am. Heart J.* 18:647, 1939.
16. Hillis D.L., Braunwald E.: Myocardial ischemia. *N. Engl. J. Med.* 296:1093–1096, 1977.
17. Hartmann J.R., Robinson J.A., Gunnar R.M.: Chemotactic activity in the coronary sinus after experimental myocardial infarction: Effects of pharmacologic intervention on ischemic injury. *Am. J. Cardiol.* 40:550, 1977.
18. Thakur M.L., Gottschalk A., Zaret B.L.: Imaging

experimental myocardial infarction with Indium-111-labeled autologous leukocytes: Effects of infarct age and residual regional myocardial blood flow. *Circulation* 60:297–305, 1979.
19. Davies R.A., Thakur M.L., Berger H.J., et al.: In-111 labeled autologous leukocytes (In WBC) for imaging inflammatory response to acute myocardial infarction (MI). *J. Nucl. Med.* 21:89, 1980.
20. Stratton J.R., Ritchie J.L., Hamilton G.W., et al.: Left ventricular thrombi: In vivo detection by Indium-111 platelet imaging and two dimensional echocardiography. *Am. J. Cardiol.* 47:874–881, 1981.
21. Ezekowitz M.D., Leonard J.C., Smith E.O., et al.: Identification of left ventricular thrombi in man using indium-111-labeled autologous platelets: A preliminary report. *Circulation* 63:803–809, 1981.
22. Buja L.M., Tofe A.J., Kulkarni P.V., et al.: Sites and mechanisms of localization of technetium-99m phosphorous radiopharmaceuticals in acute myocardial infarcts and other tissues. *J. Clin. Invest.* 60:724–740, 1977.
23. Holman B.L., Chisholm R.J., Braunwald E.: The prognostic implications of acute myocardial infarct scintigraphy with ^{99m}Tc-pyrophosphate. *Circulation* 57:320–326, 1978.
24. Rude R.E., Parkey R.W., Bonte F.J., et al.: Clinical implications of Technetium-99m stannous pyrophosphate myocardial scintigraphic "doughnut" patterns in patients with acute myocardial infarcts. *Circulation* 59:721–730, 1979.
25. Ahmad M., Logan K.W., Martin R.H.: Doughnut pattern of Technetium-99m pyrophosphate myocardial uptake in patients with acute myocardial infarction: A sign of poor long-term prognosis. *Am. J. Cardiol.* 44:13–17, 1979.
26. Olson H.G., Lyons K.P., Aronow W.S., et al.: Follow-up technetium-99m stannous pyrophosphate myocardial scintigrams after myocardial infarction. *Circulation* 56:181–187, 1977.
27. Ramanathan K.B., Bodenheimer M.M., Banker V.S., et al.: Severity of contraction abnormalities after acute myocardial infarction in man: Response to nitroglycerin. *Circulation* 60:1230–1237, 1979.
28. Stephens J.D., Dymond M.B., Sparrell R.A.J.: Radionuclide and hemodynamic assessment of left ventricular functional reserve in patients with left ventricular aneurysm and congestive heart failure: Response to exercise stress and isosorbide dinitrate. *Circulation* 61:536–542, 1980.
29. Morrison J., Coromilas J., Robbins M., et al.: Digitalis and myocardial infarction in man. *Circulation* 62:8–16, 1980.
30. Strauss H.W., Pitt B.: Common procedures for the noninvasive determination of regional myocardial perfusion, evaluation of regional wall motion, and detection of acute infarction. *Am. J. Cardiol.* 38:731–738, 1976.
31. Rigo P., Murray M., Strauss H.W., et al.: Scintigraphic evaluation of patients with suspected left ventricular aneurysm. *Circulation* 50:985–991, 1974.
32. Dymond D.S., Stephens J., Stone D., et al.: Assessment of contractile segments in patients with left ventricular aneurysms by quantitative first-pass radionuclide ventriculography: Hemodynamic correlation at rest and exercise. *Br. Heart J.* 43:125–133, 1980.
33. Dymond D.S., Jarritt P.H., Britton K.E., et al.: Detection of post infarction left ventricular aneurysms by first-pass radionuclide ventriculography using a multicrystal gamma camera. *Br. Heart J.* 41:68–78, 1979.
34. Hopkins G.B., Kan M.K., Salel A.F.: Scintigraphic assessment of left ventricular aneurysms. *J.A.M.A.* 240:2162–2165, 1978.
35. Friedman M.L., Cantor R.E.: Reliability of gated heart scintigrams for detection of left ventricular aneurysm. *J. Nucl. Med.* 20:720–723, 1979.
36. Kelly R.J., Conan R.J., Maynard C.D., et al.: Localization of 99mTc Sc pyrophosphate in left ventricular aneurysm. *J. Nucl. Med.* 18:342–345, 1977.
37. Wisneski J.A., Rollo F.D., Gertz E.W.: Correlation of 99mTc pyrophosphate myocardial accumulation with left ventricular wall motion abnormalities. *Cardiology* 66:85–101, 1980.
38. Ahmad M., Dubiel J.P., Verdon T.A., et al.: Technetium 99m stannous pyrophosphate myocardial imaging in patients with and without left ventricular aneurysm. *Circulation* 53:833–838, 1976.
39. Rigo P., Alderson P.O., Robertson R.M., et al.: Measurement of aortic and mitral regurgitation by gated cardiac blood pool scans. *Circulation* 60:306–312, 1979.
40. Sorenson S.G., O'Rourke R.A., Chandhuri T.K.: Noninvasive quantitation of valvular regurgitation by gated equilibrium radionuclide angiography. *Circulation* 62:1089–1098, 1980.
41. Bough E.W., Gandsman E.J., North D.L., et al.: Gated radionuclide angiographic evaluation of valve regurgitation. *Am. J. Cardiol.* 46:423–428, 1980.
42. Baxter R.H., Becker L.C., Alderson P.O., et al.: Quantification of aortic valvular regurgitation in dogs by nuclear imaging. *Circulation* 61:404–410, 1980.
43. Urbina A., Okada R.D., Osbakken M.D., et al.: Noninvasive detection of elevated pulmonary capillary wedge pressure from the distribution of pulmonary blood volume on the gated cardiac blood pool scan. *J. Nucl. Med.* 22:950–954, 1981.
44. Schelbert H.R., Henning H., Ashburn W.L., et al.: Serial measurements of left ventricular ejection fraction by radionuclide angiography early and late after myocardial infarction. *Am. J. Cardiol.* 38:407–415, 1976.
45. Shah P.K., Pichler M., Berman D.S., et al.: Left ventricular ejection fraction determined by radionuclide ventriculography in early states of first transmural infarction: Relation to short-term prognosis. *Am. J. Cardiol.* 45:542–546, 1980.
46. Maddahi J., Berman D.S., Matsuoka D.T., et al.:

Right ventricular ejection fraction during exercise in normal subjects and in coronary artery disease patients: Assessment by multiple-gated equilibrium scintigraphy. *Circulation* 62:133–140, 1980.
47. Slutsky R., Hooper W., Gerber K., et al.: Assessment of right ventricular function at rest and during exercise in patients with coronary heart disease: A new approach using equilibrium radionuclide angiography. *Am. J. Cardiol.* 45:63–71, 1980.
48. Okada R.D., Pohost G.M., Kirshenbaum H.D., et al.: Radionuclide determined change in pulmonary blood volume with exercise: Improved sensitivity of multigated blood pool scanning in detecting coronary artery disease. *N. Engl. J. Med.* 301:569–576, 1979.
49. Johnson L.L., McCarthy D.M., Sciacca R.R., et al.: Right ventricular ejection fraction during exercise in patients with coronary artery disease. *Circulation* 60:1284–1291, 1979.
50. Berger H.J., Johnstone D.E., Sands J.M., et al.: Response of right ventricular ejection fraction to upright bicycle exercise in coronary artery disease. *Circulation* 60:1291–1300, 1980.
51. Askenazi J., Ahnberg D.S., Korngold E., et al.: Quantitative radionuclide angiography: Detection and quantitation of left to right shunts. *Am. J. Cardiol.* 37:382–387, 1976.
52. Anderson P.A.W., Jones R.H., Sabiston D.C.: Quantitation of left to right cardiac shunts with radionuclide angiography. *Circulation* 49:512–516, 1973.
53. Boucher C.A., Ahluwalia B., Block P.C., et al.: Inhalation imaging with oxygen-15 labeled carbon dioxide for detection and quantitation of left-to-right shunts. *Circulation* 56:632–640, 1977.
54. Tamer D.M., Watson D.D., Kenny P.J., et al.: Noninvasive detection and quantitation of left-to-right shunts in children using oxygen-15 labeled carbon dioxide. *Circulation* 56:626–631, 1977.
55. Onik G., Recht L., Edwards J.E., et al.: False left ventricular aneurysm: Diagnosis by noninvasive means. *J. Nucl. Med.* 21:177–182, 1980.
56. Dymond D.S., Elliot A.T., Banim S.: Detection of a false aneurysm by first pass radionuclide ventriculography. *J. Nucl. Med.* 230:851–854, 1979.
57. Sweet S.E., Sterling R., McCormick J.R., et al.: Left ventricular false aneurysm after coronary bypass surgery: Radionuclide diagnosis and surgical resection. *Am. J. Cardiol.* 43:154–158, 1979.
58. Perkins P.J.: Radioisotopic diagnosis of false left ventricular aneurysm. *Am. J. Radiol.* 132:117–119, 1979.
59. Sabah I., Yoshikawa J., Kato H., et al.: Noninvasive diagnosis of pseudoaneurysm of the left ventricle. *Jpn. Heart J.* 20:95–103, 1979.
60. Winzelberg G.G., Miller S.W., Okada R.D., et al.: Scintigraphic assessment of false left ventricular aneurysms. *Am. J. Radiol.* 135:569–574, 1980.
61. Katz R.J., Simpson A., Dibianco R., et al.: Noninvasive diagnosis of left ventricular pseudoaneurysm: Role of two-dimensional echocardiography and radionuclide gated pool imaging. *Am. J. Cardiol.* 44:372–377, 1979.

PART VII

Mitral, Tricuspid, and Aortic Valve Prolapse

ECHOCARDIOGRAPHY

James Burke, Chin C. Chen, Daniel David, and Joel Morganroth

MITRAL VALVE PROLAPSE

IN THE 1930s, several authors suggested potential etiologies for the midsystolic nonejection click, claiming both cardiac and noncardiac sources.[1–3] In the 1960s, the click was for the first time attributed to a "chordal snap,"[4] and the late systolic murmur was thought possibly to be due to mitral value regurgitation.[5] A few years later, Barlow et al. described the mitral valve prolapse syndrome, which comprised a midsystolic click and a late systolic murmur with characteristic ECG and angiographic findings.[6, 7] Confirmation of these findings came early.[8]

One cause of the click-murmur syndrome has been postulated to be a disproportionately large mitral valve apparatus for the left ventricular cavity size. According to this proposal, the mitral valve prolapse seen in typical floppy mitral valve and in patients with the Marfan syndrome results from excessive mitral valve tissue. In contrast, the mitral valve prolapse seen in patients with atrial septal defect or idiopathic hypertrophic subaortic stenosis is thought to be due to a disproportionately small left ventricular cavity.

The current classification of mitral valve prolapse relegates the prolapse to either primary or secondary forms.[9, 10] The histologic presence of valvular myxomatous degeneration characterizes the primary or idiopathic type. An abnormal mitral valve apparatus caused by another type of cardiac disease characterizes the secondary type; possible diseases include endocarditis, cardiomyopathy, coronary or rheumatic heart disease, and calcified mitral annulus.[11]

In primary mitral valve prolapse, myxomatous degeneration causes decreased collagenous support, resulting in mitral leaflet stretching and consequent prolapse (i.e., mitral leaflet present in the left atrium during systole). Atrioventricular valve prolapse occurs in systole, while semilunar valve prolapse occurs in diastole. Compared to the normal mitral valve (Fig 13–1), the valve cusps in primary mitral valve prolapse are large, redundant, scalloped, and thickened (Fig 13–2). Annular dilation is generally present. Clinically, primary mitral valve prolapse varies from the asymptomatic state with mild mitral prolapse to the full-blown "floppy valve syndrome" with severe prolapse of several valves and severe regurgitation, often requiring prosthetic valve replacement.[12, 13]

The etiology of myxomatous degeneration has not been established. It may result from stress on the valve by perivalvular abnormalities or from a primary defect in mucopolysaccharide metabolism. Increased adrenergic tone in symptomatic patients with mitral valve prolapse suggests a more systemic process.[14] Some patients with prolapse have a primary myocardial abnormality manifested by left ventricular asynergy.[15, 16] Recent two-dimensional echocardiographic (2DE) studies have revealed segmental left ventricular dysfunction in some patients with mitral valve prolapse.[17] Abnormalities of left ventricular hemodynamics[18] and lactate metabolism[19] have also been suggested as causes of this degeneration. There have also been unconfirmed reports[20] of mitral valve prolapse

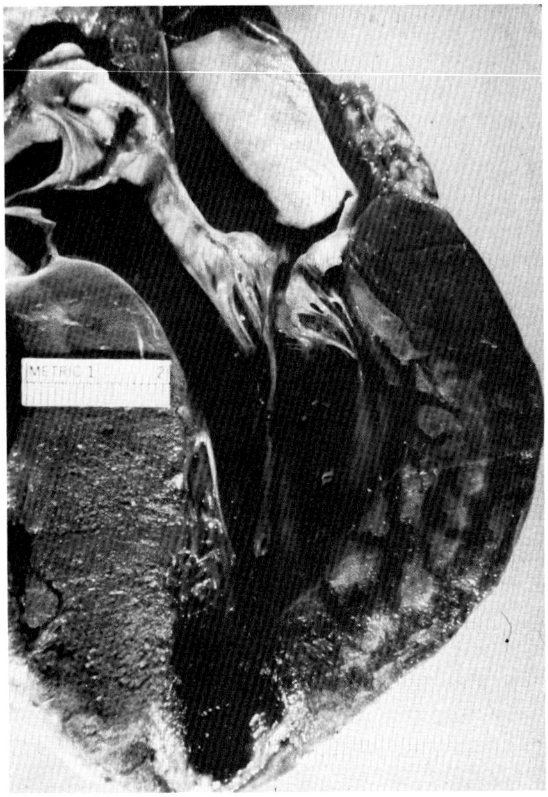

Fig 13–1.—Anatomical projection of a normal mitral valve from the frontal, cross-sectional view. (Courtesy of Jeffrey Isner, M.D., Tufts University, Boston.)

caused by underdeveloped left circumflex arteries[21] or "corkscrew" coronary vessels.[22]

Clinical Aspects

The prevalence of mitral valve prolapse in the general population is estimated at 4% (Table 13–1). Depending on the diagnostic standard employed, the prevalence of mitral valve prolapse varies from 0.4% to 21%.[23–28] Mitral valve prolapse is most common in the 20- to 50-year-old age group. Only in the age group less than 50 years old is a female preponderance noted.[29] Although the mode of inheritance remains controversial, some postulate an autosomal dominant pattern with incomplete penetrance.[30]

Chest pain, the symptom most commonly associated with mitral valve prolapse, is nonexertional and atypical of classic angina in most cases (Table 13–2).[31, 32] Although many theories, including coronary spasm,[33] have been proposed, the etiology of the chest pain remains unclear. Dyspnea, anxiety, lassitude, dizziness, palpitations, presyncope, and syncope have all been associated with mitral prolapse.[34] Arrhythmias may cause some of the symptoms, but many patients have experienced these symptoms during episodes of well-documented normal sinus rhythm.[35, 36] The association between mitral valve prolapse and tran-

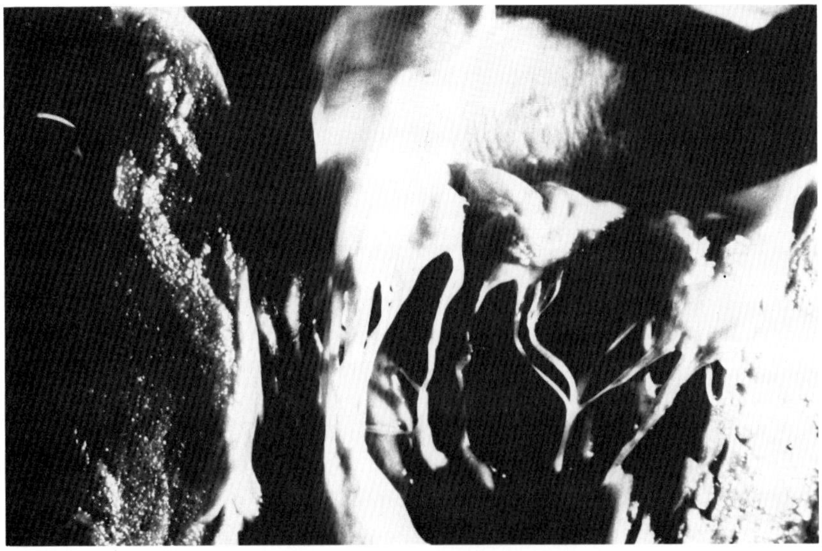

Fig 13–2.—Frontal, cross-sectional view of a mitral valve demonstrating the findings in mitral valve prolapse. Note the hooding, thickening, and prolapsing nature of this valve.

TABLE 13–1.—Prevalence of Mitral Valve Prolapse

Prevalence	
Autopsy data	5%
Auscultatory data	0.4%–17%
M-mode echocardiographic data	4.4%–21% (6%)
Most common age group	20–50 years
Female:male ratio	
Younger age group	2:1
Older age group	1:1

TABLE 13–2.—Prevalence of Clinical Symptoms in Mitral Valve Prolapse

SYMPTOM	PREVALENCE (%)
Chest pain	50–61
Dyspnea	9–60
Fatigue	9–60
Palpitations	46
Dizziness	33
Presyncope	33
Anxiety	15–38
Lassitude	15–38

TABLE 13–3.—Prevalence of Clinical Signs in Mitral Valve Prolapse

SIGN	PREVALENCE (%)
None	15–20
Systolic nonejection click	60–75
Systolic murmur	30–70
Asthenia	Common
Bony abnormalities	Common
Unusual dermatographic patterns	17
Ophthalmoplegia	Less common

sient ischemic attacks may be the result of cardiac emboli caused by adherent fibrin and blood cells breaking their attachment on a myxomatous valve.[37, 38]

Although the physical examination findings are completely normal in nearly one fifth of patients with mitral valve prolapse, the majority have a midsystolic to late systolic nonejection click (Table 13–3). Despite numerous theories, the cause of the click is uncertain.[39–41] Systolic murmurs most often occur in midsystole to late systole.[9, 32] In patients over age 50, the murmur is more likely pansystolic.[42] In addition to systolic nonejection clicks and murmurs, an early diastolic sound may also be heard.[43] Other physical findings associated with mitral valve prolapse include asthenia, bony abnormalities, characteristic dermatographic patterns, and ophthalmoplegia.[44, 45]

Electrocardiographic findings sometimes present with mitral prolapse include nonspecific repolarization abnormalities, conduction disturbances, a prolonged QT interval, and ventricular ectopy.[9, 14, 22, 26, 28, 32, 46–48] Holter monitoring is invaluable in the detection of arrhythmias. The sick sinus and Wolff-Parkinson-White syndromes as well as supraventricular and ventricular arrhythmias have been linked with mitral valve prolapse.[9, 22, 29, 35, 47, 49–51] Several explanations have been proposed to account for this increased incidence of arrhythmias, but no theory is universally accepted.[52–54] Exercise- and hyperventilation-induced ST segment changes may occur with mitral valve prolapse.[29, 55]

Diagnostic Standard for Mitral Valve Prolapse

As described below, physical examination and angiography are clearly less than optimal diagnostic standards for mitral valve prolapse. Since up to 10% of patients with the click-murmur syndrome may have normal M-mode and two-dimensional echocardiograms,[56] some consider the auscultatory finding of a click as the diagnostic standard for mitral valve prolapse.[9] Several problems make the physical examination a less than optimal standard. Nearly one fifth of patients with prolapse documented by other means have completely normal physical examination findings, including findings on cardiac auscultation.[9] The absence of a click in this syndrome is even more common (one quarter of patients). In addition, nonejection clicks are not always indicators of mitral valve prolapse. They occur in other conditions such as pneumothorax,[57] atrial myxoma,[58] intraventricular septal aneurysm,[59, 60] and idiopathic hypertrophic subaortic stenosis.[61] The systolic murmur is even less sensitive and specific.[9, 32]

Some have proposed cineangiography as the diagnostic standard for mitral valve prolapse,[62] but angiography has many shortcomings in the evaluation of prolapse.[63] The normal mitral valve has variable motion patterns on left ventricular angiography. Because of this, the angiographic criteria for mitral valve prolapse remain ill-defined and nonquantifiable.[64] The interobserver discrepancy in the angiographic detection of mitral valve prolapse is quite high.[65] The right anterior oblique left ventriculogram cannot be used to define anterior mitral valve prolapse in most cases since the valve is superimposed on the left ventricular silhouette. Regurgitant dye can also impair this assessment. Few cardiac cycles are seen on angiography compared to echocardiography. Finally, the false positive rate can be over 40%.[66] In addition, even when true prolapse of the posterior mitral leaflet is seen on angiography, both leaflets are actually involved by echocardiography.[67]

In an echocardiographic evaluation of 336 patients for mitral valve prolapse by Smith et al.,[66] the diagnostic problems of angiography were confirmed. Although only 6 of these patients had clinical evidence of the click-murmur syndrome and only 9 had the click-murmur syndrome as determined by echocardiography, nearly half of the patients had angiographic signs of mitral valve prolapse. The angiographically demonstrated prolapse was associated with a variety of cardiac disorders. Leaflet bulging was seen in 40% of patients with coronary artery disease, 32% of patients with rheumatic heart disease, 16% of those with cardiomyopathies, 42% of patients with congenital heart disease, and over half of those with chest pain and normal coronary arteries. The conclusion of the study was that end-systolic bulging of the posterior mitral leaflet is a common angiographic finding and should not be considered indicative of pathologic mitral valve function.[66]

In contrast to physical examination and angiography, echocardiography has great promise as the best diagnostic standard for the detection of mitral valve prolapse.[68] The hallmark of prolapse is the presence of mitral valve tissue in the left atrium during systole. Echocardiography seems to provide the best imaging of the location of the mitral valve with regard to the left atrium. The mitral valve ring level and mitral valve motion are generally well visualized. Multiple cardiac cycles can also be viewed with this technique.

M-Mode Echocardiography

M-mode echocardiography provides good visualization of the mitral valve. The motion of both leaflets is generally well seen in both systole and diastole (Fig 13–3). The sensitivity of M-mode echocardiography for the diagnosis of mitral valve prolapse is quite promising. Its true diagnostic ac-

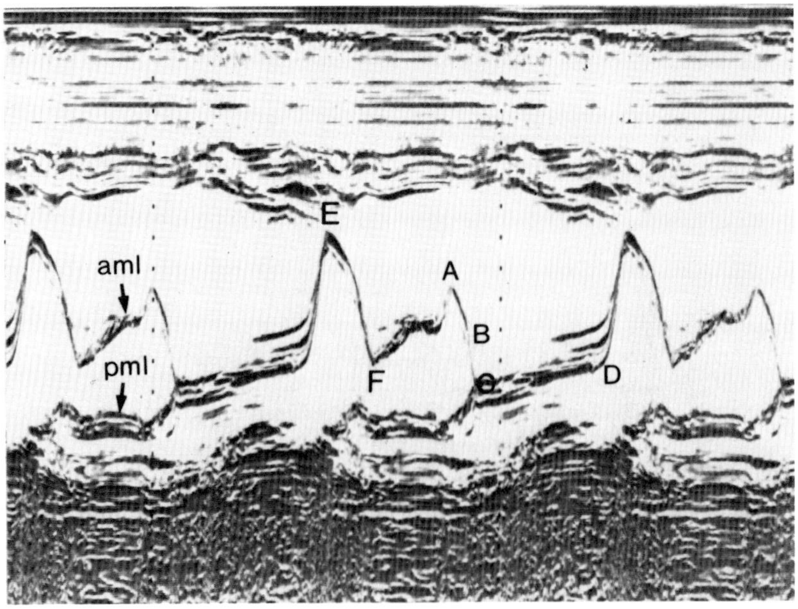

Fig 13–3.—M-mode echocardiogram at the level of the anterior mitral leaflet *(aml)* and posterior mitral leaflet *(pml)* demonstrating normal mitral valve motion in systole. Mitral valve motion during diastole is labeled at specific points.

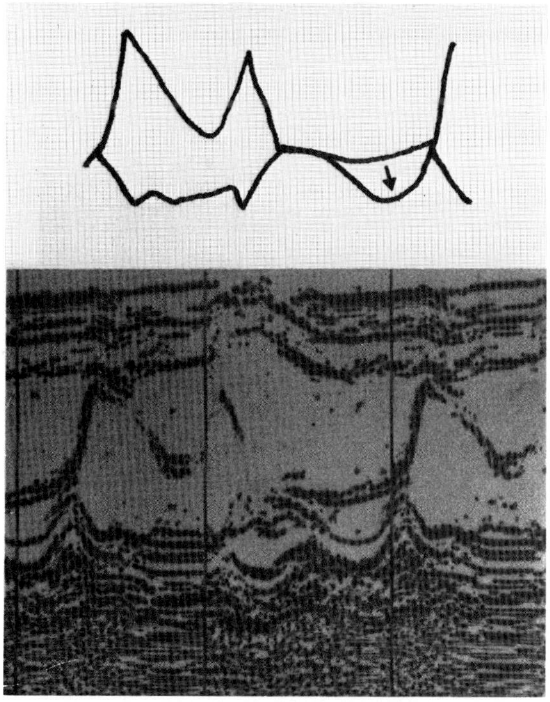

Fig 13–4.—M-mode echocardiogram from a patient with mitral valve prolapse demonstrates posterior mitral valve leaflet buckling in systole (*black arrow* in accompanying schematic). (From Morganroth J., et al.: *Am. J. Cardiol.* 46:1164–1177, 1980. Reproduced by permission.)

curacy is difficult to determine because of the lack of a diagnostic standard. Only about one fifth of patients thought to have mitral valve prolapse by auscultation are found to have prolapse on M-mode echocardiography.[65] Its correlation is slightly better when compared with left ventriculography.[26, 31, 69] These low correlations may well represent the limitations of physical examination and angiography rather than of M-mode echocardiography.

The most sensitive and specific finding for mitral valve prolapse by M-mode echocardiography is posterior midsystolic buckling of the mitral valve (Fig 13–4).[70] Technical aspects of M-mode echocardiography are critical in the detection of this finding. For example, this abnormality can be falsely produced by placing the transducer high on the chest and angling caudad (Fig 13–5, parts *A* through *C*).[26] This may create a D point posterior to the C point, with the mitral valve ring and leaflets moving perpendicularly to the echocardiographic beam and away from the transducer. This results in an apparent posterior dipping of the mitral valve. Similarly, a transducer placed low on the chest wall and angled cephalad may not visualize the posterior leaflet or may mask anterior mitral valve prolapse by locating the D point just anterior to the C point (Fig 13–5, part *D*).[26] But

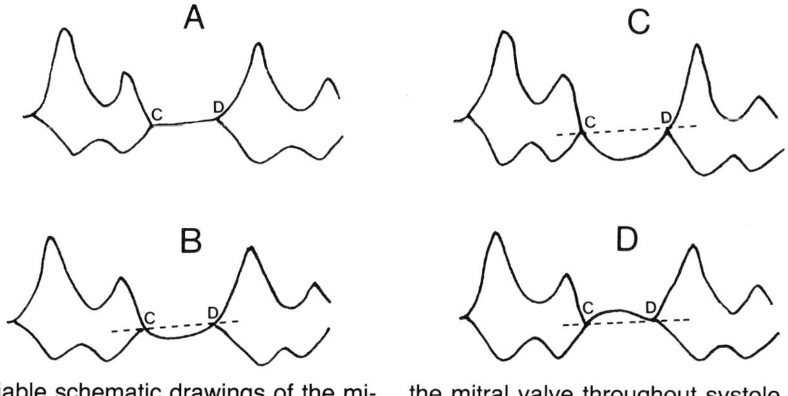

Fig 13–5.—Variable schematic drawings of the mitral valve during systole as seen on M-mode echocardiography. *A,* normal mitral valve motion between points C and D in systole. *B,* a slight posterior sagging of the mitral valve leaflets between points C and D in systole of less than 2 mm. This pattern is seen in patients with normal mitral valve in whom the echocardiographic transducer is placed high on the chest wall and angled caudad. *C,* a marked posterior sagging of the mitral valve throughout systole from points C and D of greater than 2 mm. This represents a pattern compatible with mitral valve prolapse. *D,* a false negative M-mode echocardiogram in a patient with mitral valve prolapse. The M-mode echocardiographic transducer was placed low on the chest wall and angled cephalad, producing systolic anterior motion of the mitral valve between points C and D.

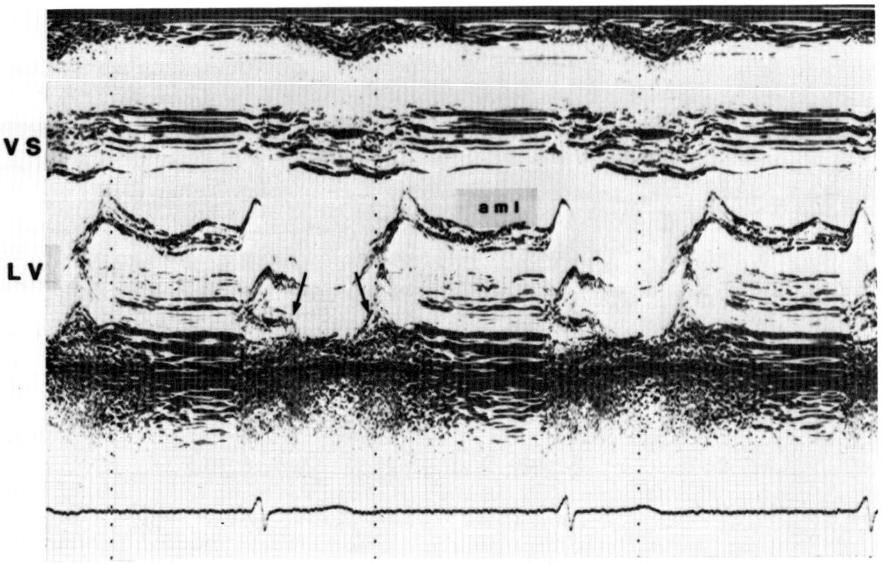

Fig 13–6.—M-mode echocardiographic recording demonstrating marked holosystolic hammocking of the mitral valve leaflets. *Arrows* point to the posterior leaflet, which has projected outside the M-mode echocardiographic view. *aml,* anterior mitral leaflet; *VS,* ventricular septum; *LV,* left ventricle.

with correct echocardiographic technique, midsystolic buckling is considered specific for mitral valve prolapse[71, 72] and diagnostic of the syndrome even in the absence of corroborative physical examination or angiographic findings.[9]

M-mode echocardiography demonstrates other findings in mitral valve prolapse. Pansystolic hammocking (Fig 13–6), though less specific for prolapse than midsystolic buckling, is another key finding.[73] The problem is to define the degree of posterior sagging which maximizes sensitivity and specificity for mitral prolapse. Though values for posterior displacement from 2 to 5 mm have been proposed,[26, 27] a 3 mm value may be optimal for diagnostic accuracy.[9] Again, beam angulation is important.[26] The two key M-mode echocardiographic features just discussed, midsystolic discrete buckling and holosystolic hammocking, can be seen in the same patient by beam angulation.[74]

Other M-mode findings are less sensitive and specific. One is increased mitral valve excursion, greater than 22 mm, with the anterior leaflet reaching the interventricular septum in early diastole.[62, 63, 65] Redundant or multiscalloped mitral leaflets in prolapse may cause more than three systolic echoes or a thickened mitral valve leaflet.[65, 75] Multiple diastolic echoes, similar to those seen with atrial myxoma, are another indicator. This finding may be caused by the posterior leaflet curling under the anterior one in diastole.[76] Redundant leaflets with multiple echo-reflective surfaces cause shaggy echoes on the mitral valve in diastole. These can be seen with or without vegetations from infective endocarditis.[77, 78] Multiple echocardiographic lines on M-mode echocardiography are caused by the ultrasonic beam intersecting the prolapsed leaflet more than once as the beam simultaneously crosses different parts of the redundant mitral leaflet. M-mode echocardiography may show posterior collapse of the mitral leaflet toward the left atrium[79] or even fragments of the mitral leaflet in the left atrium.[65] Finally, systolic anterior mitral valve motion has been reported with mitral valve prolapse. This may be caused by the chordae tendineae[80] or superimposition of echoes from the mitral annulus and the posterosuperior arching of the prolapsed leaflets.[74]

Despite the great benefits of M-mode echocardiography in the detection of mitral valve prolapse, several limitations exist. The location and extent of prolapse on M-mode echocardiography do not correlate with the degree of mitral valve regurgitation or the presence of a click or murmur on physical examination.[81] Posterior leaflet prolapse was formerly considered the most common finding by M-mode echocardiography, but after review of other techniques such as 2DE, it is now apparent that both mitral leaflets are prolapsed in the majority of cases.[75, 79, 82] False positive results may be obtained by poor technique (see Fig 13–5, parts *B* and *C*), by pericardial effusion, and by other abnormalities of the mitral valve (e.g., mitral stenosis).[83] In pericardial effusion, swinging of the heart may mimic pansystolic hammocking.[84, 85] False negative M-mode echocardiographic diagnoses of mitral valve prolapse may arise from poor technique (see Fig 13–5, part *D*) or poor-quality echocardiograms. The ice pick view obtained by M-mode echocardiography may result in incomplete visualization of the mitral valve. Also, if the prolapse occurs in a mainly superior rather than posterior direction, M-mode echocardiography can miss this type of prolapse.

Two-Dimensional Echocardiography

Two-dimensional echocardiography may well be the sought-after diagnostic standard for the detection of mitral valve prolapse. Mitral valve prolapse is defined by the presence of mitral tissue in the left atrium in systole. Two-dimensional echocardiography appears to provide the best evaluation of this abnormality. This technique has greatly expanded our knowledge of mitral valve prolapse and exposed many of the limitations of the prior diagnostic aids, particularly M-mode echocardiography. It has become clear that many false positive and false negative results on M-mode echocardiography are due to faulty transducer placement. Two-dimensional echocardiography demonstrates the superior as well as posterior direction of the prolapse of the mitral valve leaflet. The major part of the posterior leaflet may move superiorly toward the left atrium in systole while portions near the atrioventricular junction move posteriorly.[74]

Two-dimensional echocardiography has proved to be the most sensitive technique in detecting prolapse of one or both leaflets. It is now known that prolapse of both mitral leaflets is by far the most common.[67] Gilbert et al. showed that of 34 patients with mitral valve prolapse, 29 patients had both leaflets involved, 4 had isolated posterior leaflet prolapse, and only 1 had isolated anterior mitral leaflet prolapse. Thus, when isolated mitral leaflet prolapse is present, the posterior leaflet is more likely to be the one involved.[67] The short-axis view is not as useful as the apical and long-axis views in the detection of mitral valve prolapse, but it can show thickened, redundant mitral leaflets.[86] A normal 2DE long-axis view is

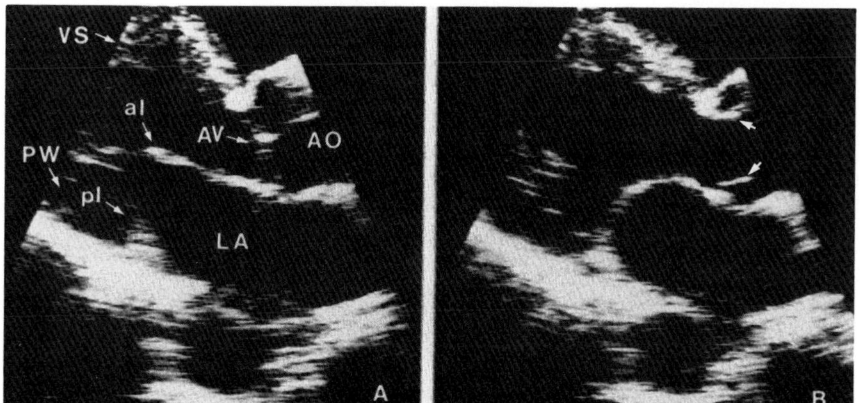

Fig 13–7.—Two-dimensional echocardiographic frames in diastole **(A)** and systole **(B)** of the parasternal long-axis left ventricular view. Note that in **B,** in systole, the mitral valve anterior and posterior leaflets lie within the left ventricular cavity. *VS,* ventricular septum; *PW,* posterior left ventricular wall; *AL,* anterior mitral leaflet; *PL,* posterior leaflet; *AV,* aortic valve; *AO,* aorta; and *LA,* left atrium. (From Morganroth J., et al.: *Am. J. Cardiol.* 46:1164–1177, 1980. Reproduced by permission.)

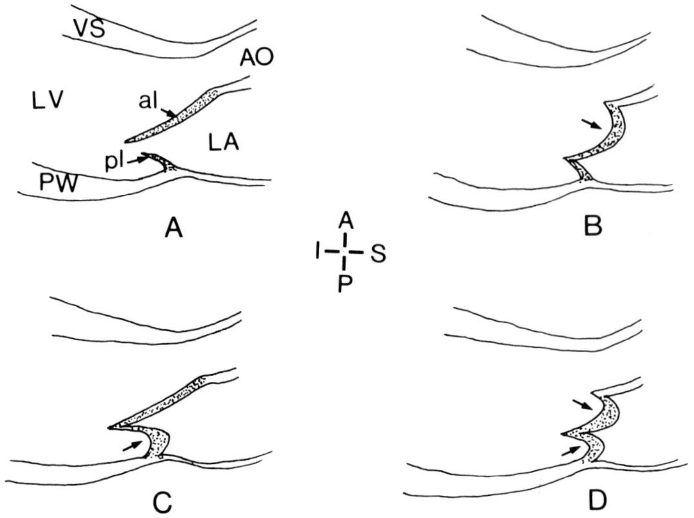

Fig 13–8.—Schematic drawings of the mitral valve as seen from a two-dimensional parasternal left ventricular long-axis view. *A,* the normal mitral valve leaflet position at end-systole. *B,* marked anterior mitral leaflet prolapse *(black arrow)* in which the anterior mitral leaflet has prolapsed into the left atrial space. *C,* posterior mitral leaflet prolapse *(black arrow)* in which the posterior mitral leaflet is in the left atrium during systole. *D,* both anterior and posterior mitral leaflet prolapse. *VS,* ventricular septum; *PW,* posterior wall; *AO,* aorta; *LV,* left ventricle; *LA,* left atrium; *AL,* anterior mitral leaflet; *PL,* posterior mitral leaflet; *A,* anterior; *P,* posterior; *I,* inferior; *S,* superior. (From Morganroth J., et al.: *Am. J. Cardiol.* 46:1164–1177, 1980. Reproduced by permission.)

shown in Figure 13–7. This should be contrasted with the findings in Figures 13–8 and 13–9. Figures 13–8 and 13–9 show the most reliable indicator of mitral valve prolapse on 2DE, namely, superior motion of the involved leaflet(s) in systole. Another finding with this technique is a displaced posterior coaptation of the leaflets.[67]

Despite the great advances in the detection of mitral valve prolapse, longitudinal cross-sectional echocardiography has specific disadvantages. Two limitations are the oblique imaging of the mitral ring and the lack of fixed adjacent landmarks. Excessive atrioventricular groove motion, which can occur in mitral prolapse, limits the study of posterior leaflet motion on the long-axis view. As with M-mode echocardiography, transducer beam angulation with medial and tangential cuts across the mitral valve can create the false picture of posterior coaptation and superior arching of the mitral valve leaflets.[68]

The use of the two-dimensional apical or four-chamber view[87] has bypassed many of the shortcomings of the long-axis view. Our recent work indicates that the apical view is better in the detection of anterior and, to a lesser extent, posterior leaflet prolapse.[88] In a study of 105 patients with mitral valve prolapse, we found that 95 had prolapse of both the anterior and posterior leaflets. The apical view revealed prolapse of the anterior mitral leaflet in 93 of 99 subjects, while the left ventricular longitudinal view demonstrated prolapse of the anterior leaflet in only 45 of 99. Of the 101 patients with prolapse of the posterior mitral valve leaflet, 84 were identified with the apical and 73 with the left ventricular longitudinal view.[88] In the apical view, the mitral ring is horizontal and perpendicular to the interventricular septum. This permits the motion of the leaflets and the coaptation point to be clearly seen in relation to the plane of the mitral valve ring. A hyperkinetic atrioventricular groove is much less pronounced on the apical view. Posterior leaflet analysis is improved because of the diminished groove motion.[68]

A grading system for the severity of mitral valve prolapse as determined by 2DE has been proposed (Table 13–4).[88] Figure 13–10 shows apical views of normal compared to severe mitral valve

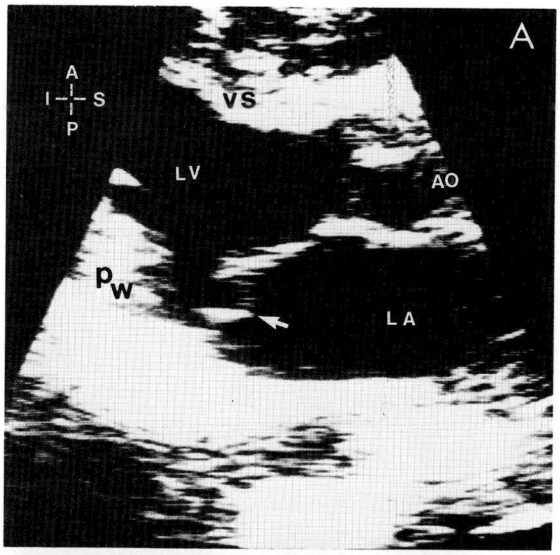

Fig 13–9.—A, two-dimensional echocardiographic view of the parasternal long-axis left ventricle demonstrating posterior mitral valve leaflet prolapse *(white arrow).* Abbreviations as in Figure 13–8. **B,** anterior and posterior mitral leaflet prolapse is depicted in this parasternal long-axis left ventricular view. The schematic at the right demonstrates the anterior mitral valve leaflet *(a)* and posterior mitral valve leaflet *(p),* which have prolapsed into the left atrium *(LA). VS,* ventricular septum; *PW,* posterior wall; *AO,* aorta.

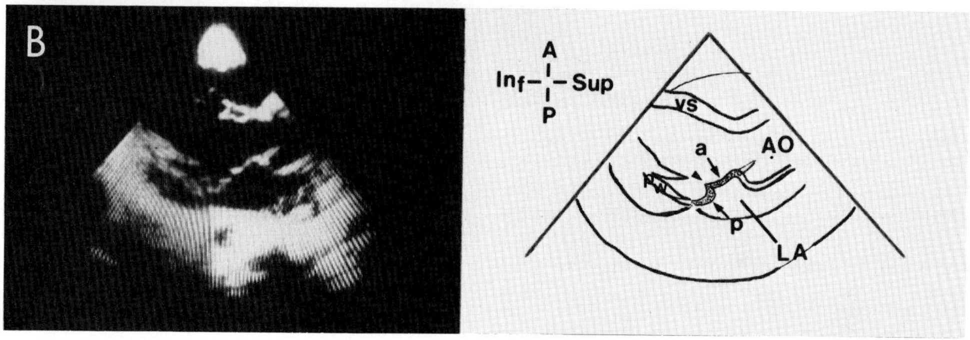

prolapse. In mild prolapse, the coaptation point of the leaflets is at the level of the mitral ring, with the leaflet(s) prolapsed toward the left atrium. In severe mitral valve prolapse, both the coaptation point and the mitral leaflet(s) are prolapsed toward the left atrium, well below the level of the mitral valve ring. Moderate prolapse yields findings between mild and severe. Mild mitral valve prolapse of both the anterior and posterior leaflets is more likely to be seen on an apical rather than a long-axis view. In our study using the apical view for mitral prolapse, the superiority of the apical view for detection of mild anterior leaflet prolapse was quite striking.[88] All 18 patients with this defect were detected when this view was used, compared with only 2 of 18 detected when the longitudinal view was used. Mild posterior leaflet prolapse was also more reliably detected with the ap-

TABLE 13–4.—GRADING SYSTEM FOR THE SEVERITY OF MITRAL VALVE PROLAPSE (TWO-DIMENSIONAL ECHOCARDIOGRAPHY)

SEVERITY	LEAFLET COAPTATION POINT	LEAFLET(S)	ANTERIOR LEAFLET PROLAPSE	POSTERIOR LEAFLET PROLAPSE
Mild	Mitral ring level	Slightly in left atrium	Apical* > long**	Apical > long
Moderate	Variable	In left atrium	Apical > long	Apical = long
Severe	Left atrium, well below mitral ring	Well into left atrium	Apical = long	Apical = long

Key: *apical four-chamber view, **left ventricular parasternal long axis; > more easily detects mitral valve prolapse than, = mitral valve prolapse detected equally as well.

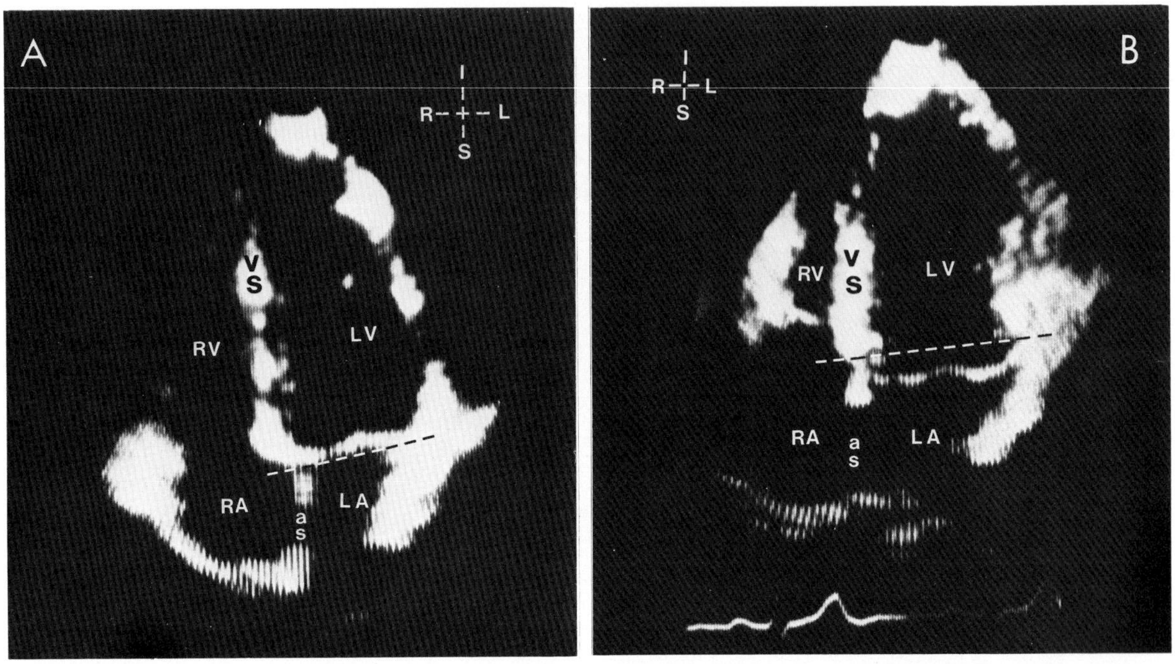

Fig 13–10.—A, two-dimensional echocardiographic apical four-chamber view demonstrating normal mitral valve position at end-systole. *Hatched line* represents the mitral annular plane. Mitral leaflets lie in the left ventricle above the mitral annular plane. *VS,* ventricular septum; *AS,* atrial septum; *RA,* right atrium; *LA,* left atrium; *RV,* right ventricle; *LV,* left ventricle. **B,** apical four-chamber two-dimensional view from a patient with moderate mitral valve prolapse of both the anterior and posterior leaflets, which are seen to lie within the left atrium at end-systole below the mitral valve ring *(hatched line).*

ical view. With moderate prolapse, both views detected posterior bowing well, but anterior leaflet prolapse is more likely to be found on an apical view. Eight of our 105 patients with mitral valve prolapse had moderate anterior mitral leaflet prolapse on the apical view that was not detected on the left ventricular longitudinal view. Both the apical and longitudinal views appear adequate to detect severe mitral valve prolapse of either or both leaflet(s).[88]

Treatment

The symptom most often reported by patients with mitral valve prolapse is chest pain. An agent such as propranolol has empirically been used to decrease the occurrence of this symptom. Betablockade may diminish left ventricular contractility and increase left ventricular volume, thus decreasing the extent of mitral valve prolapse.[89] Propranolol is generally given in doses of 40 to 80 mg/day. Larger doses are not well tolerated by many patients but may be used.[9]

The prognosis of mitral valve prolapse is generally good. A recent study confirmed the favorable prognosis in children with this syndrome.[90] Reassurance of this generally good prognosis is an important part of management. There is a small but definite rate of complications, which seems increased in patients with an associated systolic murmur.[91]

The major complications include arrhythmias followed by sudden death, bacterial endocarditis, progressive or acute severe mitral regurgitation, and transient ischemic attacks.[68] Patients with mitral valve prolapse and life-threatening arrhythmias require treatment with antiarrhythmic agents. Bacterial endocarditis occurs on the mitral valve itself,[92] but at least one case has been reported of an atrial mural endocarditis from the jet stream of mitral regurgitation.[93] Which patients with mitral valve prolapse should receive endocarditis prophylaxis remains controversial. Many physicians recommend such prophylaxis only if mitral regurgitation is present on physical examination, while others offer it to their patients whenever the diagnosis is made. Severe mitral regurgitation can occur on a chronic, progressive basis or acutely with chordal rupture. Mitral valve replacement may be required for severe mitral regurgitation, especially if it is acute. There is an increased incidence of valvular dehiscence postoperatively in these patients due to the myxomatous degeneration of the mitral annulus.

TRICUSPID VALVE PROLAPSE

Myxomatous degeneration as seen in mitral valve prolapse can involve other cardiac valves. Tricuspid valve prolapse is found in about one quarter to one half of patients with mitral valve prolapse, depending on the diagnostic standard.[38, 94–98] Patients with both mitral and tricuspid valve prolapse tend to have more severe involvement.[99] They are usually older, more symptomatic patients and more commonly have systolic clicks.[99] Isolated tricuspid valve prolapse has not been reported.[9, 98]

With M-mode echocardiography, the anterior tricuspid leaflet is visualized. M-mode echocardiography can occasionally detect tricuspid valve prolapse. The findings are similar to those of mitral valve prolapse. The limitation of M-mode echocardiography is the difficulty in always viewing well the tricuspid valve leaflets and maintaining a view of their motion throughout the cardiac cycle.

Two-dimensional echocardiography provides good visualization of the tricuspid valve in relation to the right atrium. In a prospective study of 60 patients with mitral valve prolapse,[99] we obtained good visualization of the tricuspid valve leaflets by either the right ventricular inflow longitudinal or the apical view.[87, 100] Both views were successfully obtained in over two thirds of the patients. On the right ventricular inflow view, the anterior leaflet, the larger tricuspid leaflet seen, originates from the tricuspid ring at the right ventricular free wall (Fig 13–11). The septal leaflet, the smaller one, attaches to the ventricular septum at the level of the tricuspid ring. The apical view often requires a slight modification to permit better visualization of the tricuspid valve. This adjustment is necessary because the tricuspid valve lies in a slightly different plane. With medial adjustment of the transducer, a medially located tricuspid septal leaflet and a laterally located anterior leaflet are well seen. The tricuspid ring is generally more toward the ventricular apex than the mitral valve ring.

The diagnostic finding for tricuspid valve prolapse is systolic displacement of the anterior or septal tricuspid leaflet into the right atrium (Fig 13–12). In our study of more than 60 patients with mitral valve prolapse, almost one half showed evidence of tricuspid valve prolapse on the right ventricular inflow or apical views.[99] Most of these patients had prolapse of both the anterior and septal leaflets. This study indicated that the right ventricular inflow view is slightly more sensitive than the apical view in the detection of tricuspid prolapse. Based on these findings, a classification of

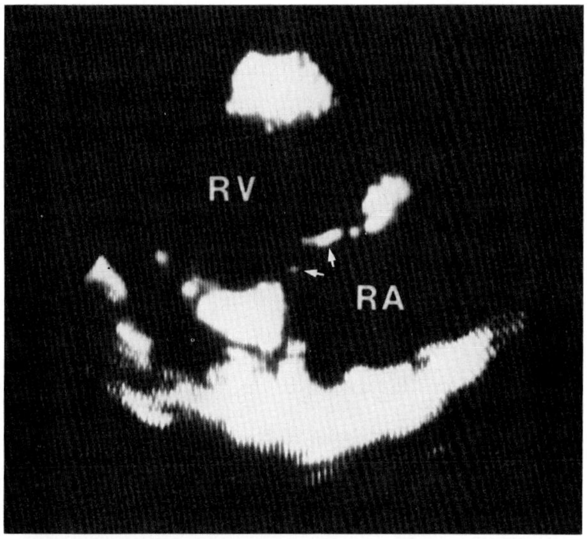

Fig 13–11.—Two-dimensional echocardiographic parasternal long-axis view of the right ventricle *(RV)* demonstrating the normal position of the anterior and septal tricuspid valve leaflets *(white arrows)*, which lie within the right ventricle at end-systole. The right atrium *(RA)* is depicted.

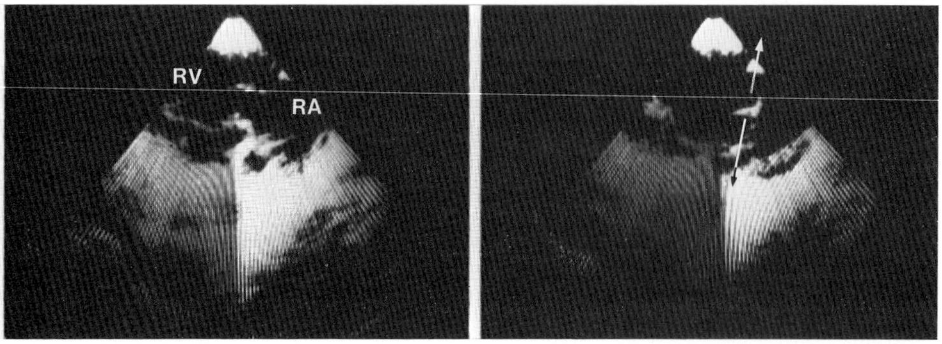

Fig 13–12.—Two-dimensional echocardiographic parasternal long-axis views of the right ventricle *(RV)* in which *(right)* a solid line has been added to demonstrate the tricuspid valve ring. Note that the anterior and septal leaflets of the tricuspid valve lie within the right atrium, thus identifying the presence of tricuspid valve prolapse.

mild, moderate, and severe tricuspid valve prolapse has been proposed with criteria analogous to those cited for mitral valve prolapse. Severe tricuspid prolapse was rarely seen in the tricuspid valve prolapse group.[99]

Tricuspid regurgitation is difficult to define by physical examination[101] and angiography. Contrast 2DE is considered by some to be the most sensitive and specific diagnostic measure of tricuspid regurgitation.[102] In a study of 45 patients, we showed that the subxiphoid echocardiographic view after peripheral vein saline injection accurately defines tricuspid regurgitation.[103] For this diagnosis to be made, microcavitations have to be identified in the hepatic veins as well as the inferior vena cava for at least three cardiac cycles (Fig 13–13). Using these criteria, the problem of superimposition of the right atrium over the inferior vena cava is overcome. With these stringent criteria, excellent sensitivity and specificity were obtained in the control groups of normal patients and patients with tricuspid regurgitation of various etiologies. With these criteria as a basis for diagnosis, there is an approximately 40% prevalence of tricuspid regurgitation with tricuspid valve prolapse.[103] This prevalence of regurgitation is similar to that reported with mitral valve prolapse.[32]

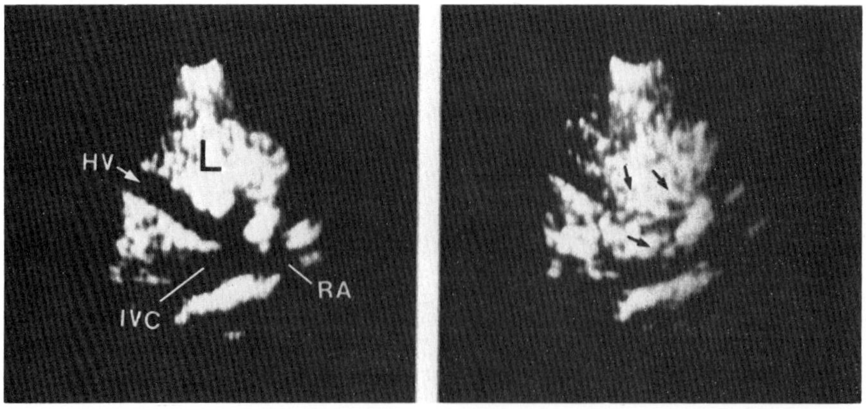

Fig 13–13.—Two-dimensional subcostal view of the liver *(L)* demonstrating the hepatic vein *(HV)*, inferior vena cava *(IVC)*, and right atrium *(RA)*. *Right,* recording made after a peripheral venous injection of saline in a patient with echocardiographically defined tricuspid valve prolapse. The *black arrows* point to microcavitation, which persisted through three cardiac cycles in both the inferior vena cava and hepatic veins, documenting the presence of tricuspid regurgitation in this patient. (From Chen C.C., et al.: *Am. J. Cardiol.* 46:983–987, 1980. Reproduced by permission.)

AORTIC VALVE PROLAPSE

Aortic valve prolapse has been found on surgical and pathologic studies.[12, 104, 105] One study suggested that up to one quarter of patients with mitral valve prolapse have aortic valve prolapse.[106] This may indicate a more extensive myxomatous process.

Causes of intact cusps with aortic valve prolapse include myxomatous degeneration, fraying of a cusp, and excessive aortic valve tissue in patients with a congenital bicuspid aortic valve.[105] Patients with myxomatous degeneration must be differentiated from those with congenital bicuspid aortic valve disease. In the latter, one cusp is usually larger and is sometimes called the "conjoined cusp."[105] The conjoined cusp may prolapse on the basis of excessive tissue relative to the distance between the two commissural attachments. The differentiation between aortic valve prolapse on the basis of the floppy valve syndrome[12] or bicuspid aortic valve disease[105] may be possible using the short-axis view on cross-sectional echocardiography. The presence of three separate aortic cusps on this view tends to exclude the presence of a bicuspid valve. Unfortunately, this finding does not entirely prove the absence of a bicuspid aortic valve, since there is an uncommon form of congenital bicuspid aortic valve in which the center of the free edge of the conjoined cusp is joined to the aortic wall by a thin strand. This might give the impression of a tricuspid aortic valve.[105]

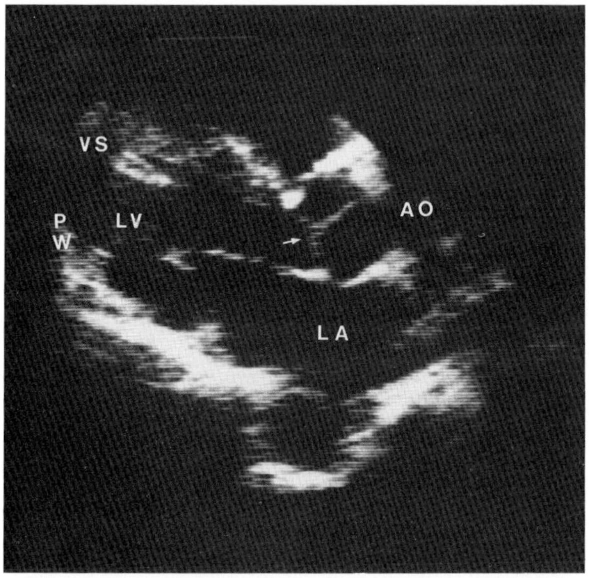

Fig 13–14.—Two-dimensional echocardiographic view of the parasternal long-axis left ventricle. The aortic valve *(arrow)* is depicted in diastole. Note that the aortic valve leaflets lie within the aorta and do not encroach upon the left ventricular outflow tract. *VS,* ventricular septum; *LV,* left ventricle; *LA,* left atrium; *AO,* aorta. (From Morganroth J., et al.: *Am. J. Cardiol.* 46:1164–1177, 1980. Reproduced by permission.)

Aortic valve prolapse is more difficult to detect by echocardiography than mitral valve prolapse. The aortic annulus is smaller and the aortic cusps are less voluminous. Normally, the aortic annulus and leaflets are less echo-reflective than the corresponding atrioventricular valve tissue.

Several findings have been cited for the M-mode echocardiographic diagnosis of aortic valve prolapse. One useful finding is eccentricity of the diastolic closure line. Aortic valve prolapse is also suggested by increased aortic valve reflections,[106] abnormal diastolic echoes in the left ventricular outflow tract, diastolic aortic leaflet fluttering,[107] aortic root dilation, or a marked aortic valve excursion pattern.[108] Aortic regurgitation, manifested by diastolic fluttering of the mitral valve on M-mode echocardiography, is associated with aortic valve prolapse less than one quarter of the time.

The normal two-dimensional aortic valve leaflets are faintly echo-reflective and have symmetric cusps. Neither the cusps nor the coaptation point show any downward or prolapsing movement toward the left ventricular outflow tract in diastole. The aortic cusps are slightly convex toward the center of the aorta at the level of their coaptation point (Fig 13–14).[106]

In an evaluation of 77 selected patients with mitral valve prolapse who had adequate aortic valve visualization, we found that 22% showed evidence of aortic valve prolapse.[106] The actual prevalence in the population is yet to be determined. Almost all patients with aortic valve prolapse showed increased echo-reflectivity of the cusp tissue. Of the 17 patients with aortic valve prolapse, 6 had eccentric aortic valve coaptation points by echocardiographic analysis. All 6 had three aortic valve

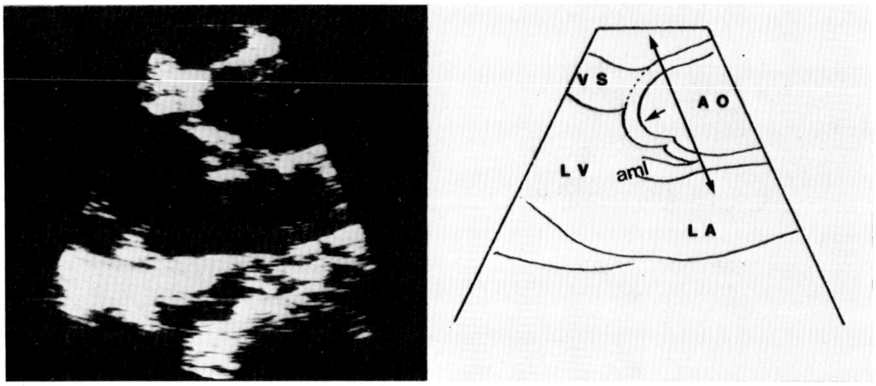

Fig 13–15.—Two-dimensional echocardiographic view of the parasternal long-axis left ventricle. Schematic shows the right coronary cusp *(arrow)* of the aortic valve prolapsing into the left ventricular outflow tract during diastole. The anterior mitral valve leaflet *(aml)* is depicted. *VS,* ventricular septum; *AO,* aorta; *LV,* left ventricle; *LA,* left atrium.

cusps demonstrated on the short-axis view. Four patients had anterior eccentricity, while 2 had posterior eccentricity. The key finding in aortic valve prolapse, however, is downward displacement or prolapse of the aortic valve cusps toward the left ventricular outflow tract in diastole (Fig 13–15).[106] Cusp redundancy is also a hallmark finding.

Two-dimensional echocardiography appears to be emerging as the diagnostic gold standard for mitral, tricuspid, and aortic valve prolapse. With 2DE, many limitations of prior diagnostic standards, such as findings on physical examination, angiography, or M-mode echocardiography, are bypassed. Though much data about valvular prolapse have been accumulated, an improved diagnostic standard, which 2DE may well provide, will aid in the revision and better definition of many aspects of the prolapse syndrome.

REFERENCES

1. Gallavardin L.: Nouvelle observation avec autopsie d'un pseudodedoublement du 2e bruit du coeur simulant le dedoublement mitral par. *Prat. Med. Franc.* 13:19, 1932.
2. White P.D.: *Heart Disease*. New York, Macmillan Publishing Co., 1931.
3. Thompson W.P., Levine S.A.: Systolic gallop rhythm: A clinical study. *N. Engl. J. Med.* 213:1021–1025, 1935.
4. Reid J.V.O.: Midsystolic clicks. *S. Afr. Med. J.* 135:353–355, 1961.
5. Humphries J.O., McKusick V.A.: The differentiation of organic and "innocent" systolic murmurs. *Prog. Cardiovasc. Dis.* 5:152–171, 1962.
6. Barlow J.B., Bosman C.K., Pocock W.A., et al.: Late systolic murmurs and non-ejection (mid-late) systolic clicks: An analysis of 90 patients. *Br. Heart J.* 30:203–218, 1968.
7. Barlow J.B., Pocock W.A., Marchand P., et al.: The significance of late systolic murmurs. *Am. Heart J.* 66:443–452, 1963.
8. Hancock E.W., Cohn K.: The syndrome associated with midsystolic click and late systolic murmur. *Am. J. Med.* 41:183–196; 1966.
9. Jeresaty R.M.: *Mitral Valve Prolapse*. New York, Raven Press, 1979.
10. Barlow J.B., Pocock W.A.: Mitral valve prolapse, the specific billowing mitral leaflet syndrome, or an insignificant non-ejection systolic click. *Am. Heart J.* 97:277–285, 1979.
11. Perloff J.K., Roberts W.C.: The mitral apparatus: Functional anatomy of mitral regurgitation. *Circulation* 46:227–239, 1972.
12. Read R.C., Thal A.P.: Surgical experience with symptomatic myxomatous valvular transformation (the floppy valve syndrome). *Surgery* 59:173–182, 1966.
13. Read R.C., Thal A.P., Wendy V.E.: Symptomatic valvular myxomatous transformation (the floppy valve syndrome): A possible forme fruste of the Marfan syndrome. *Circulation* 32:897–910, 1965.
14. Boudoulas H., Reynolds J., Mazzaferri E., et al.: Metabolic studies in mitral valve prolapse syndrome. *Circulation* 61:1200–1205, 1980.
15. Engle M.A.: The signal of apical systolic click, late systolic murmur, and abnormal T-waves. *Circulation* 39:1–2, 1969.
16. DeMaria A.N., Bogren H., Caudill C.C., et al.: Evaluation of the nonvalvular factors of cardiac performance, left ventricular contractile pattern and

coronary anatomy in the mitral valve prolapse syndrome, abstracted. *Am. J. Cardiol.* 35:132, 1975.
17. D'Cruz I., Shah S., Hirsch L., et al.: Abnormal systolic motion of the posterolateral basal left ventricle in mitral valve prolapse: A new cross-sectional echocardiographic sign. *Am. J. Cardiol.* 45(suppl.):434, 1980.
18. Gulotta S.J., Gulco L., Padmanabhan V., et al.: The syndrome of systolic click, murmur and mitral valve prolapse: A cardiomyopathy? *Circulation* 49:717–728, 1974.
19. Pasternak A., Gervais A.R., Gueret P., et al.: The systolic click syndrome: Myocardial metabolism, contraction abnormalities and ventricular performance, abstracted. *Circulation* 50(suppl. III):III-239, 1974.
20. Glassman E., Kronzon I.: Coronary artery distribution in patients with prolapse of the mitral valve, abstracted. *Circulation* 49, 50 (suppl. III): 228, 1974.
21. Gentzler R.D., Gault J.H., Liedtke A.J., et al.: Congenital absence of the left circumflex coronary artery in the systolic click syndrome. *Circulation* 52:490–496, 1975.
22. Barlow J.B., Pocock W.A.: The problem of nonejection systolic clicks and associated mitral systolic murmurs: Emphasis on the billowing mitral leaflet syndrome. *Am. Heart J.* 90:636–655, 1975.
23. Hill D.G., Davies M.J., Braimbridge M.V.: The natural history and surgical management of the redundant cusp syndrome (floppy mitral valve). *J. Thorac. Cardiovasc. Surg.* 67:519–525, 1974.
24. Pomerance A.: Ageing changes in human heart valves. *Br. Heart J.* 29:222–231, 1967.
25. Rizzon P., Biasco G., Brindicci G., et al.: Familial syndrome of mid-systolic click and late systolic murmur. *Br. Heart J.* 35:245–259, 1973.
26. Markiewicz W., Stoner J., London E., et al.: Mitral valve prolapse in one hundred presumably healthy young females. *Circulation* 53:464–473, 1976.
27. Bloch A., Vignola P.A., Walker H., et al.: Echocardiographic spectrum of posterior systolic motion of the mitral valve in the general population. *J. Clin. Ultrasound* 5:243–247, 1977.
28. Procacci P.M., Savran S.V., Schreiter S.L., et al.: Prevalence of clinical mitral-valve prolapse in 1169 young women. *N. Engl. J. Med.* 294:1086–1088, 1976.
29. Devereux R.B., Perloff J.K., Reichek N., et al.: Mitral valve prolapse. *Circulation* 54:3–14, 1976.
30. Weiss A.N., Mimbs J.W., Ludbrook P.A., et al.: Echocardiographic detection of mitral valve prolapse: Exclusion of false positive diagnosis and determination of inheritance. *Circulation* 52:1091–1096, 1975.
31. Malcolm A.D., Bonghaner D.R., Kostuk W.J., et al.: Clinical features and investigative findings in presence of mitral leaflet prolapse: Study of 85 consecutive patients. *Br. Heart J.* 38:244–256, 1976.
32. Jeresaty R.M.: Mitral valve prolapse-click syndrome. *Prog. Cardiovasc. Dis.* 15:623–652, 1973.
33. Cobbs B.W. Jr.: Clinical recognition and medical management of rheumatic heart disease and other valvular disease, in Hurst J.W., Logue R.B., Schlant R.C., et al. (eds.): *The Heart,* ed. 3. New York, McGraw-Hill Book Co., 1974, pp. 826–971.
34. Hancock E.W., Cohn K.: The syndrome associated with midsystolic click and late systolic murmur. *Am. J. Med.* 41:183–196, 1966.
35. Winkle R.A., Lopes M.G., Fitzgerald J.W., et al.: Arrhythmias in patients with mitral valve prolapse. *Circulation* 52:73–81, 1975.
36. Wigle E.G., Radowski H., Ranganathan N., et al.: Mitral valve prolapse. *Ann. Rev. Med.* 27:165–180, 1976.
37. Kostuk W.J., Barnett H.J.M., Silver M.D.: Strokes: A complication of mitral leaflet prolapse? *Lancet* 1:313–316, 1977.
38. Pomerance A.: Ballooning deformity (mucoid degeneration) of atrioventricular valves. *Br. Heart J.* 31:343–351, 1969.
39. Criley J.M., Lewis K.B., Humphries J.O., et al.: Prolapse of the mitral valve: Clinical and cine-angiocardiographic findings. *Br. Heart J.* 28:488–496, 1966.
40. Lewis H.P.: Midsystolic clicks and coronary heart disease. *Circulation* 44:493–494, 1971.
41. Craige E.: On the genesis of heart sounds. *Circulation* 53:207–209, 1976.
42. Reinke R., Higgins C., Gosink B., et al.: Significance of mitral valve prolapse, abstracted. *Circulation* 50(suppl. III):76, 1974.
43. Wei J.Y., Fortuin N.J.: The closing snap of mitral valve prolapse. *Am. J. Cardiol.* 43(suppl.):367, 1979.
44. Schwartz M.H., Herman M.V., Teichholz L.E.: Dermatoglyphic patterns in patients with mitral valve prolapse: A clue to pathogenesis. *Am. J. Cardiol.* 38:588–593, 1976.
45. Darsee J., Miklozek C., Heymsfield S., et al.: Mitral valve prolapse and ophthalmoplegia: A progressive cardioneurologic syndrome. *Ann. Intern. Med.* 92:735–741, 1980.
46. Lardani H., Moreyra A., Manubens S., et al.: Electrocardiographic findings in 125 patients with idiopathic prolapse of the mitral valve studied by angiography. *Cleveland Clin. Q.* 43:181–194, 1976.
47. Campbell R.W.F., Godman M.G., Fiddler G.I., et al.: Ventricular arrhythmias in the auscultatory electrocardiographic variant of the balloon mitral valve syndrome. *Am. J. Cardiol.* 37:126, 1976.
48. Kavey R.E., Sondheimer H., Blackman M.: Detection of dysrhythmias in pediatric patients with mitral valve prolapse. *Circulation* 62:582–587, 1980.
49. Gallagher J.J., Gilbert M., Stevenson R.H., et al.: Wolff-Parkinson-White syndrome: The problem,

evaluation and surgical correction. *Circulation* 51:767–785, 1975.
50. Schaal S.F., Fontana M.E., Wooley C.F.: Mitral valve prolapse syndrome: Spectrum of conduction defects and arrhythmias, abstracted. *Circulation* 50(suppl. III): III–97, 1974.
51. DeMaria A.N., Amsterdam E.A., Vismara L.A., et al.: Arrhythmias in the mitral valve prolapse syndrome. *Ann. Intern. Med.* 84:656–660, 1976.
52. Wit A.L., Fenoglio J.J., Wagner B.M., et al.: Electrophysiological properties of cardiac muscle in the anterior mitral valve leaflet and the adjacent atrium in the dog. *Circ. Res.* 32:731–745, 1973.
53. Shrivastava S., Guthrie R.B., Edwards J.E.: Prolapse of the mitral valve. *Mod. Concepts Cardiovasc. Dis.* 46:57–62, 1977.
54. Salazar A.E., Edwards J.E.: Friction lesions of ventricular endocardium; Relation to chordae tendineae of mitral valve. *Arch. Pathol.* 90:364–376, 1970.
55. Gardin J.M., Isner J.M., Ronan J.A., et al.: Pseudoischemic "false positive" ST segment changes induced by hyperventilation in patients with mitral valve prolapse. *Am. J. Cardiol.* 45:952–958, 1980.
56. Popp R., Rubenson D., Tucker C., et al.: Echocardiography: M-mode and two-dimensional methods. *Ann. Intern. Med.* 93:844–856, 1980.
57. Roelandt J., Willems J., van der Hauwaert L.G., et al.: Clicks and sounds (whoops) in left sided pneumothorax. *Dis. Chest* 56:31–36, 1969.
58. Martin C.E., Hufnagel C.A., deLeon A.C.: Calcified atria myxoma: Diagnostic significance of the "systolic tumor sound" in a case presenting as tricuspid insufficiency. *Am. Heart J.* 78:245–250, 1969.
59. Pickering D., Keith J.D.: Systolic clicks with ventricular septal defects: A sign of aneurysm of ventricular septum? *Br. Heart J.* 33:538–539, 1971.
60. Pieroni D.R., Bell B.B., Krovetz L.J., et al.: Auscultatory recognition of aneurysm of the membranous ventricular septum associated with small ventricular septal defect. *Circulation* 44:733–739, 1971.
61. Sze K.C., Shah P.M.: Pseudoejection sound in hypertrophic subaortic stenosis. *Circulation* 54:504–509, 1976.
62. DeMaria A.N., Mason D.T.: "Silent" mitral prolapse, letter. *Circulation* 50:1285, 1974.
63. Popp R.L., Winkle R.A.: Mitral-valve prolapse syndrome. *J.A.M.A.* 236:867–870, 1976.
64. Farry J.P., Simon A.L., Ross A.M., et al.: Quantitative angiographic assessment of the mitral annulus in the prolapsing leaflet syndrome, abstracted. *Circulation* 51(suppl. II):II–12, 1975.
65. DeMaria A.N., Neumann A., Lee G., et al.: Echocardiographic identification of the mitral valve prolapse syndrome. *Am. J. Med.* 62:819–829, 1977.
66. Smith E.R., Fraser D.B., Prudy J.W., et al.: Angiographic diagnosis of mitral valve prolapse: Correlation with echocardiography. *Am. J. Cardiol.* 40:165–170, 1977.
67. Gilbert B.W., Schatz R.A., VonRamm O.T., et al.: Mitral valve prolapse: Two-dimensional echocardiographic and angiographic correlation. *Circulation* 54:716–723, 1976.
68. Morganroth J., Jones R., Chen C., et al.: Two-dimensional echocardiography in mitral, aortic, and tricuspid valve prolapse. *Am. J. Cardiol.* 46:1164–1177, 1980.
69. Boughner D.R.: Correlation of echocardiographic and angiographic abnormalities in mitral valve prolapse. *Ultrasound Med.* 1:55–62, 1975.
70. Shah P.M., Gramiak R.: Echocardiographic recognition of mitral valve prolapse, abstracted. *Circulation* 42(suppl. III):III–45, 1970.
71. Dillon J.C., Haine C.L., Chang S., et al.: Use of echocardiography in patients with prolapsed mitral valve. *Circulation* 43:503–507, 1971.
72. Kerber R.E., Lsaeff D.M., Hancock E.W.: Echocardiographic patterns in patients with the syndrome of systolic click and late systolic murmur. *N. Engl. J. Med.* 284:691–693, 1971.
73. Feigenbaum H.: Echocardiography, ed. 3. Philadelphia, Lea & Febiger, 1976, pp. 257–260.
74. Sahn D.J., Allen H.D., Goldberg S.J., et al.: Mitral valve prolapse in children: A problem defined by real-time cross-sectional echocardiography. *Circulation* 53:651–657, 1976.
75. Popp R.L., Brown O.R., Silverman J.F., et al.: Echocardiographic abnormalities in the mitral valve prolapse syndrome. *Circulation* 49:428–433, 1974.
76. Liedtke A.J., Babb J.D., DeJoseph R.L.: Mitral valve echoes in patients with mitral valve prolapse syndrome. *Am. Heart J.* 97:286–290, 1979.
77. Chandraratna P.A.N.: Limitations of the echocardiogram in diagnosing valvular vegetations in patients with mitral valve prolapse. *Circulation* 56:436–438, 1977.
78. Wann L.S., Dillon J.C., Weyman A.E., et al.: Echocardiography in bacterial endocarditis. *N. Engl. J. Med.* 295:135–139, 1976.
79. DeMaria A.N., King J.F., Bogren H.G., et al.: The variable spectrum of echocardiographic manifestations of the mitral valve prolapse syndrome. *Circulation* 50:33–41, 1974.
80. Rakowski H., Martin R.P., Popp R.L.: Two-dimensional echocardiographic findings in mitral valve prolapse, abstracted. *Circulation* 55,56(suppl. III):III–154, 1977.
81. Dinsmore R.E., Hutter A.M., Sanders C.A.: Angiographic and clinical spectrum of mitral valve prolapse, abstracted. *Circulation* 42(suppl. III):III–149, 1970.
82. Cohen M.V.: Double mitral leaflet prolapse: Echocardiographic phonocardiographic correlation. *Am. Heart J.* 91:168–177, 1976.

83. Nichol P.M., Gilbert B.W., Kisslo J.A.: Two-dimensional echocardiographic assessment of mitral stenosis. *Circulation* 55:120–128, 1977.
84. Owens J.P., Kotler M.N., Segal B.L., et al.: Pseudoprolapse of the mitral valve in a patient with pericardial effusion. *Chest* 69:214–215, 1976.
85. Vignola P.A., Pohost G.M., Curfman G.D., et al.: Correlation of echocardiographic and clinical findings in patients with pericardial effusion. *Am. J. Cardiol.* 37:701–707, 1976.
86. Feigenbaum H.: *Echocardiography,* ed. 3. Philadelphia, Lea & Febiger, 1981, pp. 264–265.
87. Silverman H.G., Schiller N.B.: Apex echocardiography. *Circulation* 57:503–511, 1978.
88. Morganroth J., Naito M., Mardelli T.J., et al.: Apical cross-sectional echocardiography: The standard for diagnosis of mitral valve prolapse. *Chest* 79:23–28, 1981.
89. Winkle R.A., Goodman D.J., Popp R.L.: Echocardiographic evaluation of propranolol therapy for mitral valve prolapse. *Br. Heart J.* 38:129–134, 1976.
90. Bisset G., Schwartz D., Meyer R., et al.: Clinical spectrum and long-term follow-up of isolated mitral valve prolapse in 119 children. *Circulation* 62:423–429, 1980.
91. Mills P., Rose J., Hollingsworth B.A., et al.: Long-term prognosis of mitral-valve prolapse. *N. Engl. J. Med.* 297:13–18, 1977.
92. Krautz J., David D., Lewis B.S., et al.: Bacterial endocarditis on the prolapsing leaflet (Barlow's) syndrome: Report of two cases and review of the literature. *Harefuah* 92:156–161, 1977.
93. Ringer M., Feen D., Drapkin M.: Mitral valve prolapse: Jet stream causing mural endocarditis. *Am. J. Cardiol.* 45:383–385, 1980.
94. Gooch A.S., Maranhao V., Scampardonis G., et al.: Prolapse of both mitral and tricuspid leaflets in systolic murmur-click syndrome. *N. Engl. J. Med.* 287:1218–1222, 1972.
95. Scampardonis G., Yang S.S., Maranhao V., et al.: Left ventricular abnormalities in prolapsed mitral leaflet syndrome: Review of 87 cases. *Circulation* 48:287–297, 1973.
96. Maranhao V., Gooch A.S., Yang S.S., et al.: Prolapse of the tricuspid leaflets in the systolic murmur-click syndrome. *Cathet. Cardiovasc. Diagn.* 1:81–90, 1975.
97. Ainsworth R.P., Hartmann A.F., Aker U., et al.: Tricuspid valve prolapse with late systolic tricuspid insufficiency. *Radiology* 107:309–311, 1973.
98. Werner J.A., Schiller N.B., Frasquier R.: Occurrence and significance of echocardiographically demonstrated tricuspid valve prolapse. *Am. Heart J.* 96:180–186, 1978.
99. Mardelli T.J., Morganroth J., Chen C.C., et al.: Enhanced diagnosis of tricuspid valve prolapse by cross-sectional echocardiography. *Chest* 79:201–205, 1981.
100. Tajik A.J., Seward J.B., Hagler D.J., et al.: Two-dimensional real-time ultrasonic imaging of the heart and great vessels. *Mayo Clin. Proc.* 53:271–303, 1978.
101. Tavel M.E.: *Clinical Phonocardiography and External Pulse Recording,* ed. 3. Chicago, Year Book Medical Publishers, 1978, p. 139.
102. Lieppe W., Behar V.S., Scallion R., et al.: Detection of tricuspid regurgitation with two-dimensional echocardiography and peripheral vein injections. *Circulation* 57:128–132, 1978.
103. Chen C., Morganroth J., Mardelli T.J., et al.: Tricuspid regurgitation in tricuspid valve prolapse demonstrated with cross-sectional echocardiography. *Am. J. Cardiol.* 46:983–987, 1980.
104. Frable W.J.: Mucinous degeneration of the cardiac valves. *J. Thorac. Cardiovasc. Surg.* 58:62–70, 1969.
105. Carter J.B., Sethi S., Lee G.B., et al.: Prolapse of semilunar cusps as cause of aortic insufficiency. *Circulation* 53:922–932, 1971.
106. Mardelli T.J., Morganroth J., Naito M., et al.: Cross-sectional echocardiographic identification of aortic valve prolapse. *Am. Heart J.* 100:295–301, 1980.
107. Chandraratna P.A.N., Samet P., et al.: Echocardiography of the "floppy" aortic valve. *Circulation* 52:959–962, 1975.
108. Rippe J.M., Angoff G., Sloss L.J., et al.: Multiple floppy valves: An echocardiographic syndrome. *Am. J. Med.* 66:817–824, 1979.

RADIONUCLIDE IMAGING

Kenneth A. Brown and Gerald M. Pohost

RADIONUCLIDE IMAGING METHODS may be of clinical value in evaluating patients with mitral valve prolapse. The diagnosis is best established using the echocardiographic methods described in chapter 13. However, radionuclide methods are helpful in excluding coexisting coronary artery disease and in evaluating ventricular functional reserve. Both myocardial perfusion imaging and radionuclide ventriculography are of potential value.

MYOCARDIAL PERFUSION IMAGING

Chest pain is frequently associated with mitral valve prolapse.[1–9] The clinical problem is one of differentiating between coronary artery disease and mitral valve prolapse alone as the source of the pain, since chest pain can be anginal in character even in the absence of coronary disease.[1, 6–12] Furthermore, patients with mitral valve prolapse may have exercise-induced ischemic ECG changes suggesting coronary disease.[10–17] Angina pectoris and ECG changes have been hypothesized to be related to increased stress on the chordae tendineae of the mitral valve apparatus, leading to ischemia of the papillary muscles.[4, 5, 18] Because the papillary muscles have a borderline blood supply due to their intracavitary and high-pressure location,[19] ischemia might occur in the absence of coronary artery disease with only mild increases in perfusion demand. This hypothesis has been supported in part by the observation of abnormal lactate production during atrial pacing in patients with mitral valve prolapse and normal coronary arteries.[20–23]

Radionuclide myocardial perfusion imaging with thallium 201 offers insight into the regional coronary blood flow independent of oxygen supply and demand status. Several studies have investigated the relationship of myocardial distribution of radiotracer during exercise to coronary artery anatomy in patients with mitral valve prolapse and chest pain (Table 14–1). Initial reports in abstracted form gave conflicting results.[24–28] McLaughlin and colleagues found that 11 of 17 patients with mitral valve prolapse, exertional chest pain, and angiographically normal coronary arteries had perfusion defects on ^{201}Tl imaging studies with exercise.[24] Eight of the 11 also showed defects on images obtained at rest. In a similar group of patients, Padmanabhan et al. reported ^{201}Tl perfusion defects during exercise in 11 of 14 patients; no resting studies were described.[25] In addition, Soin et al. found defects on ^{201}Tl imaging in 12 of 20 patients with mitral valve prolapse. Of 9 patients with perfusion defects undergoing coronary angiography, all had normal coronary arteries.[26] However, Klein and associates found that 22 of 22 patients with mitral valve prolapse and normal coronary arteries, including 4 with typical angina, had normal exercise ^{201}Tl scans, while 6 of 7 patients with coronary artery disease associated with mitral valve prolapse had abnormal exercise perfusion images.[27] Sbarbaro et al. described normal exercise myocardial perfusion in 4 of 4 healthy medical

TABLE 14–1.—Mitral Valve Prolapse and Myocardial Perfusion Imaging

STUDY	N	CORONARY ANGIOGRAPHY	EXERCISE ECG	EXERCISE MYOCARDIAL PERFUSION IMAGING
McLauglin et al.[24]	17	Normal = 17/17	Positive = 3/17	Normal = 6/17 Defect = 11/17
Padmanabhan et al.[25]	14	Normal = 14/14	Positive = 4/14	Normal = 3/14 Defect = 11/14
Soin et al.[26]	20	Normal = 9/20 NA = 11/20	Positive = 6/20	Normal = 8/20 Defect = 12/20
Klein et al.[27]	29	Normal = 22/29	Positive = 5/22	Normal = 22/22 Defect = 0/22
		CAD = 7/29	NA	Normal = 1/7 Defect = 6/7
Sbarbaro et al.[28]	4	NA	Positive = 0/4	Normal = 4/4 Defect = 0/4
Jeresaty[29]	5	Normal = 5/5	Positive = 2/5	Normal = 5/5 Defect = 0/5
Gaffney et al.[17]	12	Normal = 3/12	Positive = 2/3	Normal = 3/3 Defect = 0/3
		CAD = 1/12	Positive = 1/1	Defect = 1/1
		NA = 8/12	Positive = 0/8	Normal = 8/8 Defect = 0/8
Massie et al.[10]	25	Normal = 19/25	Positive = 10/19	Normal = 19/19 Defect = 0/19
		CAD = 6/25	Positive = 3/6	Normal = 0/6 Defect = 6/6
Klein et al.[11]	32	Normal = 22/32	Positive = 6/22 Positive = 7/10	Normal = 22/22 Defect = 0/22
		CAD = 10/32		Normal = 1/10 Defect = 9/10
Greenspan et al.[12]	30	Normal = 30/30	Positive = 2/30	Normal = 26/30 Defect = 4/30
Combined[17, 10–12]	99	Normal = 74/99	Positive = 20/74	Normal = 70/74 Defect = 4/74
		CAD = 17/99	Positive = 11/17	Normal = 1/17 Defect = 16/17
		NA = 8/99	Positive = 0/8	Normal = 8/8 Defect = 0/8

NA, not available; CAD coronary artery disease.

students with mitral valve prolapse.[28] Furthermore, Jeresaty found normal ^{201}Tl distribution with exercise in a series of 5 patients with mitral valve prolapse and normal coronary arteries.[29] In summary, these studies yielded conflicting results, with false positive rates ranging from 0% to 100%.

More recently detailed reports[10–12, 17] have suggested that myocardial perfusion defects are highly specific for coexisting coronary artery disease in patients with mitral valve prolapse (see Table 14–1). Gaffney and colleagues described 12 patients with chest pain and mitral valve prolapse.[17] Normal exercise ^{201}Tl imaging was observed in 3 of 3 patients with angiographically documented normal coronary arteries and in 8 of 8 patients who did not undergo angiography but were believed not to have coronary artery disease, since they were women younger than 35 years of age and had normal serum lipid levels. In this group, 2 patients had exercise-induced ST segment depression suggesting ischemia. The single patient with angiographically documented coronary artery disease demonstrated an apical perfusion defect during exercise. Twenty-five patients were studied by Massie and associates.[10] Normal exercise perfusion studies were found in 19 of 19 patients with normal coronary arteries, although 10 (53%) had positive stress ECGs (Fig 14–1) and 4 had typical angina pectoris. All 6 patients with angiographically documented coronary artery disease demonstrated exercise-induced ^{201}Tl defects (Fig 14–2). Klein et al. described 32 symptomatic patients with

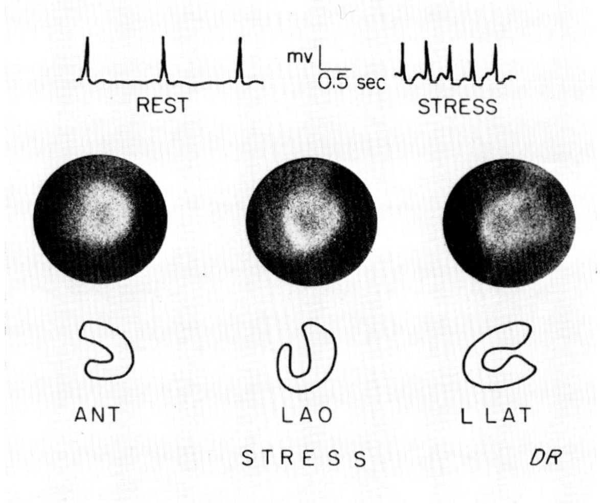

Fig 14–1.—Exercise ^{201}Tl myocardial images in a patient with mitral valve prolapse, chest pain, and normal coronary arteries. Although the exercise electrocardiogram is positive, regional ^{201}Tl myocardial uptake is normal. (From Massie B. et al.: *Circulation* 57:19–26, 1978. Reproduced by permission of the American Heart Association.)

mitral valve prolapse who underwent exercise testing.[11] They found that all 22 patients without coronary artery disease had normal exercise myocardial imaging studies, although 5 had typical angina and 6 had positive exercise ECGs. Among 10 patients with coronary artery disease, 9 demonstrated perfusion defects and 1 had a normal study. Most recently, Greenspan and colleagues reported a study of 30 patients with chest pain, mitral valve prolapse, and normal coronary arteries.[12] Twenty-six (87%) patients showed normal ^{201}Tl myocardial distribution on exercise. Two patients demonstrated defects in the anterior wall, both with exercise and at rest, that were associated with anterior hypokinesis on the rest left ventriculogram. Two additional patients had a defect on ^{201}Tl imaging with exercise but normal distribution at rest. The defects were located in the anterior wall and septum in one patient and in the posterior wall in the other. Each of these two patients also had a positive stress ECG. In the remaining 28 patients, the stress ECG was either negative or inconclusive, due to inadequate heart rate response.

The recent data summarized above demonstrate that exercise ^{201}Tl myocardial imaging is a useful means of excluding coronary artery disease in patients with mitral valve prolapse and chest pain. The combined sensitivity of the exercise ^{201}Tl studies for detecting coexisting coronary artery disease was 94% (16/17), while the combined specificity for excluding coronary artery disease was 95% (70/74). Stress ECG appears to be less useful in patients with mitral valve prolapse, with a combined sensitivity of 65% (11/17) and specificity of 73% (50/74). It is possible that false positive results with myocardial imaging in patients with mitral valve prolapse in the absence of coronary ar-

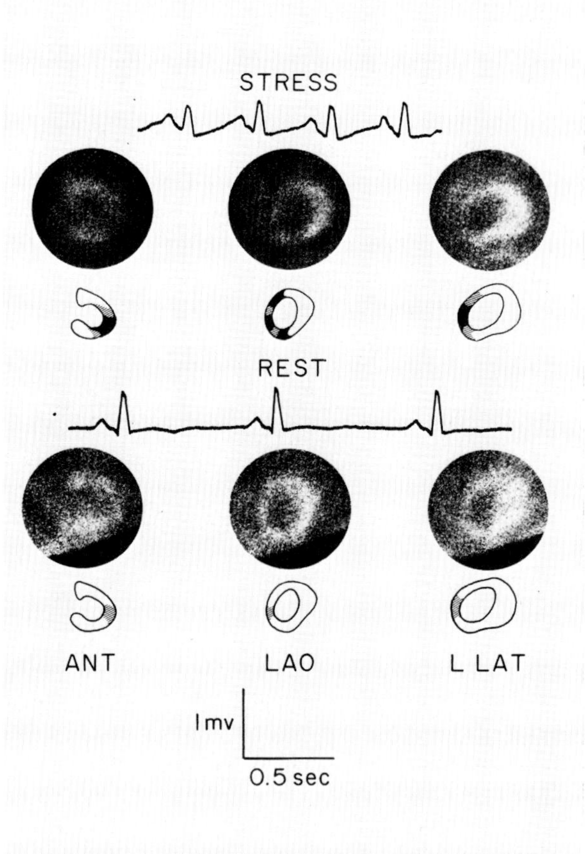

Fig 14–2.—Exercise and rest ^{201}Tl myocardial images in a patient with mitral valve prolapse and coronary artery disease. Initial perfusion defects in the apico-anterior and septal walls are much less apparent at rest, suggesting exercise-induced hypoperfusion in these regions. (From Massie B. et al.: *Circulation* 57:19–26, 1978. Reproduced by permission of the American Heart Association.)

tery disease are related to reduced perfusion to the papillary muscles due to increased tension with exercise. A second explanation of ischemia in patients with chest pain, mitral valve prolapse, and angiographically normal coronary arteries is exercise-induced coronary vasospasm. Buda and colleagues have demonstrated that patients with catheter-induced spasm have a high incidence of mitral valve prolapse.[30] In addition, Chesler et al. have described 4 young patients with mitral valve prolapse and acute myocardial infarction but normal coronary arteries.[31] The authors suggested that intermittent coronary occlusion by vasospasm might have been responsible for the myocardial infarction. Of note, however, is that Massie and associates, using ergonovine testing, failed to elicit a positive response in 10 patients with chest pain, mitral valve prolapse, and normal coronary arteries.[10] Finally, Gewirtz et al. have demonstrated that apparent apical and anterolateral defects on ^{201}Tl imaging can be observed in association with left ventricular dilation.[32] It is possible that mitral valve prolapse might lead to exercise-induced left ventricular volume overload and concomitant left ventricular dilation. This dilation could lead to an apical or anterolateral defect immediately after exercise which resolves on delayed imaging as the hemodynamic effects of exercise subside.

In summary, ^{201}Tl myocardial imaging appears to be clinically useful in evaluating patients with mitral valve prolapse and chest pain. Thallium 201 defects with exercise are highly sensitive and specific for detecting coexisting coronary artery disease. It should be emphasized that stress myocardial perfusion defects have been reported in association with symptomatic mitral valve prolapse in patients without coronary artery disease. The significance of such defects remains to be elucidated.

RADIONUCLIDE VENTRICULOGRAPHY

The observation that mitral valve prolapse is commonly associated with left ventricular contraction abnormalities in the absence of coronary artery disease has suggested that the syndrome may be associated with a cardiomyopathy.[14, 33–36] This has been supported by the demonstration of biopsy-proved interstitial or endocardial fibrosis.[23] The most consistently described wall motion abnormality is hypokinesis of the left ventricular anterolateral wall, which produces an unusually prominent convexity in this portion of the ventricle in end-systole and early diastole in 24%–70% of patients with mitral valve prolapse.[14, 33–36] In addition, abnormal resting left ventricular hemodynamics (elevated end-diastolic pressure, reduced angiographic ejection fraction, or low cardiac output) have been reported in the absence of significant mitral regurgitation.[14, 35] Failure of the cardiac index to rise appropriately with exercise was also found in many patients.[14] Some investigators, however, have reported normal resting left ventricular hemodynamics associated with mitral valve prolapse.[34]

Recently, radionuclide ventriculography has been used to evaluate resting and exercise left ventricular function in patients with mitral valve prolapse (Table 14–2).[37–39] Using equilibrium cardiac blood pool imaging, Ahmad et al. reported decreased or unchanged ejection fraction with exercise in 6 of 12 (50%) patients with normal resting ejection fraction and normal coronary arteries.[37] Similar observations were made by Gottdiener and colleagues, who found that in 10 patients with mitral valve prolapse but without coronary artery disease or significant mitral regurgitation, 1 (10%) had an abnormal resting ejection fraction and 3 (30%) had an abnormal ejection fraction response to exercise.[38] Six of 29 (21%) patients with mitral valve prolapse and no significant mitral regurgitation who did not undergo angiography also demonstrated abnormal exercise ejection fraction responses. Such findings could not be attributed to inadequate or submaximal exercise. Newman and associates, however, using first-pass radionuclide ventriculography, found normal rest and exercise wall motion and left ventricular function (including ejection fraction, end-diastolic volume, end-systolic volume, and stroke volume) in 12 patients with mitral valve prolapse, no significant mitral regurgitation, and normal coronary arteries.[39]

In patients with coronary artery disease and mitral valve prolapse, Ahmad et al. found exercise

TABLE 14–2.—MITRAL VALVE PROLAPSE AND EXERCISE RADIONUCLIDE VENTRICULOGRAPHY*

			RADIONUCLIDE ANGIOGRAPHY EJECTION FRACTION		
			Mean ±SD		
STUDY	N	PATIENT GROUP	Rest	Exercise	Abnormal Exercise Response
Ahmad et al.[37]	12	MVP + no CAD	Normal	NA	6/12†
	18	MVP + CAD	Normal	NA	17/18
Gottdiener et al.[38]	30	Normal	57 ± 1	71 ± 2	0/30‡
	39	MVP + no MR	57 + 3	64 ± 2	9/39
	8	MVP + MR	56 + 3	53 ± 4	5/8
	10	MVP + no CAD	. . .	. . .	3/10
Newman et al.[39]	11	Normal	67 ± 8	76 ± 7	1/11§
	12	MVP + no CAD + no MR	61 ± 7	71 ± 7	0/12
	11	MVP + CAD + no MR	60 ± 7	58 ± 7	6/11

*MVP, mitral valve prolapse; MR, mitral regurgitation; CAD, coronary artery disease.
†Fall or no change in ejection fraction with exercise.
‡Ejection fraction <58 or fall with exercise.
§Fall in ejection fraction with exercise.

ejection fraction reduced or unchanged compared with the resting ejection fraction in 17 of 18 (94%) patients.[37] Newman and colleagues found that of 11 patients with coronary artery disease and mitral valve prolapse, 6 (55%) had a fall in ejection fraction with exercise and 6 (55%) developed exercise-induced wall motion abnormalities.[39] Gottdiener and associates did not study patients with angiographically documented coronary artery disease but found abnormal ejection fraction responses to exercise in 5 of 8 (63%) patients with mitral valve prolapse and clinically important mitral regurgitation.[38]

The data reported by Gottdiener et al.[38] and Ahmad et al.[37] suggest that patients with mitral valve prolapse commonly have an abnormal ejection fraction response to exercise in the absence of coronary artery disease. The cause of reduced left ventricular reserve in some patients with mitral valve prolapse in the absence of coronary artery disease and mitral regurgitation is not clear. It does not appear to be related to the degree of mitral valve prolapse determined echocardiographically.[38] The possibility of exercise-induced coronary vasospasm has been discussed. Of note is that in the absence of coronary artery disease, new regional wall motion abnormalities associated with a fall in ejection fraction were reported by Ahmad and colleagues.[37] However, both Gottdiener et al.[38] and Newman et al.[39] found no focal contraction abnormalities at rest or with exercise. The abnormal ejection fraction response may be related to a more generalized left ventricular cardiomyopathy, as suggested by previous angiography[14, 33–36] and biopsy[23] studies. When chronic mitral regurgitation is present, depressed left ventricular functional reserve may reflect the effects of persistent volume overload, as previously described in patients with mitral regurgitation from other causes.

Newman et al. suggest that exercise radionuclide ventriculography may be used to predict the presence of coronary artery disease in patients with mitral valve prolapse.[39] However, the common occurrence of abnormal left ventricular ejection fraction response to exercise in patients with mitral valve prolapse but without coronary artery disease, as reported in other series,[37,38] suggests that a reduced ejection fraction response is not specific for coronary artery disease. It is possible that a new wall motion abnormality may be more specific for coexisting coronary artery disease.

In summary, exercise radionuclide ventriculography offers insight into left ventricular reserve in patients with mitral valve prolapse. Depressed left ventricular functional reserve appears to be nonspecific, occurring in a substantial number of patients with mitral valve prolapse but without coronary artery disease or chronic mitral regurgitation.

REFERENCES

1. Barlow J.B., Bosman C.K.: Aneurysmal protrusion of the posterior leaflet of the mitral valve. *Am. Heart J.* 71:166–178, 1966.
2. Hancock E.W., Cohn K.: The syndrome associated

with midsystolic click and late systolic murmur. *Am. J. Med.* 41:183, 1966.
3. Barlow J.B., Bosman C.K., Pocock W.A., et al.: Late systolic murmurs in non-ejection ("mid-late") systolic clicks. *Br. Heart J.* 30:203–218, 1968.
4. Jeresaty R.M.: Mitral valve prolapse-click murmur syndrome. *Prog. Cardiovasc. Dis.* 15:623, 1973.
5. Pocock W.A., Barlow J.B.: Etiology and electrocardiographic features of the billowing posterior mitral leaflet syndrome. *Am. J. Med.* 51:731–739, 1971.
6. Barlow J.B., Pocock W.A.: The problem of non-ejection systolic clicks and associated mitral systolic murmurs: Emphasis on the billowing mitral leaflet syndrome. *Am. Heart J.* 90:636–655, 1975.
7. Devereaux R.B., Perloff I.K., Rerchek N., et al.: Mitral prolapse. *Circulation* 54:3–14, 1976.
8. Wyle E.D., Rakowski H., Ranganathan N., et al.: Mitral valve prolapse. *Ann. Rev. Med.* 27:165–179, 1976.
9. Malcolm A.D., Boughner D.R., Kostuk W.J., et al.: Clinical features and investigative findings in presence of mitral leaflet prolapse: A study of 85 consecutive patients. *Br. Heart J.* 38:244–256, 1976.
10. Massie B., Botvinick E.H., Shames D., et al.: Myocardial perfusion scintigraphy in patients with mitral valve prolapse: Its advantage over stress electrocardiography in diagnosing associated coronary artery disease and its implications for etiology of chest pain. *Circulation* 57:19–26, 1978.
11. Klein G.J., Kostuk W.J., Boughner D.R., et al.: Stress myocardial imaging in mitral leaflet prolapse syndrome. *Am. J. Cardiol.* 42:746–750, 1978.
12. Greenspan M., Iskandrian A.S., Mintz G.S., et al.: Exercise myocardial scintigraphy with ^{201}thallium. *Chest* 77:47–52, 1980.
13. Sloman G., Wong M., Walker J.: Arrhythmias on exercise in patients with abnormalities of the posterior leaflet of the mitral valve. *Am. Heart J.* 83:312–317, 1972.
14. Gulotta S.J., Gulco L., Padmanabhan V., et al.: The syndrome of systolic click, murmur and mitral valve prolapse: A cardiomyopathy? *Circulation* 49:717–728, 1974.
15. Lobstein H.P., Horwitz L.D., Curry G.C., et al.: Electrocardiographic abnormalities and coronary arteriograms in the mitral click murmur syndrome. *N. Engl. J. Med.* 289:127–131, 1973.
16. Malcolm A.D., Ahuja S.P.: Unusual ECG response to exercise in patients with mitral prolapse, abstracted. *Circulation* 51, 52(suppl. II):II–114, 1975.
17. Gaffney P.A., Wohl A.J., Blomqvist C.G., et al.: Thallium-201 myocardial perfusion studies in patients with the mitral valve prolapse syndrome. *Am. J. Med.* 64:21–26, 1978.
18. Jeresaty R.M.: Etiology of the mitral valve prolapse-click syndrome. *Am. J. Cardiol.* 36:110–112, 1976.
19. Roberts W.C., Cohen L.D.: Left ventricular papillary muscles: Description of the normal and a survey of conditions causing them to be abnormal. *Circulation* 46:138–154, 1972.
20. Natarajan G., Nakhjavan F.K., Kahn D., et al.: Myocardial metabolism studies in prolapsing mitral leaflet syndrome. *Circulation* 52:1105–1110, 1975.
21. Duca P.R., Gottlieb R., Kasparian H., et al.: Abnormal myocardial lactate metabolism as an additional feature of the syndrome of mitral valve prolapse, abstracted. *Am. J. Cardiol.* 35:133, 1975.
22. Khullar S.C., Leighton R.F.: Mitral valve prolapse syndrome: Left ventricular function and myocardial metabolism, abstracted. *Am. J. Cardiol.* 35:149, 1975.
23. Koch F.H., Bellingham M.E., Mason J.W., et al.: Pathogenesis of the click-murmur-prolapse syndrome: Biopsy evidence supporting an underlying cardiomyopathic process, abstracted. *Am. J. Cardiol.* 38:272, 1977.
24. McLaughlin P., Huckell V.E., Staniloff H., et al.: Exercise-induced chest pain, myocardial perfusion and stress electrocardiography in patients with mitral valve prolapse, abstracted. *Circulation* 55(suppl. 3):216, 1977.
25. Padmanabhan V., Margouleff D., Binder A., et al.: Thallium-201 myocardial imaging during exercise in mitral valve prolapse, abstracted. *Circulation* 55(suppl. 3):217, 1977.
26. Soin J.S., Tresch D.D., Siegel R., et al.: Myocardial perfusion abnormalities in patients with mitral valve prolapse, abstracted. *J. Nucl. Med.* 19:736, 1976.
27. Klein G., Kostuk W.J., Chamberlain M.J.: Stress myocardial scintigraphy in patients with mitral leaflet prolapse, abstracted. *Circulation* 55(suppl. 3):217, 1977.
28. Sbarbaro J.A., Mehlman D., Wu L., et al.: A prospective study of mitral valve prolapse in young men, abstracted. *Am. J. Cardiol.* 41:433, 1978.
29. Jeresaty R.M. *Mitral Valve Prolapse*. New York, Raven Press, 1979, pp. 100–105.
30. Buda A.J., Levene D.L., Myers M.G., et al.: Coronary artery spasm and mitral valve prolapse. *Am. Heart J.* 95:457–462, 1978.
31. Chesler E., Matisonn R.E., Lakier J.B., et al.: Acute myocardial infarction with normal coronary arteries: A possible manifestation of the billowing mitral leaflet syndrome. *Circulation* 54:203–209, 1976.
32. Gewirtz H., Grötte G.J., Strauss H.W., et al.: The influence of left ventricular volume and wall motion on myocardial images. *Circulation* 59:1172–1177, 1979.
33. Gooch A.S., Vincencio F., Maranhao V., et al.: Arrhythmias and left ventricular asynergy in the prolapsing mitral leaflet syndrome. *Am. J. Cardiol.* 29:611–620, 1972.
34. Scampardonis G., Yang S.S., Maranhao V., et al.: Left ventricular abnormalities in prolapsed mitral leaflet syndrome: Review of eighty-seven cases. *Circulation* 48:287–297, 1973.
35. Nutter D.O., Wickliffe C., Gilbert C.A., et al.: The

pathophysiology of idiopathic mitral valve prolapse. *Circulation* 52:297–305, 1975.

36. Cobbs B.W. Jr., King S.B. III.: Ventricular buckling: A factor in the abnormal ventriculogram and peculiar hemodynamics associated with mitral valve prolapse. *Am. Heart J.* 93:741–758, 1977.
37. Ahmad M., Sullivan T., Harbach H., et al.: Exercise induced changes in left ventricular function in patients with mitral valve prolapse, abstracted. *Clin. Res.* 27:146A, 1979.
38. Gottdiener J.S., Borer J.S., Bacharach S.L., et al.: Left ventricular function in mitral valve prolapse: Assessment with radionuclide cineangiography. *Am. J. Cardiol.* 47:7–13, 1981.
39. Newman G.E., Gibbons R.J., Jones R.H.: Cardiac function during rest and exercise in patients with mitral valve prolapse. *Am. J. Cardiol.* 47:14–19, 1981.

COMMENT: MITRAL VALVE PROLAPSE

Joel Morganroth

Only within the last decade has the clinical recognition of mitral valve prolapse been firmly established, owing to the advent of echocardiography. Mitral valve prolapse, once thought an uncommon disorder, may be one of the most common cardiac conditions in man. Controversy still exists as to diagnostic standards, recognition and management of complications, and general facts of its natural course. Echocardiography will have a major impact on our understanding of these issues.

ETIOLOGIC DETERMINATION

It is important to differentiate between primary and secondary forms of mitral valve prolapse. Secondary mitral valve prolapse is the presence of mitral valve abnormality during systole due to conditions that secondarily affect the mitral valve apparatus. Coronary artery disease, which may affect papillary muscle function, resulting in mitral valve prolapse, is a common example of a secondary form. Rheumatic commissural fusion of the mitral valve with doming during diastole of the mitral leaflets may secondarily cause mitral valve tissue to prolapse into the left atrium during systole. Abnormalities of left ventricular wall-papillary muscle interaction such as seen in cardiomyopathy may also result in secondary systolic mitral leaflet tissue prolapsing into the left atrium. Primary dysfunction of mitral valve leaflets and chordal structures is believed to be due to myxomatous degeneration rather than abnormal left ventricular contraction abnormalities suggesting an associated form of cardiomyopathy.

The diagnosis of mitral valve prolapse depends on the ability to identify mitral leaflet tissue prolapsing, that is, being displaced from its normal left ventricular position at end-systole into left atrial space. Physical examination may detect the consequences of this prolapsing motion (click or murmur of mitral regurgitation), but such findings are secondary, variable, and nonspecific. In fact, frequently patients with mitral valve prolapse may have no abnormalities on auscultation at all. Left ventricular cineangiography poorly images the mitral leaflets and, because of the limitations of the technique, poorly identifies the precise location of mitral leaflet tissue during different phases of the cardiac cycle. Thus, cardiac catheterization is usually not warranted as a diagnostic procedure for this condition.

Obviously, echocardiography has had a major diagnostic impact on the diagnosis of this condition since it is a noninvasive and precise method by which one can identify and localize mitral leaflet tissue during any phase of the cardiac cycle. Since echocardiography primarily interrogates the anteroposterior plane and since the mitral valve's primary motion is in a superior direction during prolapse, two-dimensional echocardiography using primarily the apical four-chamber and parasternal left ventricular long-axis views has come to be the diagnostic standard for this condition. This technique, of course, can also identify the conditions that may be causing secondary mitral valve prolapse (papillary muscle dysfunction, rheumatic mitral stenosis, cardiomyopathy), and when not present, primary mitral valve prolapse is diagnosed by exclusion. Cardiac nuclear imaging does not play a role in the diagnosis of mitral valve prolapse per se.

CLINICAL CORRELATIONS

The Asymptomatic Patient

In an increasing number of patients, mitral valve prolapse may be diagnosed without cardiac symptoms. Since echocardiography as the diagnostic standard for mitral valve prolapse has only recently been defined, the clinical importance of asymptomatic mitral valve prolapse has not yet been established. If such patients are, in fact, asymptomatic and have no abnormalities on routine ECG (for example, lack of arrhythmias), we do not believe that further diagnostic workup is warranted and, in general, the patient should be reassured. Indications for the use of antibiotic prophylaxis against infective endocarditis are controversial and our own opinion is that such prophylaxis should be offered to patients who have evidence of mitral regurgitation. However, since mitral regurgitation may be intermittent, most cardiologists recommend prophylaxis in all patients with this condition.

The Symptomatic Patient

One of the common symptoms in patients with mitral valve prolapse is chest pain, which frequently may be difficult to differentiate from typical angina pectoris. The identification of possible coexisting coronary artery disease has, therefore, important therapeutic implications. Here echocardiography offers limited usefulness and cardiac nuclear imaging plays an important role. Recently, thallium perfusion exercise testing and possibly radionuclide ventriculography appeared to be highly sensitive and specific for detecting coexisting coronary artery disease in these patients. False positive tests have been identified with thallium perfusion (chest pain with abnormal perfusion but normal coronary arteriographic appearances), and the clinical importance of this finding is unknown. Progressive mitral regurgitation or acute ruptured chordae tendineae with acute severe mitral regurgitation are important complications of this disorder and the use of echocardiography in detecting these conditions and evaluating left ventricular function is well established. When echocardiographic data are equivocal or difficult to evaluate because of technical difficulties, radionuclide ventriculography may be extremely useful.

The importance of ventricular arrhythmias and the relationship to sudden cardiac death in this syndrome also remains controversial. Ambulatory (Holter) ECG monitoring is indicated in patients with symptoms of palpitations, presyncope, or syncope; and when high-frequency complex arrhythmias are present, antiarrhythmic therapy is indicated in our opinion.

Echocardiography should be performed on all patients with suspected mitral valve prolapse, not only to confirm the diagnosis but to evaluate left ventricular function and the extent of the prolapse, and to determine whether or not other cardiac valves are involved. Cardiac nuclear imaging techniques should be performed when left ventricular function cannot be assessed by echocardiography, and particularly in the differential diagnosis of chest pain in this syndrome.

SEVERITY AND PROGNOSIS

The severity of mitral valve prolapse in preliminary studies does not appear to correlate well with clinical significance or prognosis. More data on the natural history of various degrees of severity of this condition must be obtained before this issue can be settled. In general most patients have a benign prognosis, though at present we are unable to predict which patients will develop important arrhythmias or progressive or acute mitral regurgitation, which often may require mitral valve replacement, or to determine those who might develop infective endocarditis.

PART VIII

Aortic and Mitral Valve Regurgitation

ECHOCARDIOGRAPHY

Ioannis Panidis, Chin C. Chen, and Joel Morganroth

ECHOCARDIOGRAPHY IN AORTIC REGURGITATION

THE CLINICAL and hemodynamic picture of aortic regurgitation can be divided according to pathophysiologic and clinical consequences into two distinct entities: acute aortic regurgitation and chronic aortic regurgitation. The physiologic response of the left ventricle to aortic regurgitation depends mainly on the rapidity with which the regurgitation develops.[1] The gradual, slow development of aortic regurgitation (chronic state) permits the left ventricle to adapt to a progressive volume overload over time, with resultant dilation of the left ventricle and left atrium. In contrast, in acute severe aortic regurgitation the left ventricle does not have sufficient time to adapt, with the result that the left ventricular end-diastolic pressure rises dramatically, leading to left ventricular failure.

Since the echocardiographic features of these two clinical forms of aortic regurgitation are distinct, this noninvasive test may be helpful in distinguishing the two.

Acute Severe Aortic Regurgitation

Echocardiography has proved to be an invaluable noninvasive diagnostic tool in the clinical recognition of acute severe aortic regurgitation[2-5] and should be used promptly whenever this diagnosis is considered. The various causes of acute severe aortic regurgitation include infective endocarditis, a dissecting aortic aneurysm, rupture or prolapse of aortic leaflets—which can be in the form of traumatic rupture, spontaneous rupture of a myxomatous valve, spontaneous rupture of leaflet fenestrations, and sudden sagging of a "normal" leaflet—and, postoperatively, the faulty incision of a stenotic aortic valve. M-mode echocardiography and two-dimensional echocardiography (2DE) have different sensitivities for detecting each of these etiologies and for detecting different features of acute severe aortic regurgitation, as described below.

M-Mode Echocardiography

The M-mode echocardiogram identifies several important findings in acute aortic regurgitation.

Mitral valve.—Premature closure of the mitral valve is a sensitive and reliable indicator of acute severe aortic regurgitation (Fig 15–1).[3-8] Its detection requires high-quality recording and interpretation by an experienced echocardiographer. The premature closure of the mitral valve may be due to either the early diastolic elevation of left ventricular diastolic pressure, which causes the mitral valve to close prematurely, or the changing of flow characteristics around the mitral valve caused by aortic regurgitation.[9] The degree of prematurity of the closure of the mitral valve can be obscured by various factors[3]: rapid heart rates, increased left atrial pressure, and pharmacologically induced vasodilation, which reduces the regurgitant fraction. Premature mitral valve closure has also been reported in first-degree atrioventricular block[3, 10] and in mitral insufficiency.[11] In the presence of bacterial endocarditis, premature closure of the mitral valve may signal the need for immediate surgical intervention.[3–5]

Other echocardiographic features of acute severe aortic regurgitation include delayed opening of the mitral valve,[4] a decrease in EF slope,[1] diminished amplitude of opening and mid-diastolic closure of the mitral valve,[9] and minimal or no reopening of the mitral valve during atrial systole.[6] In acute severe aortic regurgitation, fluttering of the anterior leaflet (see Fig 15–1) may be present, but since it is also observed in chronic aortic regurgitation[12] it cannot be used to distinguish between the two conditions.

Left Ventricle and Left Atrium.—In addition to the changes in mitral valve motion observed in acute severe aortic regurgitation, M-mode echocardiography can be used to identify changes in the left ventricle which may help to differentiate acute from chronic aortic regurgitation (Table 15–1). Acute severe aortic regurgitation is characterized by normal to slightly increased left ventricular end-diastolic dimensions, normal or decreased septal and posterior wall motion (see Fig 15–1), and, most often, normal left atrial size,[1, 13] while in chronic aortic regurgitation the left ventricle and left atrium are dilated and the walls are hypercontractile (see Table 15–1).

TABLE 15–1.—M-MODE ECHOCARDIOGRAPHIC FEATURES OF ACUTE SEVERE AORTIC REGURGITATION*

	ACUTE	CHRONIC
Mitral valve		
Closure point	Premature	Normal
Opening point	Delayed	Normal
EF slope	Decreased	Normal
Fluttering	May be present	May be present
Left ventricle		
Internal dimension (end-diastole)	Normal	Increased
Septal and free wall thickness	Normal	Normal
Septal and free wall motion	Normal	Increased
Left ventricular mass	Normal	Increased
Aortic valve		
Premature opening	May be present	Normal
Left atrium size	Normal	Increased

*Data from Morganroth et al.[1]

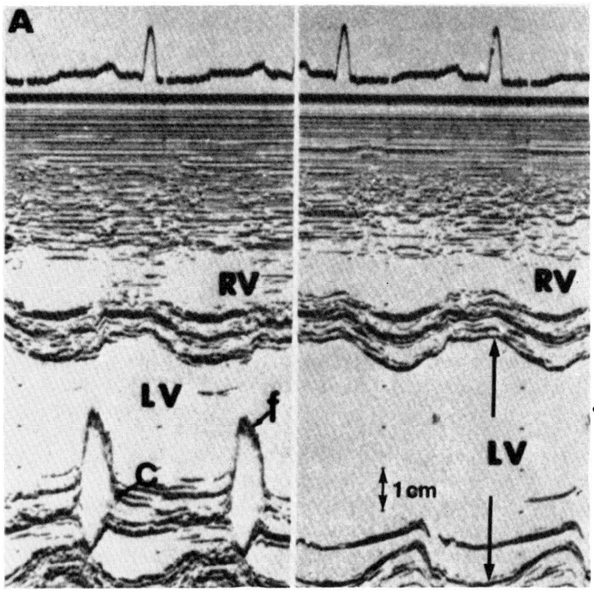

Fig 15–1.—M-mode echocardiogram showing the features of acute severe aortic regurgitation. Premature mitral valve closure is evident as the closure point of the mitral valve *(C)* precedes the R wave on the ECG. Slight left ventricular dilation, normal septal and left ventricular posterior wall motion, and fluttering of the anterior mitral valve leaflets are also seen. *RV,* right ventricle; *LV,* left ventricle; *f,* fluttering of anterior mitral valve leaflet. (From Morganroth J., et al.: *Ann. Intern. Med.* 87:223, 1977. Reproduced by permission.)

Aortic valve.—One of the most common causes of acute severe aortic regurgitation is rupture of one or more of the aortic cusps due to infective endocarditis[14-19] and, less commonly, to myxomatous degeneration.[20, 21] A flail or ruptured aortic valve leaflet is characterized by abnormal diastolic fluttering of the aortic valve, diastolic echoes in the left ventricular outflow tract, and coarse systolic oscillations of the aortic cusps (Fig 15–2).[15, 18, 22-24] Vegetations on the aortic valves are suggested by shaggy, fuzzy, or dense echoes on a normally moving aortic valve (Fig 15–3).[14, 25-29] A diameter of about 3 mm is required for the vegetations to be recorded by M-mode echocardiography[9]; therefore, M-mode echocardiography has a low sensitivity (34%) for detecting vegetations in patients with proved bacterial endocarditis.[28] Moreover, valvular vegetations are frequently difficult to differentiate from flail or rup-

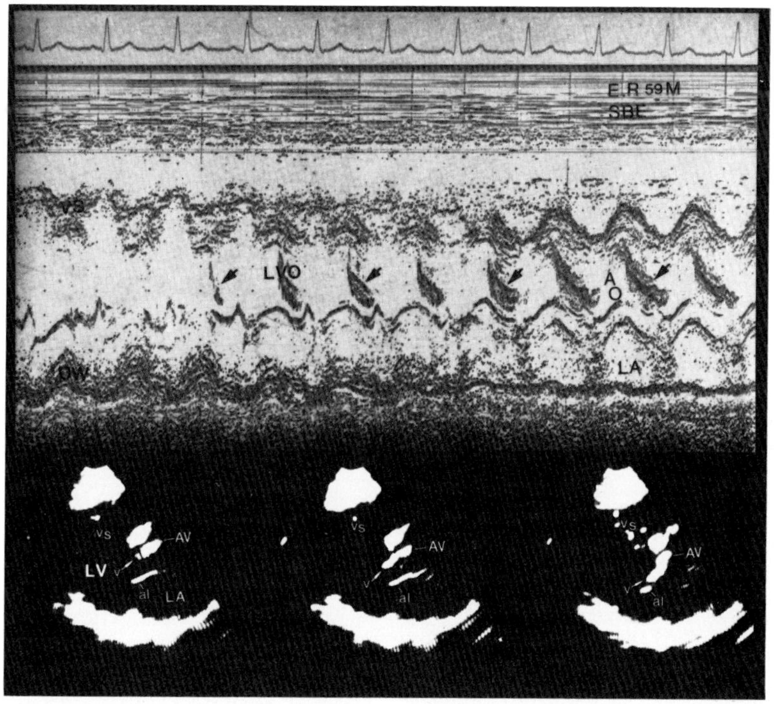

Fig 15–2.—Flail aortic valve and aortic vegetations. *Top,* M-mode echocardiogram showing diastolic echoes in the left ventricular outflow tract and on the aortic valve, compatible with aortic vegetations. *Bottom,* sequential diastolic frames of 2DE parasternal long-axis left ventricular views showing a band of echoes in the left ventricular ourflow tract emanating from the aortic valve, which represents vegetation on the aortic valve. *VS,* ventricular septum; *LV,* left ventricle; *AV,* aortic valve; *LA,* left atrium; *V,* vegetations; *al,* antrum leaflet.

tured aortic valve leaflets.[30, 31] The presence of an abnormal band of echoes extending into the left ventricular outflow tract in diastole with identical, continuous patterns on the aortic valve in diastole favors a flail aortic valve (see Fig 15–2).[15, 16, 20] However, similar echocardiographic patterns have also been reported in discrete subvalvular aortic stenosis[32] and in aneurysms of the sinus of Valsalva[33] and thus are not specific for the diagnosis of flail aortic valve. Premature opening of the aortic valve is another M-mode echocardiographic feature reported to occur, especially when the left ventricular diastolic pressure is significantly elevated.[34, 35] M-mode echocardiography may also be useful in identifying acute severe aortic regurgitation due to aortic root dissection.[36] Marked dilation of the aortic root, a double-lumen aortic root echo, and parallel motion of the separated portions of the aortic wall are echocardiographic findings that suggest aortic root dissection (Fig 15–4).[37, 38]

Two-Dimensional Echocardiography

While M-mode echocardiography serves to detect the existence of acute aortic regurgitation, the major use of 2DE is in the potential recognition of its etiology.

Two-dimensional echocardiography has been most valuable in identifying the presence of vegetations on the aortic valve due to infective endocarditis.[39–43] Vegetations appear as a discrete or irregular mass of echoes which usually do not disturb the normal motion of the aortic valve (Fig 15–5).[39–42]

Since 2DE permits simultaneous visualization of the aortic valve and the left ventricular outflow tract, it is superior to M-mode echocardiography

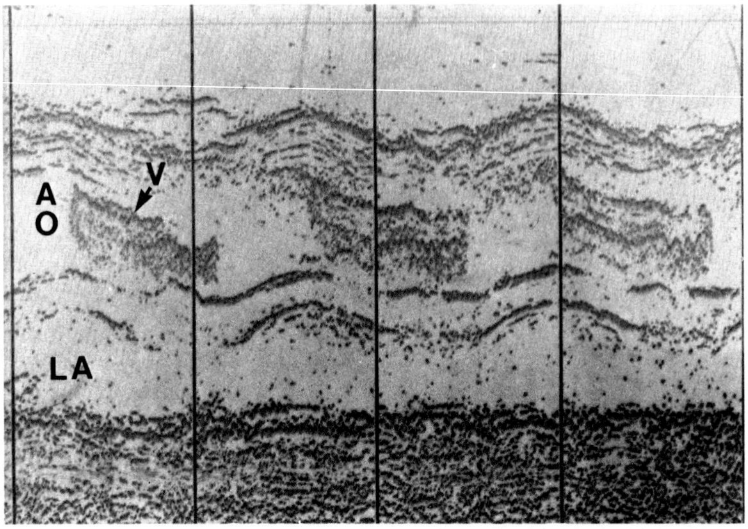

Fig 15–3.—M-mode echocardiogram demonstrating vegetations on the aortic valve. The aortic valve shows fuzzy, dense echoes in diastole; the systolic motion of the arotic valve is normal. *V,* vegetations; *AO,* aorta; *LA,* left atrium.

in the diagnosis of flail aortic valve[2, 41] and in the differentiation of flail aortic valve from vegetations.[30] The echocardiographic picture consists of abnormal echoes that move back and forth and in and out of the left ventricular outflow tract (see Fig 15–2).[2, 39] Abnormal coaptation of the aortic leaflets and left ventricular outflow tract diastolic echoes suggest a flail aortic valve, whereas increased aortic cusp echoes suggest vegetation.[2, 39, 42, 44]

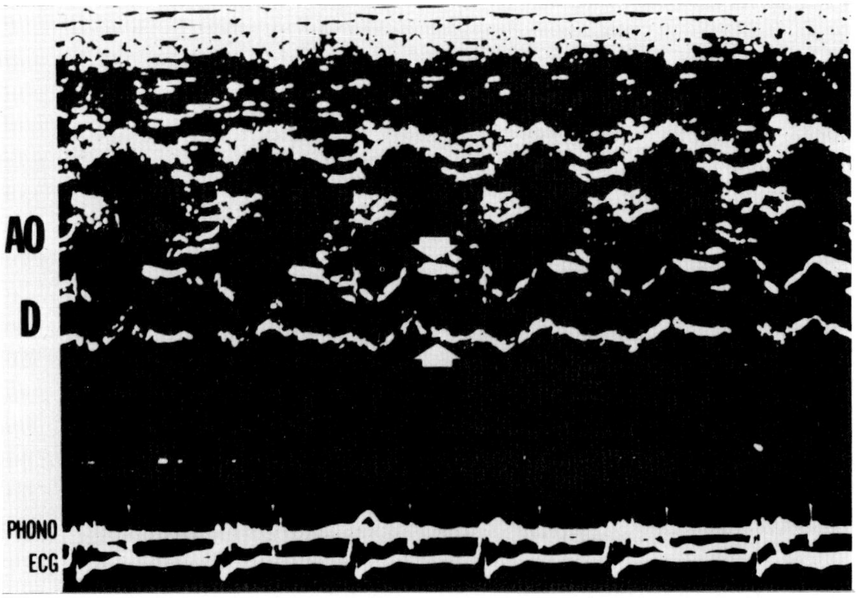

Fig 15–4.—M-mode echocardiography demonstrating aortic root dissection. White arrows identify double lumen of the posterior aortic wall. (From Nanda N.C., et al.: *Circulation* 48:506, 1973. Reproduced by permission of the American Heart Association.)

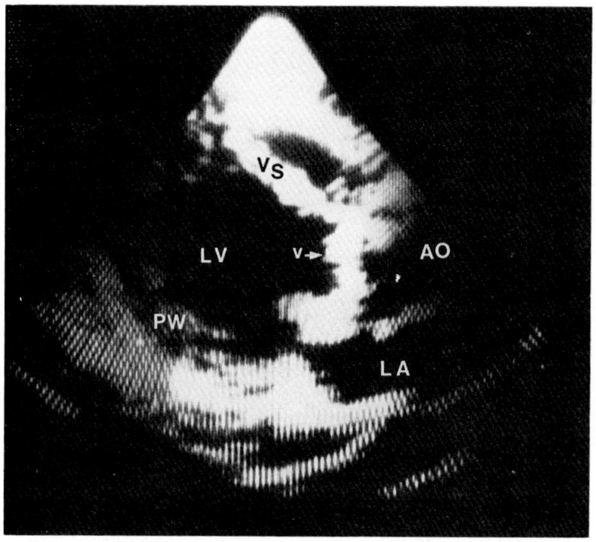

Fig 15–5.—Two-dimensional echocardiographic parasternal long-axis view of the left ventricle showing dense vegetations on the aortic valve as an irregular mass of echoes. *LV,* left ventricle; *VS,* ventricular septum; *PW,* posterior wall; *V,* vegetation; *AO,* aorta; *LA,* left atrium.

Aortic root dissection can also be reliably detected by 2DE.[45] A dilated aortic root and a double-lumen echo clearly suggest aortic root dissection (Fig 15–6).[46] However, further studies are required to determine the sensitivity and specificity of 2DE in the diagnosis of this entity.

Finally, aortic valve prolapse, which can cause acute severe aortic regurgitation, has been successfully identified by 2DE.[47]

In summary, M-mode echocardiography appears to be superior to 2DE in recognizing the presence and the severity of acute severe aortic regurgitation of any etiology, while 2DE can be used to recognize the etiology of this condition, such as vegetations on the aortic valve, and to identify a flail aortic valve and perhaps differentiate it from such vegetations.

Clinical Implications

The M-mode echocardiographic finding of premature mitral valve closure has been very useful in the clinical assessment and management of acute aortic regurgitation. The effectiveness of vasodilator treatment in acute aortic regurgitation has been echocardiographically demonstrated by the abolishment of premature mitral valve closure.[48]

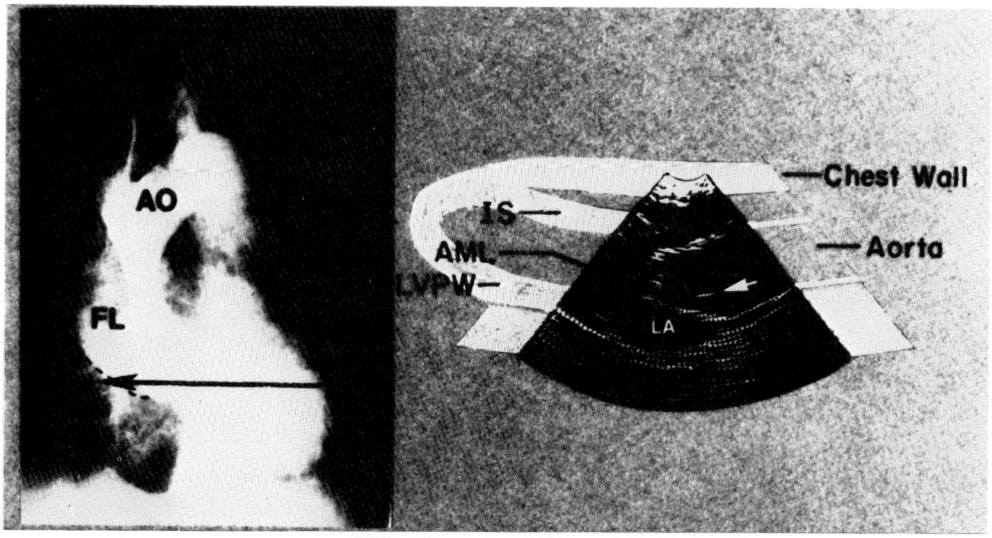

Fig 15–6.—Two-dimensional echocardiographic parasternal long-axis view of the left ventricle demonstrating the findings of aortic root dissection. Angiogram shown at left. *AML,* anterior mitral leaflet; *IS,* interatrial septum; *FL,* false lumen; *AO,* aorta; *LA,* left atrium; *LVPW,* left ventricular posterior wall. (From DeMaria A.N., et al.: *Circulation* 59:755, 1979. Reproduced by permission of the American Heart Association.)

The identification of vegetations by M-mode echocardiography or 2DE combined with the finding of an early closure of the mitral valve in the presence of clinical bacterial endocarditis is ominous prognostically[5, 40] and usually indicates that immediate surgical intervention is mandatory[3, 4, 43] The recognition of vegetations alone, however, does not necessarily indicate immediate surgical intervention, nor does estimation of size and shape of the vegetations predict the clinical outcome of the patient.[40, 43, 49]

The echocardiographic recognition of flail aortic valve in combination with premature mitral valve closure usually indicates severe hemodynamic and mechanical derangement, and operative intervention must be considered.[2, 17, 41]

Chronic Aortic Regurgitation

M-mode Echocardiography

Mitral valve.—The most common and characteristic echocardiographic finding in chronic aortic regurgitation is fluttering of the mitral valve during diastole (Fig 15–7).[50–52] This finding can be subtle and in order to be diagnostic must be confined to diastole; fine vibrations that are seen throughout the entire cardiac cycle may be artifactual. The typical diastolic oscillations of the mitral valve are usually fine and rapid, but they may sometimes appear as a mass of echoes if there is poor resolution of the recording system and thus can be misinterpreted as a thickened valve. Although fluttering is seen more frequently on the anterior leaflet, it can also be present on the posterior leaflet. Prosthetic valves do not exhibit fluttering, and detection of fluttering on fibrotic mitral valves, as in mitral stenosis, can be difficult. Mitral valve fluttering is not specific for aortic regurgitation, nor does its intensity correlate with the severity of the lesion.[9] High-flow states such as chronic anemia[53] and left-to-right shunt[54] may also cause mitral valve fluttering. Fluttering has also been reported in atrial flutter or fibrillation[55] and in mitral insufficiency due to ruptured chordae tendineae, in which case the fluttering is usually coarse.[56]

Interventricular septum.—Fluttering of the interventricular septum is another echocardiographic feature that can be found in patients with chronic aortic regurgitation (Fig 15–8).[57–60] The finding of fluttering of the ventricular septum is particularly useful in association with mitral stenosis, in which case the detection of fluttering on the thickened mitral valve might be difficult.[12] One study has shown that when fluttering of the interventricular septum occurs, the regurgitant jet passes through the proximity of the posterior or noncoronary cusp.[61]

Exaggerated motion of the interventricular septum is frequently seen in patients with chronic aortic regurgitation and may compensate for the left ventricular volume overload.[62, 63] Exaggerated septal motion is not specific for chronic aortic re-

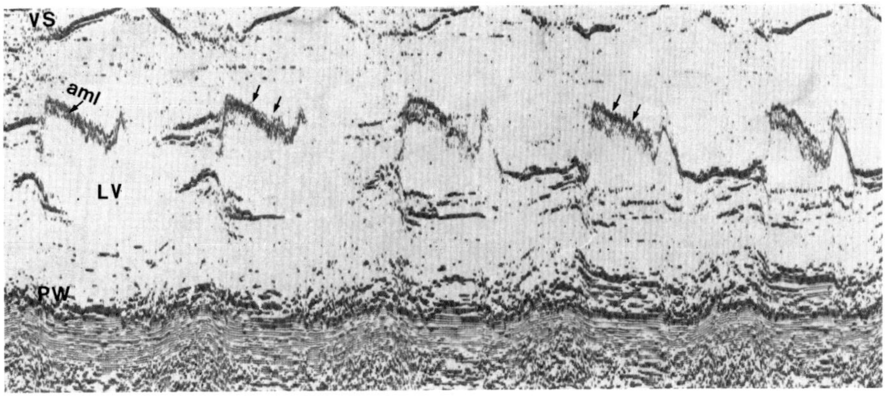

Fig 15–7.—M-mode echocardiogram showing fine fluttering of the anterior mitral leaflet *(aml)* during diastole in a patient with acute aortic regurgitation *(arrows). VS,* ventricular septum; *LV,* left ventricle; *PW,* posterior wall.

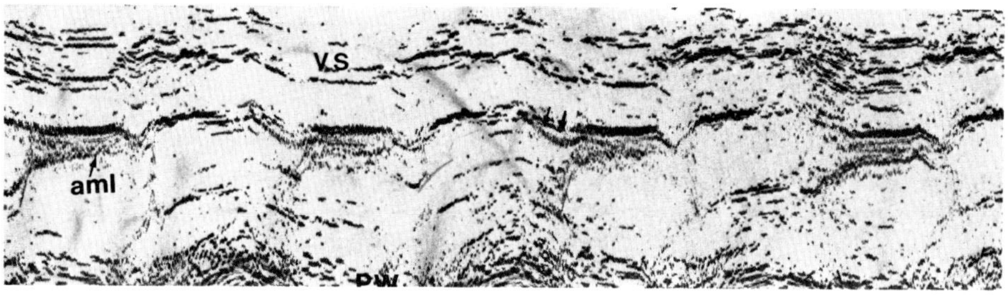

Fig 15–8.—M-mode echocardiogram of a patient with aortic regurgitation demonstrating fluttering of the interventricular septum *(VS) (arrow),* as well as the anterior mitral leaflet *(aml). PW,* posterior wall.

gurgitation; any condition causing left ventricular volume overloading can create increased amplitude of septal excursion.[62, 64, 65] A similar finding has also been observed in coronary artery disease as a "compensatory phenomenon" to abnormal segmental left ventricular free wall motion.[66] However, in patients with aortic regurgitation, an exaggerated early diastolic dip is occasionally seen.[63]

Left ventricle and left atrium.—The increased internal dimensions of the left ventricle and the exaggerated free wall motion due to volume overload, as well as the increased left atrium size, are useful echocardiographic features differentiating chronic from acute severe aortic regurgitation (Fig 15–9).[1, 13, 62]

Aortic valve.—One of the first, most logical echocardiographic signs of aortic regurgitation is diastolic separation of the aortic leaflets[67]; however, errors emanating from inherent problems of the echocardiographic beam width and point separation capability may simulate this finding and create false positive results.[9] Separation of the aortic leaflets is therefore an unreliable sign of chronic aortic regurgitation.

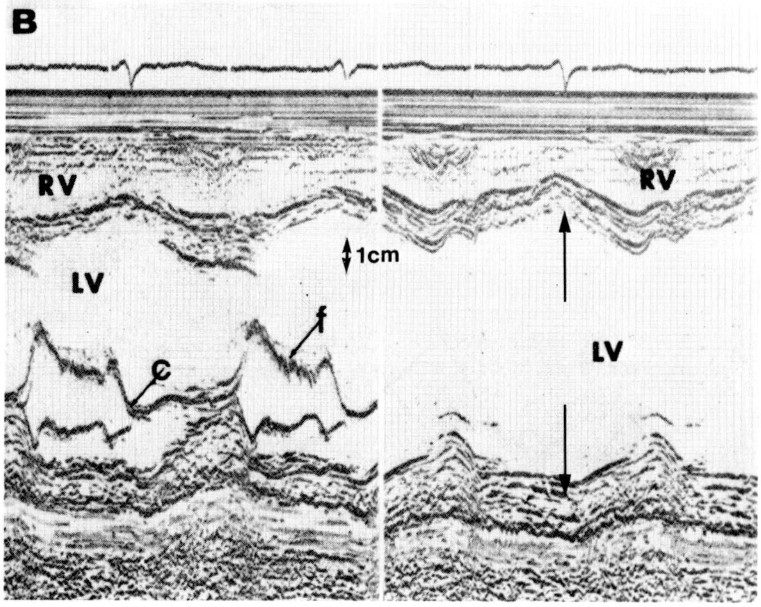

Fig 15–9.—M-mode echocardiogram showing the features of chronic aortic regurgitation. Fluttering *(f)* of the anterior mitral leaflet *(aml)* is present during diastole; the mitral valve closes at the proper time *(C).* Increased internal dimensions of the left ventricle and exaggerated wall motions are seen. *RV,* right ventricle; *LV,* left ventricle. (From Morganroth J., et al.: *Ann. Intern. Med.* 87:223, 1977. Reproduced by permission.)

Etiological echocardiographic findings.—In addition to the previously described M-mode echocardiographic findings, common in the variety of causes of chronic aortic regurgitation (Table 15–2),[68] M-mode echocardiography can be helpful in identifying bicuspid aortic valve,[69] dissection of the aortic root,[36–38] or vegetations on the aortic valve in bacterial endocarditis.[25–27] In the case of a leaking aortic prosthetic valve, the secondary signs of aortic regurgitation (e.g., fluttering of the mitral valve and exaggerated or normal septal motion) are helpful.[70, 71]

Two-Dimensional Echocardiography

As in acute severe aortic regurgitation, 2DE is less useful than M-mode echocardiography in the recognition of chronic aortic regurgitation, but it is often more useful in identifying the etiology of the aortic regurgitation.[45]

Due to lack of adequate axial resolution, 2DE is inferior to M-mode echocardiography in detecting mitral valve flutter; however, the signs of left ventricular volume overload are readily appreciable.[62] Moreover, 2DE can occasionally detect a failure of coaptation during diastole of the aortic cusps in chronic aortic regurgitation.[72, 73] The incomplete opening of the aortic valve during systole and its backward bulging into the left ventricular outflow tract during diastole may contribute to the diagnosis of aortic regurgitation,[74] although similar phenomena have been recently reported in patients with aortic valve prolapse without aortic regurgitation.[47, 75]

TABLE 15–2.—CAUSES OF CHRONIC AORTIC REGURGITATION

Congenital
Bicuspid aortic valve
Ventricular septal defect
Myxomatous degeneration of the aortic root and leaflets (Marfan syndrome)
Osteogenesis imperfecta
Hurler's syndrome
Ehlers-Danlos syndrome
Discrete subaortic membranous stenosis
Acquired
Traumatic
Infectious (e.g., rheumatic fever, syphilis, bacterial endocarditis)
Collagen diseases (e.g., rheumatoid arthritis, Reiter's syndrome, ankylosing spondylitis)
Miscellaneous
Dissection of the aorta
Severe hypertension
Chronic renal failure
Faulty prosthetic aortic valves

The main contribution of 2DE lies in the identification of the various causes of chronic aortic regurgitation.[45] These include bicuspid aortic valve,[76] a discrete subaortic membrane,[77] generalized dilatation of the aortic root,[46] prolapse of the aortic valve leaflets,[47, 75] vegetations on the aortic valve in bacterial endocarditis,[40, 41] and a defect in the function or attachment of a prosthetic aortic valve.[78, 79]

In summary, M-mode echocardiography, by identifying certain features of chronic aortic regurgitation, mainly fluttering of the mitral valve, left ventricular dilatation, and exaggerated wall motion, has been an invaluable aid in the detection, confirmation, and clinical management of chronic aortic regurgitation. Two-dimensional echocardiography has limited usefulness in the recognition of chronic aortic regurgitation but is more helpful than M-mode echocardiography in the identification of various etiologies of chronic aortic regurgitation.

Clinical Implications

Apart from its diagnostic capabilities, echocardiography has a major role in the clinical assessment of the patient suffering from aortic regurgitation.[80–84]

The critical clinical problem in these patients is knowing when to replace the aortic valve.[81, 82] This decision relies mainly on gradual changes in left ventricular function. Since echocardiography constitutes a noninvasive mode for the assessment of left ventricular function, it has become one of the most valuable instruments in the evaluation of this entity.[81, 84–88] In a serial echocardiographic study of patients with asymptomatic aortic regurgitation, Henry et al.[81] showed that early left ventricular failure is more likely to occur when end-systolic left ventricular dimensions exceed 55 mm or when the percent fractional shortening is less than 25%. On the basis of this[81] and other studies,[82, 85, 86, 89, 90] it is recommended that (1) patients with asymptomatic aortic regurgitation and left ventricular end-systolic diameter of 50 mm and less be examined once a year, (2) those with a left ventricular end-systolic diameter of 50–54 mm be examined once every 4–6 months, and (3) aortic valve replacement be considered in asymptomatic patients whose left ventricular end-systolic diameter is greater than 55 mm (Table 15–3).

Moreover, echocardiography has found its place in the evaluation of the postoperative patient.[82, 83, 91–94] Patients who do not show a marked decrease in left ventricular end-diastolic diameter (11 mm or more) in the early postoperative period after aortic valve replacement seem to have severe myocardial damage, and their prognosis is guarded.[82]

Echocardiography has some limitation in the assessment of left ventricular size and function in chronic aortic regurgitation, as stated by McDonald et al.[88] and others,[83, 84, 95] and should be used only in conjunction with other methods and a general clinical assessment.[84, 88, 90, 95]

TABLE 15–3.—CLINICAL APPLICATIONS OF M-MODE ECHOCARDIOGRAPHY IN CHRONIC AORTIC REGURGITATION

Evaluating effectiveness of medical treatment
Determining optimal time for surgical intervention in asymptomatic patients
Surgery if LVIDs* > 55 mm
4- to 6-month serial M-mode follow-up if LVIDs is 50–54 mm
Every year M-mode follow-up if LVIDs is below 50 mm
Assessing prognosis after operation in symptomatic patients
Evaluating effectiveness of surgery

*LVIDs, left ventricular internal dimension in systole.

ECHOCARDIOGRAPHY IN MITRAL REGURGITATION

Chronic mitral regurgitation may result from a multitude of abnormalities, including abnormalities of the mitral annulus, noncoaptation of the mitral valve leaflets during ventricular systole, elongation of the chordae tendineae, and dysfunction of the papillary muscles or left ventricular myocardium.[96] These clinical entities have distinct clinical, hemodynamic, and echocardiographic characteristics that distinguish them from acute mitral regurgitation or flail mitral leaflet.

Acute, Severe Mitral Regurgitation

The flail mitral valve is the major cause of acute, severe mitral regurgitation (Table 15–4), usually due to rupture of the chordae tendineae.[97] In 50%–70% of cases, chordae tendineae rupture occurs as a spontaneous isolated event in patients with no apparent heart disease.[98, 99] Other common causes of rupture are bacterial endocarditis,[100] rheumatic heart disease,[101] mitral valve prolapse,[102] and left atrial myxoma.[68] Chordal rupture has also been reported in patients with achondroplasia and coexisting atrial septal defect, Ehlers-Danlos syndrome, idiopathic hypertrophic subaortic stenosis, nonbacterial endocarditis, aortic regurgitation, and blunt chest trauma.[68] Patients with spontaneous chordal rupture more often have involvement of the posterior mitral leaflet; patients with secondary chordal rupture from other causes have equal involvement of both leaflets.[97]

TABLE 15–4.—CLASSIFICATION OF ACUTE MITRAL REGURGITATION

Rupture of chordae tendineae
Idiopathic
Bacterial endocarditis
Rheumatic heart disease
Mitral valve prolapse
Left atrial myxoma
Idiopathic hypertrophic subaortic stenosis
Aortic regurgitation
Blunt chest trauma
Achondroplasia with coexistent atrial septal defect
Ehlers-Danlos syndrome
Disorders of papillary muscles
Rupture of papillary muscle
Acute myocardial infarction, usually inferior-posterior wall infarction
Chest trauma
Bacterial endocarditis
Syphilis
Myocardial abscess
Periarteritis nodosa
Altered spatial relationships between papillary muscles and mitral leaflets (e.g., left ventricular dilation)
Intrinsic muscle dysfunction (e.g., coronary artery disease, cardiomyopathy, infiltrative diseases)
Disorders affecting mitral valve leaflets
Perforation (e.g., acute bacterial endocarditis)
Tear (e.g., blunt chest trauma)
Tumor (e.g., left atrial myxoma)
Myxomatous changes (e.g., "floppy valve" syndrome)
Drugs (e.g., methylsergide)
Dysfunction of mitral valve prosthesis

Rupture of the papillary muscles is a less common cause of flail mitral leaflet. It usually occurs as a complication of an acute myocardial infarction.[68] The incidence of this complication in patients with acute myocardial infarction is 0.5%–5%.[103, 104] Chest trauma can also cause rupture of the trabeculated tip of the papillary muscles. Among other causes of acute mitral valve regurgitation, mitral valve fenestration and prosthetic valve malfunction should be mentioned.

Patients with acute mitral regurgitation from any cause generally have severe derangement in left ventricular function and subsequent acute heart failure that usually requires urgent mitral valve replacement.[98, 99]

M-mode Echocardiography

Several M-mode echocardiographic findings suggest the diagnosis of flail mitral valve. Most specific is the occurrence of intracavitary left atrial echoes during systole.[105] These originate presumably from the flail valve or from systolic prolapse of the chordae into the left atrium (Fig 15–10).[106–109] However, similar left atrial echoes can be caused by an atrial clot or myxoma.[9] Mintz et al.,[105] in a series of 26 patients with surgically proved flail mitral valve, reported a sensitivity of 8% and specificity of 100% of left atrial echoes in defining flail mitral valve.

Systolic mitral leaflet fluttering has been reported as a very useful sign of a flail mitral valve.[110–112] This high-frequency fluttering during systole is caused by the high-velocity regurgitant flow across the freely moving leaflet restrained by the remaining intact apparatus.[110] Systolic mitral valve fluttering is characteristic of acute mitral regurgitation caused by both ruptured chordae and fenestration of the mitral valve[110, 111] but is rarely encountered in flail mitral valve caused by the rupture of a papillary muscle.[111] Mintz et al.[105] reported a sensitivity of 24% and specificity of 95% for this echocardiographic sign.

Coarse diastolic fluttering of the involved flail mitral leaflet is a common finding in chordal rupture[107–109, 113, 114] or rupture of a papillary muscle,[115] provided that the valve is pliable.[116] This finding, however, is not specific for flail mitral valve (specificity, 58%; sensitivity, 44%).[105] It is frequently observed in aortic insufficiency[55]; however, here the flutter is usually fine,[51] as opposed to the coarse flutter of the flail leaflet. Left-to-right shunt,[54] severe chronic mitral regurgitation,[105] and atrial flutter or fibrillation[55] can also create fluttering of the mitral valve leaflets.

Paradoxic systolic and diastolic motion of a flail

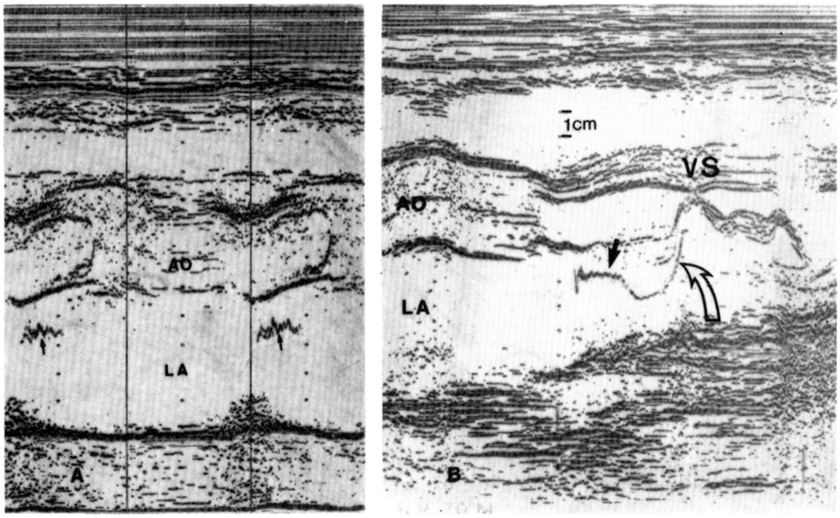

Fig 15–10.—M-mode echocardiographic findings of flail mitral valve. **A,** intracavitary left atrial echoes during ventricular systole *(small arrows);* **B,** paradoxic motion of the flail posterior mitral leaflet during systole *(black arrow)* and diastole *(white arrow). LA,* left atrium; *AO,* aorta; *VS,* ventricular septum.

posterior mitral valve leaflet[117] or chaotic diastolic motion of a flail anterior mitral leaflet[118] are additional findings observed in the setting of ruptured chordae tendineae (see Fig 15–10). When the anterior leaflet is involved, the usual finding is a chaotic, markedly irregular anterior leaflet motion during diastole, so that no two cardiac complexes show exactly the same pattern.[9, 106] When the posterior mitral leaflet is involved, it shows a rapid posterior motion during systole due to the regurgitation of the blood into the left atrium, since it is not held back by the chordae.[9, 113] This echocardiographic pattern of flail posterior mitral leaflet during systole cannot easily be distinguished from marked mitral valve prolapse by M-mode echocardiography[119, 120]; 2DE can be helpful in making this distinction,[56] as will be described later. The tendency of the flail posterior mitral leaflet to move paradoxically during diastole may be confused with the echo pattern of mitral stenosis; in that entity, however, the anterior leaflet also shows an abnormal motion pattern.

Although previous studies of patients with acute mitral regurgitation showed that at least one of the M-mode echocardiographic findings was present,[109, 121] a recent report found that the sensitivity of M-mode echocardiography is only 60% in diagnosing flail mitral valve and that 2DE is distinctly superior for this diagnosis (Table 15–5).[105]

Other echocardiographic findings in patients with acute severe mitral regurgitation are a normal left ventricular size, exaggerated intraventricular septum and posterior wall motion, a normal or only slightly increased left atrium size, and, occasionally, systolic expansion of the posterior left atrial wall.[9, 105]

In summary, the M-mode echocardiographic findings of systolic mitral valve fluttering, systolic left atrial echoes, and paradoxic motion of the involved leaflet are fairly specific but insensitive indicators of the flail mitral valve.

Two-Dimensional Echocardiography

Flair mitral valve due to ruptured chordae tendineae has been detected by 2DE.[56, 114, 116] The most dramatic finding is a characteristic motion of the tip of the affected mitral leaflet beyond the line of the mitral annulus into the left atrium during systole,[114, 122] the so-called snake tongue deformity.[123] The normal coaptation of the mitral leaflets in systole is distorted. These findings are best appreciated in the parasternal long-axis view (Fig 15–11).

Two-dimensional echocardiography is also useful in distinguishing the flail mitral leaflet from a severely prolapsed mitral valve.[56] The maximal abnormal systolic motion of the flail mitral leaflet is at its tip, which points toward the left atrium, and the normal coaptation point of the leaflets is lost (see Fig 15–11). In severe mitral valve prolapse the abnormal systolic motion is maximal at

TABLE 15–5.—STATISTICAL ANALYSIS OF M-MODE AND TWO-DIMENSIONAL ECHOCARDIOGRAPHIC FINDINGS IN FLAIL MITRAL VALVE*

	TP	TN	FP	FN	SENSITIVITY (%)	SPECIFICITY (%)
M-mode echocardiographic findings						
Systolic mitral valve flutter	6	18	1	19	24	95
Diastolic flutter of the involved mitral leaflet	11	11	8	14	44	58
Paradoxic (chaotic) posterior mitral leaflet motion	6	9	1	7	46	90
Systolic left atrium echoes	2	19	0	23	8	100
One or more findings	15	10	9	10	60	53
Two or more findings	7	18	1	18	28	95
Two-dimensional echocardiographic diagnosis	25	16	3	1	96	84

*Findings in 44 patients operated on for pure mitral valve regurgitation, 26 of whom had flail mitral valve. TP, true positive; TN, true negative; FP, false positive; FN, false negative. Data from Mintz et al.[105]

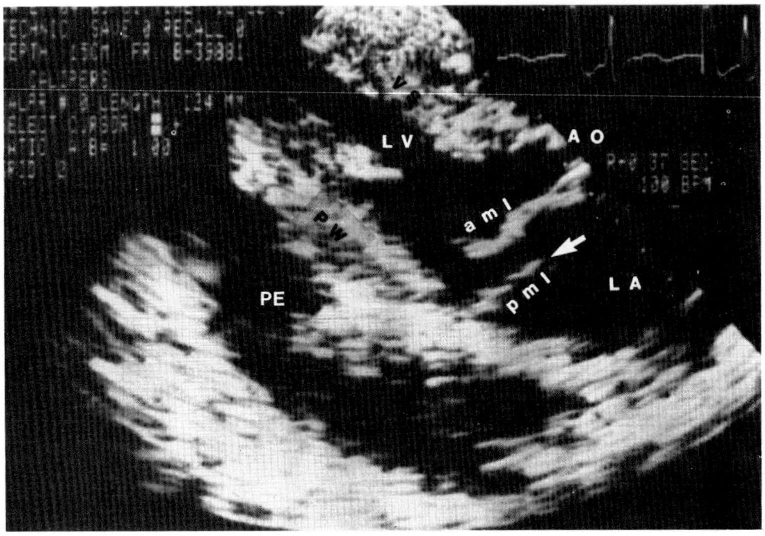

Fig 15–11.—Two-dimensional parasternal long-axis view of the left ventricle in systole showing the features of flail mitral valve. The tip *(arrow)* of the flail posterior mitral leaflet *(pml)* is located superior to the mitral annulus in the left atrial cavity and the normal coaptation point of the mitral leaflets is lost. *LV,* left ventricle; *AO,* aorta; *LA,* left atrium; *aml,* anterior mitral leaflet; *PE,* pericardial effusion.

the body of the leaflet, the tip of the leaflet points toward the left ventricle, and the coaptation of the leaflets remains intact.[56]

Furthermore, 2DE is superior to M-mode echocardiography in the identification of mitral valve vegetations in the presence of flail mitral valve[41, 116] and the detection of ruptured chordae tendineae in the presence of rheumatic heart disease.[56, 124]

Two-dimensional echocardiography has an overall higher sensitivity and specificity as compared to M-mode echocardiography in the diagnosis of flail mitral valve[105] (Table 15–5). False positive 2DE studies can occur in cases of asymmetric chordal elongation or retraction, thus giving the impression of "functionally flail" mitral valve even though the chordae are intact.

In summary, both M-mode echocardiography and 2DE are capable of detecting acute mitral regurgitation due to flail mitral leaflet. Two-dimensional echocardiography is superior to M-mode echocardiography in the detection and especially in the differentiation of the flail leaflet from severe mitral valve prolapse. Thus it provides a reliable and useful noninvasive tool for this acute clinical condition which most often requires rapid surgical intervention.[56, 98, 99]

Chronic Mitral Regurgitation

Several M-mode echocardiographic findings suggest the presence of chronic mitral regurgitation irrespective of its etiology.[9, 125] The various etiological entities of chronic mitral regurgitation can better be identified by 2DE (Table 15–6).[53, 124]

M-mode Echocardiography

A number of M-mode echocardiographic signs suggest chronic mitral regurgitation (Table 15–7).

Mitral valve.—Excessive mitral valve motion and

TABLE 15–6.—ETIOLOGY OF MITRAL REGURGITATION IN 289 PATIENTS IDENTIFIED BY TWO-DIMENSIONAL ECHOCARDIOGRAPHY*

	N	%
Rheumatic heart disease	80	28
Mitral valve prolapse	70	24
Papillary muscle dysfunction	49	17
Flail mitral leaflet	44	15
Mitral annular calcification	15	5
Unknown	12	4
Cleft anterior mitral leaflet	9	3
Idiopathic hypertrophic subaortic stenosis	5	2
Endocarditis	3	1
Left atrial myxoma	2	1

*Data from Kotler et al.[53]

TABLE 15–7.—M-MODE ECHOCARDIOGRAPHIC SIGNS OF CHRONIC MITRAL REGURGITATION COMMON TO ALL ETIOLOGIES

Mitral valve findings
- Excessive mitral valve motion
- Steep EF slope
- Separation of mitral valve leaflets during systole

Interventricular septum
- Exaggerated motion

Left ventricle
- Increased left ventricular dimensions
- Loss of isovolumic contraction—decrease in left ventricular diameter during the pre-ejection period

Left atrium
- Increased diameter
- Systolic expansion of the posterior wall

Aortic valve
- Gradual systolic or early systolic closure of the aortic valve

Aortic wall
- Steep motion of the posterior aortic wall during early systole
- Early onset of downward motion of the posterior wall in diastole

a steep EF slope have been observed in patients with chronic mitral regurgitation.[126–130] However, since this sign can be observed in a variety of other physiologic and pathologic conditions causing an increase in mitral valve flow,[131] it does not constitute a specific finding for chronic mitral regurgitation. Furthermore, in the presence of rheumatic heart disease with fibrosis and limited mitral valve motion, this sign can be abolished even in the presence of severe mitral insufficiency.[131–133]

Noncoaptation of mitral valve leaflets during systole has been occasionally observed in patients with mitral regurgitation[134, 135]; however, the difficulty of identifying the echoes originating from the edges of the mitral valve leaflets and the occasional super-imposition of the chordae tendineae on the mitral valve, in addition to the inherent technical problems of M-mode echocardiography, result in many false positive and negative results. Therefore, this echocardiographic sign is quite unreliable for the diagnosis of chronic mitral regurgitation.[9]

Since echocardiographically detectable aberrations in the motion of the mitral valve itself have not proved useful in the detection of mitral regurgitation, indirect signs of mitral regurgitation have been investigated and described and were found to be more reliable.

Interventricular septum.—Exaggerated septal motion is common in patients with chronic mitral regurgitation.[62, 136, 137] As previously discussed, this sign may also be found in patients with other causes of volume overload of the left ventricle,[64] especially in patients with aortic insufficiency.[62, 63] By observing the exact pattern of interventricular septal motion, differentiation between both entities may be possible. An early exaggerated diastolic dip in septal contraction is frequently found in patients with aortic regurgitation[63] but may be absent in mitral regurgitation.[136] The mechanism of the different septal motion pattern is unclear, and the reliability of this particular sign in distinguishing mitral regurgitation from aortic regurgitation needs further substantiation.

Left ventricle.—Chronic mitral regurgitation is marked by two major features: diastolic overload of the left ventricle and the loss of an isovolumic contraction period due to the incompetence of the mitral valve. M-mode echocardiography demonstrates both features: marked increase in left ventricular diastolic dimensions can be observed, and significant decrease in left ventricular diameter during the pre-ejection phase can be detected.[138] (In the normal heart no significant change in left ventricular diameter during the isovolumic contraction period can be detected.)

Left atrium.—A dilated left atrium and systolic expansion of the posterior left atrial wall have been proposed as useful signs of mitral regurgitation.[139–141] Unfortunately, posterior left atrial wall pulsations are infrequently seen in mitral regurgitation. They probably represent atrioventricular ring motion rather than atrial contraction and are unreliable for the diagnosis of chronic mitral regurgitation.[73] Whether exaggerated left atrial motion seen at the level of the aortic valve instead of at the atrioventricular junction is a more reliable sign of mitral insufficiency[142] is unclear; a similar finding has been noted in normal subjects and in patients with atrial septal defect.[9]

Aortic valve.—Gradual systolic or early systolic closure of the aortic valve has been reported in patients with chronic mitral regurgitation.[140, 143] A gradual closing motion of the aortic valve during systole is characteristic of conditions that entail a late systolic decrease in aortic flow and a marked decrease in cardiac output,[144] and therefore occurs mainly in the late phases of chronic mitral insufficiency. This sign must be differentiated from the abrupt midsystolic closure of the aortic valve, which is characteristic of hypertrophic subaortic stenosis.[145]

Aortic wall.—Abnormalities of the posterior aortic wall have been recently described in patients with mitral regurgitation.[140, 143, 146] A steep motion of the posterior aortic wall during the early, rapid left atrial filling phase[146] and an early onset of downward motion of the posterior aortic wall in diastole[143] have been reported to be indicative of mitral regurgitation. Moreover, by observing the aortic posterior wall[140] or aortic valve motion,[144] various authors have tried to predict the stroke volume and the regurgitant fraction.

In summary, although each of the described M-mode echocardiographic findings in itself is not specific for the diagnosis of chronic mitral regurgitation, the combination of some of these findings in conjunction with the clinical picture usually suggests the diagnosis of chronic mitral regurgitation (see Table 15–7).

Two-Dimensional Echocardiography

Only a few 2DE signs have been proposed as predictive of the actual existence of chronic mitral regurgitation. In patients with severe rheumatic mitral regurgitation, 2DE may be able to record the regurgitant mitral valve orifice in diastole.[147] The usefulness of this observation in the diagnosis of mitral regurgitation due to other causes has not been investigated.

Using the right parasternal approach, Tei et al.[148] have observed an abnormal motion and shape of the interatrial septum in patients with mitral regurgitation. Moreover, the characteristic signs of volume overload in chronic mitral regurgitation—dilated left atrium and left ventricle, hyperdynamic motion of interventricular septum and left ventricular posterior wall—can be readily identified by 2DE.

The main usefulness of 2DE, however, is in establishing the etiologic diagnosis of chronic mitral regurgitation.[45, 53, 124] The relative value and comparison of 2DE and M-mode echocardiography in the identification of the etiologic entities of chronic mitral regurgitation will be examined further.

M-Mode and 2DE Findings in Various Etiologies of Chronic Mitral Regurgitation

Rheumatic heart disease: M-mode echocardiography.—Since mitral stenosis and insufficiency often coexist in rheumatic heart disease,[125] echocardiography of the mitral valve often shows typical signs of mitral stenosis.[53, 131–133] In addition, the combination of mitral stenosis, an enlarged left atrium and left ventricle, and exaggerated motion of the interventricular septum and left ventricular posterior wall is highly suggestive of the coexistence of mitral regurgitation (Table 15–8).

Predominant mitral regurgitation may be suggested by a "ski slope" appearance of the mitral valve and a slight motion of the posterior mitral leaflet in a direction opposite to the anterior leaflet.[73, 125]

The systolic motion of the mitral valve is usually normal in rheumatic mitral regurgitation, thus distinguishing this condition from mitral valve prolapse.

Two-dimensional echocardiographic features.—Kotler et al.,[53] in a series of 80 patients with rheumatic mitral disease confirmed by cardiac catheterization and/or surgery, reported the following

TABLE 15–8.—M-MODE AND TWO-DIMENSIONAL ECHOCARDIOGRAPHIC FINDINGS IN RHEUMATIC MITRAL REGURGITATION*

M-mode echocardiography
Normal to slightly decreased amplitude of mitral valve motion
Varying EF slope ("ski-slope" EF pattern)
Thickened mitral leaflets
Parallel motion of both anterior and posterior leaflets during diastole
Enlarged left ventricle with exaggerated motion of septum and posterior wall
Enlarged left atrium
Two-dimensional echocardiography
Thickened mitral valve leaflets
Obtuse angular bend of the anterior mitral leaflet in diastole
Relatively stationary posterior mitral leaflet
Failure of mitral valve closure in systole
Enlarged left ventricle with hyperdynamic motion of the septum and posterior wall
Enlarged left atrium

*Data from Kotler et al.[53]

2DE criteria for the diagnosis of rheumatic mitral regurgitation: (1) thickened mitral valve leaflets, (2) obtuse angular bend of the anterior mitral leaflet in diastole (better observed on the parasternal long-axis view), (3) relatively immobile posterior mitral leaflet, (4) dilated left atrium and left ventricle, with hyperdynamic septal and posterior wall motion, and (5) in mild mitral regurgitation, a failure of closure of small areas of the medial or lateral aspect of the mitral valve. With respect to the last finding, in severe mitral regurgitation the mitral valve fails to close in the center.[147] Actual recording of the regurgitant mitral orifice in systole requires frame-by-frame analysis of short-axis views and good axial resolution[147]; the reliability of this particular finding for routine clinical use has not been confirmed.

Patients with pure mitral regurgitation generally have only a mild restriction of the anterior mitral leaflet motion[124] and a larger diastolic mitral valve area measurement (usually 3.0 sq cm or greater).[124, 147, 149]

It appears, therefore, that M-mode echocardiography and 2DE are equally reliable for the diagnosis of rheumatic mitral regurgitation.[45]

Mitral valve prolapse.—Although mitral valve prolapse is a common cause of clinical mitral insufficiency, only occasionally is it of hemodynamic significance. Unfortunately, 2DE cannot directly predict the severity of the mitral insufficiency in patients with mitral valve prolapse.[124]

The characteristic M-mode and 2DE criteria for the diagnosis of mitral valve prolapse[150] will be described elsewhere. However, it should be mentioned that 2DE usually can differentiate rheumatic mitral regurgitation from mitral valve prolapse. In parasternal long-axis views, there is normal coaptation of the mitral leaflets during systole in rheumatic mitral regurgitation, whereas in mitral valve prolapse an abrupt posterior and superior buckling of one or both leaflets into the left atrium in systole is observed.[53]

Papillary muscle dysfunction.—The most common cause of papillary muscle dysfunction is coronary artery disease (see chap. 7). Other causes of papillary muscle dysfunction include cardiomyopathy, any cause of left ventricular dilatation, trauma, infiltrative diseases (amyloidosis), Friedreich's ataxia, and endocardial fibrosis.[97] Injury to both papillary muscles or injury involving the left ventricular wall is usually required to cause mitral insufficiency.[151] Injury distorts the normal spatial relations of papillary muscles and thus the structural support of the mitral valve.[152] Selzer et al.[153] reported that papillary muscle dysfunction is the cause of mitral insufficiency in 11% of cases.

Diffuse or segmental abnormalities of left ventricular wall motion adjacent to and involving one or both papillary muscles have been observed on short-axis views.[124] Inferior displacement of the systolic coaptation point of the mitral leaflets into the body of the left ventricle was seen on the long-axis or four-chamber apical views in patients with papillary muscle dysfunction (Fig 15–12).[154] Recently, incomplete closure of a mitral valve leaflet due to scarring or dyskinesis of the papillary muscle has been reported in patients with ischemic heart disease and diffuse cardiomyopathy.[155, 156]

These 2DE findings cannot be used to distinguish papillary muscle dysfunction of coronary artery disease from the dysfunction of a diffuse cardiomyopathy,[124, 155, 156] and they do not necessarily imply the presence of mitral insufficiency caused by papillary muscle dysfunction.[124] They can, however, differentiate between mitral insufficiency due to left ventricular dysfunction (ischemic heart disease, cardiomyopathies) from mitral insufficiency due to valve disease,[45, 124] in which the left ventricular wall motion is usually preserved.

Therefore, the diagnosis of papillary muscle dysfunction can be made indirectly by the clinical recognition of mitral insufficiency, by the echocardiographic detection of wall motion abnormalities, and by the echocardiographic exclusion of other causes of valvular regurgitation.[73]

Mitral annular calcification.—Mitral annular calcification frequently occurs as a degenerative disorder in the aged population.[157] It has also been reported in a multitude of other clinical entities: in Marfan syndrome,[158] mucopolysaccharidosis,[159] rheumatic heart disease,[160] hypercalcemic disorders,[161] chronic renal failure requiring chronic dialysis,[162, 163] calcific valvular aortic stenosis,[164] idiopathic hypertrophic subaortic stenosis[165–167] accelerated atherosclerosis,[161] and mitral valve pro-

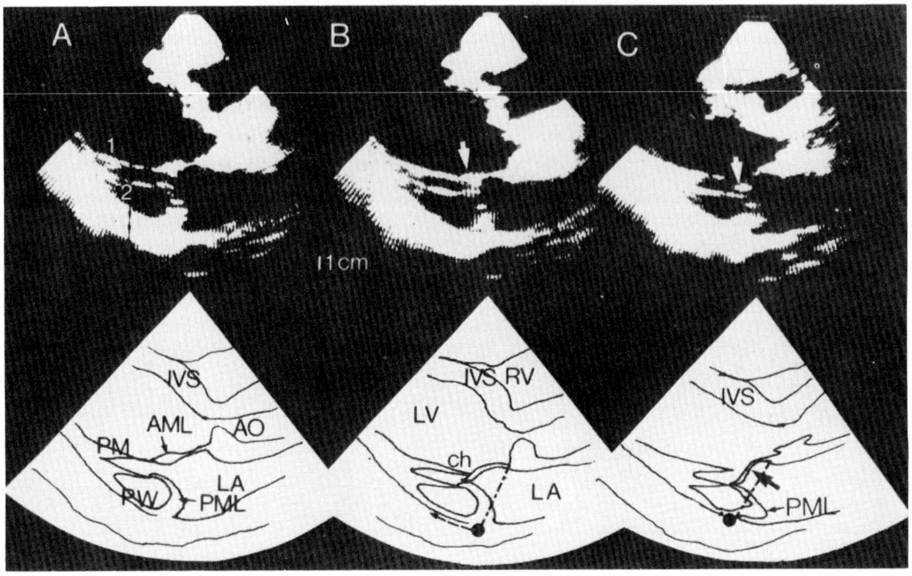

Fig 15–12.—Sequential frames from a 2DE parasternal left ventricular long-axis view and the corresponding schematic diagrams demonstrating the features of papillary muscle dysfunction. *A,* late diastole: the posteromedial papillary muscle *(pm)* and the inferoposterior left ventricular wall are akinetic. *B,* early systole: the point of mitral valve coaptation is abnormally displaced toward the left ventricular cavity *(white arrow). C,* late systole: the anterior mitral leaflet *(aml)* shows a convex bulging into the left ventricle during systole (*large black arrow* in diagram). In contrast, the posterior mitral leaflet *(PML)* prolapses into the left atrium (*small black arrow* in diagram). *IVS,* interventricular septum; *CH,* chordae; *AO,* aorta; *LV,* left ventricle; *LA,* left atrium. (From Ogawa S., et al. Cross-sectional echocardiographic spectrum of papillary muscle dysfunction. *Am. Heart J.* 97:312, 1979. Reproduced by permission.)

lapse.[168, 169] Recently it was suggested that the calcification is not actually in the mitral annulus but in the submitral region between the mitral valve and the posterior left ventricular wall.[170] The calcific process may involve the septum, causing conduction disturbances; however, involvement of the mitral leaflets is rare.[161] Mitral insufficiency is caused by the interference of the annular calcification with the normal mitral leaflet and annular motion. In the series of 289 patients with mitral regurgitation studied by Kotler et al.,[53] mitral annular calcification was the cause in 15 patients (5%).

M-mode echocardiography.—The characteristic pattern of mitral annular calcification is a dense band of echoes posterior to the mitral valve, frequently obscuring the posterior leaflet and moving in parallel to the left ventricular posterior wall.[171–174] These echoes extend from the atrioventricular junction into the body of the left ventricle. Occasionally they extend farther into the left atrium and the aortic valve region.[171] Anterior submitral calcifications are usually located anterior to the anterior mitral leaflet.

Two-dimensional echocardiography.—A dense, crescent-shaped, bright band of echoes between the posterior mitral leaflet and left ventricular posterior wall is observed in the short-axis view in patients with mitral annular calcification,[170] however, the extent of the calcification is better defined by long-axis or apical views. It occasionally extends into both the aortic valve region[171] and the root of the aorta.[175]

The described echocardiographic pattern of mitral annular calcification frequently obscures the posterior mitral leaflet and sometimes prevents a clear recording of the posterior left ventricular wall echoes; thus it can mimic and should be distinguished from pericardial effusion[171] and mitral stenosis.[175, 176] Echocardiography appears to be more sensitive than chest radiography in detecting mitral annular calcification.[172] M-mode or 2DE can be used to recognize the presence of mitral annular calcification.[45]

Cleft mitral valve.—A cleft anterior mitral leaflet is the most common form of congenital mitral insufficiency. It is usually associated with an ostium primum atrial septal defect and represents a type of partial endocardial cushion defect. The cleft mitral valve leaflet is not apparent on M-mode echocardiography. However, in patients with an associated ostium primum atrial septal defect, M-mode echocardiography shows a narrowed left ventricular outflow tract and a prolonged diastolic apposition of the anterior mitral leaflet against the septum.[53] Two-dimensional echocardiography can identify a cleft anterior mitral leaflet as well as the specific type of endocardial cushion defect.[177, 178] The systolic motion of the mitral valve is normal in patients with a cleft mitral valve. The anterior leaflet of the mitral valve, however, splits during diastole, in drawbridge fashion, into two distinct components.[53, 177] The posterior leaflet motion is normal.

Two-dimensional echocardiography is superior to M-mode echocardiography in the recognition of cleft mitral valve.[53]

Idiopathic hypertrophic subaortic stenosis.—Significant mitral regurgitation has been reported in a large percentage of patients with this type of cardiomyopathy.[125] The mechanism of mitral insufficiency is unclear. Suggested mechanisms include the systolic anterior motion of the mitral valve, the abnormal shape of the left ventricle, and misalignment of the anterior papillary muscle.

Mitral vegetations.—Mitral vegetations due to bacterial endocarditis may create chronic mitral regurgitation. The characteristic M-mode pattern of vegetations is a nonuniform, echo-producing "shaggy" mass attached to the mitral leaflet (Fig 15–13). The reported sensitivity of M-mode echocardiography in detecting valvular vegetations in patients with bacterial endocarditis, 34%–55%,[28, 179] is increased in the presence of clinical valvular insufficiency.[180] The 2DE feature of vegetation is the presence of dense, irregular, echo-producing masses attached to the mitral valve (Fig 15–14).

Two-dimensional echocardiography probably is not superior to M-mode echocardiography in the detection of vegetations on a native mitral valve without flail leaflet[43, 116]; however, neither of these two techniques can accurately differentiate between active and healed endocarditis.[53]

Left atrial myxoma.—Repeated prolapse of a left atrial myxoma through the mitral valve orifice can traumatize the mitral valve and create mitral insufficiency.[124] M-mode echocardiography identifies a large mass of echoes prolapsing into the mitral valve from the left atrium.[9] Two-dimensional echocardiography demonstrates a large echo-dense mass moving from the left atrium into the left

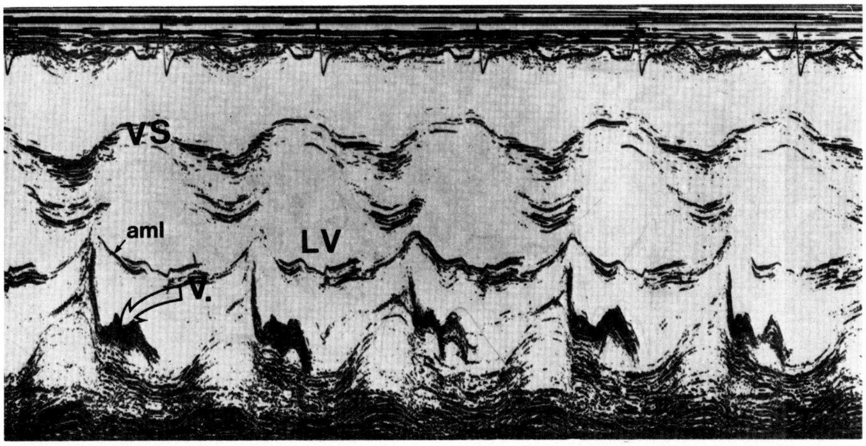

Fig 15–13.—M-mode echocardiogram demonstrating vegetations on the mitral valve *(white arrow)*. *V*, vegetations; *aml*, anterior mitral valve leaflet; *VS*, ventricular septum; *LV*, left ventricle.

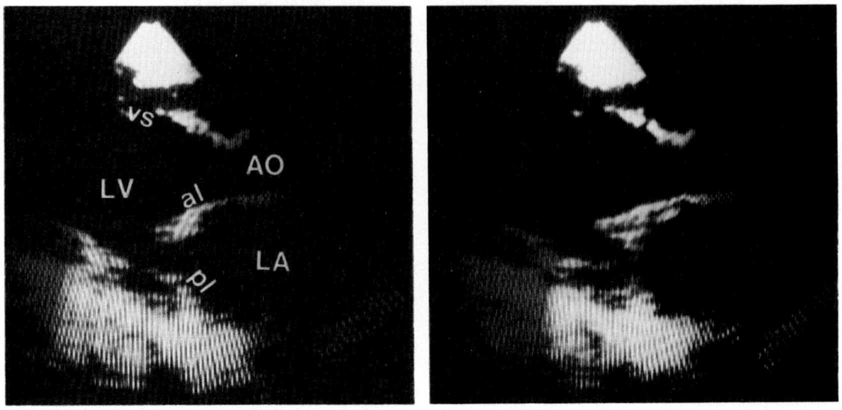

Fig 15–14.—Parasternal 2DE long-axis view of the left ventricle showing vegetations on the mitral valve. A dense, irregular echo-mass is attached to the anterior mitral leaflet *(al)*. *VS,* ventricular septum; *LV,* left ventricle; *AO,* aorta; *LA,* left atrium; *pl,* posterior mitral leaflet.

ventricular inflow tract during late diastole.[53] This technique is superior to M-mode echocardiography in detecting a left atrial myxoma.[45]

Malfunctioning prosthetic mitral valve.—A common complication of prosthetic mitral valves is mitral regurgitation due to abnormal closure of the valve or, more commonly, paravalvular leak. Several investigators have attempted to detect direct signs of mitral regurgitation due to malfunction of a prosthetic mitral valve.[181–184] The direct signs of a malfunctioning mitral prosthesis are (1) a rounding of the early diastolic motion of the disk of a Bjork-Shiley valve at the E-point in a patient with a paravalvular leak;[181] (2) fluttering of the valve leaflets in systole or diastole, or both, which may occur in patients with malfunctioning porcine xenograft valves and mitral insufficiency;[182] (3) dehiscence of a porcine valve in the mitral position with portions of the prosthesis projecting into the left atrium.[183]

The indirect M-mode echocardiographic signs of mitral regurgitation may be more reliable in the recognition of malfunctioning mitral valve prosthesis.[9] The left ventricle, and especially the interventricular septum, will show signs of left ventricular volume overload.[184] A paradoxic septal motion has been observed in most patients who undergo open heart surgery.[71, 185, 186] In patients in whom the septal motion is normal or, in some cases, even exaggerated, mitral regurgitation due to a leaking prosthetic valve should be suspected.[187] The usefulness of 2DE in the evaluation of disk or ball valve prostheses and the detection of mitral insufficiency is not well established.[73] Dislodgment of a Beall valve disk, causing acute severe mitral regurgitation, has been documented.[188] Two-dimensional echocardiography is regarded as superior to M-mode echocardiography in the general assessment of patients with bioprosthetic valves,[78] and more specifically in the detection of mitral regurgitation due to their malfunction.[182]

In summary, both M-mode echocardiography and 2DE are useful in determining the etiology of mitral regurgitation and possibly in differentiating between valvular and myocardial causes of mitral regurgitation. Two-dimensional echocardiography appears to be superior to M-mode echocardiography in the diagnosis of mitral valve prolapse, papillary muscle dysfunction, flail mitral valve, cleft mitral valve, hypertrophic cardiomyopathy, left atrial myxoma, and prosthetic mitral valve.[45, 53] The severity of mitral regurgitation is difficult to quantify with these methods.

Clinical Implications

As pointed out, echocardiography constitutes a noninvasive measure for the detection of acute and chronic mitral regurgitation. Echocardiography was successful in predicting the underlying cause and anatomy in all of 42 patients undergoing mitral valve replacement because of mitral regurgitation, as reported by Ballester et al.[189] The main clinical problem remains the timing of mitral valve replacement and the postoperative prognosis. It seems that the crucial prognostic parameter is the echocardiographically determined left ventricular diameter.[190–192] Schuler et al.[191] reported that patients who have mitral regurgitation, moderate left ventricular dilation, and a normal fractional shortening preoperatively usually have regression of myocardial hypertrophy and only minimal reduction of left ventricular fractional shortening after mitral valve replacement. In contrast, patients with mitral regurgitation who have significant left ventricular dilation (end-diastolic dimension > 70 mm, end-systolic dimension > 50 mm) and a low-normal or decreased fractional shortening preoperatively have further depression of the left ventricular fractional shortening and persistent left ventricular dilation and wall hypertrophy after mitral valve replacement.[191] This postoperative worsening of left ventricular function is due to the partial dependence of left ventricular shortening on the systolic afterload reduction.[191, 193] Cunha et al.[192] have reported similar results and a higher five-year postsurgery mortality in patients with mitral regurgitation who had an M-mode left ventricular end-diastolic dimension greater than 70 mm and end-systolic greater than 50 mm preoperatively.

Persistent left atrial dilatation with associated atrial fibrillation after mitral valve replacement for mitral regurgitation has also been found to indicate higher risk of complications (e.g., systemic emboli) and worse prognosis.[194]

In summary, M-mode echocardiography and 2DE are useful in identifying the etiology of mitral regurgitation, in evaluating left ventricular function in patients with significant mitral regurgitation, and in determining the prognosis after mitral valve replacement.

REFERENCES

1. Morganroth J., et al.: Acute severe aortic regurgitation: Pathophysiology, clinical recognition and management. *Ann. Intern. Med.* 87:223, 1977.
2. Krivokapich J., Chila J., Skorton D.: Flail aortic valve leaflets: M-mode and two-dimensional echocardiographic manifestations. *Am. Heart J.* 99:425, 1980.
3. Botvinick E., et al.: Echocardiographic demonstration of early mitral valve closure in severe aortic insufficiency. *Circulation* 51:836, 1975.
4. Pridie R.B., Benham R., Oakley C.M.: Echocardiography of the mitral valve in aortic valve disease. *Br. Heart J.* 33:296, 1971.
5. Mann T., et al.: Assessing the hemodynamic severity of acute aortic regurgitation due to infective endocarditis. *N. Engl. J. Med.* 293:108, 1975.
6. Fleuji M., et al. : Echocardiography as a method for the determination of the severity of aortic insufficiency. *Schweiz. Med. Wochenschr.* 106:1557, 1976.
7. Oki T., et al.: Echo patterns of the anterior leaflet of the mitral valve in patients with aortic insufficiency. *J. Cardiogr.* 6:307, 1976.
8. Ambrose J.A., et al.: Premature closure of the mitral valve: Echocardiographic clue for the diagnosis of aortic dissection. *Chest* 73:121, 1978.
9. Feigenbaum H.: *Echocardiography*, ed. 2. Philadelphia, Lea & Febiger, 1976.
10. Graige E., Burggraf G.: Atrioventricular valve motion and the first heart sound in complete heart block, abstracted. *Circulation* 49, 50(suppl. III):86, 1974.
11. Auger P., Wigle E.D.: Sudden severe mitral insufficiency. *Can. Med. Assoc. J.* 96:1493, 1967.
12. D'Cruz I., et al.: Flutter of left ventricular structures in patients with aortic regurgitation, with special reference to patients with associated mitral stenosis. *Am. Heart J.* 9:684, 1976.
13. McDonald I.G.: Echocardiographic assessment of ventricular function in aortic valve disease. *Circulation* 53:860, 1976.
14. DeMaria A., et al.: Echocardiography and phonography of acute aortic regurgitation in bacterial endocarditis. *Ann. Intern. Med.* 82:329, 1975.
15. Wray T.M.: Echocardiographic manifestations of flail valve leaflets in bacterial endocarditis. *Circulation* 51:832, 1975.
16. Corrigall D., Strunk B., Popp R.: Phonocardiographic and echocardiographic features of ruptured aortic valvular cusp. *Chest* 69:669, 1976.
17. Fox S., et al.: Echocardiographic diagnosis of acute aortic valve endocarditis and its complications. *Arch. Intern. Med.* 137:85, 1977.
18. Wray T.M.: The variable echocardiographic features in aortic valve endocarditis. *Circulation* 52:658, 1975.
19. Gramiak R., Waag R.C.: *Cardiac Ultrasound*. St. Louis, C.V. Mosby Co., 1975.
20. Estevez C., et al.: Echocardiographic manifestations of aortic cusp rupture in a myxomatous aortic valve. *Chest* 69:685, 1976.
21. Chandraratna P., et al.: Echocardiography of the "floppy" aortic valve. *Circulation* 52:959, 1975.
22. Lee C.C., Das G., Weissler A.: Characteristic echocardiographic manifestations in ruptured aor-

tic valve leaflet, abstracted. *Circulation* 50(suppl. III):144, 1974.
23. Whipple R., et al.: Echocardiographic manifestation of the flail aortic valve leaflet syndrome, abstracted. *Circulation* 52(suppl. II):255, 1975.
24. Gaasch W., Cleveland R.: Echocardiographic examination in aortic regurgitation, subaortic aneurysm and flail aortic leaflet. *Chest* 70:771, 1976.
25. Dillon J.C., et al.: Echocardiographic manifestations of valvular vegetations. *Am. Heart J.* 86:698, 1973.
26. Martinez E.C., Burch G.E., Giles T.D.: Echocardiographic diagnosis of vegetative aortic bacterial endocarditis. *Am. J. Cardiol.* 34:845, 1974.
27. Hirschfeld D.S., Schiller N.: Localization of aortic valve vegetations by echocardiography. *Circulation* 53:280, 1976.
28. Wann L.S., et al.: Echocardiography in bacterial endocarditis. *N.Engl. J. Med.* 295:135, 1976.
29. Roy P., et al.: Spectrum of echocardiographic findings in bacterial endocarditis. *Circulation* 53:474, 1976.
30. Whipple R.L., et al.: Echocardiographic manifestations of flail aortic valve leaflets. *J. Clin. Ultrasound* 5:417, 1977.
31. Chandraratna P.A.N., et al.: Significance of abnormal echoes in left ventricular outflow tract. *Br. Heart J.* 39:381, 1977.
32. Popp R.L., et al.: Echocardiographic findings in discrete subvalvular aortic stenosis. *Circulation* 49:226, 1974.
33. Rothbaum D.A., et al.: Echocardiographic manifestations of right sinus of valsalva aneurysm. *Circulation* 49:768, 1974.
34. Weaver W.F., et al.: Mid-diastolic aortic valve opening in severe acute aortic regurgitation. *Circulation* 55:145, 1977.
35. Pietro D.A., et al.: Premature opening of the aortic valve: An index of highly advanced aortic regurgitation. *J. Clin. Ultrasound* 6:170, 1978.
36. Nanda N.C., Gramiac R., Shah P.M.: Diagnosis of aortic root dissection by echocardiography. *Circulation* 48:506, 1973.
37. Moothart R.W., Spangler R.D., Blount S.G.: Echocardiography in aortic root dissection and dilatation. *Am. J. Cardiol.* 36:11, 1975.
38. Brown O.R., Popp R.L., Kloster F.E.: Echocardiographic criteria for aortic root dissection. *Am. J. Cardiol.* 36:17, 1975.
39. Gilbert B.W., et al.: Two-dimensional echocardiographic assessment of vegetative endocarditis. *Circulation* 55:346, 1977.
40. Wann L.S., et al.: Comparison of M-mode and cross-sectional echocardiography in infective endocarditis. *Circulation* 60:728, 1979.
41. Mintz G.S., et al.: Comparison of two-dimensional and M-mode echocardiography in the evaluation of patients with infective endocarditis. *Am. J. Cardiol.* 43:738, 1979.
42. Yoshikawa J., et al.: Cord-like aortic valve vegetation in bacterial endocarditis: Demonstration by cardiac ultrasonography. *Circulation* 53:911, 1976.
43. Martin R., et al.: Clinical utility of two-dimensional echocardiography in infective endocarditis. *Am. J. Cardiol.* 46:379, 1980.
44. Mardelli T.J., et al.: Cross-sectional echocardiographic detection of aortic ring abscess in bacterial endocarditis. *Chest* 74:576, 1978.
45. Popp R., et al.: Echocardiography: M-mode and two-dimensional methods. *Ann. Intern. Med.* 93:844, 1980.
46. DeMaria A.N., et al.: Identification and localization of aneurysms of the ascending aorta by cross-sectional echocardiography. *Circulation* 59:755, 1979.
47. Mardelli T.J., et al.: Cross-sectional echocardiographic identification of aortic valve prolapse, abstracted. *Circulation* 60(suppl. II):797, 1979.
48. Pepine C.J., et al.: Reversal of premature mitral valve closure by nitroprusside infusion in severe aortic insufficiency: Beat to beat pressure-flow and echocardiographic relationships, abstracted. *Am. J. Cardiol.* 37:161, 1976.
49. Stewart J.A., et al.: Echocardiographic documentation of vegetative lesions in infective endocarditis: Clinical implications. *Circulation* 61:374, 1980.
50. Dillon J.C., et al.: Significance of mitral fluttering in patients with aortic insufficiency, abstracted. *Clin. Res.* 18:304, 1970.
51. Winsberg F., Gabor G.E., Hernberg J.G.: Fluttering of the mitral valve in aortic insufficiency, abstracted. *Circulation* 41:225, 1970.
52. Joyner C.R., Dydra I., Reid J.M.: Behavior of the anterior leaflet of the mitral valve in patients with the Austin-Flint murmur, abstracted. *Clin. Res.* 14:251, 1966.
53. Kotler M., et al.: M-mode and two-dimensional echocardiography in mitral and aortic regurgitation: Pre- and postoperative evaluation of volume overload of the left ventricle. *Am. J. Cardiol.* 46:1144, 1980.
54. Nanda N.C., et al.: Echocardiography of the intra-atrial baffle in dextro-transposition of the great vessels. *Circulation* 51:1130, 1975.
55. Kotler M.N., et al.: Pitfalls and limitations of m-mode echocardiography. *Am. Heart J.* 94:227, 1977.
56. Mintz G.S., et al.: Two-dimensional echocardiographic recognition of ruptured chordae tendineae. *Circulation* 57:244, 1978.
57. Cope G.D., et al.: Diastolic vibration of the interventricular septum in aortic insufficiency. *Circulation* 51:589, 1975.
58. Friedewald V.E., et al.: Oscillations of the interventricular septum in aortic insufficiency, abstracted. *J.Clin. Ultrasound* 2:229, 1974.
59. Fujioka T., et al.: A clinopathological study of aortic regurgitation with septal fluttering on echocardiogram. *J. Cardiogr.* 8:697, 1978.

60. Johnson A.D., Gosink B.B.: Oscillation of left ventricular structures in aortic regurgitation. *J. Clin. Ultrasound* 5:21, 1977.
61. Nakao S., et al.: An experimental study on the mechanism of echocardiographic findings in aortic regurgitation: With special reference to the direction of regurgitant jet, abstracted. *Circulation* 60 (suppl. II):798, 1979.
62. Ajisaka R., et al.: Echocardiographic assessment of left ventricular volume overloading in aortic insufficiency and mitral insufficiency. *J. Cardiogr.* 8:209, 1978.
63. Sheikh M.V., et al.: Echocardiographic demonstration of premature notching of the interventricular septal motion in aortic incompetence, abstracted. *Clin. Res.* 26:271A, 1978.
64. Stone J.M., et al.: The use of ultrasound to detect volume overloads of the left ventricle, abstracted. *Circulation* 40(suppl. III):196, 1969.
65. Levisman J.A.: Echocardiographic diagnosis of mitral regurgitation in congestive cardiomyopathy. *Am. Heart J.* 93:33, 1977.
66. Jacobs J.J., et al.: Detection of left ventricular asynergy by echocardiography. *Circulation* 48:263, 1973.
67. Feizi O., Symons C., Yacoub M.: Echocardiography of the aortic valve: Studies of normal aortic valve, aortic stenosis, aortic regurgitation and mixed aortic valve disease. *Br. Heart J.* 36:341, 1974.
68. Hurst J.W.: Valvular heart disease, in *The Heart*, ed. 4. New York, McGraw-Hill Book Co., 1978, pp. 1022–1043.
69. Radford D.J., et al.: Echocardiographic assessment of bicuspid aortic valves. *Circulation* 53:80, 1976.
70. Salem B.I., Pachacek L.W., Leachman R.D.: Major dehiscence of a prosthetic aortic valve. *Chest* 75:513, 1979.
71. Yoshikawa J., et al.: Abnormal motion of interventricular septum of patients with prosthetic valves. *J. Clin. Ultrasound* 2:265, 1974.
72. Koda J., et al.: Diastolic aortic cusp separation in aortic regurgitation. *J. Cardiogr.* 7:163, 1977.
73. Feigenbaum H.: *Echocardiography*, ed. 3. Philadelphia, Lea & Febiger, 1980.
74. Weyman A.E., et al.: Cross-sectional echocardiography in assessing the severity of valvular aortic stenosis. *Circulation* 52:828, 1975.
75. Shahawy M., et al.: Diagnosis of aortic valvular prolapse by echocardiography. *Chest* 69:411, 1976.
76. Fowles R.E., et al.: Two-dimensional echocardiographic features of bicuspid aortic valve. *Chest* 75:434, 1979.
77. Weyman A.E., et al.: Cross-sectional echocardiography in evaluating patients with discrete subaortic stenosis. *Am. J. Cardiol.* 37:358, 1976.
78. Schapira J.N., Martin R.P., Fowles R.E.: Two-dimensional echocardiographic assessment of patients with bioprosthetic valves. *Am. J. Cardiol.* 43:510, 1979.
79. Mehta A., et al.: Two-dimensional echographic observations in major detachment of a prosthetic aortic valve. *Am. Heart J.* 101:221, 1981.
80. Wilson J., et al.: Non-invasive assessment of load reduction in patients with asymptomatic aortic regurgitation. *Am. J. Med.* 68:664, 1980.
81. Henry W.L., et al.: Observations on the optimum time for operative intervention for aortic regurgitation: Serial echocardiographic evaluation of asymptomatic patients. *Circulation* 61:484, 1980.
82. Henry W.L., et al.: Observations on the optimum time for operative intervention for aortic regurgitation: Evaluation of the results of aortic valve replacement in symptomatic patients. *Circulation* 61:471, 1980.
83. Schuler G., et al.: Serial non-invasive assessment of left ventricular hypertrophy and function after surgical correction of aortic regurgitation. *Am. J. Cardiol.* 44:585, 1979.
84. Johnson A.D., et al.: Assessment of left ventricular function in severe aortic regurgitation. *Circulation* 54:975, 1976.
85. Al-Nouri M., Hellman C., Schmidt D.H.: Echocardiographic indices predictive of early left ventricular dysfunction in patients with aortic regurgitation, abstracted. *Circulation* 60(suppl. II):137, 1979.
86. Henry W.L., et al.: Functional adaptions of the left ventricle to chronic aortic regurgitation, abstracted. *Am. J. Cardiol.* 43:412, 1979.
87. Clark C.E., et al.: Influence of ejection fraction on the results of operation in aortic regurgitation, abstracted. *Circulation* 52(suppl. II):II-169, 1975.
88. McDonald I.G., Jelinek M.V.: Serial M-mode echocardiography in severe chronic aortic regurgitation. *Circulation* 62:1291, 1980.
89. Cunha C.L.P., et al.: Surgery for aortic insufficiency: Value of m-mode echocardiography as a prognostic indicator, abstracted. *Am. J. Cardiol.* 43:406, 1979.
90. Bonow R.O., et al.: Preoperative exercise capacity in symptomatic patients with aortic regurgitation as a predictor of postoperative left ventricular function and long-term prognosis. *Circulation* 62:1280, 1980.
91. Burggraf G.W., Craige E.: Echocardiographic studies of left ventricular wall motion and dimensions after valvular heart surgery. *Am. J. Cardiol.* 35:473, 1975.
92. Gaasch W.H., Andrias W.C., Levine H.J.: Chronic aortic regurgitation: The effect of aortic valve replacement on left ventricular volume, mass and function. *Circulation* 58:825, 1978.
93. Venco A., et al.: Non-invasive assessment of left ventricular function after correction of severe aortic regurgitation. *Br. Heart J.* 38:1324, 1976.
94. Kennedy J.W., Doces J., Stewart D.K.: Left ven-

tricular function before and following aortic valve replacement. *Circulation* 56:944, 1977.

95. Abdulla A., et al.: Limitations of echocardiography in the assessment of left ventricular size and function in aortic regurgitation. *Circulation* 61:148, 1980.
96. Roberts W.C., Perloff J.K.: Mitral valvular disease. *Ann. Intern. Med.* 77:933, 1972.
97. Sanders C.A., et al.: Etiology and differential diagnosis of acute mitral regurgitation. *Prog. Cardiovasc. Dis.* 14:129, 1971.
98. Sanders C.A., et al.: Diagnosis and surgical treatment of mitral regurgitation secondary to ruptured chordae tendineae. *N. Engl. J. Med.* 276:943, 1967.
99. Luther R.R., Meyers S.N.: Acute mitral insufficiency secondary to ruptured chordae tendineae. *Arch. Intern. Med.* 134:568, 1974.
100. Roberts W.C., Braunwald E., Morrow A.G.: Acute severe mitral regurgitation secondary to ruptured chordae tendineae. *Circulation* 33:58, 1966.
101. Hwang W.S., Lam K.L.: Rupture of chordae tendineae during acute rheumatic carditis. *Br. Heart J.* 30:429, 1968.
102. Goodman D., Kimbiris D., Linhart J.W.: Chordae tendineae rupture complicating the systolic click-late systolic murmur syndrome. *Am. J. Cardiol.* 33:681, 1974.
103. Dusall J.C., Pryor R., Blount S.G.: Systolic murmur following myocardial infarction. *Am. Heart J.* 87:577, 1974.
104. Sanders R.J., Neubuerger K.T., Ravin A.: Rupture of papillary muscles: Occurrence of rupture of the posterior muscle in posterior myocardial infarction. *Dis. Chest* 31:316, 1957.
105. Mintz G.S., et al.: Statistical comparison of m-mode and two-dimensional echocardiographic diagnosis of flail mitral leaflets. *Am. J. Cardiol.* 45:253, 1980.
106. Sweatman T., et al.: Echocardiographic diagnosis of mitral regurgitation due to ruptured chordae tendineae. *Circulation* 46:580, 1972.
107. Matsukubo H., et al.: Echocardiographic findings of vegetation and ruptured chordae tendineae: Two cases of bacterial endocarditis. *Cardiovasc. Sound Bull.* 5:717, 1975.
108. Terasawa Y., et al.: Ultrasono-cardiotomogram and ultrasound cardiogram of mitral regurgitation due to ruptured chordae tendineae. *J. Cardiogr.* 8:349, 1978.
109. Humphries W.C., et al. : Echocardiographic equivalents of a flail mitral leaflet. *Am. J. Cardiol.* 40:802, 1977.
110. Meyer J.F., et al.: Systolic mitral flutter, an echocardiographic clue to the diagnosis of ruptured chordae tendineae. *Am. Heart J.* 93:3, 1977.
111. Jamal N., Winters W., Nelson J.: Echocardiographic features of flail mitral valve leaflets: Ruptured chordae tendineae versus ruptured papillary muscle, abstracted. *Circulation* 58 (suppl. II):43, 1978.
112. Sze K.C., Nanda N.C., Gramiak R.: Systolic flutter of the mitral valve. *Am. Heart J.* 96:157, 1978.
113. Duchack J.M., Chang S., Feigenbaum H.: Echocardiographic features of torn chordal tendineae, abstracted. *Am. J. Cardiol.* 29:260, 1972.
114. Nishimura T., et al.: Two-dimensional echocardiographic findings in ruptured chordae tendineae of the mitral valve. *J. Cardiogr.* 8:589, 1978.
115. Ahmad S., et al.: The echocardiographic diagnosis of rupture of a papillary muscle. *Chest* 73:232, 1978.
116. Ogawa S., Mardelli T.J., Hubbard F.E.: The role of cross-sectional echocardiography in the diagnosis of flail mitral leaflet. *Clin. Cardiol.* 1:85, 1978.
117. Burge J., et al.: Echocardiographic findings in different types of mitral regurgitation. *Circulation* 48:97, 1973.
118. Giles T.D., Burch G.E., Martinez E.C.: Value of exploratory "scanning" in the echocardiographic diagnosis of ruptured chordae tendineae. *Circulation* 49:678, 1974.
119. DeMaria A.N., et al.: The variable spectrum of echocardiographic manifestations of the mitral valve prolapse syndrome. *Circulation* 50:33, 1974.
120. Ogawa S., et al.: Flail mitral valve in rheumatic heart disease. *Chest* 74:88, 1978.
121. Child J.S., et al.: Cross-sectional and m-mode echocardiographic features of flail mitral leaflets, abstracted. *Am. J. Cardiol.* 43:411, 1979.
122. Child J.S., et al.: M-mode and cross-sectional echocardiographic features of flail posterior mitral leaflets. *Am. J. Cardiol.* 44:1383, 1979.
123. Winters W.L., et al.: Flail mitral valve leaflet: Improved diagnostic accuracy with a specific two-dimensional echocardiographic sign, abstracted. *Circulation* 60(suppl. II):25, 1979.
124. Mintz G.S., et al.: Two-dimensional echocardiographic evaluation of patient with mitral insufficiency. *Am. J. Cardiol.* 44:670, 1979.
125. DeMaria A.N., et al.: Mitral valve disease revisited. *Cardiovasc. Clin.* 9:59:84, 1978.
126. Effert S., Erkens H., Grossebrockhoff F.: Ultrasonic echo method in cardiological diagnosis. *Cerm. Med. Mth.* 2:325, 1957.
127. Edler I., et al.: Ultrasound cardiography. *Acta Med. Scand.* 370(suppl.):68, 1961.
128. Joyner C.R., Reid J.M.: Application of ultrasound in cardiology and cardiovascular physiology. *Prog. Cardiovasc. Dis.* 5:482, 1963.
129. Kim H., et al.: An attempt to correlate the mitral valve echogram with the hemodynamics of patients with pure mitral insufficiency. *Jpn. Circ. J.* 37:403, 1973.
130. Segal B.L., Likoff W., Kingsley B.: Echocardiography: Clinical application in mitral regurgitation. *Am. J. Cardiol.* 19:50, 1967.
131. Edler I.: Mitral valve function studied by the ul-

trasound endomethod, in *Diagnostic Ultrasound: Proceedings of the First International Conference*. New York, Plenum Press, 1966.
132. Winters W.L., Haler J., Soloff L.A.: Abnormal mitral valve motion as demonstrated by the ultrasound technique in apparent pure mitral insufficiency. *Am. Heart J.* 77:196, 1969.
133. Konstaninou B.A., et al.: Echocardiographic diagnosis of rheumatic mitral valve insufficiency. *Kardiologiia* 17:28, 1977.
134. Burgess J., et al.: Echocardiographic findings in different types of mitral regurgitation. *Circulation* 48:97, 1973.
135. Millward D.K., McLaurin L.P., Craige E.: Echocardiographic studies of the mitral valve in patients with congestive cardiomyopathy and mitral regurgitation. *Am. Heart J.* 85:413, 1973.
136. Fujino T., et al.: Echocardiographic abnormal motion of interventricular septum in mitral insufficiency. *J. Cardiogr.* 6:613, 1976.
137. Rosenblatt A., et al.: Echocardiographic assessment of the level of cardiac compensation in valvular heart disease. *Circulation* 54:509, 1976.
138. Chandraratna P.A.N., Ulahovich G., Aronow W.S.: Echocardiographic study of significance of left ventricular minor axis shortening during pre-ejection phase of systole. *Br. Heart J.* 41:392, 1979.
139. Patton R., et al.: The posterior left atrial echocardiogram of mitral regurgitation. *Circulation* 57:1134, 1978.
140. Yorozu T., et al.: Echocardiographic estimation of stroke volume and mitral regurgitant volume using new parameter from aortic posterior wall motion. *J. Cardiogr.* 8:473, 1978.
141. Sasse L.: Echocardiography of left atrial wall. *J.A.M.A.* 228:1667, 1974.
142. Anonymous: Ultrasound cardiography in the diagnosis of mitral insufficiency. *China Med. J.* 3:164, 1973.
143. Reeves W.C., Nanda N.C., Gramiak R.: The relationship between aortic valve closure and aortic root motion. *Radiology* 127:751, 1978.
144. Yeh H.C., Winsberg F., Mercer E.M.: Echocardiographic aortic valve orifice dimension: Its use in evaluating aortic stenosis and cardiac output. *J. Clin. Ultrasound* 1:182, 1973.
145. Shah P.M., et al.: Role of echocardiography in diagnostic and hemodynamic assessment of hypertrophic subaortic stenosis. *Circulation* 44:891, 1971.
146. Hall R.J.C., Clarke S.E., Brown D.: Evaluation of posterior aortic wall echogram in diagnosis of mitral valve disease. *Br. Heart J.* 41:522, 1979.
147. Wann L.S., et al.: Cross-sectional echocardiographic detection of rheumatic mitral regurgitation. *Am. J. Cardiol.* 41:1258, 1978.
148. Tei C., et al.: Real-time cross-sectional echocardiographic evaluation of the interatrial septum by right atrium-interatrial septum-left atrium direction of ultrasound beam. *Circulation* 60:539, 1979.
149. Nimura Y., et al.: Causes of mitral regurgitation and ultrasonocardiotomographic approaches. *J. Cardiogr.* 6:237, 1976.
150. Gilbert B.W., et al.: Mitral valve prolapse: Two-dimensional echocardiographic and angiographic correlation. *Circulation* 54:716, 1976.
151. Mittal A.K., et al.: Combined papillary muscle and left ventricular wall dysfunction as a cause of mitral regurgitation. *Circulation* 44:174, 1971.
152. Burch G.E., DePasquale N.P., Phillips J.H.: The syndrome of papillary muscle dysfunction. *Am. Heart J.* 75:399, 1968.
153. Selzer A., Katayama F.: Mitral regurgitation: Clinical patterns, pathophysiology and natural history. *Medicine* 51:337, 1972.
154. Ogawa S., et al.: Cross-sectional echocardiographic spectrum of papillary muscle dysfunction. *Am. Heart J.* 97:312, 1979.
155. Godley R.W., et al.: Patterns of mitral leaflet motion in patients with probable papillary muscle dysfunction, abstracted. *Am. J. Cardiol.* 43:411, 1979.
156. Godley R.W., et al.: Relation of incomplete mitral leaflet closure to the site of dyssynergy in patients with papillary muscle dysfunction, abstracted. *Circulation* 60 (suppl. II):204, 1979.
157. Simon M.A., Liu S.F.: Calcification of the mitral annulus and its relation to functional valvular disturbance. *Am. Heart J.* 48:497, 1954.
158. Crossman M., Knott A.P., Jacoby W.J.: Calcified annulus fibrosus with mitral insufficiency with Marfan's syndrome. *Arch. Intern. Med.* 121:561, 1968.
159. Schieken R.M., et al.: Cardiac manifestation of the mucopolysaccharides. *Circulation* 43:700, 1975.
160. Cruickshank B.: Heart lesions in rheumatic disease. *J. Pathol. Bacteriol.* 76:223, 1958.
161. Roberts W.G., Dangel J.C., Bulkley B.H.: Nonrheumatic valvular cardiac disease. *Cardiovasc. Clin.* 5:333–466, 1973.
162. Schott C.R., et al.: Echocardiographic spectrum in chronic renal failure. *Circulation* 54 (suppl. II):221, 1976.
163. Terman D.S., et al.: Cardiac calcification in uremia: A clinical biochemical and pathologic study. *Am. J. Med.* 50:744, 1971.
164. Roberts W.C., Perloff J.K., Constantinos R.: Severe valvular aortic stenosis in patients over 65 years of age: A clinicopathologic study. *Am. J. Cardiol.* 27:497, 1971.
165. Tajik A.J., et al.: Mitral valve and/or annulus calcification associated with idiopathic hypertrophic subaortic stenosis (IHSS). *Circulation* 46(suppl. II):228, 1972.
166. Tajik A.J., et al.: Idiopathic hypertrophic subaortic stenosis: Long-term surgical follow-up. *Am. J. Cardiol.* 34:815, 1974.

167. Kronzon I., Classman E.: Mitral ring calcification in idiopathic hypertrophic subaortic stenosis. *Am. J. Cardiol.* 42:60, 1978.
168. McLean J., et al.: The echocardiographic association of mitral valve prolapse and mitral annulus calcification. *Clin. Cardiol.* 2:220, 1979.
169. Fulkerson P.K., et al.: Calcification of the mitral annulus: Etiology, clinical associations, complications, and therapy. *Am. J. Med.* 66:967, 1979.
170. D'Cruz I., et al.: Submitral calcification or sclerosis in elderly patients: M-mode and two-dimensional echocardiography in "mitral annulus calcification." *Am. J. Cardiol.* 44:31, 1979.
171. Dashkoff N., et al.: Echocardiographic features of mitral annulus calcification. *Am. Heart J.* 94:585, 1977.
172. Schott C.R., et al.: Mitral annular calcification: Clinical and echocardiographic correlations. *Arch. Intern. Med.* 137:1143, 1977.
173. Howard P.F., et al.: The echocardiographic diagnosis of calcified mitral annulus. *Am. J. Med.* 273:267, 1977.
174. Curati W.L., Petitclerc R., Winsberg F.: Ultrasonic features of mitral annulus calcification: A report of 21 cases. *Radiology* 122:215, 1977.
175. Gabor G.E., et al.: Echocardiographic and clinical spectrum of mitral annular calcification. *Am. J. Cardiol.* 38:836, 1976.
176. D'Cruz I.A., et al.: Clinical manifestations of mitral annulus calcification, with emphasis on its echocardiographic features. *Am. Heart J.* 94:367, 1977.
177. Hagler D.J., et al.: Real-time phased array 80° sector echocardiography: Atrioventricular canal defects, abstracted. *Circulation* 56(suppl. III):42, 1977.
178. Fisher D.J., et al.: Evaluation of endocardial cushion defects by phased array sector scanner. *Am. J. Cardiol.* 41:353, 1978.
179. Thompson K., Nanda N., Gramiak R.: The reliability of echocardiography in the diagnosis of infective endocarditis, abstracted. *Circulation* 54(suppl. II):11–112, 1976.
180. Andy J.J., et al.: Echocardiographic observation in opiate addicts with active infective endocarditis. *Am. J. Cardiol.* 40:17, 1977.
181. Bernal-Ramirez J.A., Phillips J.H.: Echocardiographic study of malfunction of the Bjork-Shiley prosthetic heart valve in the mitral position. *Am. J. Cardiol.* 40:449, 1977.
182. Alam M., et al.: M-mode and two-dimensional echocardiographic features of porcine valve dysfunction. *Am. J. Cardiol.* 43:502, 1979.
183. Brown J.W., et al.: Late spontaneous disruption of a porcine xenograft mitral valve: Clinical, hemodynamic, echocardiographic, and pathological findings. *J. Thorac. Cardiovasc. Surg.* 75:606, 1978.
184. Miller H.C., Gibson D.G., Stephen J.D.: Role of echocardiography and phonocardiography in the diagnosis of mitral paraprosthetic regurgitation with Starr-Edwards prostheses. *Br. Heart J.* 35:1217, 1973.
185. Kerber R.E., Doty D.B.: Abnormalities of interventricular septal motion following cardiac surgery: Cross-sectional echocardiographic studies. *Am. J. Cardiol.* 41(suppl. II):96, 1978.
186. Yoshikawa J., et al.: Abnormal motion of interventricular septum in patients with prosthetic valve. *Cardiovasc. Sound Bull.* 5:211, 1976.
187. Miller H.C., Stephens J.D., Gibson D.G.: Echocardiographic features of mitral Starr-Edwards paraprosthetic regurgitation. *Br. Heart J.* 35:560, 1973.
188. Chen C.C., Pauletto F.J., Morganroth J.: Real-time echocardiographic identification of an embolized disc from a ball mitral valve prosthesis. *Chest* 81:108, 1982.
189. Ballester M., et al.: Two-dimensional echocardiographic (2DE) findings with surgical correlation in mitral regurgitation, abstracted. *Circulation* 62:III–19, 1980.
190. McDonald I.G.: Echocardiographic assessment of left ventricular function in mitral valve disease. *Circulation* 53:865, 1976.
191. Schuler G., et al.: Temporal response of left ventricular performance to mitral valve surgery. *Circulation* 59:1218, 1979.
192. Cunha C.L.P., et al.: Preoperative m-mode echocardiography as a predictor of surgical results in chronic mitral insufficiency, abstracted. *Am. J. Cardiol.* 45:442, 1980.
193. Wong C.Y.H., Spotnitz H.M.: Systolic and diastolic properties of the human left ventricle during valve replacement for chronic mitral regurgitation. *Am. J. Cardiol.* 47:40, 1981.
194. Sherrid M.V., Clark R.D., Cohn K.: Echocardiographic analysis of left atrial size before and after operation in mitral valve disease. *Am. J. Cardiol.* 43:171, 1979.

RADIONUCLIDE IMAGING

Richard A. Wilson and Charles A. Boucher

RADIONUCLIDE ANGIOGRAPHY is a noninvasive way to assess ventricular size and function in patients with aortic or mitral valve regurgitation, or both. Blood pool imaging is particularly well suited for studying these patients because the structures with large blood pools—aorta, left ventricle, and left atrium—in left ventricular volume overload are clearly visualized. Because of their size, these blood pools may be difficult to image in their entirety using ultrasound and contrast angiographic methods. This chapter reviews the use of radionuclide angiography in these disorders in terms of qualitative findings, quantitation of the volume overload, quantitation of left ventricular function, and the clinical utility of radionuclide imaging.

Aortic and mitral regurgitation differ from valvular stenosis in the variety of etiologies that may produce the regurgitation.[1, 2] As a result, the time course of the regurgitation may vary considerably from patient to patient. There may be acute regurgitation due to endocarditis or there may be chronic rheumatic regurgitation. Acute regurgitation differs from chronic regurgitation in clinical findings, hemodynamic findings, patient management, and radionuclide findings. Although this chapter does not examine the clinical and pathologic findings of valvular regurgitation, an appreciation of the numerous possible etiologies and variable chronicity of regurgitation is important in understanding its hemodynamic effects and must be considered when interpreting radionuclide images.

QUALITATIVE FINDINGS

Aortic Regurgitation

In most patients with aortic regurgitation, the left ventricle is dilated and thickened. An example of a blood pool scan in a patient with aortic regurgitation is shown in Figure 16–1. Hypertrophy appears as an area of diminished activity surrounding the left ventricular blood pool. Although this silhouette may be due to either a thickened myocardial wall or a pericardial or left pleural effusion, thickening of the septum in the left anterior oblique view is specific for left ventricular hypertrophy.

The total stroke volume (more precisely, stroke counts) of the left ventricle is strikingly larger than the stroke volume of the right ventricle (assuming no left-to-right shunting or tricuspid or pulmonary valve regurgitation). This increased stroke volume is necessary to maintain an adequate net forward cardiac output[3] and reflects the magnitude of the regurgitation. The end-diastolic volume also enlarges in response to the volume overload, and therefore stroke volume relative to end-diastolic volume (ejection fraction) is usually normal or depressed.[3]

In aortic regurgitation the ascending aorta may appear dilated. Dilation may be secondary to the valve disorder or may be primary if an aortic root

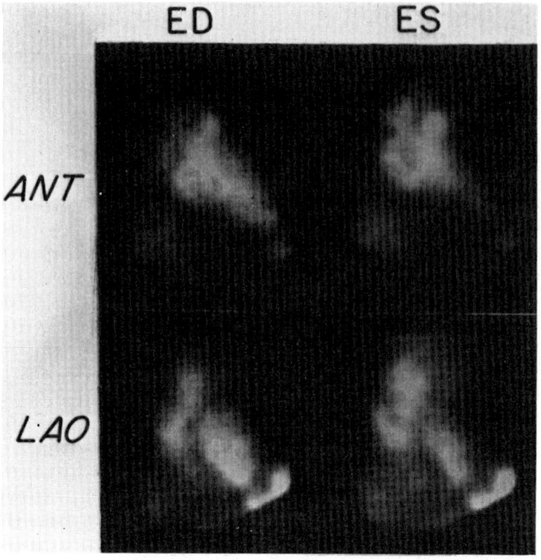

Fig 16–1.—Anterior *(ANT)* and left anterior oblique *(LAO)* end-diastolic *(ED)* and end-systolic *(ES)* views in a 54-year-old woman with severe aortic regurgitation.

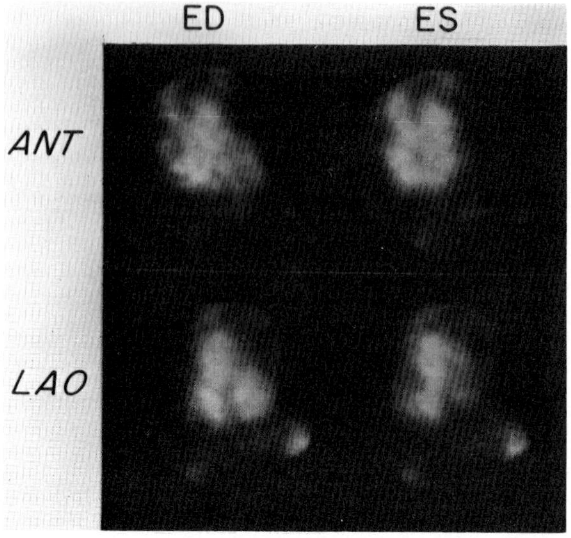

Fig 16–2.—Anterior *(ANT)* and left anterior oblique *(LAO)* end-diastolic *(ED)* and end-systolic *(ES)* views in a 65-year-old man with severe mitral regurgitation.

disease such as cystic medial necrosis, giant cell aortitis, syphilis, Marfan syndrome, or aortic dissection is present. Because the extent and pattern of the aortic dilation are easily appreciated on the scan and are different in primary and secondary regurgitation, the scan may suggest a particular cause for the aortic regurgitation. In addition, the pulsatile motion of the ascending aorta may be prominent on the gated blood pool images and so may aid in the assessment of the severity of the aortic regurgitation.

Mitral Regurgitation

There are unique findings in mitral regurgitation on the blood pool images (Fig 16–2). As in aortic regurgitation, a large, dilated, but normally contracting left ventricle is usually present. The stroke volume is elevated and the ejection fraction is usually normal.[4, 5] The left ventricular wall thickness may be increased, but hypertrophy is usually not as dramatic as in aortic regurgitation.[6]

Increased left atrial size often accompanies chronic mitral regurgitation. The appendage of an enlarged left atrium may be seen on the conventional anterior or left anterior oblique views, but since the left atrium is a posterior structure, it is best appreciated on the left posterior oblique view. And since elevated left atrial pressure may impose a burden on the right ventricle, the right heart may also be affected in mitral regurgitation. The right ventricle and pulmonary artery may be dilated, and right ventricular contraction may be reduced. Occasionally there is secondary tricuspid regurgitation, which is visualized on a gated first-pass radionuclide study as systolic reflux into the inferior vena cava during right ventricular systole.[7]

The findings in either aortic or mitral regurgitation tend to be less dramatic when the valvular regurgitation is acute. There is little time for aortic or left atrial dilation. The left ventricle tends to be only moderately dilated and the contraction almost always remains vigorous because the left ventricle is relatively noncompliant. Such patients will present in severe congestive heart failure before there is reduction in left ventricular contraction.

Occasionally, severe left ventricular dysfunction develops in a patient with left ventricular volume overload, evident as a large, round, poorly contracting left ventricle on the scan.[8] In these patients, regional left ventricular wall motion abnormalities, particularly at the left ventricular apex, may be seen in chronic left ventricular volume overload, without coronary artery disease.[9] Thallium 201 imaging may be useful in identifying previous myocardial infarction in this setting.

QUANTITATION OF THE VOLUME OVERLOAD

Quantitation of the severity of the left ventricular volume overload may be possible using radionuclide angiography.[10–15] Rigo et al.[10] suggested that the severity of aortic and mitral valve regurgitation may be determined from the left anterior oblique equilibrium gated blood pool image by quantitating the relative left-to-right ventricular stroke volumes (left ventricular end-diastolic minus end-systolic counts/right ventricular end-diastolic minus end-systolic counts). Assuming that there is no tricuspid or pulmonic regurgitation or left-to-right shunting, the difference in stroke counts between left and right ventricles should reflect the regurgitant volume. An alternative way of expressing the left and right ventricular stroke counts inequality is by the regurgitant fraction (left ventricular stroke counts minus right ventricular stroke counts/left ventricular stroke counts).

All methods of determining right and left ventricular stroke counts use a left anterior oblique (40–45 degree) projection. This view permits separation of the right and left ventricles. In one technique, regions of interest are drawn over the left and right ventricle by visual inspection, with special attention given to exclusion of areas which increase activity during ventricular systole, such as the atria, aorta, and pulmonary artery. The end-systolic and end-diastolic frames are selected separately for the right and left ventricle, based on the individual time-activity curves. A fixed region of interest is used for both systole and diastole, and since only absolute change in counts is of interest, background subtraction is not performed.

There are several methodological problems with this approach. These include a different degree of atrial overlap for the two ventricles and difficulty in defining the ventricular edges next to the atria and great vessels. In one study, Bough et al. used a 30-degree slant-hole collimator in an attempt to improve atrial and ventricular separation.[11] These authors also used a frame subtraction method to assist in delineation of ventricular borders: subtraction of end-systolic from end-diastolic frames produced a ventricular stroke volume image, and to delineate atrial volume changes, the end-diastolic frame was subtracted from the end-systolic frame. These two subtraction images—ventricular stroke volume and atrial volume—were then superimposed to obtain a composite functional image that improved definition of atrioventricular borders and ventricular regions, especially the right ventricular conus. This composite image was then used as a guide for drawing the right and left ventricular regions of interest. In another study, Lam et al. used a caudal tilt of the camera to improve atrioventricular separation, as well as a subtraction method similar to that used by Bough et al., with the addition of simultaneous display of end-diastolic, end-systolic, and subtraction images and a double cursor technique for outlining the ventricle.[12] The extent to which these adjustments overcome the methodological problems remains unclear.

Table 16–1 summarizes the previously reported studies of the quantitation of the left ventricular overload. All investigators used a left anterior oblique projection and few subtracted background in determining relative right and left ventricular stroke counts. Imaging techniques varied slightly among the studies. In these studies the mean value for regurgitant index in normal subjects was above the true value of unity. These systematically higher values were due to either underestimation of right ventricular stroke counts or overestimation of left ventricular stroke counts, or both. Relatively more attenuation of counts within the right ventricle may be partially responsible, although there are other potential artifacts, such as (1) inclusion of more atrial counts in the right ventricular than in the left ventricular region of interest (especially within a fixed region of interest throughout the cardiac cycle) and (2) exclusion of a portion of the right

TABLE 16–1.—GATED RADIONUCLIDE ANGIOGRAPHIC QUANTITATION OF MITRAL AND AORTIC REGURGITATION BY REGURGITANT INDEX*

STUDY	COLLIMATOR	CAUDAL TILT	RANGE OF NORMAL VALUES	2 SD UPPER LIMIT OF NORMAL	RANGE OF REGURGITANT VALUES	SENSITIVITY†	SPECIFICITY‡	CORRELATION WITH CATHETERIZATION
Rigo et al.[10]	Parallel-hole	No	. . .	1.45	1.36–5.30	18/19 (95%)	. . .	. . .
Bough et al.[11]	30-degree slant-hole	No	. . .	1.20	1.13–3.49	24/25 (95%)	18/18 (100%)	0.87
Lam et al.[12]	Parallel-hole	Yes	0.9–2.9	1.94	0.90–12.00	. . .	. . .	. . .
Urquhart et al.[13]	Parallel-hole	No	0.99–1.49	1.62	1.84–6.73	10/10 (100%)	. . .	0.95
Kress et al.[14]	Parallel-hole	No	1.07–1.49	1.66	1.18–6.55	. . .	. . .	0.75
Sorensen et al.[15]	Parallel-hole	No	0.84–1.23	1.30	1.22–5.56	28/30 (93%)	19/20 (95%)	0.85

*Regurgitant index (stroke index ratio; stroke volume ratio) = LV stroke counts/RV stroke counts = LV end-diastolic − LV end-systolic counts/RV end-diastolic − RV end-systolic counts.

†Number of patients with regurgitation with values above the 2 SD upper limit of normal.

‡Number of normal subjects with values below the 2 SD lower limit of values in patients with regurgitation.

ventricular outflow tract. On the other hand, inclusion of counts due to left atrial enlargement (as could be seen in mitral regurgitation) would tend to decrease the left ventricular stroke counts, since the left atrium increases in counts during left ventricular systole. This effect, although more marked in mitral regurgitation, may also be a source of error in aortic regurgitation or in the normal left ventricle.[7] A more precise measurement of stroke volume index may be possible with transverse section imaging because this method may overcome some of the atrial contamination and background problems inherent in the two-dimensional approach.

The 2 SD range of regurgitant index values in normal subjects is large enough so that there is significant overlap with values in patients with left-sided volume overload, particularly mild regurgitation. Therefore the regurgitant index is not a reliable way to detect patients with mild left ventricular volume overload. Although quantitation of the volume overload by radionuclide angiography correlates with quantitative assessment at cardiac catheterization, and although there are significant differences in mean regurgitant index values in patients with different grades of severity of left ventricular volume overload, there is considerable overlap in these values. Therefore, there may be difficulties in comparing one patient to another. A more precise application of this technique is the serial evaluation of the same patient because systematic errors in the calculation of the regurgitant index are likely to be constant for an individual patient. This approach may be useful in identifying patients with residual left-sided regurgitation after valve replacement.[13] Intraobserver and interobserver variability using these techniques appear to be low, despite the time and expertise required to derive these values.[10, 13]

Thus, the clinical role of radionuclide quantitation of left ventricular volume overload includes confirmation of the presence of severe left ventricular overload and detection of changes in severity of left-sided regurgitation. Although these findings may be of interest and may provide important physiologic information, their importance in terms of clinical management remains to be demonstrated.

QUANTITATION OF VENTRICULAR FUNCTION

Since aortic or mitral valve regurgitation has an important impact on left ventricular function, assessment of left ventricular function is the most useful aspect of radionuclide imaging in patients with aortic and mitral regurgitation. Although patients with acute regurgitation tend to have well preserved function, some patients with chronic regurgitation develop a severe reduction in function, even after apparently successful valve surgery, which has important prognostic implications.[16] This section reviews the changes in ventricular function to be anticipated in valvular regurgitation and analyzes the effects of two interventions, exercise and valve replacement, on ventricular function as assessed by radionuclide angiography.

The increased stroke volume in chronic aortic or mitral regurgitation is maintained by an increase in end-diastolic volume (preload) and the Starling effect. As a result, the ejection fraction is usually normal and rarely above normal.[4–5, 9, 17–20] The ventricular enlargement is associated with a change in the pressure-volume relationship of the left ventricle.[18–27] End-diastolic pressure is often normal despite the increased end-diastolic volume, suggesting increased left ventricular compliance. In chronic aortic regurgitation, signs and symptoms of pulmonary congestion associated with increased end-diastolic volume or pressure are present only when a reduction in left ventricular ejection fraction has occurred.[18, 28–30] In contrast, in the setting of acute volume overload, compliance changes have not yet occurred, and end-diastolic pressure rises dramatically even with a normal ejection fraction.[6, 31–34] Patients with acute (symptoms for less than three months) valve regurgitation due to infectious endocarditis tend to manifest pulmonary congestive symptoms at lower regurgitant volumes than patients with more chronic regurgitation, because the left ventricle is less compliant in the former.

In contrast to aortic regurgitation, congestive pulmonary symptoms appear earlier in mitral regurgitation as a result of increased left atrial pressure directly due to the regurgitation.[19, 35–37] Pulmonary congestion may be present before the development of left ventricular dysfunction. Although changes in left ventricular compliance do occur with mitral regurgitation, a more important determinant of left atrial pressure is left atrial compliance.[35–38] Acute mitral valve regurgitation is associated with normal sinus rhythm and a normal-sized left atrium, but a markedly increased left atrial pressure. Chronic mitral valve regurgitation is associated with a dilated left atrium, less severe atrial pressure elevation, and onset of atrial fibrillation.[5] In extreme left atrial enlargement, the left atrial pressure may even be normal.[39]

In addition to changes in compliance, another major compensatory mechanism that occurs in left ventricular volume overload is an increased wall thickness as the left ventricle dilates. The ratio of wall thickness to chamber radius remains constant. This phenomenon is termed "eccentric hypertrophy" and tends to normalize wall stress.[25, 37, 40–43] The ventricle also changes shape, from ellipsoidal to spherical, which also tends to normalize wall stress. This change to spherical shape parallels the development of left ventricular dysfunction.[18–19, 25, 40]

Hypertrophy is greater in aortic than in mitral regurgitation because the afterload on the left ventricle is greater in aortic than in mitral regurgitation.[21, 44] In mitral regurgitation, ejection occurs into a low-pressure chamber, the left atrium. Nearly half of the regurgitation occurs before aortic valve opening (isovolumic contraction),[9, 37] and therefore afterload is low. In aortic regurgitation, there is ejection of a large volume against a higher pressure, and therefore afterload is above normal. Because of the larger afterload in aortic regurgitation, end-diastolic volume is larger and the ejection fraction is lower for a given severity or duration of regurgitation.[6] Both eccentric hypertrophy and degenerative changes are minimal in chronic mitral regurgitation unless severe left ventricular dysfunction is present.[45]

The ejection fraction in aortic or mitral regurgitation varies inversely with acute changes in outflow resistance (afterload).[46] Such changes in afterload may be produced pharmacologically, and resultant changes in left ventricular contraction in both aortic and mitral regurgitation have been documented.[47–50] The ejection fraction tends to fall with angiotensin administration and rise with hydralazine administration. Radionuclide angiography offers a noninvasive means of assessing the effects of drugs and other interventions on the ejection fraction and regurgitant fraction.

Exercise

Because patients with chronic aortic regurgitation tend to become symptomatic only with advanced left ventricular dysfunction, radionuclide angiography, both at rest and on exercise, has been proposed as a means of detecting early left ventricular dysfunction not evident clinically. Delay in recognition of such an abnormality may allow potentially irreversible left ventricular dysfunction to progress, resulting in a less optimal surgical outcome.[51] Borer et al.,[52] studied the ejection fraction response to exercise in 22 patients with aortic regurgitation. Eight patients with symptomatic aortic regurgitation who were generally considered candidates for valve replacement all demonstrated a decrease in ejection fraction during maximal supine bicycle exercise. Of 21 patients with asymptomatic aortic regurgitation, all but 1 had a normal (> 0.45) resting ejection fraction. With maximal exercise, however, 16 had a subnormal and 6 had a normal ejection fraction response to exercise. An exercise ejection fraction of 0.55 or more was considered a normal response.

The 16 patients with an abnormal ejection fraction response were thought to have exercise-induced left ventricular dysfunction, which suggested that earlier valve replacement might have been indicated. However, it may not be possible to compare ejection fraction values in patients with aortic regurgitation with values in normal subjects. The normal left ventricle responds to exercise by increasing ejection fraction, but exercise is a complex intervention involving changes in sympathetic state, preload, afterload, and heart rate.[53, 54] In severe aortic regurgitation, the left ventricle is substantially larger due to the regurgitant volume, which may contribute as much as three fourths of diastolic filling. With exercise, heart rate increases and diastolic filling per beat and peripheral resistance decrease.[55, 56] As a result, the regurgitant volume per beat falls substantially. This dramatic fall in preload may affect the anticipated ejection fraction response. Furthermore, in disease not due to regurgitation, stroke volume usually fails to increase and there is an exercise-induced increase in end-diastolic volume. As a result, there is a fall in ejection fraction. In contrast, a subnormal ejection fraction response to exercise in patients with aortic regurgitation is usually associated with a decrease in end-diastolic volume[52] because of the large decrease in total stroke volume (Fig 16–3). Forward stroke volume may actually increase with exercise as regurgitant volume falls.[56] For this reason a decreasing or unchanging ejection fraction with exercise is a common finding in severe aortic regurgitation and may not necessarily imply worsening left ventricular dysfunction alone. The degree to which a fall in ejection fraction may be attributable to altered loading conditions has not been determined.

The ejection fraction response to exercise in patients with mitral regurgitation was similar to the response of patients with aortic regurgitation.[57] Borer et al.[57] studied 20 patients with mitral valve regurgitation and found that 10 (50%) had a decrease in ejection fraction with exercise. However, a faster heart rate does not appear to affect the regurgitant fraction in mitral regurgitation as it does in aortic regurgitation. Because of the usual earlier clinical presentation of patients with mitral regurgitation and the marked effect of the reduced afterload on contraction, changes in left ventricular contraction on exercise radionuclide studies may not provide clinically useful information.

Postoperative Studies

Numerous studies have evaluated the effect of surgical correction of aortic and mitral regurgitation on left ventricular function.[17, 58–60] Despite a generally favorable clinical response, angiographic assessments of left ventricular function in this setting have yielded varying data.

The immediate effect of valve replacement in patients with left ventricular volume overload is correction of the volume overload state and reduction of the stroke volume. End-systolic vol-

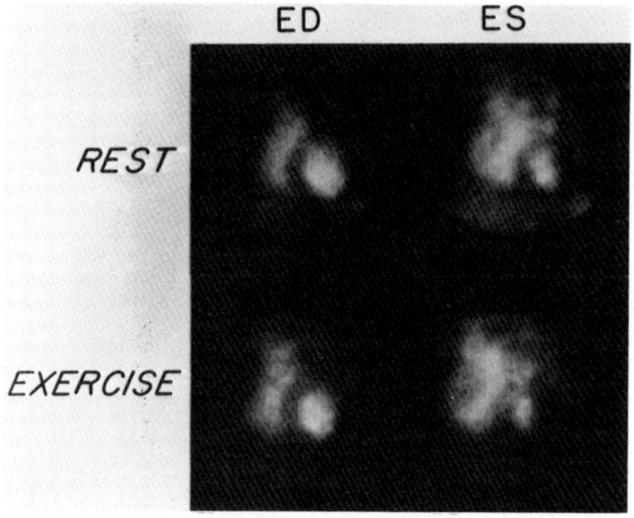

Fig 16–3.—Rest and peak exercise end-diastolic *(ED)* and end-systolic *(ES)* views in a 29-year-old man with asymptomatic aortic regurgitation. Ejection fraction at rest was 65% and at peak exercise was 70%. Note the smaller end-diastolic and end-systolic volumes on the peak exercise images.

ume changes very little and the ejection fraction decreases.[11] Several mechanisms have also been proposed to explain this fall in ejection fraction early after valve replacement: (1) The abnormal septal motion may contribute to a decrease in systolic left ventricular function.[61–62] Nearly all patients demonstrate paradoxic septal motion postoperatively.[61–62] The mechanism and significance of this finding are unknown. (2) Perioperative myocardial damage.[64–66] (3) Altered loading conditions,[63–65] especially the reduction in preload secondary to elimination of the regurgitant volume. However, after valve replacement, increased afterload may be present due to a residual systolic pressure gradient across currently available aortic prosthetic valves[67–69] or to the elimination of the low-pressure blow-off after mitral valve replacement.

Changes that occur late after valve replacement appear to differ in aortic versus mitral regurgitation. In patients with aortic regurgitation, most of the reduction in end-diastolic volume after aortic valve replacement appears to occur early, within two to four weeks postoperatively, although there is an additional reduction in end-diastolic volume subsequently (Fig 16–4).[63] The late decrease in end-diastolic volume after aortic valve replacement appears to be associated with a significant fall in end-systolic volume and a rise in the ejection fraction toward preoperative levels. These late changes are consistent with late regression of hypertrophy and realignment of fibers resulting from a reduction of increased afterload after valve replacement. As a result, there is no overall change in ejection fraction after correction of aortic regurgitation.[57, 70–72]

After valve replacement for mitral regurgitation, there is removal of the low-impedence ejection pathway in the left atrium[73] and apparently no further late decrease in end-diastolic volume or end-systolic volume, so that the late postoperative ejection fraction remains below the preoperative value.[63, 65, 71, 74] Despite the decrease in ejection fraction postoperatively, there is an excellent postoperative improvement in functional class of most patients with mitral regurgitation. Thus the functional significance of the reduction in ejection fraction remains uncertain.[74–75]

Assessment of the change in ejection fraction with exercise postoperatively in aortic regurgitation patients has been suggested for unmasking abnormalities of left ventricular function postoperatively. However, no study to date has reported postoperative rest and exercise ejection fraction measurements in aortic regurgitation patients who were asymptomatic preoperatively. Borer et al.[76]

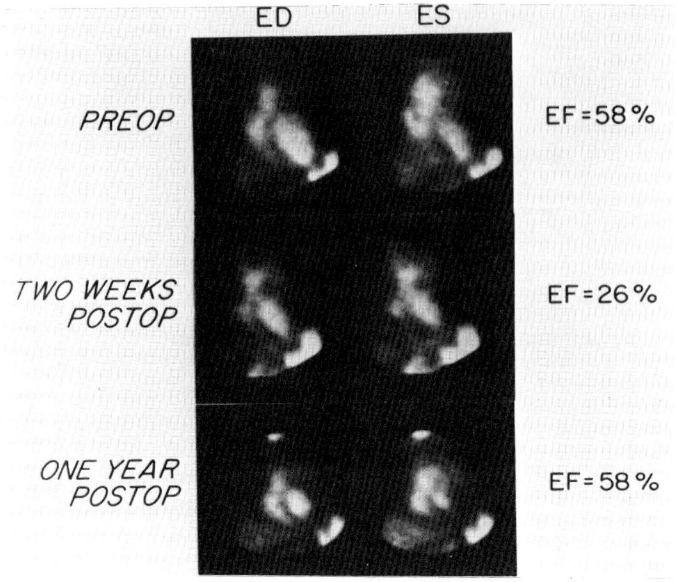

Fig 16–4.—Preoperative and early and late postoperative end-diastolic *(ED)* and end-systolic *(ES)* images after aortic valve replacement for severe aortic regurgitation in a 54-year-old woman.

recently reported rest and exercise ejection fraction responses in 16 patients with symptomatic aortic regurgitation. Of the 10 patients with normal resting ejection fractions preoperatively, 9 had abnormal ejection fractions with exercise preoperatively and 4 continued to have an abnormal exercise ejection fraction postoperatively. All 6 patients with abnormal resting ejection fraction preoperatively had abnormal ejection fraction responses to exercise both preoperatively and postoperatively. These findings are consistent with a component of irreversible myocardial damage present preoperatively as a result of chronic volume overload.[77]

CLINICAL UTILITY

The clinical value of radionuclide angiography in left ventricular overload is still evolving. Following are some situations in which it appears to be particularly useful:

1. To assist in the detection of volume overload of the left ventricle when the diagnosis is in question, for example, if murmurs suggest mitral regurgitation and aortic regurgitation (Austin-Flint murmur). The scan may also identify the volume overload as a cause of heart failure.

2. To provide accurate baseline information on the severity of the volume overload and left ventricular function. This permits the clinician to objectively and noninvasively follow a patient serially, which may help determine the time for and necessity of catheterization and valve replacement.

3. To assess the possibility of a paravalvular leak postoperatively.

4. To evaluate persistent symptoms postoperatively and to determine the degree to which they may be a result of left ventricular dysfunction.

In summary, radionuclide angiography appears to have an important role in the evaluation and management of patients with aortic or mitral regurgitation. This role is likely to increase as further improvements in scan data analysis become available which will separate intrinsic contractile function from the effect of altered loading conditions on contraction and will more precisely separate the regurgitant from the net forward stroke volume.

REFERENCES

1. Schlant R.C., Nutter D.O.: Heart failure in valvular heart disease. *Medicine* 50:421–451, 1971.
2. Hildner F.J., Javier R.P., Cohen L.S., et al.: Myocardial dysfunction associated with valvular heart disease. *Am. J. Cardiol.* 30:319–326, 1972.
3. Rackley C.E., Hood W.P. Jr.: Quantitative angiographic evaluation and pathophysiologic mechanisms in valvular heart disease. *Prog. Cardiovasc. Dis.* 15:427–447, 1973.
4. Kennedy J.W., Twiss R.D., Blackmon J.R., et al.: Quantitative angiocardiography: III. Relationships of left ventricular pressure, volume, and mass in aortic valve disease. *Circulation* 38:838–845, 1968.
5. Kennedy J.W., Yarnall S.R., Murray J.A., et al.: Quantitative angiocardiography: IV. Relationship of left atrial and ventricular pressure and volume in mitral valve disease. *Circulation* 41:817–824, 1970.
6. Mason D.T.: Regulation of cardiac performance in clinical heart disease. *Am. J. Cardiol.* 32:437–448, 1973.
7. Winzelberg G.G., Boucher C.A., McKusick K.A., et al.: Right ventricular function in aortic and mitral valve disease: Relation of gated first pass radionuclide angiography to clinical and hemodynamic findings. *Chest* 79:520–528, 1981.
8. Wexler L., Silverman J.F., DeBusk R.F., et al.: Angiographic features of rheumatic mitral regurgitation. *Circulation* 44:1080–1086, 1971.
9. Bolen J.L., Alderman E.L.: Ventriculographic and hemodynamic features of mitral regurgitation of cardiomyopathic, rheumatic and non-rheumatic etiology. *Am. J. Cardiol.* 39:177–183, 1977.
10. Rigo P., Alderson P.O., Robertson R.M., et al.: Measurement of aortic and mitral regurgitation by gated cardiac blood pool scans. *Circulation* 60:306–312, 1979.
11. Bough E.W., Gandsman E.J., North D.L., et al.: Gated radionuclide angiographic evaluation of valve regurgitation. *Am. J. Cardiol.* 46:423–428, 1980.
12. Lam W., Pavel D., Byron E., et al.: Radionuclide regurgitant index: Value and limitation. *Am. J. Cardiol.* 47:292–298, 1981.
13. Urquhart J., Patterson R.E., Packer M., et al.: Quantification of valve regurgitation by radionuclide angiography before and after valve replacement surgery. *Am. J. Cardiol.* 47:287–291, 1981.
14. Kress P., Geffers H., Stauch M., et al.: Evaluation of aortic and mitral regurgitation by radionuclide ventriculography: Comparison with the method of Sandler and Dodge. *Clin. Cardiol.* 4:5–10, 1981.
15. Sorensen S.G., O'Rourke R.A., Chaudhuri T.K.: Noninvasive quantitation of valvular regurgitation by gated equilibrium radionuclide angiography. *Circulation* 62:1089–1098, 1980.
16. Ross J., Morrow A.G., Mason D.R., et al.: Left ventricular function following replacement of the aortic valve. *Circulation* 33:507–516, 1966.
17. Gould K.L., Lipscomb K., Hamilton G.W., et al.: Relation of left ventricular shape, function and wall stress in man. *Am. J. Cardiol.* 34:627–634, 1974.
18. Henry W.L., Bonow R.O., Borer J.S., et al.: Observations on the optimum time for operative intervention for aortic regurgitation: 1. Evaluation of the result of aortic valve replacement in symptomatic patients. *Circulation* 61:47–83, 1980.
19. Miller G.H., Kirklin J.W., Swan H.J.C.: Myocardial function and left ventricular volumes in acquired valvular insufficiency. *Circulation* 31:374–384, 1965.
20. Eckberg D.L., Gault J.H., Bouchard R.L., et al.: Mechanics of left ventricular contractions in chronic severe mitral regurgitation. *Circulation* 47:1252–1259, 1973.
21. Urschel C.W., Covell J.W., Sonnenblick E.H., et al.: Myocardial mechanics in aortic and mitral valvular regurgitation: The concept of instantaneous impedance as a determinant of the performance of the intact heart. *J. Clin. Invest.* 47:867–883, 1968.
22. Taylor R.R., Covell J.W., Ross J. Jr.: Left ventricular function in experimental aorto-caval fistula with circulation congestion and fluid retention. *J. Clin. Invest.* 47:1333–1342, 1968.
23. McCullagh W.H., Covell J.W., Ross J. Jr.: Left ventricular dilatation and diastolic compliance changes during chronic volume overloading. *Circulation* 45:943–951, 1972.
24. Ross J.Jr., McCullagh W.H.: Nature of enhanced performance of the dilated left ventricle in the dog during chronic volume overloading. *Circ. Res.* 30:549–556, 1972.
25. Taylor R.R., Hopkins B.E.: Left ventricular response to experimentally induced chronic regurgitation. *Cardiovasc. Res.* 6:404–414, 1972.
26. Cooper G. IV, Puga F.J., Zujko K.J., et al.: Normal myocardial function and energetics in volume-overloaded hypertrophy in the cat. *Circ. Res.* 32:140–148, 1973.
27. Papadimitriou J.M., Hopkins B.E., Taylor R.R.: Regression of left ventricular dilatation and hypertrophy after removal of volume overload. *Circ. Res.* 35:127–135, 1974.
28. Kreulen R.H., Bove A.A., McDonough M.T., et al.: The evaluation of left ventricular function in man. *Circulation* 51:677–688, 1975.
29. Gewirtz H., Grotte G., Strauss H.W., et al.: The influence of left ventricular volume and wall motion on myocardial images. *Circulation* 59:1172–1177, 1979.
30. Osbakken M., Bove A., Spann J.: Left ventricular function in chronic aortic regurgitation with reference to end-systolic pressure, volume and stress relations. *Am. J. Cardiol.* 47:193–198, 1981.
31. Gunning J.F., Copper G. IV, Harrison C.E., et al.: Myocardial oxygen consumption in experimental hypertrophy and congestive heart failure due to pressure overload. *Am. J. Cardiol.* 32:427–436, 1973.

32. Welch G.H. Jr., Braunwald E., Sarnoff S.J.: Hemodynamic effects of quantitatively varied experimental aortic regurgitation. *Circ. Res.* 5:546–551, 1957.
33. Mann T., McLaurin L., Grossman W., et al.: Assessing the hemodynamic severity of acute aortic regurgitation due to infectious endocarditis. *N. Engl. J. Med.* 293:108–113, 1975.
34. Morganroth J., Perloff J.K., Zeldis S.M., et al.: Acute severe aortic regurgitation. *Ann. Intern. Med.* 87:223–232, 1977.
35. Braunwald E.: Mitral regurgitation: Physiologic, clinical and surgical considerations. *N. Engl. J. Med.* 281:425–433, 1969.
36. Lewis B.S., Gotsman M.S.: Left ventricular function during systole and diastole in mitral incompetence. *Am. J. Cardiol.* 34:635–643, 1974.
37. Yoran C., Yellin E.L., Becker R.M., et al.: Dynamic aspects of acute mitral regurgitation: Effects of ventricular volume, pressure and contractility on the effective regurgitant orifice area. *Circulation* 60:170–176, 1979.
38. Klughaupt M., Flamm M.D., Hancock W.E., et al.: Non-rheumatic mitral insufficiency: Determination of operability and prognosis. *Circulation* 39:307–316, 1969.
39. Braunwald E., Awe W.C.: The syndrome of severe mitral regurgitation with normal left atrial pressure. *Circulation* 27:29–35, 1963.
40. Grossman W., Jones D., McLaurin L.P.: Wall stress and patterns of hypertrophy in the human left ventricle. *J. Clin. Invest.* 56:56–64, 1975.
41. Fischl S.J., Gorlin R., Herman M.V.: Cardiac shape and function in aortic valve disease: Physiologic and clinical implications. *Am. J. Cardiol.* 39:170–176, 1977.
42. Gaasch W.H.: Left ventricular radius to wall thickness ratio. *Am. J. Cardiol.* 43:1189–1194, 1979.
43. Ross J. Jr.: Adaptations of the left ventricle to chronic volume overloading. *Circ. Res.* 35(suppl. II):II–64–70, 1974.
44. Rapaport E.: Natural history of aortic and mitral valve disease. *Am. J. Cardiol.* 35:221–227, 1975.
45. Fuster V., Danielson M.A., Robb R.A., et al.: Quantitation of left ventricular myocardial fiber hypertrophy and interstitial tissue in human hearts with chronically increased volume and pressure overload. *Circulation* 55:504–508, 1977.
46. Reeve R., Sakal F.J., Kennedy J.W., et al.: Ejection fraction and varying afterload, abstracted. *Am. J. Cardiol.* 39:284, 1977.
47. Braunwald .E., Welch G.H. Jr., Sarnoff S.J.: Hemodynamic effects of quantitatively varied experimental mitral regurgitation. *Circ. Res.* 5:539–545, 1957.
48. Bolen J.L., Holloway E.L., Zener J.C., et al.: Evaluation of left ventricular function in aortic regurgitation using afterload stress. *Circulation* 53:132–136, 1976.
49. Chatterjee K., Parmley W.W., Swan H.J.C., et al.: Beneficial effects of vasodilator agents in severe mitral regurgitation due to dysfunction of subvalvular apparatus. *Circulation* 48:684–690, 1973.
50. Harshaw C.W., Grossman W., Munro A.B., et al.: Reduced systemic vascular resistance as therapy for severe mitral regurgitation of valvular origin. *Ann. Intern. Med.* 83:312–316, 1975.
51. Rahimtoola S.H.: Early valve replacement for preservation of ventricular function, editorial. *Am. J. Cardiol.* 40:472–475, 1977.
52. Borer J.S., Bacharach S.L., Green M.V., et al.: Exercise-induced left ventricular dysfunction in symptomatic and asymptomatic patients with aortic regurgitation: Assessment with radionuclide cineangiography. *Am. J. Cardiol.* 42:351–357, 1978.
53. Krayenbuehl H.P., Hess O.M., Turina J.: Assessment of left ventricular function. *Cardiovasc. Med.* 3:883–908, 1978.
54. Ross J. Jr.: Afterload mismatch and preload reserver: A conceptual framework for the analysis of ventricular function. *Prog. Cardiovasc. Dis.* 18:255–264, 1976.
55. Judge T.P., Kennedy J.W., Bennet L.J., et al.: Quantitative hemodynamic effects of heart rate in aortic regurgitation. *Circulation* 44:355–367, 1971.
56. Ettinger P.O., Frank M.J., Levinson G.E.: Hemodynamics at rest and during exercise in combined aortic stenosis and insufficiency. *Circulation* 45:267–276, 1972.
57. Borer J.S., Gottdiener J.S., Rosing D.R., et al.: Left ventricular function in mitral regurgitation: Determination during exercise, abstracted. *Circulation* 60(suppl. II):II-38, 1979.
58. Thompson R., Yacoub M., Ahmed M., et al.: Influence of preoperative left ventricular function on results of homograft replacement of the aortic valve for aortic stenosis. *Am. J. Cardiol.* 43:929–938, 1979.
59. Kennedy J.W., Twiss R.D., Blackmon J.R., et al.: Hemodynamic studies one year following homograft aortic valve replacement. *Circulation* 37(suppl. II)II–110–7, 1968.
60. Boucher C.A., Bingham J.B., Okada R.D., et al.: Early changes in left ventricular volumes following correction of chronic left ventricular volume overload, abstracted. *Circulation* 60(suppl. II):II-241, 1979.
61. Burggraf G.W., Craige E.: Echocardiographic studies of left ventricular wall motion and dimension after valvular heart surgery. *Am. J. Cardiol.* 35:473–480, 1975.
62. Vignola P., Boucher C.A., Curfman G.D., et al.: Abnormal interventricular septal motion following surgery: Clinical, surgical, echocardiographic and radionuclide correlates. *Am. Heart J.* 97:27–34, 1979.
63. Boucher C.A., Bingham J.B., Osbakken M.D., et al.: Early changes in left ventricular size and function following correction of left ventricular volume overload. *Am. J. Cardiol.* 47:991–1004, 1981.

64. Smith N., McAnulty J.H., Rahimtoola S.H.: Severe aortic stenosis with impaired left ventricular function and clinical heart failure: Results of valve replacement. *Circulation* 58:255–264, 1978.
65. Schuler G., Peterson K.L., Johnson A., et al.: Temporal response of left ventricular performance to mitral valve surgery. *Circulation* 59:1218–1231, 1979.
66. Seabra-Gomes R., Sutton R., Parker D.J.: Left ventricular function after aortic valve replacement. *Br. Heart J.* 38:491–496, 1976.
67. Pantely G., Morton M.J., Rahimtoola S.H.: Effects of successful uncomplicated valve replacement on ventricular hypertrophy, volume and performance in aortic stenosis and aortic incompetence. *J. Thorac. Cardiovasc. Surg.* 75:383–391, 1978.
68. Morton M.J., McAnulty J.H., Rahimtoola S.H.: "Ventricular function curve" from a single diagnostic left ventriculogram: Technique, results and value. *Am. J. Cardiol.* 41:710–717, 1978.
69. Rahimtoola S.H.: The problem of valve prosthesis-patient mismatch. *Circulation* 58:20–24, 1978.
70. O'Toole J.D., Geiser E.A., Reddy P.S., et al.: Effect of preoperative ejection fraction on survival and hemodynamic improvement following aortic valve replacement. *Circulation* 58:1175–1184, 1978.
71. Kennedy J.W., Doces J., Stewart D.K.: Left ventricular function before and following aortic valve replacement. *Circulation* 56:944–950, 1977.
72. Schuler G., Peterson K.L., Johnson A.D., et al.: Serial noninvasive assessment of left ventricular hypertrophy and function after surgical correction of aortic regurgitation. *Am. J. Cardiol* 44:585–594, 1979.
73. Kennedy J.W., Doces J.G., Stewart D.K.: Left ventricular function before and following surgical treatment of mitral valve disease. *Am. Heart J.* 97:592–598, 1979.
74. Phillips H.R., Levine F.H., Carter J.E., et al.: Mitral valve replacement for isolated mitral regurgitation: Analysis of clinical course and late postoperative left ventricular ejection fraction. *Am. J. Cardiol.*, to be published.
75. O'Rourke R.A., Crawford M.H.: Timing of valve replacement in patients with chronic aortic regurgitation, editorial. *Circulation* 61:493–495, 1980.
76. Borer J.S., Rosing D.R., Kent K.M., et al.: Left ventricular function at rest and during exercise after aortic valve replacement in patients with aortic regurgitation. *Am. J. Cardiol.* 44:1297–1304, 1979.
77. Maron B.K., Ferrans V.J.: Ultrastructural features of hypertrophied ventricular myocardium. *Prog. Cardiovasc. Dis.* 21:207–238, 1978.

COMMENT: AORTIC AND MITRAL VALVE REGURGITATION

Joel Morganroth

ONE of the most difficult decisions in adult cardiology is to judge the proper timing for valve replacement in patients with chronic mitral or aortic regurgitation. In addition, the identification of acute severe aortic or mitral regurgitation which present as surgical emergencies must not be overlooked, since providing medical therapy alone usually results in disaster. The advent of noninvasive cardiac testing has allowed the recognition of these cardiac conditions and provides guidelines for surgical intervention.

ETIOLOGIC CONSIDERATIONS

Echocardiography is a direct way to determine the cause of acute or chronic mitral or aortic regurgitation. Acute valvular regurgitation due to infective endocarditis with perforation of a valve cusp or rupture of chordae tendineae may be easily identified by two-dimensional (2DE) and/or M-mode echocardiography. Dissection of the aorta with secondary aortic regurgitation can also be distinguished. Chronic valvular regurgitation due to congenital or acquired disease, such as congenital bicuspid aortic valve or valvular prolapse syndrome, can be precisely identified. Recognition of the etiology has important therapeutic implications. Radionuclide imaging has limited impact on determination of the etiology of valvular regurgitation.

CLINICAL CONSIDERATIONS

The Symptomatic Patient

The patient suffering from acute severe mitral or aortic regurgitation usually presents with acute pulmonary edema. Echocardiographic criteria for acute severe aortic regurgitation are well defined and include early closure of the mitral valve on M-mode echocardiography. Acute severe mitral regurgitation often presents with a hyperkinetic but only modestly dilated left ventricle and left atrium, and the cause of the acute regurgitation is often immediately apparent on the echocardiogram (e.g., vegetation or ruptured chord). Patients with chronic regurgitation who develop symptoms of left ventricular failure or angina should be evaluated by echocardiography to determine the degree of left ventricular dysfunction, size of the left atrium, size of the aortic root, and left ventricular outflow tract. These physiologic parameters help guide the surgeon in the proper selection of a valvular prosthesis and in delineating associated lesions. Radionuclide imaging is also useful in assessing left ventricular function in such cases and can be used when echocardiographic data are equivocal or unobtainable.

The Asymptomatic Patient

The proper timing for valve replacement in patients with asymptomatic mitral or aortic regurgitation remains controversial. Most clinicians agree that if the beginning of left ventricular dysfunction in such patients can be detected, valvular replacement should take place before the damage becomes irreversible. Echocardiographic studies have suggested criteria for aortic valve replacement in asymptomatic patients with aortic regurgitation based on a decrease in the shortening fraction of the left ventricle. Similar suggestions have been made using radionuclide ventriculography, particularly during exercise, which may prove to be a more sensitive technique. At present we recommend either echocardiography or exercise radionuclide angiography, or both, as a means of determining in a serial fashion changes in left ventricular performance. When left ventricular function begins to deteriorate in patients with chronic valvular regurgitation, even in asymptomatic patients, we recommend surgical intervention.

The use of echocardiography in patients after aortic and mitral valve replacement may have important prognostic implications. Patients who do not have a decrease in left ventricular size may have irreversible myocardial damage, and their prognosis is guarded. Radionuclide imaging can provide similar information.

Echocardiography should be routinely done on all patients after aortic and mitral valve replacement to establish a baseline study of the prosthetic valve and left ventricular function that can be later used for comparison if complications or changes in the clinical state develop. The use of echocardiography to detect valvular prosthetic dysfunction, perivalvular regurgitation, and the development of left ventricular clot, among other complications, has important therapeutic implications. Echocardiographic evaluation of left atrial size in patients with mitral valve disease who have atrial fibrillation may have an important prognostic implication in terms of the rate of success for cardioversion to normal sinus rhythm.

PART IX

Aortic and Mitral Valve Stenosis

ECHOCARDIOGRAPHY

Masahito Naito, Chin C. Chen, Daniel David, and Joel Morganroth

MITRAL STENOSIS

MITRAL STENOSIS is almost always a late complication of rheumatic fever. Congenital mitral stenosis is relatively uncommon and is usually associated with other cardiac lesions. However, the echocardiographic features of these two forms are quite similar.

Since the advent of two-dimensional echocardiography (2DE), the assessment of mitral stenosis has been the best indication of the utility of this technique, since the mitral valve orifice size can be measured directly by using the short-axis view rather than indirectly by predicting the area with hemodynamic equations. Confirmation of the severity of mitral stenosis using the parasternal long-axis view of the mitral valve, which can demonstrate the segmental anatomy, has been reported.

The Normal Mitral Valve

M-mode Echocardiography

The M-mode echocardiographic examination usually begins with recording of the anterior leaflet of the mitral valve. The echo of this structure is among the easiest identified, since the movement of the leaflet during diastole is perpendicular to the ultrasound beam. In normal subjects, the posterior leaflet of the mitral valve can also be detected quite easily. It moves in a direction opposite to that of the anterior leaflet and with less amplitude during diastole.

The normal mitral valve presents a thin echo complex, and the normal anterior leaflet provides the distinctive M-shaped configuration during diastole. Figure 17–1 shows the commonly used nomenclature for the anterior mitral leaflet. *A* is the point of maximal opening occurring with atrial systole. The *B* point occurs at the beginning of ventricular systole and may not always be distinctive on the AC slope of the anterior leaflet. Valve closure motion begins immediately after atrial systole, and two leaflets come together as the mitral valve is closed by the following ventricular systole. The point of closure is termed the *C* point. The *D* point indicates the onset of mitral valve opening during diastole. During systole (CD segment) the closed mitral valve moves gradually anteriorly, probably as a result of the mitral annulus drawing toward the base of the heart.

When diastole begins, the two valve leaflets rapidly open to their maximal excursion, the *E* point. This initial opening occurs during the rapid filling phase of the left ventricle. Both leaflets then return to a position of partial closure, corresponding to the *F* point. This EF slope is normally rapid ($\geq$ 80 mm/second). Following the ECG P wave, the valve again opens with atrial systole, and the cycle is repeated. If diastole is sufficiently long, a low-amplitude, mid-diastolic opening is sometimes seen before the next atrial systole. The normal leaflets usually demonstrate an excursion (DE amplitude) of greater than 20 mm.

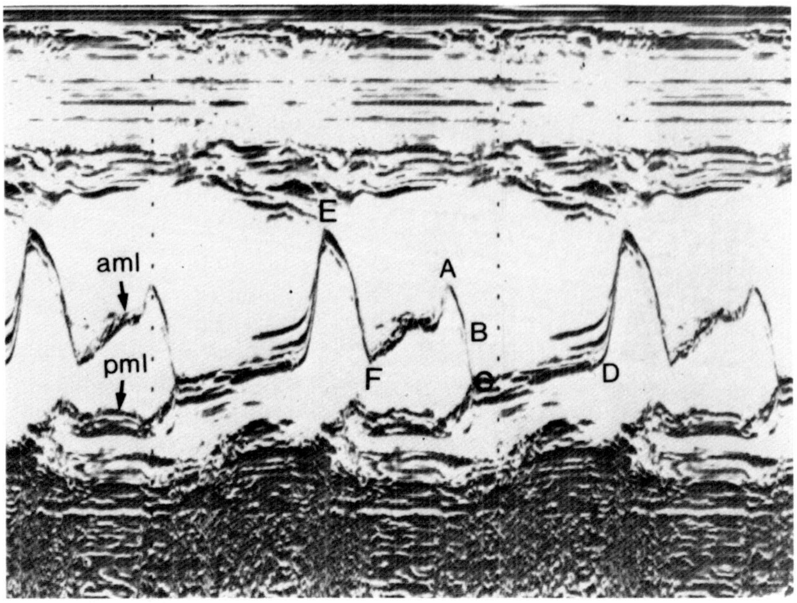

Fig 17–1.—M-mode echocardiogram of a normal mitral valve. The anterior *(aml)* and posterior *(pml)* mitral leaflets separate abruptly at point *D*. The point of maximal excursion *(E)* is followed by early diastolic closure (*EF* slope). Following atrial contraction, the leaflets reopen *(A)* and begin a presystolic closing motion which ends at the mitral coaptation point *(C)*. During systole the mitral valve shows a gradual anterior movement.

Two-Dimensional Echocardiography

Long-axis view.—The long-axis view of the left ventricle (Fig 17–2) allows visualization of the anterior and posterior leaflets of the mitral valve along with their chordal and papillary muscle attachments. The anterior leaflet is longer than the posterior leaflet. Both are thin and usually produce uniform echoes. With the onset of diastole, the tip of the anterior mitral leaflet approximates the left ventricular septal surface, moves posteriorly to lie in a mid-open position during mid-diastole, and reopens with atrial systole. The posterior mitral leaflet has a similar motion but smaller excursion than the anterior leaflet.

During systolic ejection, the mitral valve leaflets coapt at a point inferior (toward the apex) to the posterior atrioventricular groove and the papillary muscles contract. The slight arching of the bodies of both mitral valve leaflets is somewhat more apparent in late systole.

Short-axis view.—Figure 17–3 shows the mitral anterior and posterior leaflets in cross sectional. The mitral valve orifice has a fishmouth shape during diastole when imaged near the edge of the leaflets.

Apical four-chamber view.—As shown in Figure 17–4, the mitral valve ring is normally slightly more superior (toward the left atrial root) than the tricuspid valve ring. The anterior mitral leaflet inserts into the left atrioventricular sulcus, whereas the septal leaflet of the tricuspid valve inserts near the mid-portion of the membranous septum. This results in a lower position of the tricuspid valve (toward the cardiac apex) compared with the mitral valve.

Rheumatic Mitral Stenosis

Rheumatic fever may cause mitral commissural fusion, leaflet thickening, and chordal fusion, leading to mitral valvular stenosis. Because of interchordal fusion, the secondary orifices are obliterated, and the commissural fusion causes a reduction of the size of the principal orifice. Echocardiography has made possible an enormous in-

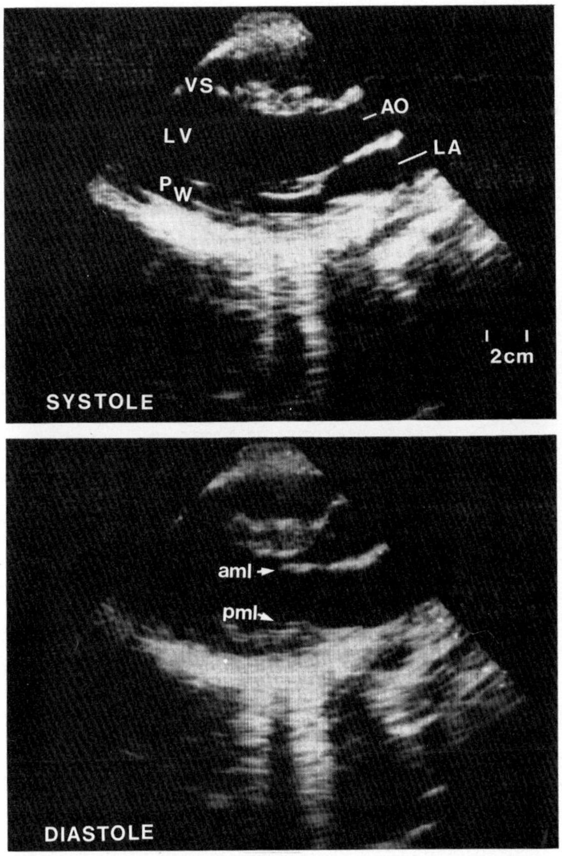

Fig 17–2.—Normal parasternal long-axis 2DE obtained in systole *(top)* and diastole *(bottom)*. The tip of the anterior mitral leaflet *(aml)* approximates the ventricular septum *(VS)* in diastole. *LV,* left ventricle; *PW,* left ventricular posterior wall; *AO,* aorta; *LA,* left atrium; *pml,* posterior mitral leaflet.

crease in our ability to evaluate patients with mitral stenosis. However, some characteristic echocardiographic features are based solely on secondary changes in mitral valve motion, and both physiologic and anatomical information must be integrated to understand the alterations in the mitral apparatus.

M-mode Echocardiography

Historically, the first clinical application of echocardiography was the detection of mitral stenosis and utilized the recording of an echo from the anterior mitral leaflet.[1] Although the mechanical abnormality in patients with mitral stenosis consists of the inability of the mitral leaflets to open sufficiently to provide an adequate orifice for atrioventricular flow in diastole, the diagnostic abnormality on the echocardiogram recognized in this disorder was a marked reduction in the early diastolic closure slope of the anterior mitral leaflet, or EF slope (Fig 17–5).[2–7] Other M-mode echocardiographic features of mitral stenosis include anterior motion of the posterior mitral leaflet, thickened mitral leaflet (multiple echoes), decreased mitral excursion, and separation of the two leaflets.[7]

Several initial studies[4–8] have shown good correlation between the EF slope and the mitral valve area as estimated at surgery or necropsy. However, this finding is not highly specific and can be observed in patients with reduced left ventricular compliance,[7] since the EF slope is a function of the rate of filling of the left ventricle. Cope et al.[9] found poor correlation ($r = 0.51$) between the EF slope on the echocardiogram and the calculated mitral valve area.

Subsequently it became clear that an abnormal anterior motion of the posterior mitral leaflet in diastole is the main diagnostic hallmark of mitral stenosis[3] and results from commissural fusion. However, Levisman et al.[10] have found that the posterior mitral leaflet can move posteriorly (in 16 of 167 cases) in patients with very mild mitral stenosis (Fig 17–6). Assessment of the severity of mitral orifice reduction in patients with mitral stenosis has also been attempted by analysis of valvular thickening and decreased opening excursion on the echocardiogram.[9, 11] Although these two parameters may determine whether patients with mitral stenosis can undergo successful commissurotomy, they have not been entirely useful in predicting valve orifice area. Multiple discrete linear echoes or amorphous thick conglomerate echoes within the mitral valve complex suggest significant calcification. In such a setting, mitral valve replacement is usually necessary (Fig 17–7).[11]

Two-Dimensional Echocardiography

In 2DE, the mitral valve can be imaged in long-axis, short-axis, and apical four-chamber views (see Figs 17–2 through 17–4). In the past, most investigators assessed mitral valve orifice size by using the short-axis view.[12–16] Less information is available with the long-axis view.[13, 17, 18]

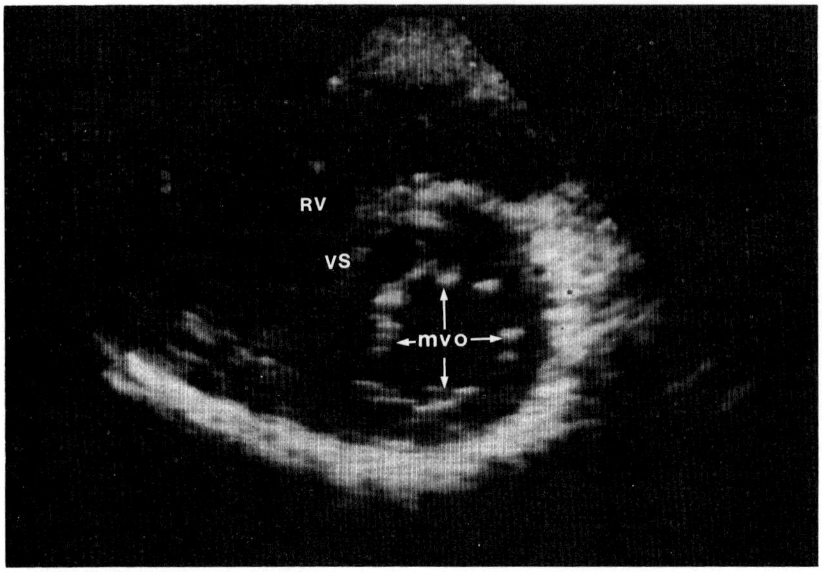

Fig 17–3.—Normal short-axis 2DE of the left ventricle at the level of the mitral valve. Note the area of the mitral valve orifice *(mvo)*. *RV,* right ventricle; *VS,* ventricular septum.

Long-axis view.—Nichol et al.[13] described the 2DE findings in 25 patients with pure mitral stenosis (Table 17–1). They also demonstrated arching of the anterior mitral leaflet in diastole and found that the valve leaflets were more thickened and immobile at the leaflet tip while maximum mobility was in the leaflet's body. Chandraratna et al.[17] found further that all patients with mitral valve arching in diastole had an opening snap on auscultation, whereas patients with heavy calcification of the mitral anterior leaflet's tip and body had no opening snap.

Recently, Naito et al.,[18] using the left ventricular long-axis view, observed three predominant patterns of anterior mitral leaflet motion in mitral stenosis. The 2DE analysis using the long-axis view could demonstrate the pliability and degree of doming of the anterior mitral leaflet, providing information for the estimation of the severity of mitral stenosis (Table 17–2 and Figs 17–8 through

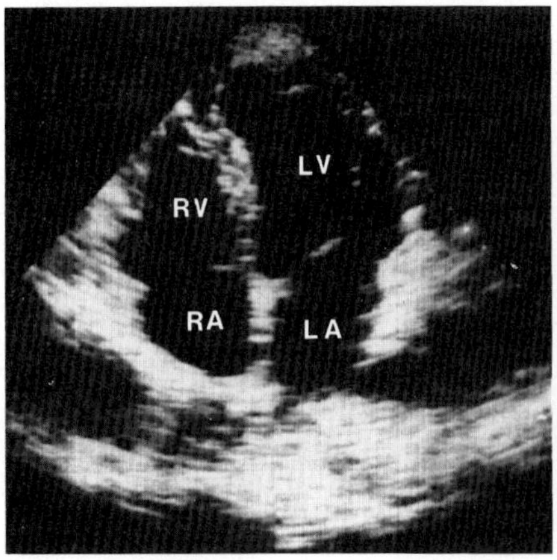

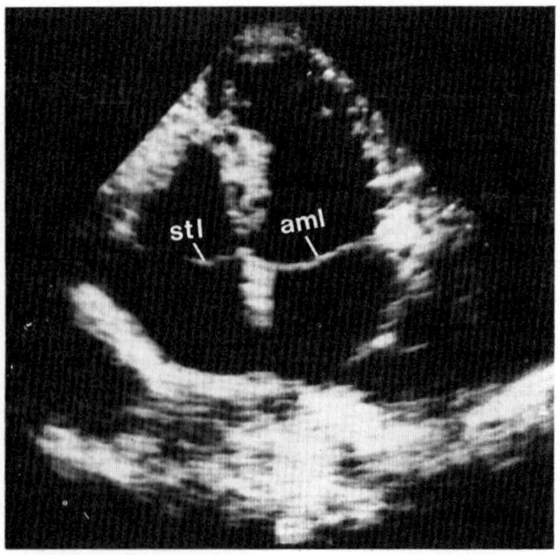

Fig 17–4.—Normal 2DE of an apical four-chamber view in diastole *(left)* and systole *(right)*. Note that the septal leaflet of the tricuspid *(stl)* valve is located more apically than the anterior leaflet of the mitral valve *(aml)*. *RV,* right ventricle; *LV,* left ventricle; *RA,* right atrium; *LA,* left atrium.

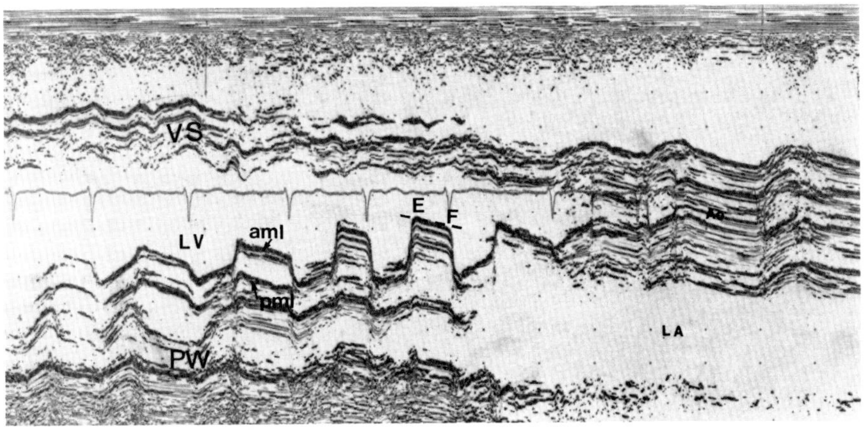

Fig 17–5.—M-mode echocardiographic scan from the left ventricular cavity *(LV)* to the aorta *(Ao)* in a patient with combined rheumatic mitral and aortic valve stenosis. Note the multiple echo lines and poor separation of the cusps of the aortic valve. The EF slope of the mitral valve is reduced, the posterior mitral leaflet *(pml)* moves anteriorly in early diastole, and the leaflets are thickened. *aml,* anterior mitral leaflet; *VS,* ventricular septum; *PW,* left ventricular posterior wall; *LA,* left atrium.

17–10). Nichol et al.[13] and Naito et al.[18] observed a prolapse motion of the anterior mitral leaflet into the left atrium in systole (Fig 17–11). Naito et al.[18] suggested that this mitral valve prolapsing motion may require a pliable anterior leaflet with severe commissural fusion and doming, and that the presence of mitral valve prolapse pattern may be associated with hemodynamically severe mitral stenosis. Of course, there is a chance of the two distinct entities of rheumatic mitral stenosis and

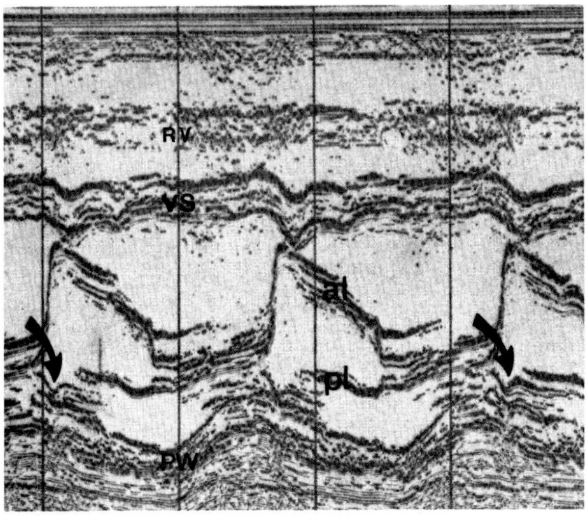

Fig 17–6.—M-mode echocardiographic recording of a patient with rheumatic mitral stenosis. Note the posterior motion of the posterior mitral leaflet *(pl, arrows)* in early diastole, signifying very mild mitral stenosis. *al,* anterior mitral leaflet; *VS,* ventricular septum; *PW,* left ventricular posterior wall; *RV,* right ventricle.

TABLE 17–1.—Mitral Stenosis: Two-Dimensional Echocardiographic Features

LONG-AXIS VIEW	SHORT-AXIS VIEW
Increased echoes from the margins of the thickened deformed valve leaflets	Thickened leaflets
Doming of the anterior mitral leaflet into the left ventricular outflow tract during diastole	Decreased mobility
Narrowed diameter of valve orifice at peak separation	Direct recording of the mitral valve orifice area
Fixed or poorly moving posterior mitral leaflet	
Dilated left atrium	

TABLE 17–2.—Correlation of the Pattern of Anterior Mitral Leaflet Motion and Severity of Mitral Stenosis

PATTERN BY CROSS-SECTIONAL LONGITUDINAL VIEW	SEVERITY BASED ON CATHETERIZATION FINDINGS: Mild	Moderate	Severe
Pattern A (N = 8)			
Mild to moderate doming (N = 2)	1	1	0
Severe doming (N = 6)	2	2	2
Pattern B (N = 8)	0	1	7
Pattern C (N = 5)	0	0	5

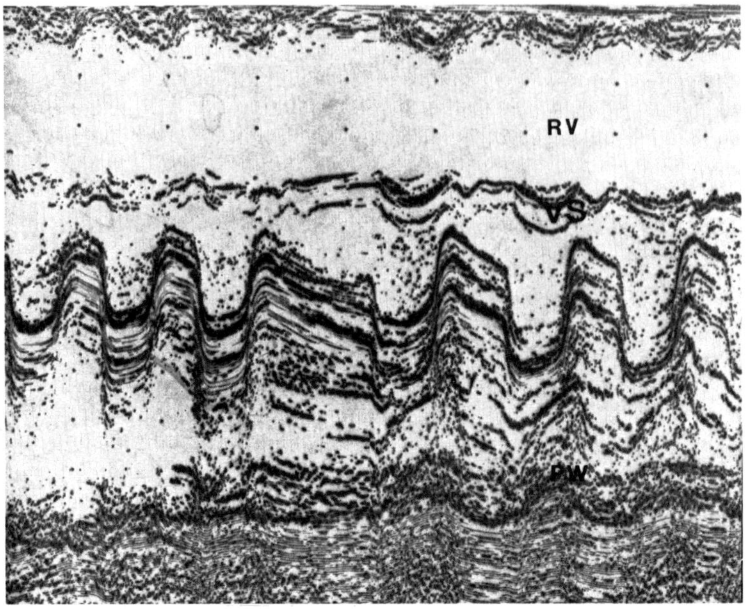

Fig 17–7.—M-mode echocardiographic recording from a patient with severe mitral stenosis and a calcified mitral valve. Note the multiple echo lines within the mitral valve. *VS,* ventricular septum; *PW,* left ventricular posterior wall; *RV,* right ventricle.

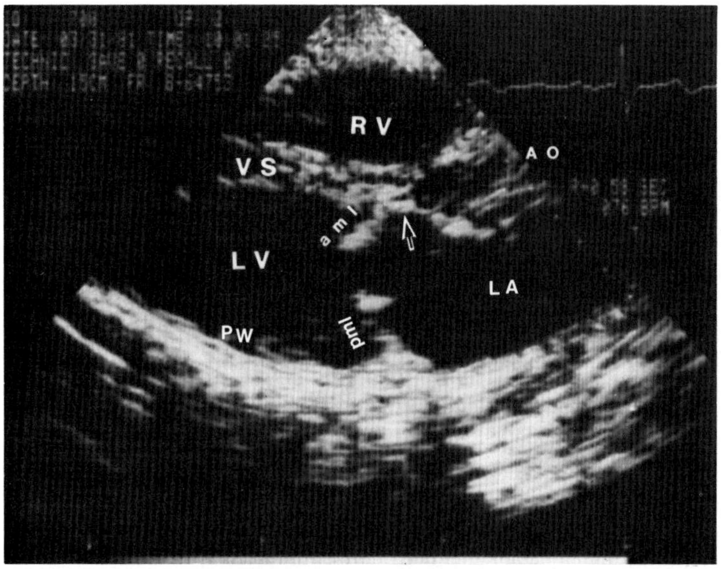

Fig 17–8.—Left ventricular parasternal longitudinal 2DE view in a patient with mild mitral stenosis. Note the restricted motion of the leaflet's tip with marked doming *(arrow). aml,* anterior mitral leaflet; *pml,* posterior mitral leaflet; *RV,* right ventricle; *VS,* ventricular septum; *LV,* left ventricle; *PW,* left ventricular posterior wall; *AO,* aorta; *LA,* left atrium.

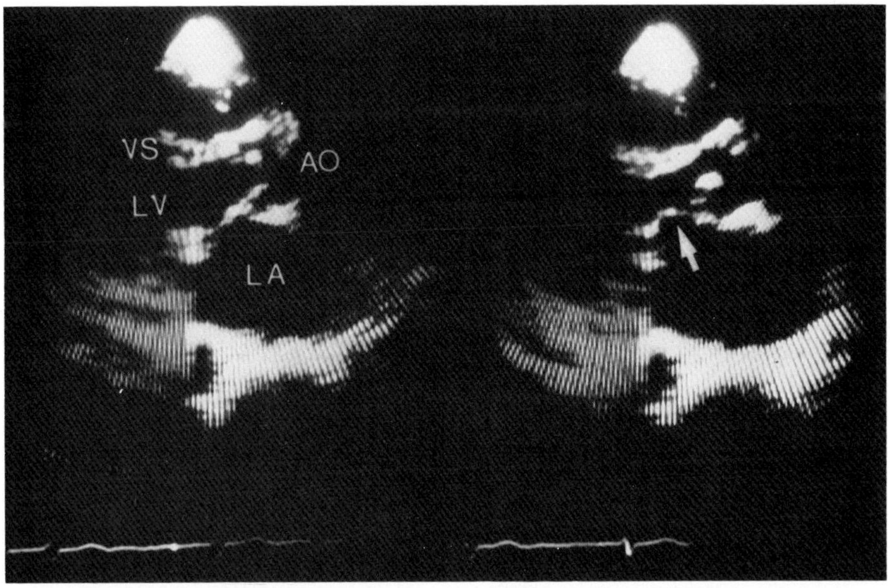

Fig 17–9.—Left ventricular parasternal longitudinal 2DE view in a patient with moderate mitral stenosis. Note the restricted motion of the body and tip of the anterior mitral leaflet with a moderate degree of doming *(arrow). AO,* aorta; *VS,* ventricular septum; *LV,* left ventricle; *LA,* left atrium.

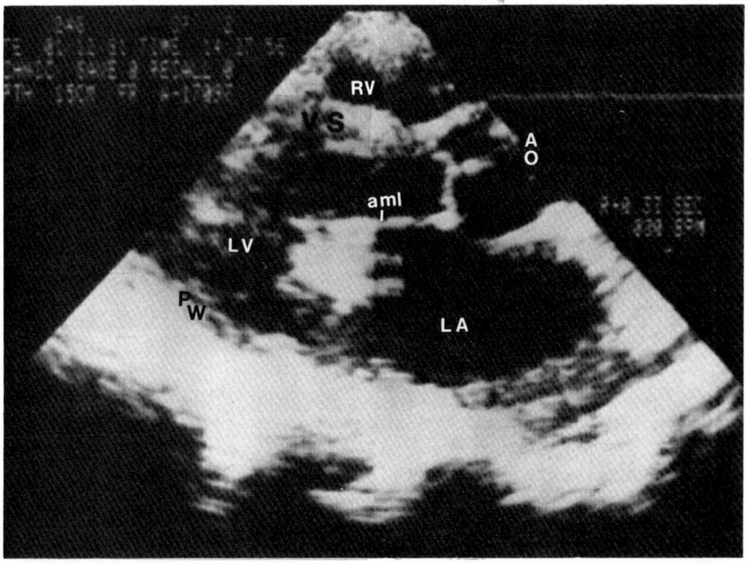

Fig 17–10.—Left ventricular parasternal longitudinal 2DE view in a patient with severe mitral stenosis. Note the severely restricted leaflet motion with almost no doming and the heavily calcified mitral valve. *aml,* anterior mitral leaflet; *RV,* right ventricle; *VS,* ventricular septum; *LV,* left ventricle; *AO,* aorta; *PW,* left ventricular posterior wall; *LA,* left atrium.

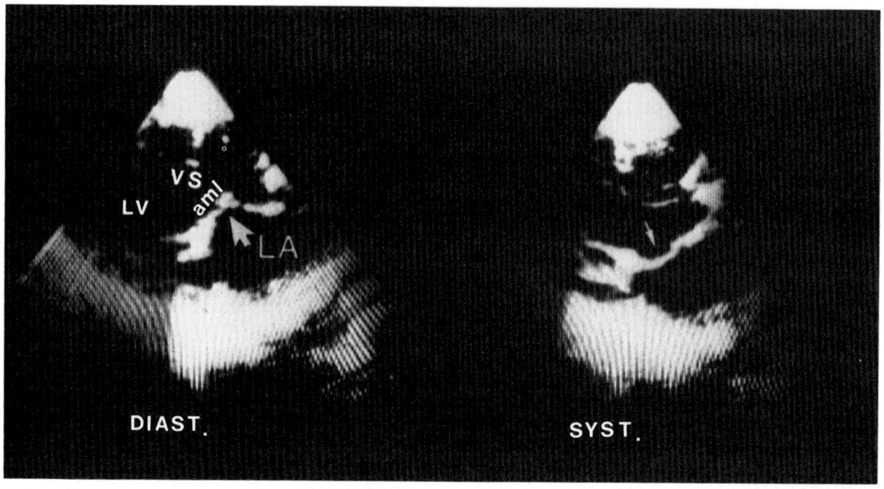

Fig 17–11.—Left ventricular parasternal longitudinal 2DE view of a patient with moderate mitral stenosis. In diastole *(left),* there is doming of the anterior mitral leaflet *(aml) (large white arrow),* whereas in systole *(right),* a prolapse pattern of the aml *(small white arrow)* is seen as a rebound phenomenon. *VS,* ventricular septum; *LV,* left ventricle; *LA,* left atrium. (From Naito M., et al.: Rheumatic mitral stenosis: Cross-sectional echocardiographic analysis. *Am. Heart J.* 100:34-40, 1980. Reproduced by permission.)

idiopathic mitral valve prolapse occurring coincidentally together in the same patient, as Weinrauch et al.[19] have suggested.

Finally, some investigators have emphasized the measurement of the space between the mitral valve and the interventricular septum in judging the size of the left ventricular outflow tract.[20] This measurement is felt to be important in judging whether the ventricle can accommodate a ball valve prosthesis or whether a low-profile or disk prosthetic valve will be necessary. Two-dimensional echocardiography using the long-axis view can provide this information, since it clearly demonstrates the anatomical structures involved.

Short-axis view.—Henry et al.[12] were the first to find an excellent correlation between the mitral valve orifice size measured on 2DE of the left ventricular short-axis view and that measured at cardiac surgery (Fig 17–12). Mitral valve orifice size measured by echocardiography may be superior to that obtained at the time of cardiac catheterization by means of the Gorlin formula, particularly in the presence of concomitant mitral regurgitation. Nevertheless, Wann et al.[14] found a good correlation between the mitral valve orifice size measured on the short-axis view and that calculated by Gorlin's method at cardiac catheterization. Nichol et al.[13] demonstrated that the mitral valve orifice size determined by planimetry of the stop-frame videotape images from the phased array 2DE system compares favorably with the mitral valve orifice size determined by cardiac catheterization (Fig 17–13). Weyman et al.,[15] however, pointed out the technical difficulties in determining this measurement and the importance of proper gain settings. They reported that the mitral valve orifice size as determined on 2DE overestimates the cardiac catheterization measurement by a mean of 0.2 $cm.^2$ This was to be expected, since in 2DE one measures just the orifice seen, whereas the hemodynamic estimation is based on mitral valve flow, which may be altered by subvalvular stenosis and other factors. Weyman et al. also suggested that the mitral valve orifice size measured on the short-axis view correlates very well with that obtained at cardiac catheterization in patients with severe mitral stenosis but less well in patients with mild mitral stenosis.

There are several limitations to the assessment of mitral stenosis by 2DE, especially using the short-axis view. Two-dimensional echocardiograms of 17% of the original 30 patients assessed by Nichol et al.[13] were inadequate for evaluation because of poor sound transmission qualities caused

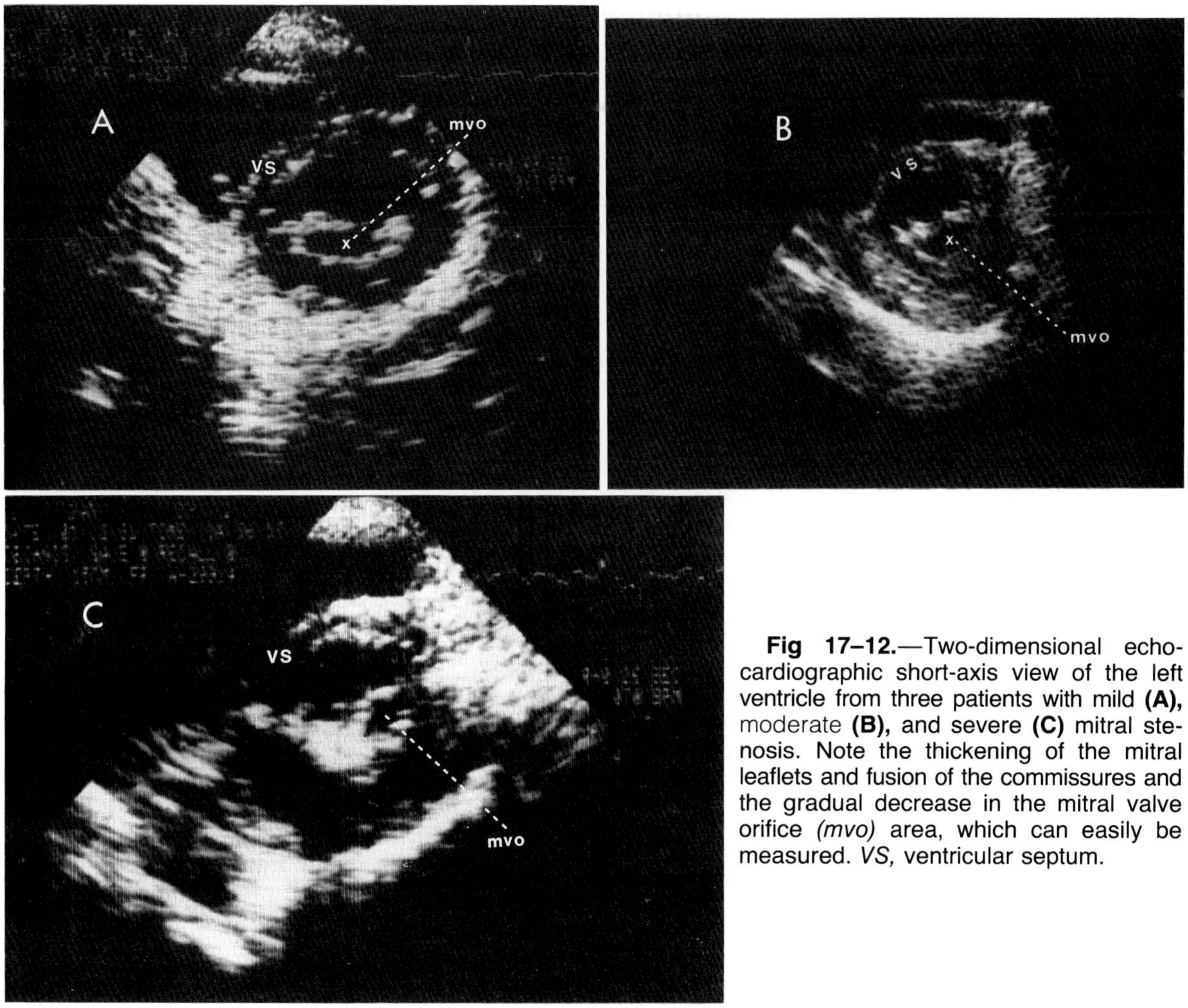

Fig 17–12.—Two-dimensional echocardiographic short-axis view of the left ventricle from three patients with mild **(A)**, moderate **(B)**, and severe **(C)** mitral stenosis. Note the thickening of the mitral leaflets and fusion of the commissures and the gradual decrease in the mitral valve orifice *(mvo)* area, which can easily be measured. *VS*, ventricular septum.

by abnormal chest wall configuration, patient age, and the presence of interposed lung. The quality of mitral valve orifice images depends on (1) the inherent resolution properties of the imaging system and (2) the gain control setting, which varies for each individual patient. In mitral stenosis, rather bright echoes are reflected from a thickened and often calcified valve. As a result, the gain setting should be lower for assessing mitral stenosis than for other cardiac structures. It should also be noted that loss of echo targets (dropout) when the structure being studied is parallel to the echo beam is most commonly seen in the commissural areas when the stenotic orifice is seen on a short-axis view. Therefore, a careful technique is mandatory. Other aspects of 2DE that have been pointed out by Martin et al.[16] likely to be problematic are determination of true orifice location (Fig 17–14), timing of orifice measurement in mid- to late diastole, and the optimal method of drawing the imaged mitral valve orifice.

Apical view.—Kushner et al.[21] evaluated the role of the apical view in patients with mitral stenosis. Using a 30-degree mechanical sector scanner, they measured right atrial size in one dimension and were able to detect right atrial involvement before right ventricular dilation began in patients with pulmonary hypertension due to mitral stenosis.

Patients with rheumatic mitral stenosis can de-

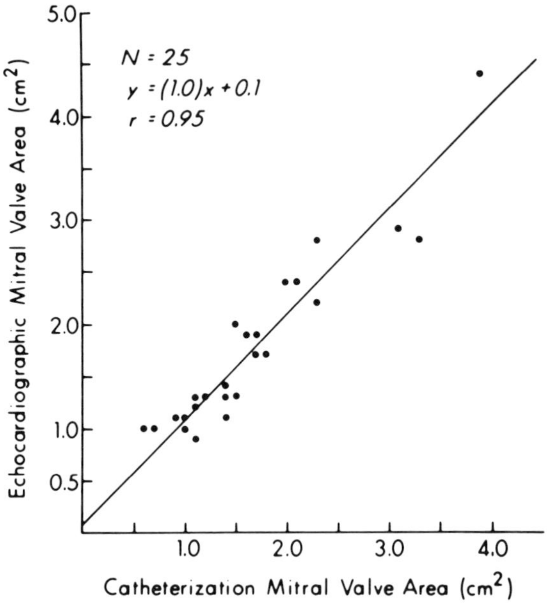

Fig 17–13.—Graph showing an excellent correlation between the mitral valve area derived from cardiac catheterization and the mitral valve orifice area measured on the two-dimensional echocardiogram. (From Nichol P.M., et al.: Two-dimensional echocardiographic assessment of mitral stenosis. *Circulation* 55:120-128, 1977. Reproduced by permission of the American Heart Association.)

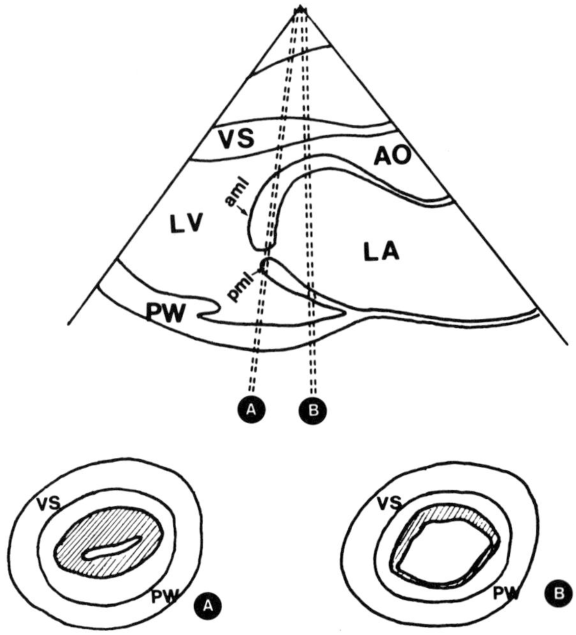

Fig 17–14.—Schematic diagrams showing the importance of accurate mitral valve orifice determination using 2DE. *Top,* a schematic parasternal long-axis left ventricular view in early diastole. *Bottom left,* short-axis view of beam A intersecting the mitral valve at its tip. The mitral leaflets appear to be thick and the orifice small. *Bottom right,* the short-axis view of beam B which intersects the valve on the atrial side of the true orifice. The mitral orifice has a falsely larger appearance. *aml,* anterior mitral leaflet; *pml,* posterior mitral leaflet; *AO,* aorta; *VS,* ventricular septum; *LV,* left ventricle; *PW,* left ventricular posterior wall; *LA,* left atrium.

velop left atrial thrombi; however, detection by 2DE is still uncertain and difficult (Fig 17–15).

Calcified Mitral Annulus

Calcified mitral annulus is frequently encountered at autopsy in persons over age 65 years. Although the precise etiology of this lesion has not been resolved, it apparently is degenerative in nature. Echocardiography appears to be more sensitive than chest x-ray studies in detecting this condition, although it may sometimes be difficult to distinguish mitral annular calcification from massive mitral valvular calcification in patients with rheumatic heart disease.

The characteristic pattern of mitral annular calcification on the M-mode echocardiogram consists of a uniform dense band of echoes beneath the posterior mitral leaflet (Fig 17–16).[22–24] D'Cruz et al.,[25] however, described 12 patients with calcification within the left ventricle anterior to the plane of the anterior mitral leaflet. They called this presentation "anterior submitral calcification," as opposed to "mitral annular calcification of the posterior submitral calcification." They also found that 2DE demonstrated localization of mitral annular calcification more clearly than M-mode echocardiography. Posterior submitral calcifications were usually seen to be quite separate from the posterior wall of the left ventricle and left atrium on both long- and short-axis views. Anterior submitral calcifications and their anatomical relationship to the aortic root, aortic valve, and mitral valve were also well demonstrated. Mitral stenosis solely due to inhibition of mitral leaflet motion from a calcified mitral annulus can occur.

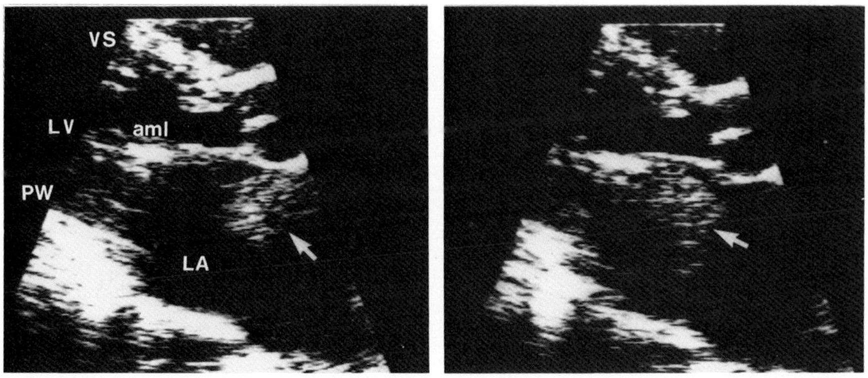

Fig 17–15.—Parasternal long-axis 2DE view of the left ventricle in a patient with mitral stenosis. *Arrow* indicates a left atrial thrombus that was confirmed at surgery. Note the dilated left atrium *(LA)*. *VS,* ventricular septum; *LV,* left ventricle; *aml,* anterior mitral leaflet; *PW,* left ventricular posterior wall.

Congenital Mitral Stenosis

The echocardiographic appearance of classic congenital valvular mitral stenosis is almost identical to that seen in adults as a result of rheumatic mitral valve disease.[26, 27] On the long-axis view the fused leaflets bulge inferiorly into the left ventricular outflow tract in diastole, and short-axis real-time imaging provides an estimate of the mitral valve orifice as measured by planimetry. The 2DE long-axis view can also visualize a congenital membrane within the left atrium in patients with supravalvular mitral ring and cor triatriatum. However, Snider et al.[27] reported that these two abnormalities could not be easily differentiated on echocardiography.

Another form of mitral valvular stenosis in children is the parachute deformity of the mitral valve, characterized by a complex of chordal and papillary fusions and poor development of the mitral valve leaflets themselves. On the long-axis view the poorly mobile, shortened mitral leaflets sometimes appear tethered to a single enlarged papillary muscle, and the whole apparatus moves poorly in real time.

Summary

Thus, both M-mode echocardiography and 2DE provide the qualitative and quantitative information necessary for the detection of mitral stenosis. These techniques have proved to be extremely reliable, and they can also be used to determine the degree of severity of associated lesions. Long-term evaluation of patients with mitral stenosis, especially after surgical intervention, is feasible. Heger et al.[28] evaluated long-term changes in the mitral valve area after commissurotomy and found 2DE

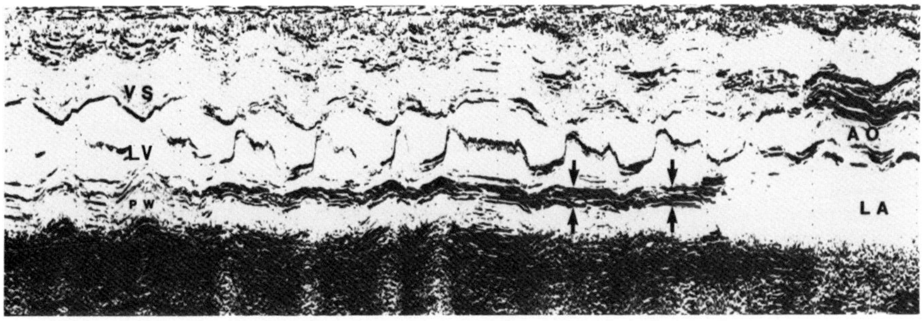

Fig 17–16.—M-mode echocardiogram from a patient with posterior submitral calcification *(black arrows)*. Scan was from the left ventricle *(LV)* to the aorta *(AO)*. *VS,* ventricular septum; *PW,* left ventricular posterior wall; *LA,* left atrium.

to be useful for long-term follow-up. The process of mitral restenosis after commissurotomy can also be followed by serial echocardiography.[28] When the characteristic echocardiographic findings are present in a patient with the clinical manifestations of mitral stenosis, useful information can be obtained. Size of the left ventricular outflow tract, left ventricular function, size of left atrium, and size of right atrium and right ventricle are useful parameters in the assessment of the severity of mitral stenosis, degree of pulmonary hypertension, function of the left ventricle, and type of treatment (e.g., type of prosthesis) required.

AORTIC STENOSIS

Aortic valvular stenosis has multiple etiologies. Congenital etiologies include a unicuspid or bicuspid aortic valve and subvalvular or supravalvular aortic stenosis; etiologies of acquired aortic stenosis include rheumatic valvulitis and degenerative calcification. The severity of the lesion is difficult to determine noninvasively, since only small changes in the valve orifice area may make the difference between a lesion of subclinical importance and one causing critical hemodynamic impairment. Thus, assessment of aortic valvular stenosis is more complicated and associated with more potential errors than assessment of mitral stenosis.

Three methods to estimate the severity of aortic valvular stenosis by 2DE have been described: (1) the measurement of the maximal aortic cusp separation compared to the aortic root diameter on the long-axis view, (2) direct measurement of aortic valve orifice area on the short-axis view, and (3) an indirect method of predicting peak left ventricular pressure using the end-systolic relative wall thickness ratio.

The Normal Aortic Valve

M-mode echocardiography

Recording of the aortic valve is often difficult because the leaflets present a relatively small tar-

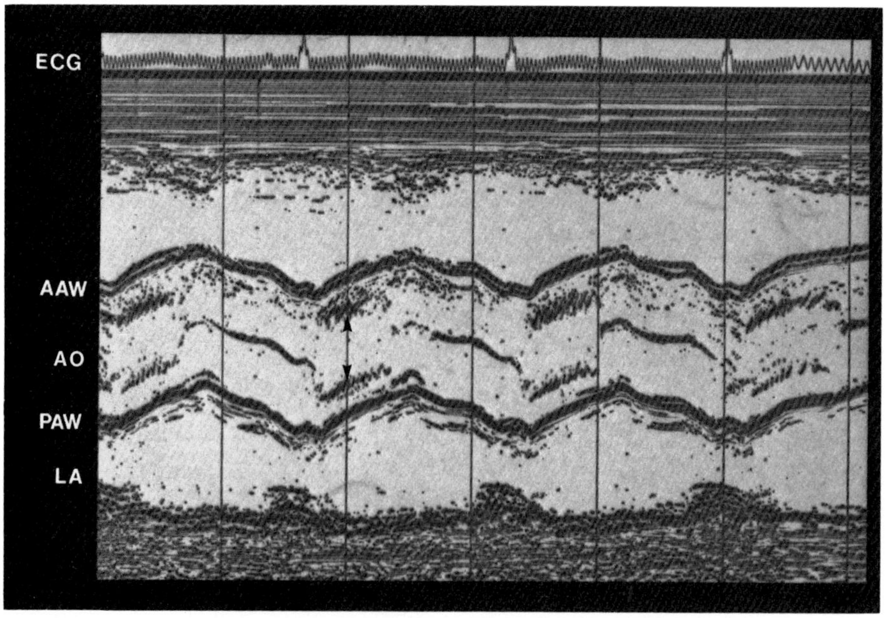

Fig 17–17.—M-mode echocardiogram of a normal aortic valve. Note the box-like pattern *(arrowheads)* during systole and a thin band echo during diastole. *AAW,* anterior aortic wall; *AO,* aorta; *PAW,* posterior aortic wall; *LA,* left atrium.

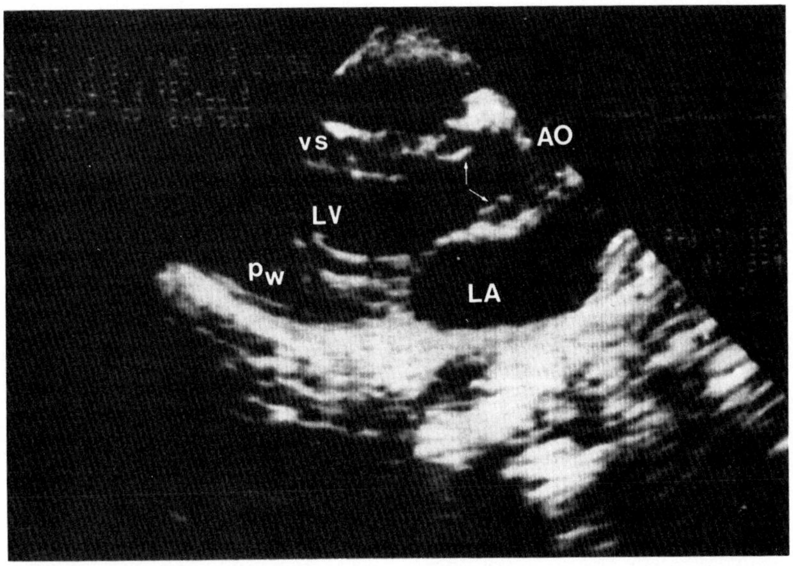

Fig 17–18.—Normal parasternal long-axis 2DE view of the aortic valve in systole. Note the thin echoes of the normal aortic leaflet *(arrows). VS,* ventricular septum; *LV,* left ventricle; *PW,* left ventricular posterior wall; *AO,* aorta; *LA,* left atrium.

get for the ultrasound beam. However, since the aortic walls are among the easiest structures to record consistently throughout the cardiac cycle, they provide a landmark to search for the aortic valve.

Figure 17–17 is an echocardiogram of a normal aortic valve. During diastole the normal aortic valve leaflets are recognized as a single echo or a thin band of echoes situated approximately in the center of the aortic root. During systole, aortic valve echoes present a box-like appearance. The anterior leaflet echoes originate from the right coronary cusp, and the posterior leaflet echoes most likely originate from the noncoronary cusp. Each of these demonstrate as a single thin echo adjacent to and parallel with the aortic walls. The separation between the anterior and posterior leaflets remains constant throughout systole and ranges from 1.7 to 2.1 cm in adults. The duration of opening of the aortic cusps during systole corresponds to the duration of the left ventricular ejection period. Aortic valve closure at the end of systole is rapid and may be difficult to record; it occurs while the aortic root is moving anteriorly. In normal individuals, fine oscillations of the aortic leaflets can be seen, representing a pliable, thin valve leaflet.

Two-Dimensional Echocardiography

Long-axis view.—The long-axis view of the left ventricle allows the visualization of the aortic root and aortic valve leaflets (Fig 17–18). A slight dilation of the aorta marks the sinuses of Valsalva and the position of the aortic valve. The aortic valve leaflets appear thin, and they coapt during diastole. The coapted aortic valve forms a single or double ultrasonic signal in the midline of the aortic root. At the onset of ejection, the aortic valve echoes move abruptly toward the aortic walls and appear almost to merge with them. The normal aortic valve leaflets show a rapid lateral mobility in real-time presentation.

Short-axis view.—On the short-axis view at the level of the great arteries, the aorta appears as a circle with a tri-leaflet aortic valve that has the appearance of the letter *Y* during diastole (Fig 17–19).

Acquired Aortic Stenosis

M-Mode Echocardiography

Mild aortic stenosis, such as frequently coexists with rheumatic mitral stenosis, is characterized by

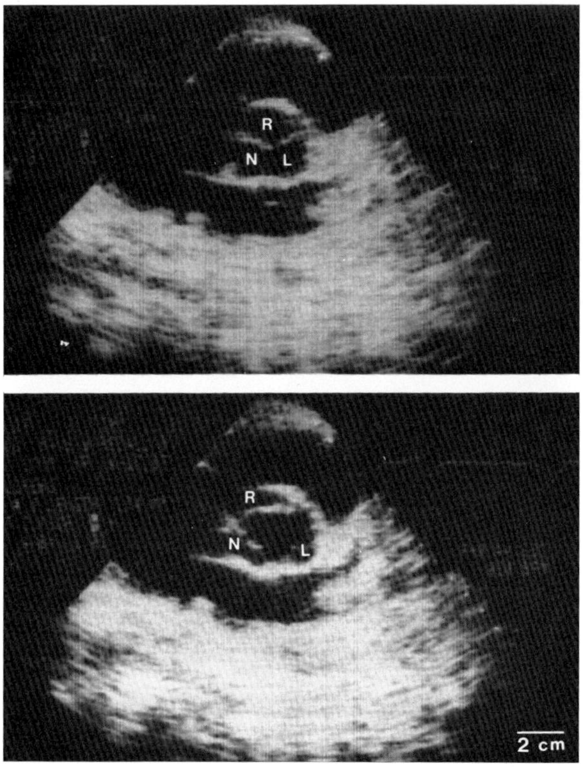

Fig 17–19.—Short-axis 2DE view of the aorta and aortic valve leaflets at the level of the great arteries during diastole *(top)* and systole *(bottom)*. Note the "tricuspid" appearance of the aortic valve during diastole. *R*, right coronary cusp; *L*, left coronary cusp; *N*, noncoronary cusp.

slight thickening of the valve with restriction of cusp motion (Fig 17–20). Severe acquired aortic stenosis in the adult is seldom associated with a normal aortic valve echogram.[7, 29] Almost all patients with mild aortic stenosis are 40 years old or older and have echocardiographic signs of aortic valve calcification. The echocardiographic appearance of calcium is an increase in echo density and increased width and smudging of the individual echo lines.[7] Technical factors, including the characteristics of different echocardiographic recorders and gain settings, vary significantly, so each laboratory should initially standardize its criteria for increased thickness. A heavily calcified aortic valve of any etiology shows marked restriction of cusp motion, and dense echoes may be recorded in systole and diastole. However, not all calcified valves are severely stenotic. If thin, discrete aortic valve echograms are obtained with a normal valve motion in an elderly patient, significant aortic stenosis can be excluded.

If heavy calcification is not present and rheumatic or acquired aortic stenosis is present, then the closure line in diastole is not eccentric, as may be seen in congenital bicuspid aortic stenosis.[30, 31]

The aortic orifice size can be affected by the aortic flow and the cardiac output.[32] In patients with poor cardiac output, the aortic valve will not open fully and may close prematurely. An increase in cardiac output (e.g., by the use of dopamine) can reinstitute normal aortic valve dimension and movement.

Other indirect echocardiographic parameters such as concentric hypertrophy of the left ventricle and decreased diastolic closure slope of the mitral valve may be useful in the assessment of patients with aortic stenosis.[33, 34]

Quantitation of the severity of acquired aortic stenosis in the adult based on M-mode aortic valve echocardiogram has been attempted in a number of laboratories.[35–41] However, neither aortic valve dimension nor severity of aortic valve calcification is a reliable predictor of the severity of obstruction.

Two-Dimensional Echocardiography

Weyman et al.[35] have used 2DE to determine the quantitative severity of aortic stenosis in 28 patients, many of whom had acquired aortic stenosis. They observed that 2DE long-axis views of the left ventricle were readily obtained (Fig 17–21), but true short-axis views of the valve orifice were technically difficult to reproduce. Nonetheless, the 2DE images distinguished between severe stenosis (orifice dimension, 4–11 mm) and mild stenosis (orifice dimension, 14–20 mm) (Fig 17–22) more accurately than M-mode echocardiography. In addition, M-mode echocardiographic aortic orifice dimensions could be determined in only 75% of patients in whom 2DE images and accurate measurements could be obtained. Evidently, 2DE significantly improves echocardiographic quantitation of acquired aortic stenosis.

Recently, Leo et al.[42] reported a good correlation ($r = 0.92$) between the aortic valve area obtained by the 2DE long- and short-axis views and

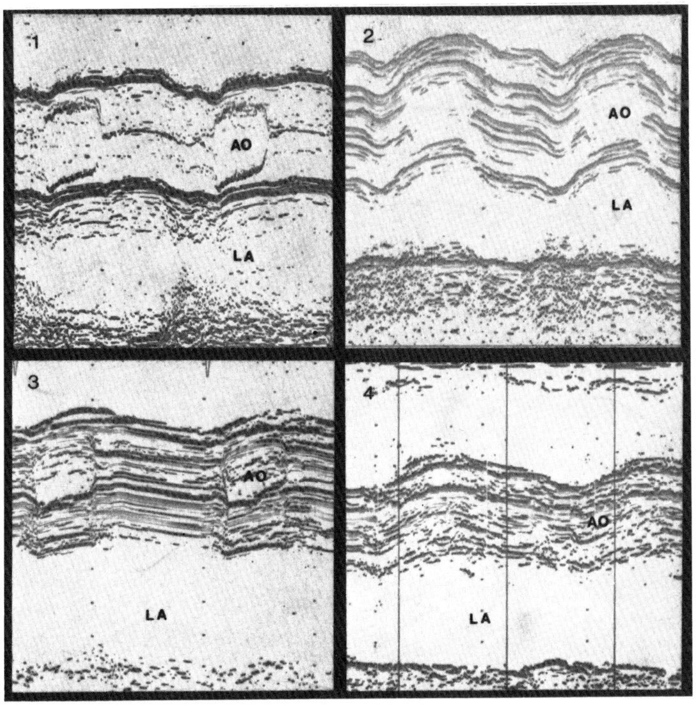

Fig 17–20.—M-mode echocardiograms from a normal subject *(1)* and three patients with various degrees of severity of aortic stenosis *(2–4)*. Note the multiple dense echoes during diastole and systole and reduced orifice size as the degree of aortic stenosis increases. *AO,* aorta, *LA,* left atrium.

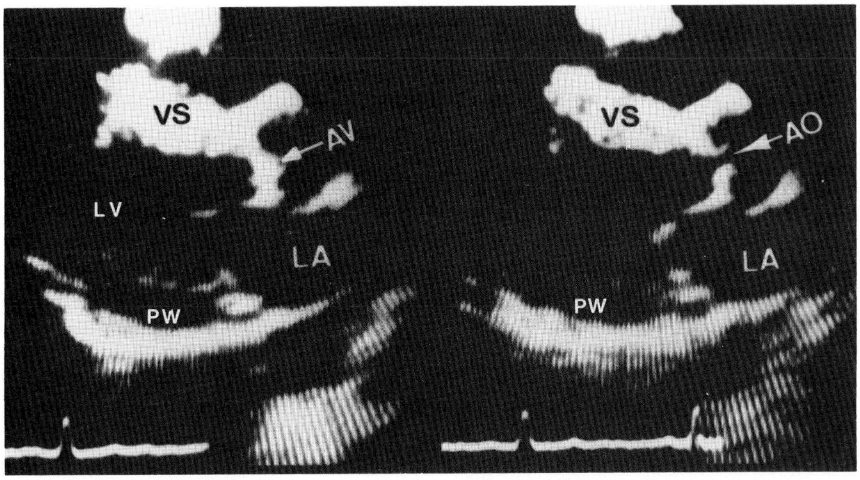

Fig 17–21.—Left ventricular parasternal long-axis 2DE view from a patient with aortic stenosis during diastole *(left)* and systole *(right)*. Note the thickened aortic leaflets with restricted opening during systole. *VS,* ventricular septum; *AV,* aortic valve; *LV,* left ventricle; *LA,* left atrium; *PW,* left ventricular posterior wall.

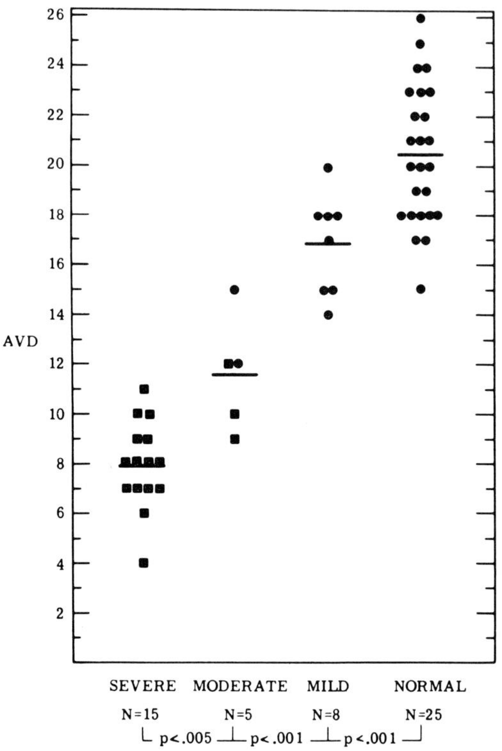

Fig 17–22.—Graphic relationship between aortic valve orifice diameter as determined on 2DE to the severity of aortic stenosis as determined on cardiac catheterization. Note that there is no overlap between severe cases and mild cases but some overlap of moderate cases. (From Weyman A.E., et al.: Cross-sectional echocardiography in assessing the severity of valvular aortic stenosis. *Circulation* 52:828–834, 1975. Reproduced by permission of the American Heart Association.)

measurements derived from catheterization data. These authors emphasize the importance of gain setting to avoid overestimation or underestimation of orifice size. DeMaria et al.[43] have tried to quantitate valvular aortic stenosis using long-axis, short-axis, and apical views. They obtained technically adequate echograms in 72 (85%) of 85 patients with aortic stenosis and found that echocardiography tended to overestimate the severity of aortic stenosis. In addition, the correlation between aortic leaflet separation and aortic gradient was poor (Fig 17–23).

In addition to these direct echocardiographic examinations of the aortic valve, an indirect method of predicting peak left ventricular pressure might be useful. When the left ventricle is under chronic pressure load, it compensates by cencentric left ventricular hypertrophy with usually symmetric thickening of the left ventricular wall. The prominent physiologic feature of this concentric left ventricular hypertrophy is that wall stress is maintained within a constant narrow range.

Wall stress is expressed as force per unit of cross-sectional area of myocardium, and force is directly proportional to left ventricular diameter, conveniently measured as left ventricular internal dimension (LVID) on the echocardiogram. The ratio of wall thickness (h) to LVID (h/LVID) increases in parallel with the degree of left ventricular hypertrophy.

Bennett et al.[33] used this approach to develop an echocardiographic method for predicting peak left ventricular pressure. According to their calculations, peak left ventricular systolic pressure (P) $= 225 \times (h/\text{LVID})$ ($r = 0.91$). Therefore, by subtracting cuff blood pressure from the calculated peak left ventricular pressure in patients with aortic stenosis, a reasonable estimate of the actual

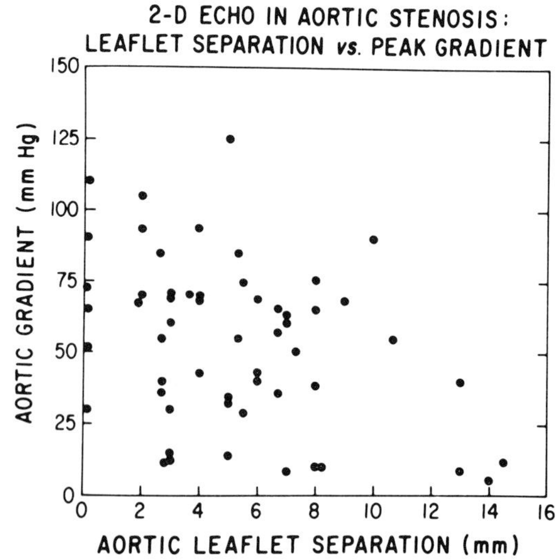

Fig 17–23.—Graph showing the lack of correlation between the aortic valve gradient as determined on cardiac catheterization and the maximal aortic leaflet separation as determined on 2DE. (From DeMaria A.N., et al.: Value and limitations of cross-sectional echocardiography of the aortic valve in the diagnosis and quantification of valvular aortic stenosis. *Circulation* 62:304-312, 1980. Reproduced by permission of the American Heart Association.)

pressure gradient across the stenotic valve can be obtained ($r = 0.87$).

Schwartz et al.[34] have also reported that 30 of 44 patients with aortic stenosis had their aortic gradient accurately estimated by the echocardiogram ($r = 0.75$). However, in patients with poor left ventricular systolic function, left ventricular pressure and aortic gradient could not be accurately estimated using this method. Thus, this echocardiographic method to examine the effects of aortic stenosis on the left ventricle can be used as a screening procedure to select those who should undergo cardiac catheterization and to identify those with insignificant left ventricular outflow obstruction.

Congenital Aortic Stenosis

M-Mode Echocardiography

The congenitally stenotic aortic valve may be unicuspid, bicuspid, or tricuspid. In children and young adults, congenitally stenotic valves usually do not show the M-mode echocardiographic signs typical for aortic stenosis.[7] This is because many such valves dome in systole. Thus, despite narrowing of the valve orifice, the leaflets may be normally separated along much of the valve's length.

Nanda et al.[44] have described the echocardiographic features of aortic stenosis associated with a bicuspid aortic valve. They demonstrated marked eccentricity of the aortic valve cusp echoes in diastole. Employing an eccentricity index (½ aortic luminal diameter/minimum distance of the diastolic aortic echo from the nearest aortic margin), they were able to differentiate patients with tricuspid aortic valves from those with bicuspid aortic valves. Generally, patients with bicuspid aortic valves had an eccentricity index above 1.5–1.6, and those with tricuspid aortic valves had an index as low as 1.0–1.25. In approximately half of the patients with bicuspid aortic valves, multilayered diastolic echoes were demonstrated.

Radford et al.[29] found that an eccentricity index greater than 1.3 was present in 74% of 31 patients with nonobstructed bicuspid aortic valves. However, the central aortic leaflet echoes occurred in the remaining 26% of patients. Therefore, a normal finding does not exclude a bicuspid aortic valve. Thus, the sensitivity of echocardiography in the diagnosis of bicuspid aortic valve appears to be about 75%.

Two-Dimensional Echocardiography

Recently, 2DE features of congenitally stenotic aortic valve have been characterized and found helpful in its diagnosis.[45] Theoretically, a true short-axis view of the aortic orifice could be obtained with this method and planimetry could be used to measure valve area; however, these methods have proved extremely difficult. It is, however, feasible to obtain a long-axis view of the domed valve and measure the cusp separation at the orifice. To correct for the wide range of body size encountered in the pediatric population, Hurwitz et al.[45] have suggested that the ratio of cusp separation to aortic dimension be used as an index of stenosis, rather than absolute cusp separation itself. Using this approach, they observed in 12 subjects with moderate to severe aortic stenosis a cusp separation-aortic dimension ratio of 40% or less, while patients with mild stenosis had ratios of 42% to 63% and normal subjects had ratios of 63% or more.

Weyman et al.[46] have also reported 2DE findings in 28 patients with congenital aortic stenosis. Findings were similar to those in acquired aortic stenosis, i.e., an increase in echo production by the thickened aortic valve leaflets, abnormal motion pattern, and good correlation between maximum aortic cusp separation and aortic valve area. An example of such a valve is shown in Figure 17–24. The cusp separation-aortic dimension ratios were 53% in patients with mild aortic stenosis and 30% in patients with moderate to severe aortic stenosis.

The congenitally bicuspid aortic valve may be functionally normal throughout life, intrinsically stenotic, or develop late acquired stenosis or incompetence. Two-dimensional echocardiographic evaluation of the valve orifice and M-mode assessment of the left ventricle can lead to an accurate appraisal of the functional status of the bicuspid valve. Fowles et al.[30] correctly identified anatomy in 18 (95%) of 19 patients with bicuspid aortic valve using the 2DE short-axis view. The criteria used were the number of cusps seen in real-time mo-

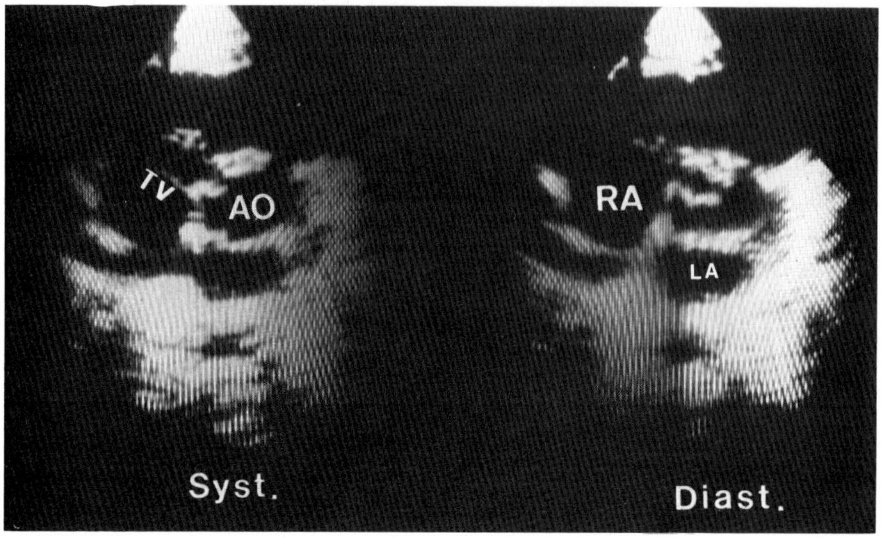

Fig 17–24.—Two-dimensional short-axis view of a bicuspid aortic valve. In systole *(left)* the leaflets open widely, whereas in diastole *(right)* the bicuspid leaflets are closed in a redundant curvilinear pattern. *TV,* tricuspid valve; *AO,* aorta; *RA,* right atrium; *LA,* left atrium.

tion, the irregularity or folding of cusp margins, and the location of commissural insertions; using the M-mode technique alone they were able to identify only 14 (74%) of these 19 patients using the eccentricity index. Because of variation in aortic valves and technical problems, there was a variability in eccentricity index (Fig 17–25).

Supravalvular Aortic Stenosis

Usher et al.[47] and Bolen et al.[48] have reported that supravalvular aortic stenosis can be identified echocardiographically by comparison of the aortic root dimension at the level of the aortic valve leaflets with that seen by scanning the aorta above the valve level on a continuous strip chart sweep.

A recent report by Feigenbaum et al.[49] indicates that 2DE from the suprasternal notch may be a useful method for identifying supravalvular aortic stenosis.

Discrete Subaortic Stenosis

Discrete subvalvular aortic stenosis can be divided into three types: stenosis due to a discrete membranous lesion (the most common type), stenosis of the fibromuscular collar, and stenosis of the fibromuscular tunnel. M-mode echocardiographic features of subaortic stenosis due to a membranous lesion include early systolic closure of the aortic valve, abnormal echoes within the left ventricular outflow tract, and left ventricular hypertrophy.[50, 51] The abnormal pattern of aortic

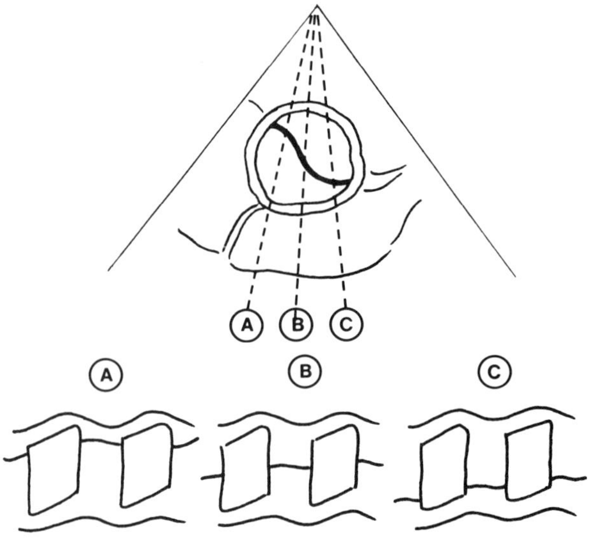

Fig 17–25.—Diagram showing the varying diastolic eccentricity index on the M-mode echocardiogram in a patient with bicuspid aortic valve. As the M-mode echocardiographic beam intersects the closed cusps at varying points *(A, B, C),* a different eccentricity index results.

valve motion produces a spike-and-plateau contour to the systolic aortic valve echogram (Fig 17–26). This spike-and-plateau configuration is similar to that seen in idiopathic hypertrophic subaortic stenosis, but in the latter condition the aortic valve leaflets stay open slightly longer than in discrete subvalvular aortic stenosis. In idiopathic hypertrophic subaortic stenosis the leaflets partially close in mid-systole before reopening in late systole.

The other two types of discrete subaortic stenosis include the fibromuscular collar and the fibromuscular tunnel varieties, which are rare lesions. Weyman et al.[52] have described the 2DE appearance of discrete subaortic stenosis of the membranous and fibromuscular collar types. Two

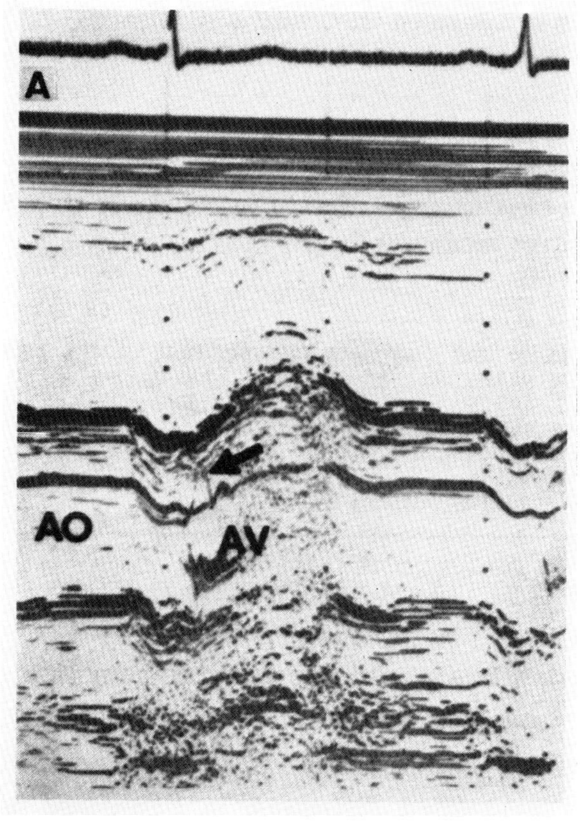

Fig 17–26.—M-mode echocardiogram of a patient with discrete fibromembranous subaortic stenosis. Note the early partial closure of the aortic valve. (From Greenspan A.M., et al.: Discrete fibromembranous aortic stenosis in middle age. *Cardiology* 64:306-316, 1979. Reproduced by permission of S. Karger AG, Basel.)

patients with a discrete membrane showed distinct linear echoes within the outflow tract which showed dynamic motion during the cardiac cycle. Five subjects with fibromuscular collar lesions showed diffuse or shell-like narrowing of the outflow tract. Three subjects with prior surgical palliation of subvalvular stenosis showed residual areas of outflow tract narrowing. Thus, 2DE may be more sensitive in differentiating these conditions; however, more experience with this technique is needed.[53, 54]

Summary

The assessment of aortic valvular stenosis is not as good as that of mitral valvular stenosis from the quantitative standpoint. The maximum aortic cusp separation-aortic root ratio can be used for distinguishing cases of mild and moderate to severe stenosis in children but is less applicable to adults. The presence of hypertrophy of the septum and left ventricular posterior wall helps to confirm outflow obstruction. Since the ratio of wall thickness to left ventricular diameter increases in parallel with left ventricular hypertrophy, peak left ventricular systolic pressure calculated using this ratio might be also used for a screening procedure to distinguish between cases of mild and moderate to severe stenosis, especially in children.

REFERENCES

1. Edler I., Gustafson A.: Ultrasonic cardiogram in mitral stenosis. *Acta Med. Scand.* 159:85–90, 1957.
2. Zaky A., Nasser W.K., Feigenbaum H.: A study of mitral valve action recorded by reflected ultrasound and its application in the diagnosis of mitral stenosis. *Circulation* 37:789–799, 1968.
3. Duchak J.M., Chang S., Feigenbaum H.: The posterior mitral valve echo and the echocardiographic diagnosis of mitral stenosis. *Am. J. Cardiol* 29:628–632, 1972.
4. Segal B.L., Likoff W., Kingsley B.: Echocardiography: Clinical application in mitral stenosis. *J.A.M.A.* 195:161–166, 1965.
5. Edler I.: Ultrasound cardiography in mitral valve stenosis. *Am. J. Cardiol.* 19:18, 1967.
6. Effert S.: Pre- and postoperative evaluation of mitral stenosis by ultrasound. *Am. J. Cardiol.* 19:59, 1967.
7. Feigenbaum H.: *Echocardiography*. Philadelphia, Lea & Febiger, 1981.
8. Gustafson A.: Correlation between ultrasound cardiography, hemodynamics and surgical findings in

mitral stenosis. *Am. J. Cardiol.* 19:32–41, 1967.
9. Cope G.D., Kisslo J.A., Johnson M.L., et al.: A reassessment of the echocardiogram in mitral stenosis. *Circulation* 52:664–670, 1975.
10. Levisman J.A., Abbasi A.S., Pearce M.L.: Posterior mitral leaflet motion in mitral stenosis. *Circulation* 51:511–514, 1975.
11. Nicolosi G.L., Atkins F., Dunn M.: Echocardiographic evaluation of mitral stenosis in predicting mitral valve replacement vs commissurotomy. Relation to hemodynamic measurements. *Chest* 77:147–154, 1980.
12. Henry W.L., Griffith J.M., Michaelis L.L., et al.: Measurement of mitral orifice area in patients with mitral valve disease by real-time, two-dimensional echocardiography. *Circulation* 51:827–831, 1975.
13. Nichol P.M., Gilbert B.W., Kisslo J.A.: Two-dimensional echocardiographic assessment of mitral stenosis. *Circulation* 55:120–128, 1977.
14. Wann L.S., Weyman A.E., Feigenbaum H., et al.: Determination of mitral valve area by cross-sectional echocardiography. *Ann. Intern. Med.* 88:337–341, 1978.
15. Weyman A.E., Wann L.S., Rogers E.W., et al.: Five-year experience in correlating cross-sectional echocardiographic assessment of the mitral valve area with hemodynamic valve area determinations, abstracted. *Am. J. Cardiol.* 43:386, 1979.
16. Martin R.P., Rakowski H., Kleiman J., et al.: Reliability and reproducibility of two-dimensional echocardiographic measurement of the stenotic mitral valve orifice area. *Am. J. Cardiol.* 43:560–568, 1979.
17. Chandraratna P.A.N., Aronow W.S., Lurie M., et al.: Cross-sectional echocardiographic observations on the mechanism of preservation of the opening snap in calcific mitral stenosis, abstracted. *Circulation* 59, 60 (suppl. II):II–79, 1979.
18. Naito M., Morganroth J., Mardelli T.J., et al.: Rheumatic mitral stenosis: Cross-sectional echocardiographic analysis. *Am. Heart J.* 100:34–40, 1980.
19. Weinrauch L.A., McDonald D.G., DeSilva R.A., et al.: Mitral valve prolapse in rheumatic mitral stenosis. *Chest* 72:752–756, 1977.
20. Nanda N.C., Gramiak R., Shah P.M., et al.: Echocardiographic assessment of left ventricular outflow width in the selection of mitral valve prosthesis. *Circulation* 48:1208–1214, 1973.
21. Kushner F.G., Lam W., Morganroth J.: Apex sector echocardiography in evaluation of the right atrium in patients with mitral stenosis and atrial septal defect. *Am. J. Cardiol.* 42:733–737, 1978.
22. Hirshfeld D.S., Emilson B.B.: Echocardiogram in calcified mitral annulus. *Am. J. Cardiol.* 36:354, 1975.
23. D'Cruz I.A., Cohen H.C., Prabhu R.: Clinical manifestations of mitral annulus calcification, with emphasis on its echocardiographic features. *Am. Heart J.* 94:367, 1977.
24. Dashkoff N., Karacuschansky M., Come P.C.: Echocardiographic features of mitral annulus calcification. *Am. Heart J.* 94:585, 1977.
25. D'Cruz I.A., Panetta F., Cohen H., et al.: Submitral calcification or sclerosis in elderly patients: M-mode and two-dimensional echocardiography in "mitral annulus calcification." *Am. J. Cardiol.* 44:31–38, 1979.
26. Collins-Nakai R.L., Rosenthal A., Castaneda A.R., et al.: Congenital mitral stenosis: A review of 20 years' experience. *Circulation* 56:1039–1046, 1977.
27. Snider A.R., Roge C.L., Schiller N.B., et al.: Congenital left ventricular inflow obstruction evaluated by two-dimensional echocardiography. *Circulation* 61:848–855, 1980.
28. Heger J.J., Wann L.S., Weyman A.E., et al.: Long-term changes in mitral valve area after successful mitral commissurotomy. *Circulation* 59:443–448, 1979.
29. Radford D.J., Bloom K.R., Izukawa T., et al.: Echocardiographic assessment of bicuspid aortic valves: Angiographic and pathological correlates. *Circulation* 53:80–85, 1976.
30. Fowles R.E., Martin R.P., Abrams J.M., et al.: Two-dimensional echocardiographic features of bicuspid aortic valve. *Chest* 75:434–440, 1979.
31. Gramiak R., Shah P.M.: Echocardiography of the normal and diseased aortic valve. *Radiology* 96:1–8, 1970.
32. Winsberg F.: Aortic valve, in Gramiak R., (ed.):*Cardiac Ultrasound*. St. Louis, C.V. Mosby Co., 1972.
33. Bennett D.H., Evans D.W., Raj M.V.J.: Echocardiographic left ventricular dimensions in pressure and volume overload: Their use in assessing aortic stenosis. *Br. Heart J.* 37:971–977, 1975.
34. Schwartz A., Vignola P.A., Walker H.J., et al.: Echocardiographic estimation of aortic-valve gradient in aortic stenosis. *Ann. Intern. Med.* 89:329–335, 1978.
35. Weyman A.E., Feigenbaum H., Dillon J.C., et al.: Cross-sectional echocardiography in assessing the severity of valvular aortic stenosis. *Circulation* 52:828–834, 1975.
36. Chang S., Clements S., Chang J.: Aortic stenosis: Echocardiographic cusp separation and surgical description of aortic valve in 22 patients. *Am. J. Cardiol.* 39:499–504, 1977.
37. Gewitz M.H., Werner J.C., Kleinman C.S., et al.: Role of echocardiography in aortic stenosis: Pre- and postoperative studies. *Am. J. Cardiol.* 43:67–73, 1979.
38. Henry W.L., Bonow R.O., Borer J.S., et al.: Evaluation of aortic valve replacement in patients with valvular aortic stenosis. *Circulation* 61:814–825, 1980.
39. Voelkel A.G., Kendrick M., Pietro D.A., et al.: Noninvasive tests to evaluate the severity of aortic

stenosis: Limitations and reliability. *Chest* 77:155–160, 1980.
40. Kirkman J., Hagan A.D., DiSessa T.G., et al.: Selection criteria for echocardiographic assessment of left ventricular pressure and peak gradient in patients with valvular aortic stenosis, abstracted. *Am. J. Cardiol.* 45:471, 1980.
41. Richards K., Crawford M., Cannon S., et al.: Quantification of aortic stenosis by doppler, M-mode and two-dimensional echocardiography, abstracted. *Circulation* 62:III–99, 1980.
42. Leo L.R., Barrett M.J., Leddy C.L., et al.: Determination of aortic valve area by cross-sectional echocardiography, abstracted. *Circulation* 59, 60(suppl. II):II–203, 1979.
43. DeMaria A.N., Bommer W., Joye J., et al.: Value and limitations of cross-sectional echocardiography of the aortic valve in the diagnosis and quantification of valvular aortic stenosis. *Circulation* 62:304–312, 1980.
44. Nanda N.C., Gramiak R., Manning J., et al.: Echocardiographic recognition of the congenital bicuspid aortic valve. *Circulation* 49:870–875, 1974.
45. Hurwitz R.A., Weyman A.E., Feigenbaum H., et al.: Cross-sectional echocardiographic assessment of severity of aortic stenosis in children, abstracted. *Am. J. Cardiol.* 37:144, 1976.
46. Weyman A.E., Feigenbaum H., Hurwitz R.A., et al.: Cross-sectional echocardiographic assessment of the severity of aortic stenosis in children. *Circulation* 55:773–778, 1977.
47. Usher B.W., Goulden D., Murgo J.P.: Echocardiographic detection of supravalvular aortic stenosis. *Circulation* 49:1257–1259, 1974.
48. Bolen J.L., Popp R.L., French J.W.: Echocardiographic features of supravalvular aortic stenosis. *Circulation* 52:817–822, 1975.
49. Feigenbaum H., Weyman A.E., Dillon J.C., et al.: Cross-sectional echocardiographic detection of aortic obstruction, abstracted. *Circulation* 54(suppl. II):221, 1976.
50. Popp R.L., Silverman J.F., French J.W., et al.: Echocardiographic findings in discrete subvalvular aortic stenosis. *Circulation* 49:226–231, 1974.
51. Davis R.H., Feigenbaum H., Chang S., et al. Echocardiographic manifestations of discrete subaortic stenosis. *Am. J. Cardiol* 33:277–280, 1974.
52. Weyman A.E., Feigenbaum H., Hurwitz R.A., et al.: Cross-sectional echocardiography in evaluating patients with discrete subaortic stenosis. *Am. J. Cardiol* 37:358–365, 1976.
53. Nanda N.C., Gramiak R.: Two-dimensional echocardiographic features of discrete subaortic stenosis, abstracted. *Circulation* 59,60(suppl. II):II–26, 1979.
54. Wilcox W.D., Seward J.B., Hagler D.J., et al.: Discrete subaortic obstruction: Two-dimensional echocardiographic features, abstracted. *Am. J. Cardiol.* 45:434, 1980.

RADIONUCLIDE IMAGING

James Rothendler and Robert D. Okada

PATIENTS with aortic or mitral stenosis may develop abnormalities in the size and function of one or more cardiac chambers. Radionuclide blood pool imaging done with technetium 99m has been useful in characterizing these abnormalities and studying their association with the severity of disease, symptomatology, prognosis, and postoperative results. Thallium 201 myocardial perfusion imaging has been used in evaluating the presence of associated coronary artery disease.

AORTIC STENOSIS

Pathophysiology

The normal response of the left ventricle to outflow obstruction due to aortic stenosis is the development of concentric hypertrophy. The increased wall thickness tends to counterbalance the increased intracavitary pressure and keep wall tension in the normal range.[1] When left ventricular hypertrophy is adequate for the degree of increased left ventricular systolic pressures, end-diastolic volume and ejection fraction remain near normal, although the left ventricular mass to volume ratio and the end-diastolic pressures are generally increased.[2] In some patients with aortic stenosis, the ejection fraction is above normal, possibly secondary to excessive hypertrophy.[3] A depressed ejection fraction and elevation of end-diastolic volume may be due to either inadequate hypertrophy or an intrinsic depression of contractility caused by long-standing and severe aortic stenosis, associated cardiomyopathy, or coronary artery disease. When a depressed ejection fraction is due to inadequate hypertrophy alone, the left ventricular ejection fraction may be very dependent on afterload. Valve replacement surgery in these patients should promote a significant increase in the ejection fraction. On the other hand, patients with a depressed ejection fraction due to intrinsic depression of contractility will probably show less improvement after surgery.[4, 5]

Patients with aortic stenosis may be subject to myocardial ischemia, even in the absence of significant coronary artery disease, due to an imbalance in oxygen supply and demand. Oxygen demand is increased by the presence of myocardial hypertrophy and elevated left ventricular systolic pressures. Oxygen supply, especially to the subendocardial region, may be decreased by a combination of factors. The systolic ejection time increases since the left ventricle is ejecting blood through an obstruction, and so there is a decrease in the diastolic time period during which most of coronary artery flow occurs. In addition, concentric left ventricular hypertrophy leads to an increase in diastolic left ventricular intramural pressure relative to coronary artery perfusion pressure.[6] This may compromise myocardial perfusion, especially to the deeper subendocardial layers.

Although aortic stenosis affects predominantly the left ventricle, other chambers may be affected as well. A mild to moderate degree of left atrial enlargement is not uncommon, especially in association with left ventricular failure. The development of atrial fibrillation may precipitate more severe failure due to loss of the atrial "kick." Right ventricular enlargement is infrequent but may develop in association with secondary pulmonary hypertension.[7] Finally, poststenotic dilation of the ascending aorta may be present in long-standing aortic stenosis.

Gated Blood Pool Imaging

Figure 18–1 shows gated blood pool images obtained in the anterior and left anterior oblique views in a patient with aortic stenosis. The left ventricle is only moderately enlarged. Left ventricular hypertrophy is suggested by a prominent photon-deficient halo around the left ventricle, the result of greater than normal separation between the blood pool in the ventricle and that in the lung. In addition, there may be an increased separation between the blood pools in the right and left ventricles on the left anterior oblique view due to septal hypertrophy. The halo effect can be seen on both anterior and left anterior oblique views, but it is difficult to quantitate and may occasionally be confused with pericardial effusions. It may be that left ventricular hypertrophy can be distinguished from effusion by determining whether the outer border of the halo contracts during systole and also by looking for evidence of septal hypertrophy. However, these findings have not been evaluated in prospective studies. Poststenotic dilation of the ascending aorta, also shown in Figure 18-1, is best seen on the anterior view.

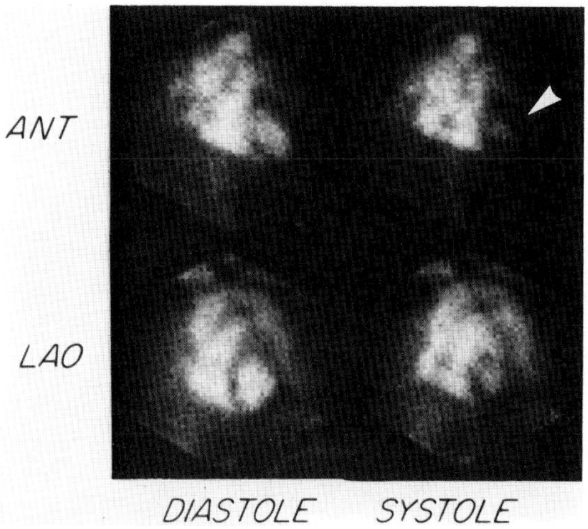

Fig 18–1.—Cardiac gated blood pool images in end-diastole and end-systole in a patient with aortic stenosis. *ANT,* anterior; *LAO,* left anterior oblique. The ascending aorta is prominent and there is a wide halo *(arrow)* surrounding the left ventricle, suggesting the possibility of hypertrophy.

Left ventricular size and ejection fraction can be readily evaluated with the gated blood pool technique. As noted previously, the ejection fraction may be normal, increased, or decreased. In studies in which wall stress was not specifically measured, the ejection fraction alone (as determined by contrast angiography) did not correlate well with functional class, postsurgical survival, valve area, cardiac index, or peak systolic gradient.[8, 9] However, Carabello et al.[10] identified a subgroup of patients with aortic stenosis and depressed ejection fraction in whom the calculated left ventricular wall stress was lower than expected, suggesting an intrinsic decrease in contractility. These patients appeared to have a poorer postoperative prognosis than patients with aortic stenosis, low ejection fractions, and "appropriate" wall stress. Therefore, although the resting left ventricular ejection fraction may be of limited value when used by itself, there may be a subset of patients with depressed ejection fractions and reduced contractility who may have a poorer prognosis, even after corrective surgery.

The response of left ventricular function to stress in aortic stenosis has been studied with Isuprel infusions[11] and with supine exercise testing.[12] The normal response to exercise is an increase in left ventricular ejection fraction. Many patients with aortic stenosis fail to demonstrate such a normal response. However, although exercise testing may detect an early abnormality in left ventricular function in patients with aortic stenosis, the prognostic and therapeutic implications of such a finding have not been determined. Furthermore, inducing stress in patients with severe aortic stenosis may be dangerous, and the routine use of exercise testing cannot be recommended.

Determination of left ventricular ejection fraction following aortic valve surgery may be useful in certain cases. In patients with depressed ejection fractions preoperatively this parameter usually returns to normal, particularly if the initial abnormality was caused by "inadequate" hypertrophy.[8, 9, 13–16] Studies suggest that normalization occurs very soon after surgery.[17] Figure 18–2 shows preoperative and 10-day postoperative end-diastolic and end-systolic images obtained in a patient with aortic stenosis. The ejection fraction increased from 30% preoperatively to 55% postoperatively.

In patients who develop congestive heart failure after aortic valve replacement, determination of ejection fraction may be useful in recognizing surgically correctable cases. Goldman et al.[18] found that an ejection fraction of greater than 50% in the setting of heart failure was highly predictive of correctable conditions, usually aortic or mitral insufficiency. Patients with ejection fractions less than or equal to 50% usually had congestive heart failure due to myocardial failure, and surgery did not improve their condition.

Thallium 201 Imaging

Bailey et al.[19] reported the possible utility of thallium 201 imaging at rest and exercise in identifying those patients with aortic stenosis who also had associated coronary artery disease. Twenty-two patients were studied, 11 with significant coronary stenosis (>70% diameter narrowing) in at least one vessel and 11 without significant coronary artery disease (<30% stenosis). Of the 11 patients with significant coronary disease, 4 had focal ^{201}Tl defects on resting studies preoperatively and 7 had defects on exercise. In addition, 8 of these 11 patients had a pattern of ^{201}Tl uptake during exercise compatible with diffuse wall thinning. In the 11 patients without significant coronary artery disease (of whom 6 had some degree of diameter narrowing up to 30%), one patient had a resting focal defect while 6 had focal defects with exercise. Six patients were also noted to have a pattern of exercise-induced thinning. Although there was a greater percentage of resting focal defects in the patients with significant coronary disease, the difference was not statistically significant owing to the small number of patients studied. The studies obtained during exercise failed to add to the diagnostic accuracy. Although the studies suggesting focal defects in the patients without significant coronary disease may be labeled false positives, the basis for the defects may still be a relative decrease in blood flow to the particular area. As noted earlier, patients with aortic stenosis may develop myocardial ischemia in the absence of coronary artery disease. Furthermore, a 30% coronary artery lesion, while not normally significant hemo-

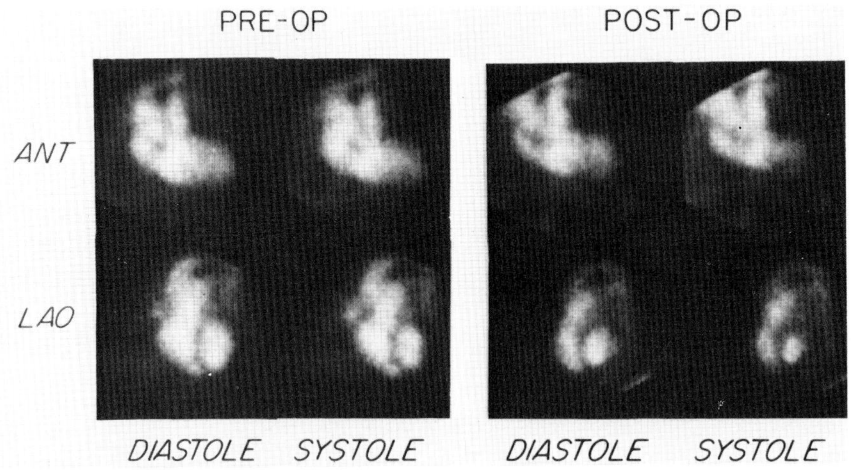

Fig 18–2.—Preoperative and postoperative cardiac gated blood pool images in diastole and systole in the anterior and left anterior oblique projections. In the postoperative images there has been a decrease in size of the left ventricle in both diastole and systole, and the ejection fraction has increased from 30% to 55%.

dynamically in the absence of aortic stenosis, may cause a relative flow deficit when demands are particularly high, as when a patient with left ventricular hypertrophy and aortic stenosis exercises. Finally, increases in left ventricular volume on exercise may cause apparent defects to occur in the anterior wall and apex due to geometric factors alone, despite the absence of ischemia.[20] Such a change in volume might be expected in patients with severe aortic stenosis.

MITRAL STENOSIS

Pathophysiology

Inflow obstruction to the left ventricle due to mitral valve stenosis causes an elevation in the left atrial pressure and subsequent left atrial enlargement. The elevated left atrial pressure in turn raises pulmonary venous and pulmonary capillary pressures. Right ventricular chamber size and function may remain normal during mild to moderate pressure overload as long as adequate hypertrophy develops.[21, 22] However, severe, long-standing pulmonary hypertension may lead to right ventricular chamber enlargement, a depressed right ventricular ejection fraction, and enlargement of the main pulmonary artery segment. Right atrial enlargement is a frequent accompaniment of depressed right ventricular function with elevated filling pressures. Tricuspid regurgitation may also be present, either secondary to right ventricular dilation or as a result of rheumatic involvement of the valve.

Although left ventricular function is generally not severely affected in mitral stenosis without concomitant mitral regurgitation or aortic valve disease, a decrease in ejection fraction is not uncommon.[22] One hypothesis for this reduced ejection fraction is chronic underfilling of the ventricle with a markedly reduced preload. Others have hypothesized left ventricular dysfunction on the basis of a rigid "mitral complex" immobilizing the posterobasal area of the left ventricle.[23] Residual scarring due to either the acute episode of rheumatic fever or chronic rheumatic myocarditis has also been proposed as a possible etiology for the depressed left ventricular ejection fraction.[24]

Blood Pool Imaging

Figure 18–3 shows a gated blood pool image obtained in a patient with mitral stenosis. The left atrium, right ventricle, right atrium, and main pulmonary artery all are enlarged. The left atrium is best seen on the left posterior oblique view, the right atrium and main pulmonary artery on the anterior view, and the right ventricle on the anterior and left anterior oblique views. In mitral stenosis the right ventricular ejection fraction is decreased but the left ventricular function is normal. Right and left atrial sizes may not change significantly between diastole and systole, a reverse of what is found in atrial fibrillation.

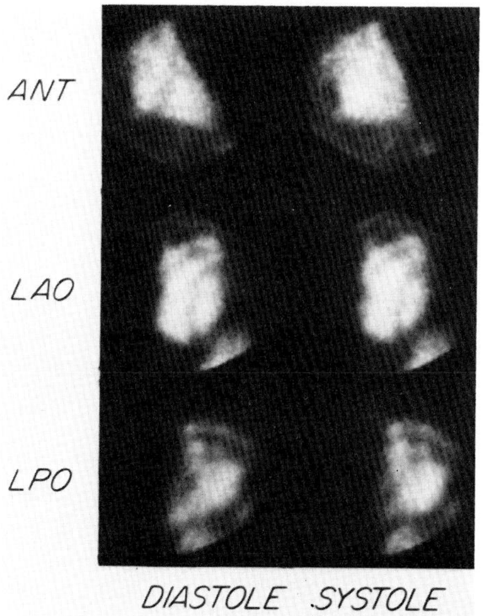

Fig 18–3.—Cardiac gated blood pool images in diastole and systole in a patient with mitral stenosis. *ANT,* anterior; *LAO,* left anterior oblique; *LPO,* left posterior oblique. The right ventricle is enlarged and poorly contracting. The left atrium, best seen on the LAO and LPO views, is markedly enlarged. The main pulmonary artery is prominent. The left ventricle is normal in size and function.

Imaging of the first-pass transit of isotope as it enters the right side of the heart after injection into the arm may be a sensitive method of detecting even mild degrees of tricuspid regurgitation when present in association with mitral stenosis and right ventricular failure.[21] Characteristically, activity may be seen refluxing into the inferior vena cava or hepatic vein during ventricular systole. In cases of severe regurgitation, the stroke count relationship between the right and left ventricles may be useful.

That many patients with mitral stenosis are in atrial fibrillation may create a problem for gated blood pool imaging. Since the R-R intervals are continually varying, and since the duration of ventricular systole depends on the preceding R-R interval, the end-systoles will not exactly coincide. Further, there is often a dropoff in counts in late frames in the composite gated image owing to some cycles ending early. These factors tend to degrade image quality. Nevertheless, the averaged gated image produced in this manner probably yields an ejection fraction that reflects the ventricular function better than a contrast ventriculogram, which samples only a few beats. A possible solution to problems encountered with averaged cycles may be the use of high-efficiency nonimaging probes.[25] These devices may be useful in assessing beat-to-beat variability and allowing more accurate evaluation of the effect of filling time on cardiac performance in these patients. Another solution is list mode acquisition.

Right ventricular ejection fraction has not correlated well with early surgical prognosis in mitral stenosis,[22] although DiCola et al. have found that it does seem to correlate with preoperative mitral valve area.[26] When right ventricular ejection fraction is depressed prior to surgery, there is frequently a significant improvement shortly after valve replacement.[27] The degree of left ventricular functional impairment does not appear to correlate with the degree of stenosis present.[28]

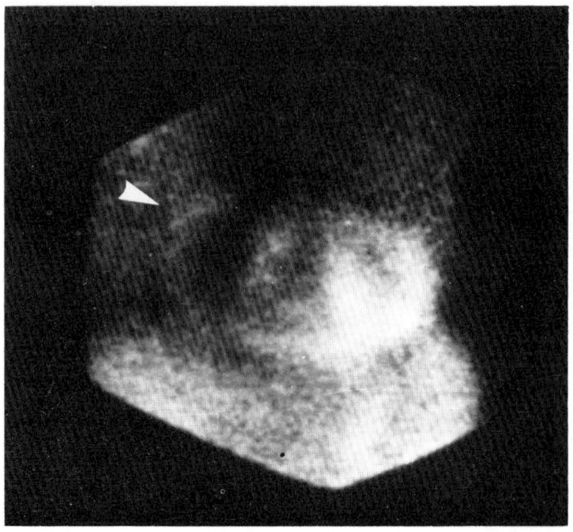

Fig 18–4.—Thallium image of the heart in a patient with mitral stenosis, taken in the left anterior oblique projection. There is an area of increased uptake *(arrow)* anterior to the right ventricle, probably representing the right atrium.

Thallium 201 Imaging

Thallium 201 imaging has not been extensively used in evaluating the presence of associated coronary artery disease in patients with mitral stenosis because of the danger of precipitating pulmonary edema with exercise. However, several reports have documented an increase in the right ventricular uptake of ^{201}Tl in the setting of pulmonary hypertension.[29, 30] Although not specific for mitral stenosis, the technique appears to be fairly sensitive. Similarly, visualization of the right atrial appendage has been reported in association with right ventricular pressure overload.[31, 32] Figure 18–4 shows a ^{201}Tl image in the left anterior oblique view in a patient with mitral stenosis in whom right ventricular uptake is increased and right atrial uptake is present. Adachi et al.[32] proposed that the most important factor in visualization of the right atrium may be rotation of the right atrium to a more anterior position in these patients, bringing the right atrial appendage closer to the chest wall and decreasing attenuation and scatter.

TRICUSPID AND PULMONIC STENOSIS

Tricuspid stenosis is usually rheumatic in origin and is rarely an isolated lesion, often being accompanied by mitral or aortic involvement. Although not specific for tricuspid stenosis, right atrial enlargement is frequently present and may be easily appreciated in the anterior or right anterior oblique view using the gated blood pool technique. Other cardiac chamber abnormalities may be due to associated lesions of the mitral or aortic valve, especially those resulting from mitral stenosis.

Pulmonic stenosis is usually congenital in origin but may also be due to rheumatic or carcinoid involvement. Pathologic changes caused by right ventricular pressure overload may be present, and both gated blood pool and ^{201}Tl imaging may be useful in clinical evaluation.

REFERENCES

1. Sasayama S., Ross J.Jr., Franklin D., et al.: Adaptions of the left ventricle to chronic pressure overload. *Circ. Res.* 38:172, 1976.
2. Dodge H.T., Kennedy J.W., Peterson J.L.: Quantitative angiocardiographic methods in the evaluation of valvular heart disease. *Prog. Cardiovasc. Dis.* 16:1–23, 1973.
3. Hasin Y., Rod J.L., Friedman G.: Co-existing aortic stenosis and secondary hypertrophic cardiomyopathy manifested by an hourglass left ventricle. *Chest* 76:232–234, 1979.
4. Gunther S., Grossman W.: Determinants of ventricular function in pressure-overload hypertrophy in man. *Circulation* 59:679–688, 1979.
5. Schwarz F., Flameng W., Schaper J., et al.: Myocardial structure and function in patients with aortic valve disease and their relation to postoperative results. *Am. J. Cardiol.* 41:661–669, 1978.
6. Vincent W.R., Buckberg G.D., Hoffman J.I.E.: Left ventricular subendocardial ischemia in severe valvar and supravalvar aortic stenosis. *Circulation* 59:326–333, 1974.
7. Gould L., Venkataramen U., Goswami M., et al.: Right-sided heart failure in aortic stenosis. *Am. J. Cardiol.* 31:381–383, 1973.
8. Thompson R., Yacomb M., Ahmed M., et al.: Influence of preoperative left ventricular function on results of homograft replacement of the aortic valve for aortic stenosis. *Am. J. Cardiol.* 43:929–938, 1979.
9. Schwarz F., Flameng W., Langebartels F., et al.: Impaired left ventricular function in chronic aortic valve disease: Survival and function after replacement by Björk-Shiley prosthesis. *Circulation* 60:48–58, 1979.
10. Carabello B.A., Green L., Cohn L.H., et al.: Prognosis of valve replacement in aortic stenosis with low ejection fraction, abstracted. *Circulation* 60:II–192, 1979.
11. Schwarz F., Flameng W., Thormann J., et al.: Cardiac reserve during isoproterenol stress in patients with aortic valve disease before and after corrective surgery. *Am. Heart J.* 95:146–153, 1978.
12. Borer J.S., Bacharach S.L., Green M.V., et al.: Left ventricular function in aortic stenosis: Response to exercise and effects of operation, abstracted. *Am. J. Cardiol.* 41:382, 1978.
13. Smith N., McAnulty J.H., Rahimtoola S.H.: Severe aortic stenosis with impaired left ventricular function and clinical heart failure: Results of valve replacement. *Circulation* 58:255–264, 1978.
14. O'Toole J.D., Gelser E.A., Reddy S., et al.: Effect of preoperative ejection fraction on survival and hemodynamic improvement following aortic valve replacement. *Circulation* 58:1175–1184, 1978.
15. Crake R.P., Pifarre R., Sullivan H., et al.: Reversal of advanced left ventricular dysfunction following aortic valve replacement for aortic stenosis. *Ann. Thorac. Surg.* 24:38–43, 1977.
16. Pantely G., Morton M., Rahimtoola S.H.: Effects of successful, uncomplicated valve replacement on ventricular hypertrophy, volume, and performance in aortic stenosis and aortic incompetence. *J. Thorac. Cardiovasc. Surg.* 75:383–391, 1978.
17. Carabello B.A., Wynne J., Holman B.L.: Assessment of left ventricular function early after aortic valve replacement, abstracted. *Circulation* 60:II–193, 1979.
18. Goldman M.R., Boucher C.A., Block P.C., et al.: Value of gated blood pool scan in assessing development of heart failure following aortic valve replacement, abstracted. *Circulation* 60:II–193, 1979.
19. Bailey I.A., Come P.C., Kelly D.T., et al.: Thallium-201 myocardial perfusion imaging in aortic valve stenosis. *Am. J. Cardiol.* 40:889–899, 1977.
20. Gewirtz H., Grötte G.J., Strauss H.W., et al.: The influence of left ventricular volume and wall motion on myocardial images. *Circulation* 59:1172–1177, 1979.
21. Winzelberg G.G., Boucher C.A., McKusick K.A., et al.: Right ventricular function in aortic and mitral valve disease: Relation of gated first pass radionuclide angiography to clinical and hemodynamic findings. *Chest* 79:520–528, 1981.
22. Wroblewski E., James F., Spann F., et al.: Right ventricular performance in mitral stenosis. *Am. J. Cardiol.* 47:51–55, 1981.
23. Heller S.J., Carleton R.A.: Abnormal left ventricular contraction in patients with mitral stenosis. *Circulation* 42:1099–1110, 1970.
24. Ahmed S.S., Regan T.J., Fiore J.J., et al.: The state of the left ventricular myocardium in mitral stenosis. *Am. Heart J.* 94:28–36, 1977.
25. Schneider J., Berger H., Sands M.J., et al.: The relationship of mean ejection fraction to beat-to-beat function in atrial fibrillation, abstracted. *Circulation* 62:III–102, 1980.
26. DiCola V.C., Boucher C.A., Shea W.H., et al.: Right and left ventricular performance before and after correction of mitral stenosis, abstracted. *Am. J. Cardiol.* 47:424, 1981.

27. Levine F.H., Lappas D.L., Pohost G.M., et al.: Radionuclide and hemodynamic assessment of pulmonary hypertension and right ventricular function after mitral valve replacement, abstracted. *Am. J. Cardiol.* 43:406, 1979.
28. Kennedy J.W., Yarwell S.R., Murray J.A., et al.: Quantitative angiocardiography: IV. Relationships of left atrial and ventricular pressure and volume in mitral valve disease. *Circulation* 41:817–832, 1970.
29. Cohen H.A., Baird M.G., Rouleau J.R., et al.: Thallium-201 myocardial imaging in patients with pulmonary hypertension. *Circulation* 54:790–795, 1976.
30. Kondo M., Kubo A., Yamazuki H., et al.: Thallium-201 myocardial imaging for evaluation of right ventricular overloading. *J. Nucl. Med.* 19:1197–1203, 1978.
31. Cowley M.J., Coughlan H.C., Logic J.R.: Visualization of atrial myocardium with thallium-201: Case report. *J. Nucl. Med.* 18:984–986, 1977.
32. Adachi H., Torii Y., Kamide T., et al.: Visualization of right atrial appendix by thallium-201 myocardial scintigraphy. *J. Nucl. Med.* 21:914–918, 1980.

COMMENT: AORTIC AND MITRAL VALVE STENOSIS

Joel Morganroth

THE RECOGNITION of clinically important aortic and mitral valvular stenosis remains an important challenge to the clinician. Failure to recognize these conditions often results in inappropriate medical therapy and progressive deterioration of the patient's condition. While physical examination remains the principal means of clinical recognition and detection, confirmation of examination findings by noninvasive cardiac testing, especially in the patient with obscure disease, is often mandatory.

ETIOLOGIC DETERMINATION

Echocardiography is the major noninvasive diagnostic tool in the recognition and etiologic determination of mitral and aortic stenosis. Echocardiography can be used not only to image valvular tissue, but also, because of its fine resolution, to determine whether congenitally bicuspid or acquired atherosclerotic aortic valvular stenosis is present. Mitral stenosis in adults is almost invariably due to rheumatic heart disease, though severe annular calcification with obstruction to mitral valve flow can also be detected by echocardiography. Other conditions obstructing normal diastolic transmitral valvular blood flow such as left atrial myxoma or left atrial thrombus can be detected as well. Cardiac nuclear imaging plays no important role in etiologic determination.

CLINICAL CONSIDERATION

Mitral Stenosis

Two-dimensional echocardiography (2DE) has a major role in the detection and determination of severity of mitral valvular stenosis. Short-axis 2DE measurement of the mitral orifice area has become a standard diagnostic technique and in many institutions has eliminated the need for cardiac catheterization for this determination. The estimation of valve pliability helps to determine the surgical procedure (e.g., commissurotomy vs. valve replacement) and the estimation of the left ventricular outflow tract size guides the cardiac surgeon in the type of prosthesis to implant. The importance of the echocardiographic evaluation of left ventricular function and possible associated valvular lesions is obvious. In patients in whom echocardiographic evaluation is limited or equivocal, cardiac nuclear imaging can predict the state of left ventricular function and the presence of right ventricular hypertrophy suggesting concomitant pulmonary hypertension. However, at present cardiac nuclear imaging in patients with mitral stenosis has limited utility.

Aortic Stenosis

Unfortunately, echocardiographic assessment of the severity of aortic valvular stenosis is markedly limited compared to its use in mitral stenosis. However, here as well as in mitral stenosis echocardiography is helpful since normal or only slightly impaired aortic valve motion on echocardiography virtually excludes the presence of clinically significant aortic stenosis. Thus, many patients with prominent systolic ejection murmurs who are suspected of having severe aortic valvular stenosis should not undergo diagnostic cardiac catheterization if echocardiography reveals a mobile aortic valve without evidence of heavy calcification. The reverse, however, is more difficult. The presence of aortic valvular calcification may often mask the true mobility of aortic leaflet tissue and may eliminate the possibility of determining whether or not clinically significant aortic valvular stenosis is present. The presence of left ventricular hypertrophy without coexisting hypertension or other causes for such hypertrophy may be an important clue in identifying clinically important aortic stenosis in such cases. The potential use of doppler techniques in conjunction with echocardiography may help define the degree of aortic stenosis. Radionuclide imaging techniques are indicated in the evaluation of patients with suspected aortic stenosis only when echocardiographic estimation of left ventricular function and thickness is equivocal or not feasible. Exercise thallium perfusion scans to detect coronary artery disease in patients with concomitant aortic stenosis and chest pain appear to have poor predictability. In the elderly patient with an abnormal echocardiogram in whom aortic stenosis is suspected, it is still frequently necessary to resort to diagnostic cardiac catheterization.

ASSESSMENT OF PROGNOSIS

Echocardiography is an easy, noninvasive means of following patients with aortic or mitral stenosis, particularly after surgical intervention. Valvular prosthesis dysfunction, changes in left ventricular performance, postcommissurotomy changes, restenosis, and associated conditions such as left atrial thrombus formation can all be detected with this technique. We usually recommend echocardiography in all patients after valvular replacement to determine a baseline record of cardiac prosthetic motion and to evaluate left ventricular size and performance. When complications occur, repeat echocardiography is frequently useful in diagnosis and management. The use of radionuclide angiography to evaluate ventricular size and function or the presence of associated regurgitant lesions is an alternative approach when echocardiography is equivocal or technically difficult.

PART X

Intracardiac Masses

ECHOCARDIOGRAPHY

Daniel A. Pietro and Alfred F. Parisi

PRIOR TO the widespread use of echocardiography, evaluation of masses within the heart cavities was limited to direct inspection or cardiac angiography with its associated risks, cost, and limitations. The availability of echocardiography, first M-mode and more recently the two-dimensional (2DE) technique, now permits cardiac chambers and structures to be scrutinized with ease, at no risk, and as frequently as required. As a result, previously unrecognized intracavitary lesions can now be diagnosed and treated or followed serially. Information on the natural history of intracardiac mass lesions and their response to therapeutic approaches is rapidly increasing. The information provided by echocardiography thus promises to shape further the management of patients with these conditions.

INTRACARDIAC TUMORS

By virtue of their location, intracardiac tumors are associated with a high degree of morbidity and mortality, regardless of their composition. Within the heart, they may produce inflow or outflow tract obstruction. If they embolize to the systemic or pulmonary circulation they can produce target organ infarction. The intracardiac tumors may be primary (cardiac) or secondary (metastatic) in origin.

Primary Tumors

The most common primary cardiac tumor is the myxoma, although it is still infrequent (1 in 4,000 autopsy cases).[1] Its recognition is especially important because it can be cured surgically, with dissolution of the presenting constitutional symptoms of fever, malaise, and weight loss, removal of the intracardiac obstruction, and a reduction in the risk of embolism and sudden death. The morphological characteristics of the myxoma made it an appropriate candidate for detection in the early days of echocardiography. Myxomas were first detected in Germany in 1952 by M-mode echocardiography,[2] and so had an important role in demonstrating the clinical potential for this new diagnostic tool.

The myxoma is a gelatinous disarray of tissue which has a high acoustic impedance. Four characteristics—size, location, peduncular shape, resulting in characteristic motion, and high acoustic reflectance—all enhance its detection by echocardiography.

It is generally a large, bulky, pedunculated tumor and is usually attached by a stalk to the atrial wall, most frequently at the interatrial septum.

The location—left atrial in 75% of the cases—is important because the M-mode technique readily examines this chamber.[3] Presently 2DE can be used to examine all four cardiac chambers, in particular the right atrium, thus increasing the sensitivity of echocardiography for tumor detection in locations other than the left atrium.

The characteristic motion of the left atrial

myxoma relates to its peduncular attachment. This allows the myxoma to travel with the flow of blood into the funnel-shaped inflow tract of the left ventricle and around the mitral leaflets during diastole. The tumor typically interferes with mitral leaflet motion and produces a characteristic pattern of echoes. During systole, the left atrial myxoma is expelled back into the left atrium and can be seen as a mass of echoes in the left atrium during this part of the cardiac cycle (Figs 19–1

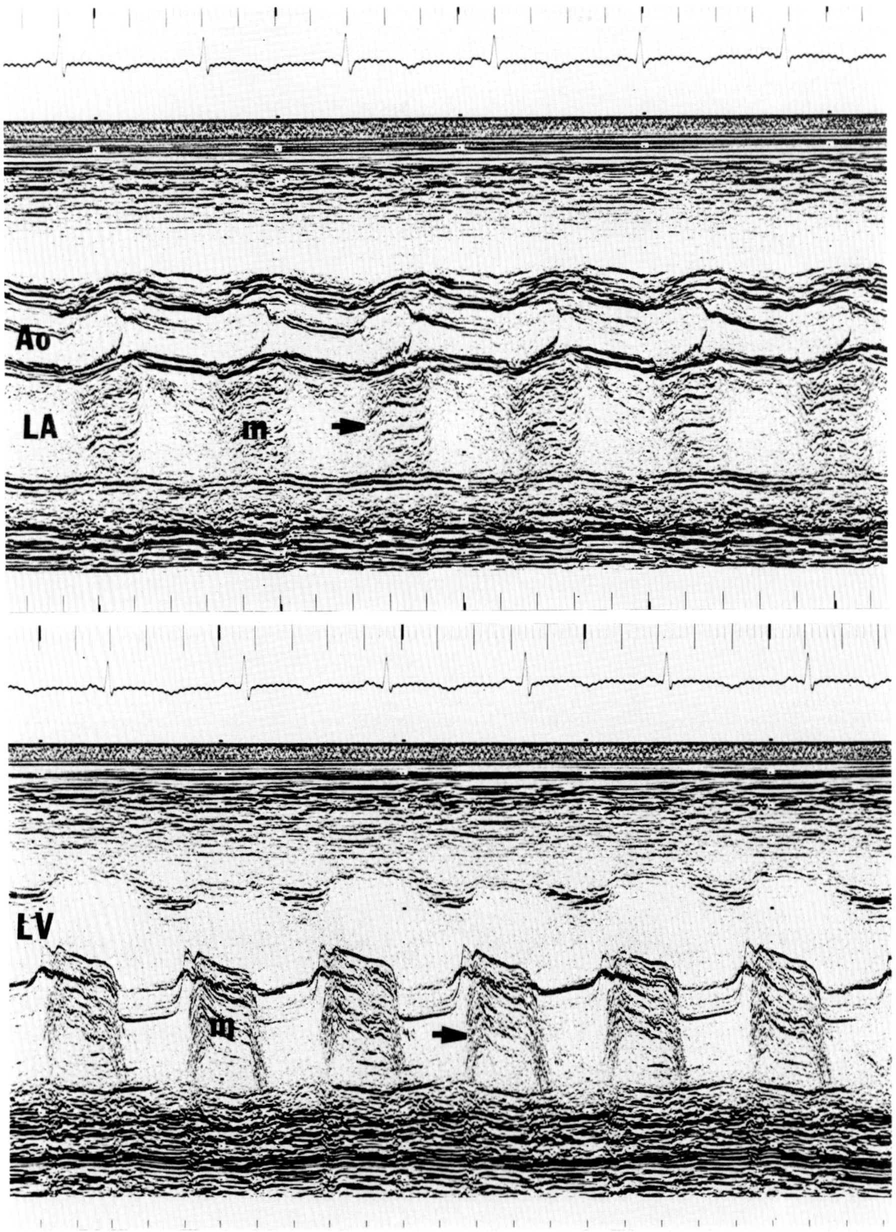

Fig 19–1.—Left atrial myxoma is represented by the mass of echoes in the left atrium during systole *(arrow, top panel)* and behind the anterior mitral valve leaflet *(arrow, bottom panel)* during diastole. Note the temporal separation between DE excursion of the anterior mitral leaflet and the appearance of the tumor mass. *Ao,* aorta; *m,* myxoma; *LA,* left atrium; *LV,* left ventricle.

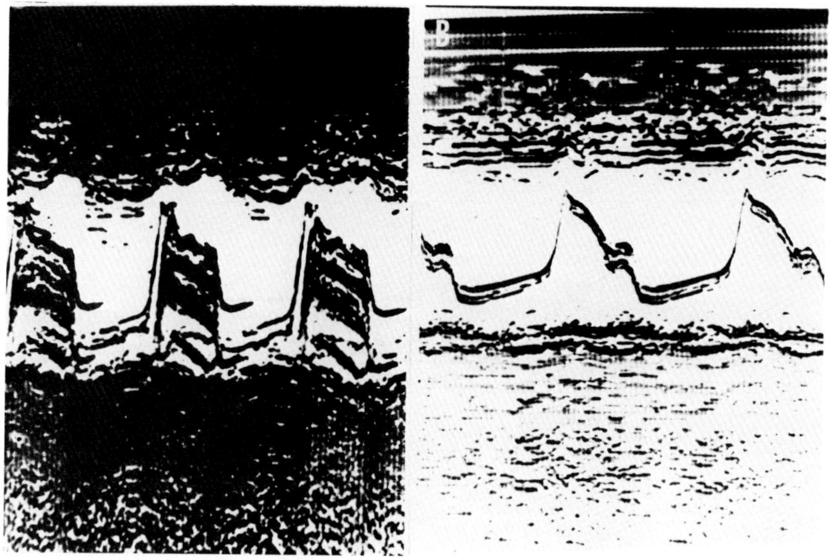

Fig 19–2.—Preoperative *(left)* and postoperative *(right)* echocardiograms of a patient with a left atrial myxoma. On the preoperative echocardiogram, note the mass of echoes behind the anterior mitral valve leaflet, interfering with its motion. Postoperatively the mass behind the mitral leaflet is no longer present and there is more normal motion of the valve.

and 19–2). It is this systolic-diastolic motion and its relation to the mitral valve that assists in distinguishing myxoma from other intracavitary lesions such as thrombus, vegetation, or annular calcification. Approximately 20%–25% of myxomas are located in the right atrium and have similar characteristic findings associated with the tricuspid valve. Some 1%–2% are located in the ventricles and can mimic the findings of left or right outflow tract obstruction (Figs 19–3 and 19–4).[4–10]

Compared with other imaging techniques, which most commonly silhouette intracardiac structures, 2DE provides a better indication of size and attachment and increases the ability to detect multiple myxomas, the most common being biatrial. Two-dimensional echocardiography can be used to define the size and attachment of myxomas with such confidence that further invasive evaluation prior to surgical intervention is rarely necessary.

While most myxomas have a high acoustic reflectance and are detectable by echocardiographic examination, some highly vascularized myxomas that escape detection by ultrasonic techniques have been reported.[11] These highly vascular tumors are thought to have acoustic reflectant properties similar to blood and therefore are not well imaged by the echo beam.

Secondary Tumors

The most frequent manifestation of metastatic or secondary spread of malignancy to the heart is a pericardial effusion. However, reports of echocardiographic detection of mural metastatic tumor masses as well as contiguous spread of tumors, compressing cardiac chambers[12, 13] or filling venous inflow tracts, are increasing in frequency (Fig 19–5). This is attributable to the increased availability of 2DE with its broad spatial field providing the ability to examine such areas as the inflow tracts of the right heart, right atrium, and right ventricle. Mural metastatic involvement may present with signs of valvular obstruction, valvular insufficiency, pulmonary or peripheral embolization, arrhythmia, conduction abnormalities, or congestive heart failure.

The list of malignancies metastatic to intracardiac locations detected by echocardiography include carcinoma of the colon[14] and cervix,[15] malignant melanoma,[16] bronchogenic carcinoma,[17] renal cell carcinoma,[18] testicular carcinoma,[15] and angiosar-

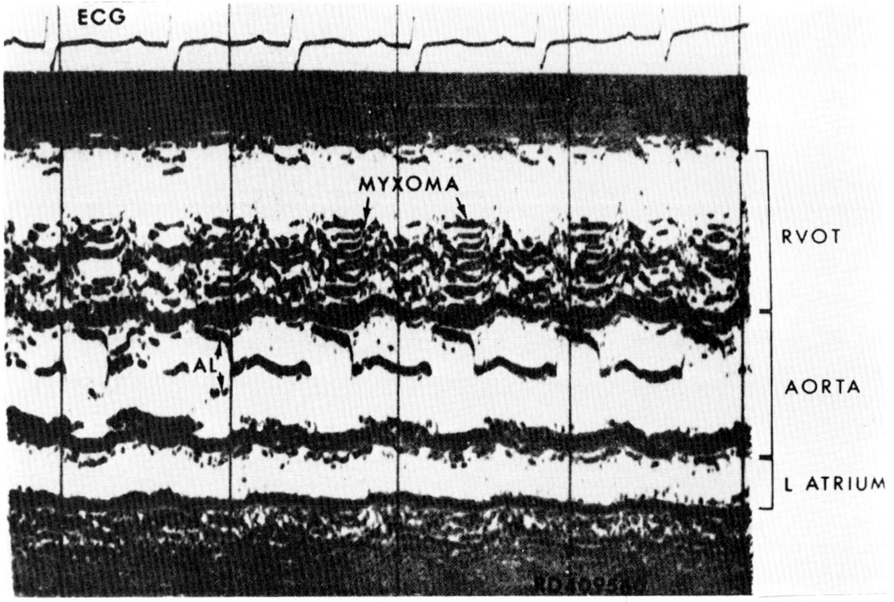

Fig 19–3.—Echocardiogram shows mass of echoes located anterior to the aortic root in the right ventricular outflow tract, representing a right heart myxoma. *RVOT,* right ventricular outflow tract; *AL,* aortic leaflet. (From De Maria A.N. et al.[5] used by permission.

coma.[19] Unlike the pedunculated and mobile masses of myxoma, these metastatic lesions are sessile and contiguous with the cardiac wall and therefore quite difficult to distinguish from normal cardiac wall.

However, mural involvement of the myocardium can change the acoustic and functional properties of the cardiac wall and can produce an increase in wall thickness, wall motion abnormalities, partial obliteration of cardiac chambers, and

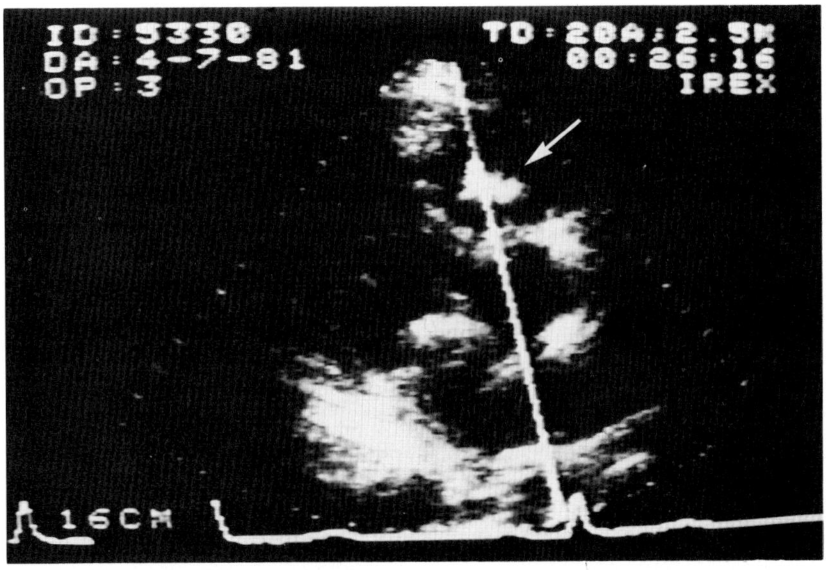

Fig 19–4.—Right ventricular outflow tract mass is demonstrated on the two-dimensional echocardiogram, short-axis view at the aortic root level. Note dense echo mass pierced by radial sector line anterior to the aortic root *(arrow).*

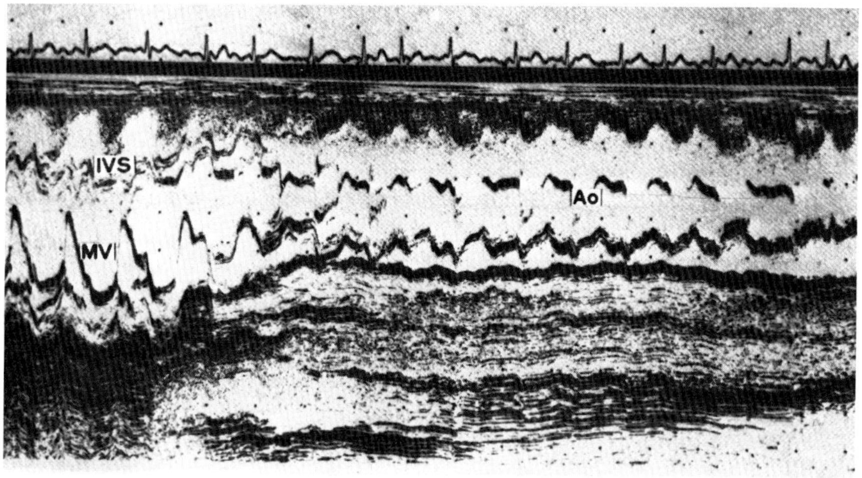

Fig 19–5.—The left atrium is compressed or filled by a mass of echoes representing an esophageal carcinoma. Intrinsic involvement of the left atrial wall cannot be distinguished from extrinsic compression in this example. *IVS,* interventricular septum; *Ao,* aortic root; *MV,* mitral valve. (From Yoshikawa J. et al.[13] Used by permission.)

multilayered echoes of increased density adjacent to "normal" myocardium. These findings have most frequently been noted in the right ventricular anterior wall, left ventricular posterior wall, and interventricular septum, but involvement of any cardiac structure is possible. Tumors in the interventricular septum have been mistaken for asymmetric septal hypertrophy (Fig 19–6).[20]

Progress in the diagnosis of intracavitary tumors initiated by M-mode echocardiography has been dramatically advanced by 2DE, which allows a simultaneous and more comprehensive view of contiguous areas of the cardiac wall and structures for comparison. With further refinement in equipment and growing experience in examining the heart from different transducer locations, more frequent reports of cardiac involvement by tumor are predicted.

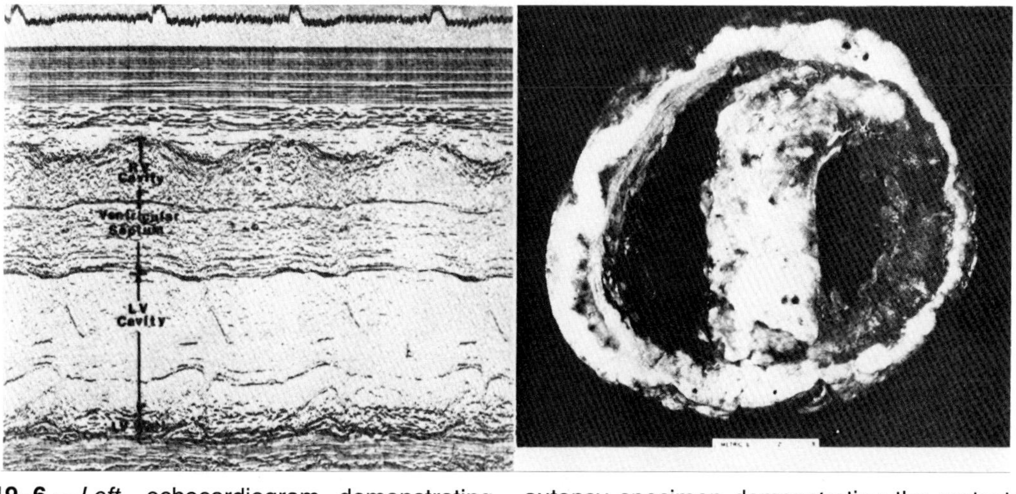

Fig 19–6.—*Left,* echocardiogram demonstrating marked thickening of interventricular septum. Appearance of the echocardiogram could be mistaken for asymmetric septal hypertrophy. *Right,* cross-section of autopsy specimen demonstrating the metastatic infiltration of the interventricular septum responsible for the echocardiographic presentation. (From Esner J. et al.[20] Used by permission.)

VEGETATIVE ENDOCARDITIS

The role of echocardiography in the evaluation of infective endocarditis continues to evolve. The initial description of the echocardiographic findings of an infective vegetation was published in 1973.[21] Echocardiographic detection of vegetation now is used to identify a subgroup of patients with a higher risk of emboli, congestive heart failure, and more frequent need for surgical intervention.

The echocardiographic findings of endocarditis relate to the characteristics of the vegetation itself as well as to the hemodynamic effects of valvular incompetence and valvular destruction.

Vegetations associated with endocarditis have been detected by direct visual inspection in approximately 55% of patients with positive blood cultures who subsequently undergo surgery or autopsy.[22, 23] These vegetations may involve the cardiac valves, the ventricular or atrial walls, chordae, or papillary muscles. Most vegetations are small, 1–3 mm in size, and not infrequently occur on previously calcified and diseased valves. Since 30%–45% of patients with bacterial endocarditis do not have vegetations detectable by direct inspection, the inability to detect a vegetation by echocardiography is not at all surprising. The resolution of echocardiography is in the range of 1–2 mm and a significant proportion of vegetations cannot be identified because they are beyond the lower limits of ultrasonic resolution.[24] Finally, a valve that has had significant thickening, calcification, or deformity prior to the onset of endocarditis makes it more difficult to separate out echoes related to new vegetations.

These problems indicate significant limitations to the use of echocardiography in establishing a diagnosis of vegetative endocarditis, and therefore the diagnosis should never be excluded on the basis of a negative echocardiographic examination. Nevertheless, echocardiography has an important role in the assessment of the patient with infective endocarditis.

Valvular vegetations are often described as "smudgy" or "shaggy" nonuniform echoes that are usually intimately involved with the valve leaflets (Figs 19–7 and 19–8). They move with the valve leaflets in systole and diastole since their attachments arise from the valve structures. In more destructive lesions, flailing of the leaflets or a long

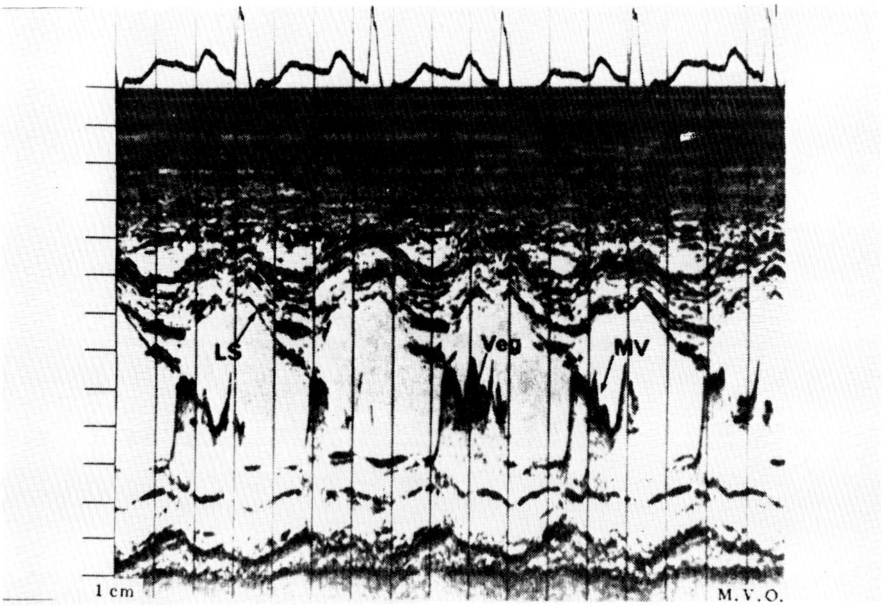

Fig 19–7.—"Smudgy" echo densities involving the anterior leaflet of the mitral valve due to vegetative endocarditis. *Veg,* vegetation; *MV,* mitral valve; *LS,* left side of interventricular septum. (From Dillon J.C.: *Amer. J. Med.* 62:856, 1977. Used by permission.)

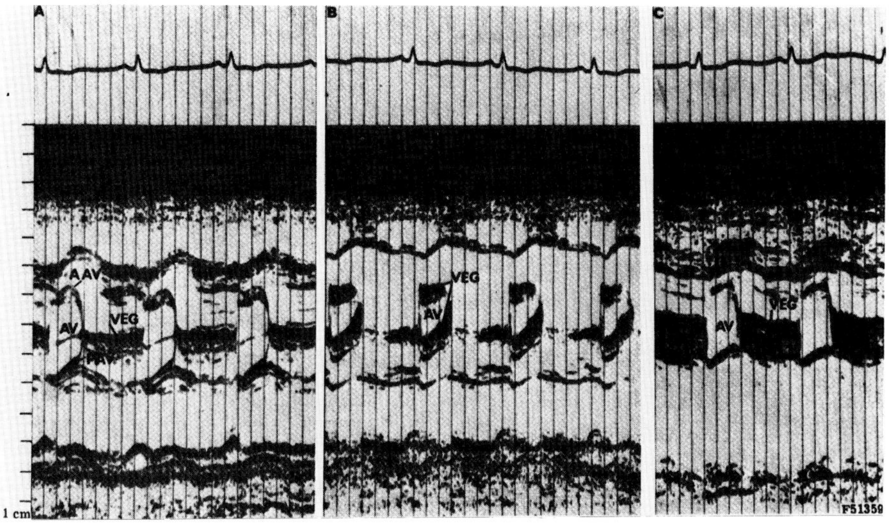

Fig 19–8.—M-mode echocardiogram in three views of a patient with vegetative endocarditis involving the aortic valve. Note the smudgy density intimately involved with the aortic leaflets. *AAV,* anterior aortic valve leaflet; *AV,* aortic valve; *PAV,* posterior aortic valve leaflet; *Veg,* vegetations. (From Wray T.M.: *Circulation* 52:658, 1975. Used by permission.)

tail-like vegetation will be indicated by a chaotic echo moving in and out of the inflow or outflow tract.(Figs 19–9 and 19–10).

The ability of M-mode echocardiography to detect vegetations has been well documented and will continue to be important in assessment of endocarditic lesions. However, 2DE facilitates detection by providing a wider field of view with increased ability to examine right heart valves and by allowing better assessment of prosthetic valves (Figs 19–11 and 19–12).[25] The 2DE technique more readily characterizes size, location, and morphology of the vegetations and complications such as chordae rupture, flail valve leaflets, and the more unusual myocardial abscess formation and sinus of Valsalva aneurysms (Fig 19–13).

The combined use of M-mode echocardiography and 2DE can also assess left ventricular function and the hemodynamic importance of such conditions as aortic insufficiency. In a clinical setting of endocarditis, surgical interventions can often be recommended solely on the basis of clinical picture and echocardiographic findings.

Echocardiographic findings associated with aortic valvular insufficiency in vegetative endocarditis include diastolic fluttering of the anterior mitral leaflet, premature mitral valve closure, and, rarely, premature aortic valve opening as indicators of increasing severity of aortic insufficiency.[26] Premature mitral valve closure (before the onset of left ventricular systole) implies severe aortic in-

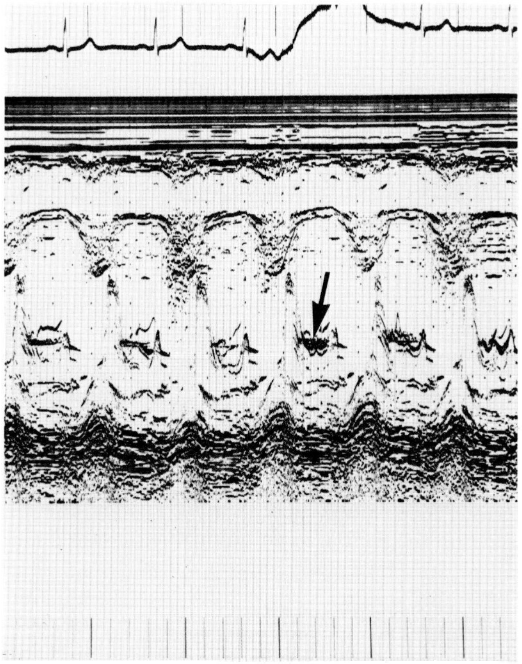

Fig 19–9.—Flail anterior mitral chord secondary to endocarditis. Note the random motion of flail mitral chord, indicated by the *arrow.*

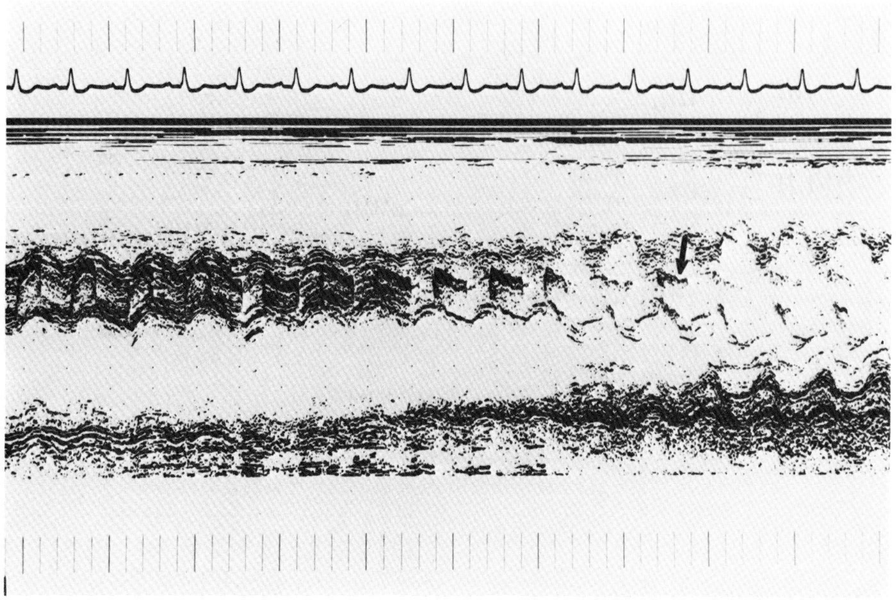

Fig 19–10.—Vegetative endocarditis with flailing of aortic valve. Note the echo-dense mass *(arrow)* in the LV outflow tract which is present during diastole but ejected into aortic root during systole.

sufficiency with a left ventricular end-diastolic pressure of greater than 20 mm Hg. Premature aortic valve opening occurs only in the most extreme cases of aortic regurgitation, when there is equilibration of left ventricular end-diastolic and aortic diastolic pressures (Table 19–1).

The specificity of combined M-mode echocardiography and 2DE for identifying vegetations is quite good when compared to findings at surgery or autopsy. Therefore, all patients suspected of having endocarditis or with the clinical diagnosis of endocarditis should have an ultrasonic examination to identify vegetations, to determine the number of valves involved, to assess the degree of valvular destruction, and to categorize the hemodynamic effect of the associated valvular incompetence.

The echocardiographic detection of vegetations identifies a subgroup of patients at higher risk for congestive heart failure, embolism, or death and a greater need for valve replacement.[27, 28] However, the inability of echocardiography to detect vegetations does not preclude the subsequent development of these complications. Although ultra-

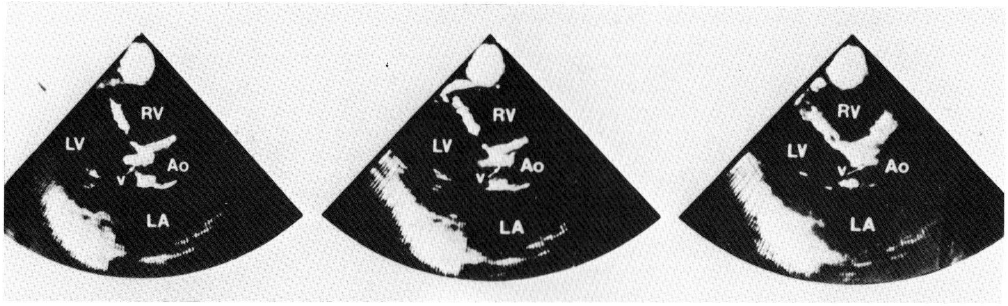

Fig 19–11.—Two-dimensional long-axis parasternal view of an endocarditic vegetation and flailing of the aortic valve. *Left,* note echo-dense mass during diastole, located in the left ventricular *(LV)* outflow tract below level of the aortic leaflets. As LV contraction starts *(center),* echo mass moves toward aorta. *Right,* during peak systole the vegetation and flail valve are now pushed against anterior aortic wall. *RV,* right ventricle; *Ao,* aortic root; *LA,* left atrium; *V,* vegetation.

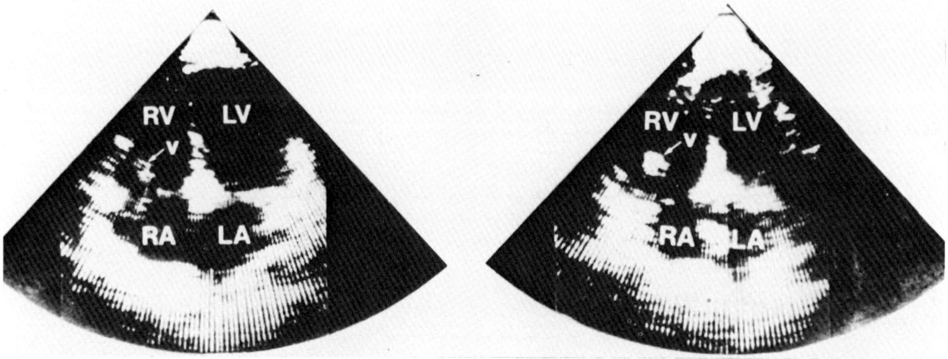

Fig 19–12.—Two-dimensional echocardiogram, four-chamber apical view, of patient with bacterial endocarditis involving the tricuspid valve. Note the large vegetation *(V)* attached to the tricuspid leaflet. *RV,* right ventricle; *RA,* right atrium; *LV,* left ventricle; *LA,* left atrium.

sonic definition of vegetations has been rewarding, serial evaluations of vegetations as an indication of activity or response to therapy has generally been disappointing. Vegetations may increase or decrease in size unrelated to appropriate antibiotic therapy and irrespective of the clinical course of the patient. The size and morphology have not reliably predicted clinical course or risk of embolization in individual patients. This should not detract from the echocardiographic ability to define a high-risk subgroup of patients or to reduce the need for cardiac catheterization in a subgroup of patients with definable vegetative lesions and evidence of severe hemodynamic problems.[29] Although the specificity is good, there will continue to be occasional false positives due to myxomatous valve degeneration, mitral valve prolapse, valve or annular calcification, and tumors.

THROMBI

The formation of an intracardiac thrombus is most often associated with identifiable abnormalities in cardiac contraction or blood flow patterns. Intracardiac thrombosis occurs in such conditions as myocardial infarction, with or without ventricular aneurysm, cardiomyopathy, and mitral valve disease, especially if associated with atrial fibrillation. However, atrial fibrillation without mitral

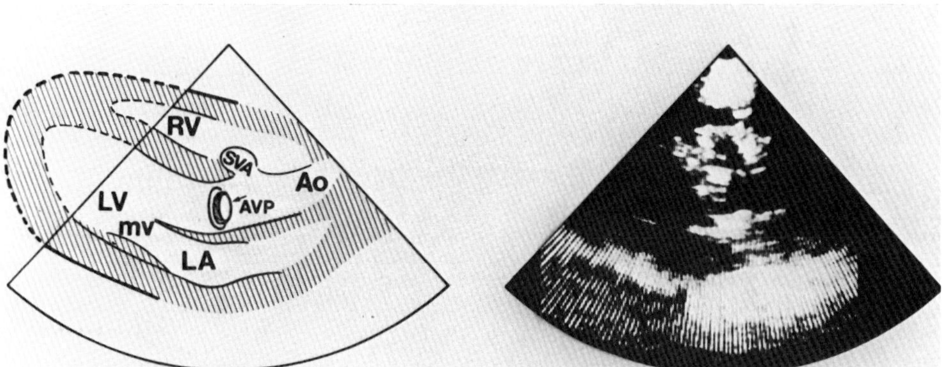

Fig 19–13.—*Right,* two-dimensional echocardiogram, parasternal long-axis view of left ventricle and aortic root. Note circular echo-free area anterior to aortic root and prosthetic valve. This represents a sinus of valsalva aneurysm *(SVA). Left,* schematic representation. *AVP,* aortic valve prosthesis; *Ao,* aortic root; *MV,* mitral valve; *LV,* left ventricle; *LA,* left atrium; *RV,* right ventricle.

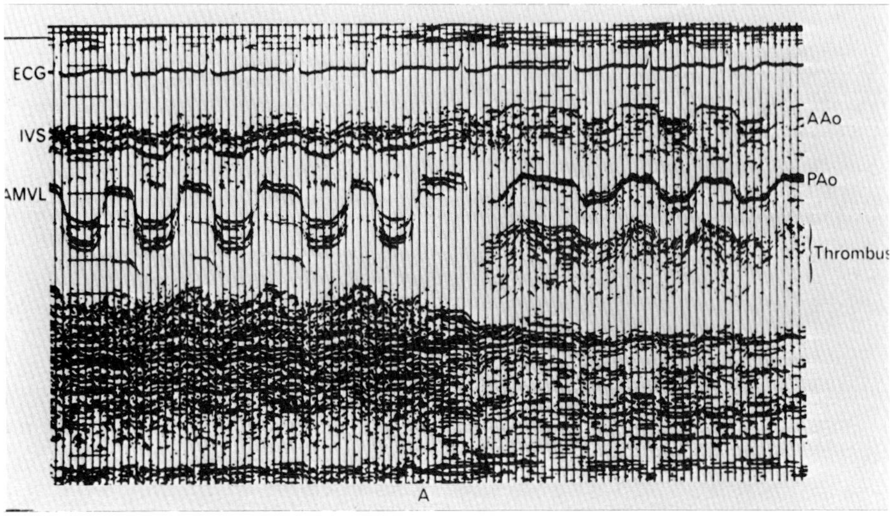

Fig 19–14.—M-mode echocardiogram of a patient with mitral stenosis and persistent linear echoes in the left atrium due to a left atrial thrombus. *AAo,* anterior aortic wall; *PAo, posterior aortic wall; IVS,* interventricular septum; *AMVL,* anterior mitral valve leaflet. (From Spangler R.D. et al.: Chest 67:716, 1975.)

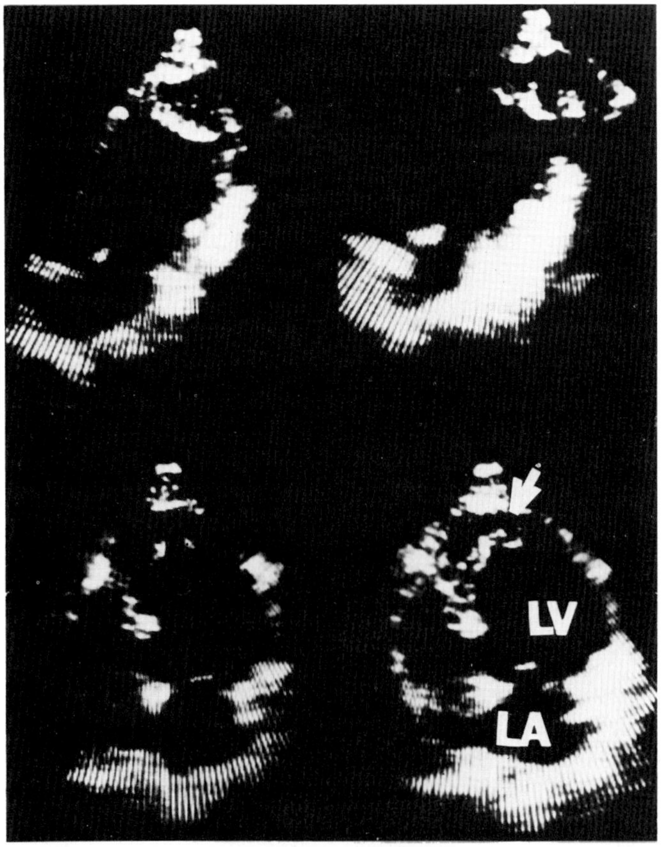

Fig 19–15.—Skewed two-dimensional echocardiogram, two-chamber apical view, demonstrating an apical aneurysm with echo-reflectant thrombus located in the aneurysm *(arrow). LV,* left ventricle; *LA,* left atrium.

TABLE 19–1.—LEFT HEART PRESSURES ASSOCIATED WITH ECHOCARDIOGRAPHIC FINDINGS IN AORTIC INSUFFICIENCY

ECHOCARDIOGRAPHIC FINDING	PULMONARY CAPILLARY WEDGE PRESSURE (mm Hg)	LEFT VENTRICLE END DIASTOLE PRESSURE (mm Hg)
Premature mitral valve closure	10–25	16–45
Premature aortic valve opening	20–30	40–50
Diastolic fluttering of the anterior mitral valve leaflet	Does not correlate with hemodynamic parameters of aortic insufficiency	

valve disease is also associated with an increased risk of thrombus formation and peripheral embolization.

Based on autopsy series, the frequency of thrombus formation in the damaged area of the ventricle in myocardial infarction is 20%–60%.[30–32] In spite of this large number noted on direct visual examination, the ability to identify these clots without direct inspection has remained limited.

Angiography has been the method of choice, yet it identifies at most only 50%–60% of infarct-related thrombi found at autopsy or surgery.[32] The first echocardiographically demonstrated intracardiac thrombus was reported in 1959 by Effert and Domanig.[33] However, only recently with the increasing availability of 2DE have investigators been able to demonstrate evidence of intracardiac thrombi.[34] Two-dimensional echocardiography has been shown to predict accurately the presence of left ventricular thrombus in 75%–80% of patients with demonstrable clot at surgery or autopsy and now is the preferred method for diagnosis.[35] The great majority of left ventricular thrombi occur in apical infarcts and aneurysms, with associated thrombus formation in these areas. Additionally, cardiomyopathic left ventricles also tend to form thrombi in the apical segments of the ventricular cavity. Two-dimensional echocardiography readily images the left ventricular apex and can be used to identify intracavitary and mural clot in that region.

The posterior wall is the second most frequent location of a left ventricular thrombus which is associated with posterior wall infarction, yet this is significantly less frequent than an apical thrombus formation. Left atrial thrombi are associated with mitral stenosis, atrial fibrillation, and prosthetic mitral valves; the thrombi are frequently located in the left atrial appendage (Fig 19–14). The predictive accuracy of echocardiography in detecting left atrial thrombi does not approach its accuracy in detecting left ventricular apical thrombi, possibly relating to its inability to locate and image the left atrial appendage.

Because of their frequent apical locations, left ventricular thrombi are most often seen on the apical four-chamber or two-chamber 2DE views (Fig 19–15). The echocardiographic appearance of the thrombi is determined by shape, attachment, and degree of fibrosis, calcification, and organization. Most left ventricular thrombi have shaggy, irregular cavitary borders and adhere to the apex. The more organized and, therefore, the more echo reflectant the thrombus, the denser the echo image. The echocardiographic image, however, may be quite variable, and descriptions have ranged from dust-like linear shadows to unusual thickening of cardiac walls to a discrete mass of echoes with chaotic motion. Obviously, this variability makes the specificity of ultrasonic detection somewhat less than desired, yet it is the most sensitive noninvasive test available. Recognition of intracavitary thrombosis with echocardiography also provides us with a means of assessing response to therapy. Future studies with echocardiography will undoubtedly allow a further definition of the natural history of intracardiac thrombi and their response to treatment.

MISCELLANEOUS CONDITIONS AND ARTIFACTS

Although echocardiography has added a great deal to the detection and recognition of a variety of intracardiac lesions, increasing utilization of the technique has resulted in detecting a number of conditions which appear as intracardiac masses. These include prosthetic devices such as temporary and permanent pacing wires (Fig 19–16),[35] right heart pressure catheters, and prosthetic heart

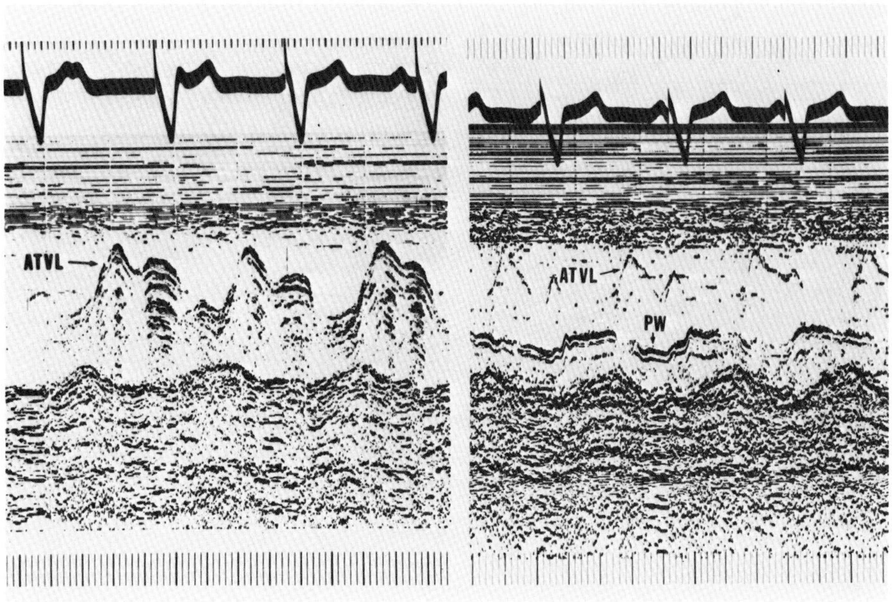

Fig 19–16.—*Left,* mass of echoes behind the anterior tricuspid leaflet *(ATVL)* simulating a right atrial myxoma but actually due to a redundant permanent pacing wire. *Right,* wire has been pulled taut. Note pacing wire *(PW)* echo and disappearance of mass of echo consistent with right atrial myxoma.

valves. Mitral annular calcification (Fig 19–17), prominent trabeculae, and calcification of chordal or papillary muscle regions are not infrequent and can also result in a misleading echocardiographic examination, especially if the M-mode technique alone is used. The two-dimensional examination and assessment of the clinical setting significantly reduce the misinterpretation of these miscellaneous causes of echocardiographic masses.

The most important cause of false positive re-

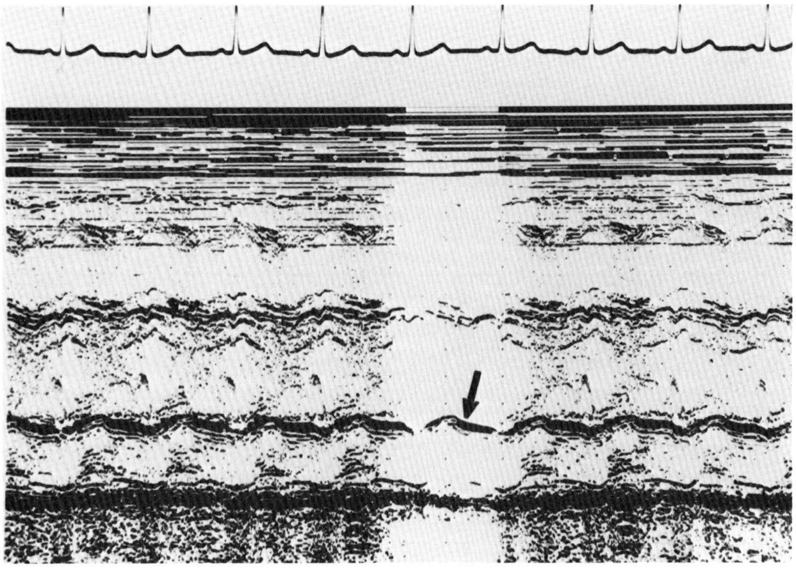

Fig 19–17.—Markedly echo-dense mass of echoes behind the posterior mitral valve leaflet but separate from the posterior left ventricular wall is due to mitral annular calcification *(arrow).* Such calcification frequently extends into the posterior aortic wall and can be demonstrated with an M-mode scan.

sults remains artifact due to improper use of receiver gain and reject settings and the production of side lobes from dense or calcified cardiac structures. The two-dimensional technique, particularly with phased array systems, is more apt to cause these artifacts, probably because of a lower signal to noise ratio and more limited lateral resolution.

In spite of these shortcomings, several approaches and clues can be used to minimize artifactual production of intracardiac masses. Most important is the reduction of receiver gain settings and reject adjustments to minimize artifacts due to overload of receiver crystals. True intracardiac masses are attached to the cardiac structures; otherwise they would be expelled from the chamber. Therefore, this attachment should be demonstrable. The demonstration of the mass in the same anatomical region through several echocardiographic windows supports the diagnosis of a true intracardiac mass. The mass usually will display some motion unless the overlying cardiac wall is akinetic, as is the case with mural thrombus associated with myocardial infarction. This akinesis is pertinent in that mural thrombus is unlikely to be located beyond a region of wall motion abnormality. Careful scrutiny is required, but with experience and attention to the clinical presentation and instrument settings these artifacts can be minimized.

Echocardiography has continued to expand its role in clinical cardiology. In the few years since its introduction it has become the method of choice in diagnosing pericardial effusion and mitral stenosis and has opened up the area of intracardiac mass detection. It is the noninvasive method of choice for detection of myxoma and intracardiac thrombosis and adds significantly to the evaluation of patients with endocarditis. Its role will undoubtedly grow in pace with increased experience and technical improvements that are already on the horizon.

REFERENCES

1. Heath D.: Pathology of cardiac tumors. *Am. J. Cardiol.* 21:315, 1968.
2. Goldberg H.P., Glen F., Dotter C.T., et al.: Myxoma of the left atrium: Diagnosis made during life with operative and postmortem findings. *Circulation* 6:672, 1952.
3. Meller J., Teichholz L.E., Pichard A.D., et al.: Left ventricular myxoma: Echocardiographic diagnosis and review of the literature. *Am. J. Med.* 63:816, 1977.
4. Chandraratna P.A.N., San Pedro S., et al.: Echocardiographic, angiographic, and surgical correlation in right ventricular myxoma simulating valvular pulmonic stenosis. *Circulation* 55:619, 1977.
5. DeMaria A.N., Vismara L.A., et al.: Unusual echocardiographic manifestations of right and left heart myxomas. *Am. J. Med.* 59:713, 1975.
6. Horgan J.H., Beachley M.C., et al.: Primary and secondary right atrial tumors detected by echocardiography. *J. Clin. Ultrasound* 5:92, 1977.
7. Levisman J.A., MacAlpin R.N., et al.: Echocardiographic diagnosis of a mobile, pedunculated tumor in the left ventricular cavity. *Am. J. Cardiol.* 36:957, 1975.
8. Meller J., Teichholz L.E., Pichard A.D., et al.,: Left ventricular myxoma: Echocardiographic diagnosis and review of the literature. *Am. J. Med.* 63:816, 1977.
9. Nanda N.C., Barold S.S., Gramiak R., et al.: Echocardiographic features of right ventricular outflow tumor prolapsing into the pulmonary artery. *Am. J. Cardiol.* 40:272, 1977.
10. Ports T.A., Schiller N.B., Strunk B.L.: Echocardiography of right ventricular tumors. *Circulation* 56:439, 1977.
11. Stewart J.A., Warnia J.W., Kirk M.E., et al.: Left atrial myxoma: False negative echocardiographic findings in a tumor demonstrated by coronary angiography. *Am. Heart J.* 98:228, 1979.
12. Horgan J.H., Beachley M.C., et al.: Primary and secondary right atrial tumors detected by echocardiography. *J. Clin. Ultrasound* 5:92, 1977.
13. Yoshikawa J., Sabah I., Yanagihara K., et al.: Cross-sectional echocardiographic diagnosis of large left atrial tumor and extracardiac tumor compressing the left atrium. *Am. J. Cardiol.* 42:853, 1978.
14. Birmingham C., Peretz D.: Metastatic carcinoma presenting as obstruction to the right ventricular outflow tract. *Am. Heart J.* 97:229, 1979.
15. Krivokapich J., Warren E.W., Child J.S., et al.: M-Mode and cross-sectional echocardiographic diagnosis of right ventricular cavity masses. *J. Clin. Ultrasound* 9:5, 1981.
16. Ports T.A., Schiller N.B., Strunk B.L.: Echocardiography of right ventricular tumors. *Circulation* 56:439, 1977.
17. Kocwaya Y., Yoshiharu K., Yasuhiko O., et al.: Echocardiographic detection of metastatic cardiac mural tumor. *J. Clin. Ultrasound* 8:443, 1980.
18. Horgan J.H., Beachley M.C., et al.: Primary and secondary right atrial tumors detected by echocardiography. *J. Clin. Ultrasound* 5:92, 1977.
19. Panella J., Page M., Vutu T., et al.: Angiosarcoma of the heart. *Chest* 76:221, 1979.
20. Esner J., Falcone M., Virmani R., et al.: Cardiac

sarcoma causing "ASH" and simulating coronary heart disease. *Am. J. Med.* 66:1025, 1979.
21. Dillon J.C., Feigenbaum H., et al.: Echocardiographic manifestations of valvular vegetations. *Am. Heart J.* 86:698, 1973.
22. Buchbinder N., Roberts W.: Left-sided active infective endocarditis: A study of forty-five necropsy patients. *Am. J. Med.* 53:20, 1972.
23. Arnett E., Roberts W.: Active infective endocarditis: A clinicopathologic analysis of 137 necropsy patients. *Curr. Probl. Cardiol.* 1(7), 1976.
24. Wann L.S., Dillon J.C., Weyman A.E., et al.: Echocardiography in bacterial endocarditis. *N. Engl. J. Med.* 295:135, 1976.
25. Martin R., Meltzer R., Chia B., et al.: Clinical utility of two-dimensional echocardiography in infective endocarditis. *Am. J. Cardiol.* 46:379, 1980.
26. Pietro D.A., Parisi A.F., Harrington J.J., et al.: Premature opening of the aortic valve: An index of highly advanced aortic regurgitation. *J. Clin. Ultrasound* 6:170, 1978.
27. Wann L.S., Dillon J.C., Weyman A.E., et al.: Echocardiography in bacterial endocarditis. *N. Engl. J. Med.* 295:135, 1976.
28. Stewart J., Silimperi D., Harris P., et al.: Echocardiographic documentation of vegetative lesions in infective endocarditis: Clinical implications. *Circulation* 61:374, 1980.
29. Strom J., Becker R., Davis R., et al.: Echocardiographic and surgical correlations in bacterial endocarditis. *Circulation* 62(suppl. I): I–164, 1980.
30. DeMaria A.N., Bommer W., et al.: Left ventricular thrombi identified by cross-sectional echocardiography. *Ann. Intern. Med.* 90:14, 1979.
31. Jordan R., Miller R., Edwards J., et al.: Thromboembolism in acute and in healed myocardial infarction. *Circulation* 6:1, 1952.
32. Ruder G., Tajik A., Seward J.: Left ventricular mural thrombus: Two-dimensional echocardiographic diagnosis. *Mayo Clin. Proc.* 56:82, 1981.
33. Effert S., Domanig E.: The diagnosis of intra-atrial tumor and thrombi by ultrasonic echo method. *German Med. Monatschr.* 4:1, 1959.
34. DeMaria A.N., Bommer W., et al.: Left ventricular thrombi identified by cross-sectional echocardiography. *Ann. Intern. Med.* 90:14, 1979.
35. Kendrick M.H., Harrington J.J., et al.: Illustrative echocardiogram. *Chest* 72:649, 1977.

RADIONUCLIDE IMAGING

Samuel Z. Goldhaber and Gerald M. Pohost

IN THIS CHAPTER, we shall discuss the role of radionuclide imaging in diagnosing intracardiac tumor, bacterial endocarditis, intracardiac thrombus, coronary artery and carotid thrombus, and venous thromboembolism. The radioisotopic imaging procedures used to study these conditions vary widely in their accuracy and acceptance as routine diagnostic aids. Perhaps the most established scanning procedure for any of these disorders is the conventional ventilation-perfusion lung scan. One of the most recently introduced procedures is the radioisotope-labeled platelet scan, whose utility for assessing many different thromboembolic disorders is under investigation.

INTRACARDIAC TUMOR

The diagnosis of atrial myxoma by ungated cardiac blood pool scanning was first reported in 1967 by Bonte and Curry, using ^{99m}Tc human serum albumin.[1] The scan demonstrated an intracardiac oval defect that did not correspond to any abnormality on the chest roentgenogram. The differential diagnosis included thrombus or tumor. At operation, a tumor mass occupied most of the right atrial cavity and extended into the right ventricle without attachment to the tricuspid valve or right ventricular wall. The tumor weighed 160 gm, measured 9.5 × 4.5 × 4.8 cm, and was identified histologically as a myxoma.

In 1972, Zaret and associates reported the radioisotopic diagnosis of an intracardiac mass by both ungated radionuclide angiocardiography and ECG gated cardiac imaging.[2] As anticipated, the tumor was more clearly defined in the gated study. It was detected within the left ventricle during end diastole but not during ventricular systolc. Thc tumor was not clearly detected in the left atrium during gated end-systolic imaging, probably because of intense overlying radioisotopic activity in the aortic root and pulmonary vasculature in the right anterior oblique position. Subsequently, cardiac surgery and histologic evaluation confirmed the diagnosis of left atrial myxoma.

To study the utility of the gated cardiac blood pool scan in the diagnosis of left atrial myxoma, Pohost and associates performed gated blood pool scanning in seven patients with left atrial tumors demonstrated by echocardiography or contrast ventriculography.[3] Technetium 99m-labeled human serum albumin was used as the tracer. In four of the seven patients, a multigated study dividing the cardiac cycle into eight equal intervals was obtained. Figure 20-1 illustrates an eight-frame study, the first multigated scan to be published in the cardiac literature.

An abnormal region of diminished radioisotopic activity was identified within the cardiac blood pool in six of the seven patients with left atrial myxoma. In these six patients, the abnormal region was observed in the 30-degree RAO projection. In four of these six patients, the intracardiac mass was also identified in the LAO projection. The characteristic motion of the filling defect distinguished it from other possible abnormalities. The tumor was observed to move into the left ventricle in diastole and into the left atrium in systole. However, in one patient, no filling abnormality could be identified by gated scan. In this patient, the right atrial and ventricular blood pools were the largest among the seven patients and contributed to the difficulty in defining this tumor.

Thus, the gated radionuclide cardiac blood pool scan is helpful in demonstrating atrial myxoma and can assess its position, excursion, and size. In addition, ^{201}Tl defects have been observed in patients with primary or secondary neoplastic involvement of the myocardium. Thus radionuclide studies provide a noninvasive technique for detecting intracardiac tumor, and the gated blood pool scan can demonstrate the size and motion of these tumors. A limitation is that a large tumor, filling nearly the entire cardiac chamber, may not be detected. Such tumors, however, will always generate abnormal echocardiograms. Perhaps the most practical use for radionuclide assessment of potential intracardiac tumors is to evaluate patients in whom technically satisfactory echocardiograms cannot be obtained.

INTRACARDIAC THROMBUS

Several radionuclide approaches to detecting intracardiac thrombus have been reported.[4–10] The first approach, reported in 1967 by investigators at the National Institutes of Health, utilized radioiodinated (^{131}I) antifibrinogen (RIAF) antibody as the tracer in 12 patients suspected clinically of having intracardiac thrombi.[4] Imaging with a single-probe rectilinear scanner demonstrated cardiac activity in only one of the 12 patients. This patient had had a traumatic left ventricular aneurysm resected 10 months before scanning. Postoperatively, the patient experienced multiple cerebral and peripheral arterial emboli. The RIAF scan demonstrated increased radioactivity in the left ventricular apex. However, the patient's debilitated conditon precluded further surgery, and death occurred 8 weeks after RIAF scanning. At postmortem examination, a large, friable thrombus was found. Two other patients in this series with mitral valvular disease had large left atrial thrombi excised surgically, despite negative scans. These thrombi had presumably developed slowly over many years and were pathologically distinct from the clot that formed acutely in the patient who was scanned after cardiac trauma. The investigators concluded that RIAF is effectively concentrated within fresh intracardiac thrombi but is not taken up by chronic, highly organized thrombi.

In 1976, results of a study in 20 preoperative surgical patients using ^{131}I fibrinogen were more encouraging for detecting intracardiac clot.[5] Surveys for intracardiac thrombus were undertaken at 5 minutes, 3 hours, 24 hours, and 2–6 days after ^{131}I fibrinogen administration, using gamma camera imaging or rectilinear scanning. Of 11 patients with negative scans, none had thrombus at surgery. Of nine patients with scans demonstrating tracer uptake in the region of the heart, eight of the nine patients had intracardiac thrombi confirmed at surgery. Four patients had ventricular aneurysms, two had mitral stenosis, and two had prosthetic aortic valves. There was one false positive scan. The smallest active thrombus detected by scanning weighed 1.1 gm and was attached to a larger, organized thrombus that did not accumulate radioactivity. Unfortunately, the relatively poor resolution from high-energy gamma photons of ^{131}I has limited its general clinical applicability.

Because gamma-camera imaging after administration of ^{111}In-labeled platelets[6] is now being used to detect intravascular thrombus, we shall briefly review some technical aspects of this particular isotope. Before the introduction of ^{111}In platelet labeling, ^{51}Cr was utilized. However, ^{51}Cr did not label platelets efficiently and therefore required a large volume of blood (200–500 ml) to accumulate sufficient numbers of tagged structures needed for platelet survival studies. Chromium 51 cannot be used as an imaging tracer, since it has a relatively long physical half-life (27.7 days) and a low yield of gamma photons (10% at 320 keV). Indium 111 has several advantages over ^{51}Cr. Indium 111 has a half-life of 2.8 days, and the two gamma photons it emits (90% at 172 keV and 94% at 247 keV) make it acceptable for external imaging. When ^{111}In is chelated with 8-hydroxyquinoline (oxine), a lipid-

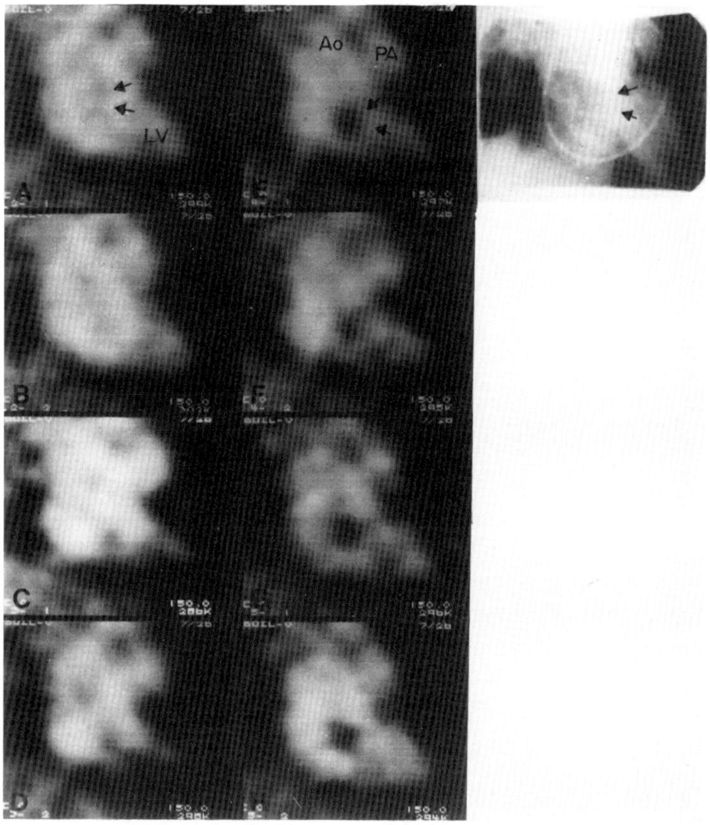

Fig 20–1.—Eight-frame multigated acquisition cardiac blood pool imaging study, 30-degree RAO projection, in a patient with a left atrial myxoma. **A,** left ventricle *(LV)* is illustrated in early systole. Frames appear sequentially (**A** through **H**). The myxoma appears as a large round defect displacing blood pool activity in late systole **(E)** through end diastole **(G, H).** The tumor characteristically moves toward the left ventricle during diastole and left ventricular filling. End-diastolic frame of the left ventricular cineangiogram *(upper right)* faintly depicts the myxoma *(arrows)* in inflow region of left ventricle. Aorta *(AO)* and pulmonary artery *(PA)* are also labeled.

soluble complex is formed which labels platelets efficiently and without adversely affecting their survival or ability to participate in active thrombosis.[7] A 45-minute method for labeling human platelets has recently been described and requires only 26 ml of blood.[8]

Ezekowitz and associates recently investigated the identification of left ventricular thrombus in 29 patients using ^{111}In-labeled platelets.[9] Twenty-one had documented left ventricular aneurysms—20 by contrast ventriculography and one by radionuclide ventriculography. All 21 had previous myocardial infarction. Seven of these 21 patients had experienced previous transient cerebral ischemic episodes or peripheral emboli. In an evaluation that included contrast ventriculography, the remaining eight patients had no evidence of left ventricular aneurysm. Images were obtained daily or on alternate days for 5–8 days. All patients were imaged in the anterior, 45-degree LAO, and left lateral positions. In most patients, an additional 30-degree RAO image was obtained. In 17 patients, examination of the left ventricle for clot was undertaken either at surgery (16) or at autopsy (1). On day 1, gamma-camera images demonstrated blood pool activity in the heart and great vessels in all patients (Fig 20–2). Nine of the 29 patients developed areas of increased activity within the cardiac blood pool, first evident at 60–96 hours (Fig 20–3). Five of these nine had tissue confir-

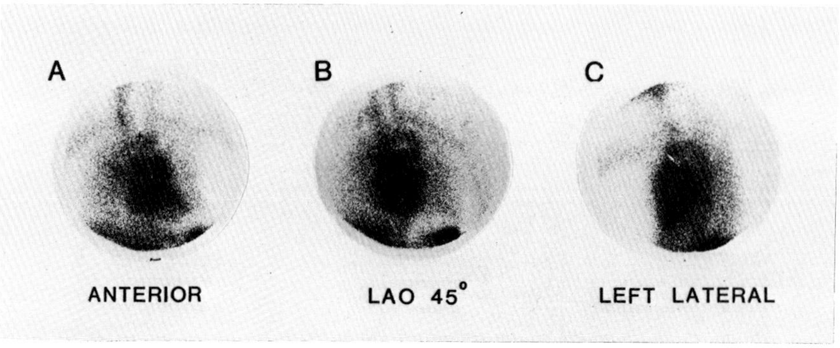

Fig 20–2.—Indium-III scintiphoto 6 hours after injection of platelet suspension. Images are oriented with top of figure cephalad. Increased activity in right lower quadrant of each frame is due to the spleen. Activity in left lower quadrant in frames **A** and **B** is from the liver. Both the cardiac blood pool and blood pool from the great vessels are clearly delineated. (Figure kindly supplied by Michael D. Ezekowitz, M.D.)

mation of clot (Fig 20–4) at surgery (4) or autopsy (1). The remaining four patients did not undergo surgery, and therefore the accuracy of the positive platelet scans could not be checked. Twelve of the 20 patients without cardiac accumulation of ^{111}In activity underwent surgery and had no evidence of left ventricular thrombus. Surgical confirmation of negative scans was obtained in six of 12 patients with left ventricular aneurysms and in six of eight patients without left ventricular aneurysms. Thus, the diagnostic accuracy of platelet scanning in this series was 100%.[9] Indeed, ^{111}In-labeled platelet scanning may be better than contrast ventriculography for identifying patients with left ventricular thrombus. A recent report from the Mayo Clinic evaluated the role of contrast angiography in diagnosing mural thrombus in 100 consecutive patients undergoing left ventricular aneurysectomy.[10] The study found that angiography had a sensitivity of only 31%, specificity of 75%, and relatively low overall predictive accuracy of 54%. Low angiographic sensitivity in diagnosing left ventricular clot is due principally to three factors: (1) failure of contrast material to mix well in dyskinetic areas, (2) obscuring of filling defects by overlying dense contrast material, (3) difficulty in distinguishing small clots from prominent trabecular patterns. With contrast ventriculography, the silhouette of an intracardiac clot is obtained. With platelet scanning, a "hot-spot" image of platelets being incorporated into thrombus is obtained. Theoretically, ventriculography may be more spe-

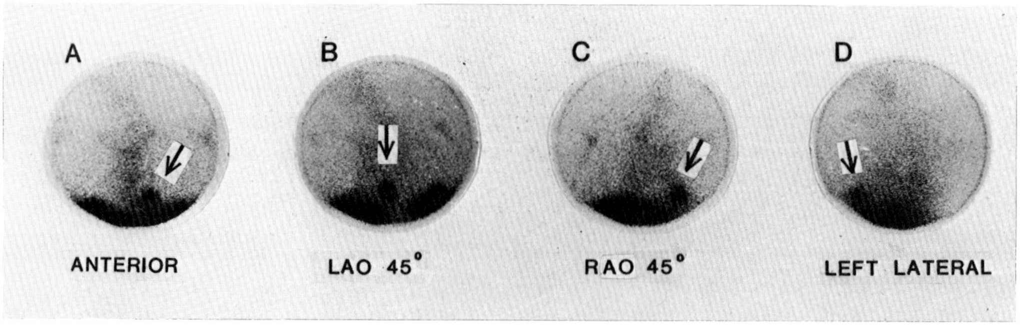

Fig 20–3.—Scintiphoto obtained 96 hours after injection of platelet suspension. Orientation of images is similar to Figure 20–1. An additional RAO 45-degree image **(C)** shows the liver superimposed on the spleen and occupying the lower zone of the frame. All four views depict a round homogenous area of increased and abnormal ^{111}In activity *(arrows)*, which represents an active thrombus within a large anteroseptal left ventricular aneurysm. Note the markedly decreased blood pool activity compared to Figure 20–1. (Figure kindly supplied by Michael D. Ezekowitz, M.D.)

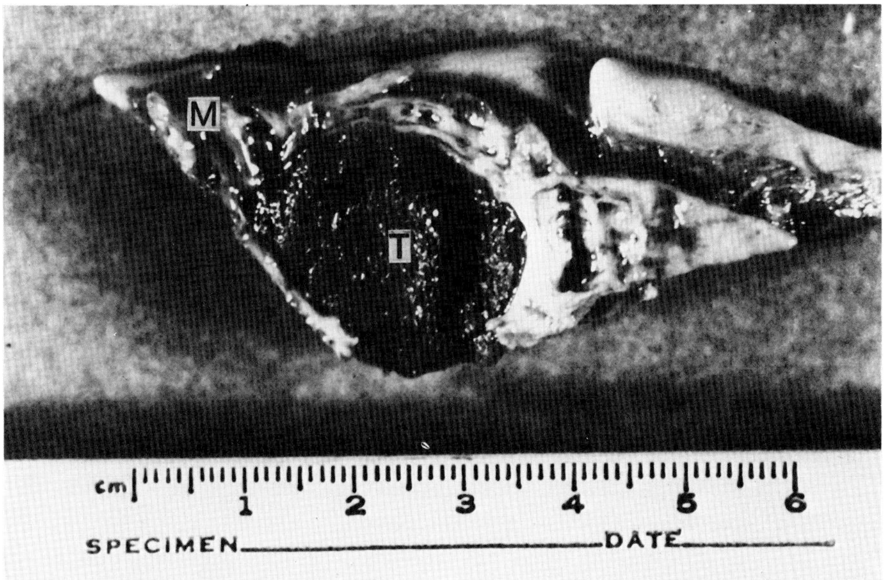

Fig 20–4.—Pathologic specimen from an aneurysm removed at surgery. Rounded thrombus *(T)* within a sacular component of the aneurysm is typical of the lesion identified by platelet scintigraphy and described in Figure 20–2. *M* represents myocardium involved in the aneurysm but without adherent thrombus. (Figure kindly supplied by Michael D. Ezekowitz, M.D.)

cific and more reliable than platelet scanning in patients with chronic inactive thrombus that is no longer actively incorporating platelets. In the future, ^{111}In-labeled platelet scanning might be used as a noninvasive method to identify patients with active thrombus formation. Clinically, such scanning would be useful to follow serially patients at risk of developing left ventricular thrombus, such as those with acute myocardial infarction or left ventricular aneurysm. In patients who have suffered a thromboembolic stroke without a clear-cut source for the thrombus, platelet scanning might detect otherwise unsuspected left ventricular thrombus. Finally, in patients undergoing anticoagulation or antiplatelet therapy for established left ventricular thrombus, platelet scanning might be useful to assess the effectiveness of therapy.

BACTERIAL ENDOCARDITIS

Gallium-67 citrate has been used as a radiotracer to study patients with bacterial endocarditis because it concentrates in areas of acute inflammation. In one report by Wiseman and coworkers,[11] 10 patients underwent gamma-camera scanning 2–7 days after intravenous administration of 3 mCi of ^{67}Ga. Six of the 10 patients with clinical bacterial endocarditis had ^{67}Ga uptake. The scans were positive in four of five patients with culture-proved *Staphylococcus aureus* endocarditis. In two patients with positive scans, bacterial endocarditis was confirmed at postmortem examination. A fifth scan was positive in a patient with Micrococcus. The sixth scan was positive in a patient with negative blood cultures who had developed acute mitral regurgitation and who improved following a 6-week course of antibiotic therapy. In patients with positive scans, the location of the affected valve could not be determined with certainty. Unfortunately, follow-up scans were not obtained in any patients after antibiotic therapy and clinical improvement.

In another report, a patient with staphylococcal endocarditis underwent ^{67}Ga scanning and was found to have a focal abnormality of ^{67}Ga uptake, which was the first indication of a myocardial abscess.[12] Three days after injection of ^{67}Ga, a discrete area of abnormal isotope accumulation was identified in the basal portion of the left ventricle. Technetium 99m pyrophosphate and thallium 201 myocardial imaging studies in this patient were both normal. A radionuclide angiocardiogram revealed an enlarged left atrium, increased left ventricular ejection fraction (both consistent with mitral regurgitation), but no regional wall motion abnormalities. At surgery, a myocardial abscess in the left ventricle, inferior to the mitral annulus, was identified and drained.

Riba and associates studied radioisotopic imaging of experimental bacterial endocarditis with technetium 99m pyrophosphate (Tc 99m PYP)[13] and with ^{111}In-labeled platelets.[14] They established aortic valve infective endocarditis in rabbits by abrading the aortic valvular endocardium with a 1-mm polyethylene catheter, followed several days later by an intravenous injection of approximately 10 million colony-forming units of *Streptococcus sanguis*. With Tc 99m PYP scanning, these experimental lesions were detectable within 2 hours. With ^{111}In platelet imaging, the 24-hour image showed only the cardiac blood pool. By 72 hours, blood pool activity had cleared and abnormal ^{111}In uptake was visualized in the region of the aortic valve in all animals. Imaging was also attempted in five animals with ^{111}In-labeled leukocytes; but no abnormal or focal aortic valvular uptake was seen, despite the presence of extensive vegetations at post mortem. The disadvantage of ^{111}In-labeled platelets compared to Tc 99m PYP was the 48–72 hours required for adequate images. The advantages of ^{111}In-labeled platelet imaging over Tc 99m PYP were a much greater concentration of the tracer by the lesion, better quality of images, and lack of competing uptake in the bony thorax.

It must be emphasized that these studies were performed in laboratory animals with fulminant endocarditis resulting in large aortic valvular lesions. Clinical imaging trials need to be undertaken before any statement regarding clinical utility can be made. Furthermore, these experimental studies have not determined whether healed or subacute bacterial endocarditis valvular lesions will concentrate platelets and to what extent antibiotic therapy affects platelet deposition.[13]

Although radionuclide imaging to detect and evaluate the extent of bacterial endocarditis appears promising, more clinical trials are necessary before radionuclide diagnosis can be recommended for clinical application. At this time, however, it seems reasonable to utilize ^{67}Ga imaging to help detect myocardial abscess when it is suspected clinically.

ARTERIAL THROMBUS

In addition to imaging left ventricular thrombus, ^{111}In-labeled platelets have been used to evaluate experimental thrombosis in native canine coronary arteries and in canine coronary artery bypass grafts. Indium 111 platelet scanning readily detected acute coronary artery thromboses in dogs but failed to detect 24-hour-old thrombi.[15] Indium 111 platelets were imaged in the study of canine bypass grafts 8 and 32 hours after surgery. It is uncertain whether the early deposition of platelets was a transient response to graft endothelial injury or a continuous process that could lead to occlusion of the graft.[16] In a follow-up study of canine coronary artery bypass grafts, treating dogs perioperatively with aspirin and dipyridamole led to considerably less ^{111}In platelet deposition.[17]

Indium 111-labeled platelet scanning also detects atherosclerotic lesions in the carotid arteries.[18] In 23 patients with suspected cerebrovascular disease, platelet scanning was compared with contrast angiography. The sensitivity of platelet scanning was 75% (12 positive scans out of 16 positive angiograms) with one false positive scan out of seven angiographically normal carotid studies. Angiography demonstrated 33 extracranial atherosclerotic lesions. Indium 111 platelets accumulated at 20 of these 33 sites (61%) and at three other sites without definite angiographic abnormalities. Platelet imaging has become an area of active investigation and may provide a clinically useful means of evaluating the activity of an atherosclerotic lesion. Digital subtraction angiography (discussed later in this chapter) may also be a useful noninvasive method of detecting carotid atherosclerotic lesions.

VENOUS THROMBOSIS

Considerable effort has been devoted to developing a radioisotopic substitute for contrast venography and pulmonary angiography. In the early 1970s, ^{125}I fibrinogen scanning was reported to be useful in the diagnosis of deep venous thrombosis.[19] A careful study of ^{125}I fibrinogen scanning in postoperative patients who underwent total hip replacement demonstrated a 50% sensitivity and 86% specificity, using venography as the gold standard.[20] Further studies suggested that ^{125}I fibrinogen scanning could not distinguish between superficial and deep venous thrombosis. This assertion is an important clinical distinction because deep venous thrombosis is much more likely than superficial venous thrombosis to cause pulmonary embolism. Consequently, with deep venous thrombosis, treatment usually consists of systemic anticoagulation, despite the risks of iatrogenic hemorrhage, whereas superficial venous thrombosis is usually treated only symptomatically, with heat and elevation of the affected leg. Another drawback to ^{125}I fibrinogen scanning is its lack of reliability in detecting femoral vein thrombi and thrombi above the inguinal ligament.[21, 22] Such thrombi, if present, are in the deep venous system and can embolize to the pulmonary arteries. The disadvantages of ^{125}I fibrinogen scanning may be due to the very low gamma energy of ^{125}I. Iodine-123, a more powerful gamma emitter, might provide a more effective fibrinogen label and might result in fibrinogen scans more sensitive to thrombi in the large and deep leg veins. However, ^{123}I is not widely available.

Investigators from Hamilton, Ontario have advocated the combined use of ^{125}I fibrinogen scanning to detect venous calf thrombi and impedance plethysmography to detect more proximal venous thrombi as an alternative to venography in the diagnosis of venous thrombosis.[23, 24] Sasahara and coworkers have stressed the accuracy of electrical impedance plethysmography alone in detecting clinically significant deep venous thrombosis leading to pulmonary embolism.[25] It must be stressed that impedance plethysmography requires specialized expertise which may only be available in certain medical centers. Until sufficient personnel are trained in this technique, venography will remain the routine approach to definitive diagnosis of deep venous thrombosis.

In several small experimental[26] and clinical[27, 28] studies, ^{111}In-labeled platelet scanning appears promising for diagnosis of venous thrombosis. We will continue to look with interest at the radionuclide approaches for detecting venous thromboses. Since the accuracy of these methods is somewhat limited, the new angiographic approach, using intravenous contrast injected into the antecubital fossa with digital subtraction (see p. 356), may obviate the need for them.

PULMONARY EMBOLISM

Ventilation-perfusion lung scans have been used clinically since the early 1970s to diagnose pulmonary embolism (PE) noninvasively. Perfusion scans can be performed with ^{99m}Tc-iron hydroxide aggregates of human serum albumin and ventilation scans with ^{133}Xe.[29] When such scans satisfy criteria for a high probability of PE,[30, 31] the diagnosis is very accurate, and pulmonary angiography is usually unnecessary. Nevertheless, there remains a substantial group of patients with abnormal chest roentgenograms who may have nonspecific abnormalities on lung scanning. In such patients, the diagnosis of PE by lung scanning may be equivocal.[32] Furthermore, a recent autopsy study has shown that, despite the availability of lung scans and pulmonary angiograms, patients who have pneumonia or congestive heart failure in addition to PE are at high risk for not having their PEs diagnosed ante mortem.[33] In such patients, the clinician was frequently satisfied with the single diagnosis of pneumonia or congestive heart failure and often did not pursue the diagnosis of PE with lung scanning or pulmonary angiography. However, if lung scanning or pulmonary angiography was ordered, the accuracy of clinical diagnosis was greatly enhanced.

To improve the state of the art for noninvasive diagnosis of PE, other radionuclide approaches have been developed and evaluated. Experimentally induced small pulmonary ischemic lesions have been imaged in dogs after cyclotron-produced ^{11}C labeled carbon monoxide inhalation, using a standard gamma camera fitted with a medium-energy tungsten collimator.[34] Sequential positron imaging after inhalation of cyclotron-produced radioactive ^{15}O-labeled carbon dioxide has also been used to image experimental PEs in dogs[35] and clinical PEs in humans.[36] In the clinical study, both sensitivity and specificity for inhalation imaging were superior to conventional ventilation-perfusion lung scanning. However, a major practical limitation is the need for a nearby cyclotron to generate ^{15}O (T 1/2 = 2.1 minutes) and a positron camera, although a standard gamma camera equipped with a medium- or high-energy collimator may allow reasonable imaging. As with other intravascular thromboemboli, ^{111}In-labeled platelets have been used in experimental[37] and clinical studies[38, 39] for imaging PEs. The ^{111}In platelet approach may enhance the accuracy of PE detection; however, further studies are necessary. Digital subtraction angiography (next section) may ultimately replace pulmonary angiography.

DIGITAL SUBTRACTION ANGIOGRAPHY

A new method of cardiovascular diagnosis using a computerized radiographic approach after intravenous injection of radiopaque contrast medium (see last chapter) has recently been described.[40–43] If initial studies can be confirmed, this process may eventually obviate the need for certain radionuclide methods, as well as conventional angiography, in many clinical settings. A relatively expensive computer system is integrated with existing fluoroscopic cine radiographic apparatus to collect and store background and angiographic images. Imaging is begun just before injecting 40–70 ml of contrast material into an antecubital vein. Satisfactory images have been obtained of cervicocerebral arteries, aortic and abdominal arteries, pulmonary arteries, cardiac chambers, coronary artery bypass grafts, and arteries of the extremities. Digital subtraction angiography is an exciting diagnostic procedure which appears certain to have considerable impact on radionuclide and standard catheterization approaches. Obvious disadvantages include the expense of equipment and the need for large doses of contrast medium.

Radionuclide imaging can be used to evaluate a wide range of cardiovascular disorders, including intravascular tumor, valvular vegetation, and clot, particularly when active platelet deposition is present. In combination with other noninvasive procedures, the radioisotopic scans we have described can often diagnose or exclude pathologic conditions without the morbidity and cost of contrast angiography. Furthermore, the impact of therapy for these disorders can be assessed noninvasively with serial radionuclide scans.

REFERENCES

1. Bonte F.J., Curry T.S. III: Technetium-99m HSA blood pool scan in diagnosis of an intracardiac myxoma. *J. Nucl. Med.* 8:35–39, 1967.
2. Zaret B.L., Hurley P.J., Pitt B.: Noninvasive scintiphotographic diagnosis of left atrial myxoma. *J. Nucl. Med.* 13:81–84, 1972.
3. Pohost G.M., Pastore J.O., Mckusick K.A., et al.: Detection of left atrial myxoma by gated radionuclide cardiac imaging. *Circulation* 55:88–92, 1977.
4. Kramer R.S., Ashburn W.L., Vasko J.S., et al.: Detection of intracardiac thrombi using radio-iodinated antifibrinogen (RIAF) and precordial scanning: experimental and clinical studies. *Ann. Surg.* 166:173–182, 1967.
5. Frisbie J.H., Tow D.E., Sasahara A.A., et al.: Noninvasive detection of intracardiac thrombosis: I-131 fibrinogen cardiac survey. *Circulation* 53:988–991, 1976.
6. Thakur M.L., Welch M.J., Joist J.H., et al.: Indium-111 labeled platelets: studies on preparation and evaluation of in vitro and in vivo functions. *Thromb. Res.* 9:345–357, 1976.
7. Heaton W.A., Davis H.H., Welch M.J., et al.: Indium-111: a new radionuclide label for studying human platelet kinetics. *Br. J. Haematol.* 42:613–622, 1979.
8. Hawker, R.J., Hawker L.M., Wilkinson A.R.: Indium (In-11)-labelled human platelets: optimal method. *Clin. Sci.* 58:243–248, 1980.
9. Ezekowitz M.D., Leonard J.C., Smith E.O., et al.: Identification of left ventricular thrombi in man using indium-111 labeled autologous platelets: a preliminary report. *Circulation* 63:803–810, 1981.

10. Reeder G.S., Lengyel M., Tajik A.J., et al.: Mural thrombus in left ventricular aneurysm. Incidence, role of angiography, and relation between anticoagulation and embolization. *Mayo Clin. Proc.* 56:77–81, 1981.
11. Wiseman J., Rouleau J., Rigo P., et al.: Gallium-67 myocardial imaging for the detection of bacterial endocarditis. *Radiology* 120:135–138, 1976.
12. Spies S.M., Meyers S.N., Barresi V., et al.: A case of myocardial abscess evaluated by radionuclide techniques: case report. *J. Nucl. Med.* 18:1089–1090, 1977.
13. Riba A.L., Downs J., Thakur M.L., et al.: Technetium-99m stannous pyrophosphate imaging of experimental infective endocarditis. *Circulation* 58:111–119, 1978.
14. Riba A.L., Thakur M.L., Gottschalk A., et al.: Imaging experimental infective endocarditis with indium-111-labeled blood cellular components. *Circulation* 59:335–343, 1979.
15. Riba A.L., Thakur M.L., Gottschalk A., et al.: Imaging experimental coronary artery thrombosis with indium-111 platelets. *Circulation* 60:767–775, 1979.
16. Dewanjee M.K., Fuster V., Kaye M.P., et al.: Imaging platelet deposition with In-111-labeled platelets in coronary artery bypass grafts in dogs. *Mayo Clin. Proc.* 53:327–331, 1978.
17. Fuster V., Dewanjee M.K., Kaye M.P., et al.: Noninvasive radioisotopic technique for detection of platelet deposition in coronary artery bypass grafts in dogs and its reduction with platelet inhibitors. *Circulation* 60:1508–1512, 1979.
18. Davis H.H. II, Siegal B.A., Sherman L.A., et al.: Scintigraphic detection of carotid atherosclerosis with indium-111-labeled autologous platelets. *Circulation* 61:982–988, 1980.
19. Kakkar V.V.: The diagnosis of deep venous thrombosis using the I-125 fibrinogen test. *Arch. Surg.* 104:152–159, 1972.
20. Harris W.H., Salzman E.W., Athanasoulis C., et al.: Comparison of I-125 fibrinogen count scanning with phlebography for detection of venous thrombi after elective hip surgery. *N. Engl. J. Med.* 292:665–667, 1975.
21. Hirsh J.: Venous thromboembolism: diagnosis, treatment, prevention. *Hosp. Prac.* 10:53–62, 1975.
22. Hirsh J., Gallus A.S.: I-125-labeled fibrinogen scanning: use in the diagnosis of venous thrombosis. *J.A.M.A.* 233:970–973, 1975.
23. Hull R., Hirsh J., Sackett D.L., et al.: Combined use of leg scanning impedance plethysmography in suspected venous thrombosis: an alternative to venography. *N. Engl. J. Med.* 296:1497–1500, 1977.
24. Hull R., Hirsh J., Sackett D.L., et al.:Replacement of venography in suspected venous thrombosis by impedance plethysmography and I-125 fibrinogen leg scanning. *Ann. Intern. Med.* 94:12–15, 1981.
25. Sasahara A.A., Sharma G.V.R.K., Parisi A.F.: New developments in the detection and prevention of venous thromboembolism. *Am. J. Cardiol.* 43:1214–1224, 1979.
26. Knight L.C., Primeau J.L., Siegel B.A., et al.: Comparison of In-111-labeled platelets and iodinated fibrinogen for the detection of deep vein thrombosis. *J. Nucl. Med.* 19:891–894, 1978.
27. Fenech A., Dendy P.P., Hussey J.K., et al.: Indium-111 labelled platelets in diagnosis of leg-vein thrombosis: preliminary findings. *Br. Med. J.* 280:1571–1573, 1980.
28. Davis H.H. II, Siegel B.A., Sherman L.A., et al.: Scintigraphy with In-111-labeled autologous platelets in venous thromboembolism. *Radiology* 136:203–207, 1980.
29. McNeil B.J., Holman L, Adelstein J.: The scintigraphic definition of pulmonary embolism. *J.A.M.A.* 227:753–756, 1974.
30. McNeil B.J.: A diagnostic strategy using ventilation-perfusion studies in patients suspect for pulmonary embolism. *J. Nucl. Med.* 17:613–616, 1976.
31. McNeil B.J.: Ventilation-perfusion studies and the diagnosis of pulmonary embolism: concise communications. *J. Nucl. Med.* 21:319–323, 1980.
32. Cheely R., McCartney W.H., Perry J.R., et al.: The role of noninvasive tests versus pulmonary angiography in the diagnosis of pulmonary embolism. *Am. J. Med.* 70:17–22, 1981.
33. Goldhaber S.Z., Hennekens C.H. Evans D.A., et al.: Factors influencing the correct ante mortem diagnosis of major pulmonary embolism. *Am. J. Med.* In press, 1982.
34. Taplin G.V., Chopra S.K., MacDonald N.S., et al.: Imaging small pulmonary ischemic lesions after radioactive carbon monoxide inhalation. *J. Nucl. Med.* 17:866–871, 1976.
35. Nichos A.B., Cochavi S., Moore R.H., et al.: Detection of experimental pulmonary emboli in dogs by sequential positron imaging after inhalation of O–15–carbon dioxide. *Circ. Res.* 42:53–63, 1978.
36. Nichols A.B., Cochavi S., Hales C.A., et al.: Scintigraphic detection of pulmonary emboli by serial positron imaging of inhaled O–15–labeled carbon dioxide. *N. Engl. J. Med.* 299:279–284, 1978.
37. McIlmoyle G., Havis H.H., Welch M.J., et al.: Scintigraphic diagnosis of experimental pulmonary embolism with In-111-labeled platelets. *J. Nucl. Med.* 18:910–914, 1977.
38. Goodwin D.A., Bushberg J.T., Doherty P.W., et al.: Indium-111-labeled autologous platelets for location of vascular thrombi in humans. *J. Nucl. Med.* 19:626–634, 1978.
39. Ezekowitz M.D., Smith E.O., Cox A.C., et al.: The feasibility of using indium-111 platelet scintigraphy in the study of thrombo-embolic disease: a report of 100 consecutive studies. *Clin. Res.* 29:494A, 1981.
40. Crummy A.B., Strother C.M., Sackett J.F., et al.: Computerized fluoroscopy: digital subtraction for intravenous angiocardiography and arteriography. *AJR* 135:1131–1140, 1980.

41. Ovitt T.W., Christenson P.L., Fisher H.D. III, et al.: Intravenous angiography using digital video subtraction: X-ray imaging system. *AJR* 135:1141–1144, 1980.
42. Christenson P.C., Ovitt T.W., Fisher H.D. III, et al.: Intravenous angiography using digital video subtraction: intravenous cervicocerebrovascular angiography. *AJR* 135:1145–1152, 1980.
43. Meaney T.F., Weinstein M.A., Buonocore E., et al.: Digital subtraction angiography of the human cardiovascular system. *AJR* 135:1153–1160, 1980.

COMMENT: INTRACARDIAC MASSES

Alfred F. Parisi

THE ABILITY to detect intravascular and intracardiac masses by ultrasonic and radionuclide methods represents a historic breakthrough in cardiovascular diagnosis. Prior to the development of either of these techniques, masses were detected only through invasive procedures and often quite fortuitously, either at cardiac catheterization or at cardiac surgery. Clinically, masses were usually suspected only after an embolic event. In cases of pulmonary and cerebral embolism, the consequences were often so devastating at the time of the diagnosis that they frustrated the physican's attempt to intervene in a meaningful way with the underlying disorder.

Left atrial myxoma, though a rare disease, perhaps exemplifies best the important advances made by modern noninvasive imaging techniques which are capable of demonstrating filling defects and masses *within* the cardiac chambers, an accomplishment previously achieved only by contrast angiography. Atrial myxomas present in one of several ways. First, the disorder may masquerade as mitral disease, usually mitral stenosis, with respiratory symptoms that are the result of pulmonary venous hypertension. Second, peripheral embolism, perhaps suggesting the diagnosis of bacterial endocarditis, is also encountered fairly frequently as friable material breaks loose from the gelatinous intra-atrial mass. Third, a wasting, usually febrile illness, simulating malignant disease, is a possible manifestation. Because atrial myxoma is considerably rarer than any of the disorders it mimics, it is quite understandable why historically this disorder, which could not be approached directly, was often misdiagnosed or undiagnosed until postmortem examination. Occasionally, the diagnosis of left atrial myxoma was made by histopathologic examination of embolic tissue which was retrieved after the patient had survived a peripheral embolic event. The ability to image left atrial myxomas directly, both by echocardiography and radionuclide angiography, has completely changed the outlook for the patient with this disease. While previously having a grim future, the patient with myxoma can now be routinely identified and surgical cure can be effected without delay. Indeed, in most adequately equipped and staffed hospital settings today, the noninvasive detection of an appropriate mass in the left atrium usually constitutes adequate reason for performing cardiac surgery without cardiac catheterization in patients who meet the other criteria for this syndrome.

The important differences relating to the ability of echocardiography and nuclear methods to detect cardiac masses are defined in terms of two inherently different properties of each technique. The first difference is the *superior spatial resolution of echocardiography*. The second difference is the *intrinsic versatility of nuclear methods*, which allows radiolabels to interact with a number of different pathologic processes. These properties make one or the other technique more advantageous in a given clinical setting and underlie their mutual complementarity in evaluating the vast majority of patients who have problems related to intravascular and intracardiac mass lesions.

Two-dimensional echocardiography has a resolution two to five times greater than that achievable by radionuclide methods. Thus, echocardiography is able to detect smaller space-occupying lesions. In particular, it can identify low-profile sessile masses which minimally infringe on the confines of cardiac chamber cavities. The superior resolution of echocardiography also allows intimate anatomical localization of masses with respect to the structures they involve, e.g., vegetations affecting specific cardiac valves in bacterial endocarditis. Despite these theoretical advantages, echocardiograpy is not applicable to diagnosis of most intravascular, as opposed to intracardiac, masses. It is not a practical technique to detect most forms of venous thrombosis, and it cannot be used at all to detect pulmonary embolism. That echocardiographic evaluations are difficult in some patients is also a limitation.

Radionuclide angiography is an extremely useful technique in recognizing *large* intracavitary cardiac masses which present as "cold spot" filling defects. Furthermore, radionuclide methods can detect any intravascular or intracardiac mass that concentrates radiolabel with a high enough avidity so that it is detectable by external means. And because radiation is unaffected by transmission through air, radionuclides are especially useful in recognizing the malperfusion patterns characteristic of pulmonary embolism. The ability to detect specific radiolabels that interact with pathologic processes involving inflammatory responses and fibrin deposition also makes radionuclide imaging a versatile method for detecting deep venous thrombosis and bacterial infections of the heart. However, radionuclide angiography and "hot spot" labeling methods cannot provide the anatomical details of cardiac structure afforded by echocardiography. Thus, while radionuclide imaging might detect an infected mass within the confines of the cardiac silhouette, it may not be able to localize the mass to the mitral or aortic valve. Certainly radionuclide methods are unlikely to show the aortic valve prolapse which can result from leaflet destruction or to demonstrate the severity of aortic regurgitation, as can be done by examining the timing of mitral valve closure by echocardiography.

When the techniques are used properly, there is very little competitive overlap between radionuclide and echocardiographic methods for the spectrum of diseases which present with intravascular or intracardiac masses. In selected patients, echocardiography is the method of choice for detecting intracardiac masses. In patients suspected of having extracardiac masses, particularly venous thrombosis and pulmonary embolism, radionuclide imaging is the method of choice. In addition, radionuclide methods are useful in detecting large cardiac masses in patients who are not well suited to ultrasonic examination.

PART XI

Congenital Heart Disease

ECHOCARDIOGRAPHY

Peter Bloomfield and Alfred F. Parisi

THIS CHAPTER does not attempt to provide a definitive account of echocardiograhic findings in congenital heart disease, since there are several excellent textbooks on this subject.[1–3] Instead, this chapter outlines the general principles that apply to pediatric echocardiography. Congenital anomalies more likely to be seen by the adult cardiologist are described in greater detail, while less common anomalies are described only briefly. Rather than the usual division of congenital disease into cyanotic and acyanotic forms, anomalies are described in terms of alteration of structure as they appear to the echocardiographer. Thus, shunt lesions, lesions causing obstruction to ventricular outflow, and lesions due to malalignment of chambers and great vessels are described separately.

SHUNT LESIONS

An abnormal communication between the right and left side of the heart permits abnormal blood flow from left to right, and vice versa. In the case of an atrial septal defect, if the defect is small, there may be a pressure gradient of several mm Hg between the left and right atria; if the defect is large the mean pressure in both atria is identical. Blood flows from left atrium to right atrium not only because of a pressure difference (if one exists) but also because of the greater compliance or distensibility of the right-sided chambers. In patients with dominant left-to-right shunts, a small right-to-left shunt may occur with respiratory variation in intrathoracic pressure and may be accentuated by the Valsalva maneuver. Should pulmonary hypertension develop and right-sided pressures exceed those on the left, shunt reversal occurs, with abnormal blood flow becoming predominantly right to left.

Since chambers and major blood vessels carrying a higher blood flow may respond by dilating, the diagnosis of shunt lesions by M-mode echocardiography is largely deductive, based on changes in relative chamber size. Two-dimensional echocardiography (2DE) now allows direct visualization of the defects responsible for intracardiac shunts, facilitates assessment of relative chamber sizes, and, by the simple technique of a contrast "bubble" injection, can often demonstrate flow through an abnormal communication. This last technique, known as contrast echocardiography, followed from an observation made by early investigators performing echocardiography in the catheterization laboratory in order to correlate cardiac anatomy with the echocardiogram. They noticed that indocyanine green dye injected through a catheter appeared as a mass of echo-dense material because the ultrasound waves were reflected from mircobubbles within the injected dye.[4] It was subsequently found that injection of any freshly mixed solution such as saline into a peripheral vein is followed by the appearance of echo-dense material in the right side of the heart. Right-to-left shunts can be demonstrated by the passage of bubbles from the right to left side of the heart.[5] In left-to-right shunts a streaming effect with displacement of the bubbles within the right side by shunted but nonopacified blood, the so-called negative contrast effect, can be seen.[6]

Atrial Septal Defect

The anatomical sites of interatrial defects are shown in Figure 21–1. The ostium secundum type is the most common. It is midseptal in location in the region of the fossa ovalis. Defects of the sinus venosus type are high in the atrial septum, near the entry of the superior vena cava, and are frequently associated with anomalous drainage of the pulmonary veins from the right lung into the right atrium. Ostium primum defects lie immediately adjacent to the atrioventricular valves, either of which may be deformed or incompetent when associated with this type of defect.

With an abnormal communication through the interatrial septum, an increased volume of blood flows through the left atrium, both right-sided chambers of the heart, and the pulmonary veins. With the increased flow all of these structures usually dilate, with the exception of the left atrium, presumably because the increased flow into this chamber can pass either into the right atrium via the defect or across the mitral valve. The left ventricle and aorta, which do not receive shunted blood, remain normal in size.

The characteristic M-mode findings in atrial septal defect are thus a dilated right ventricle with normal left atrial, aortic root, and left ventricular sizes (Fig 21–2).[7] Right ventricular size has been shown to correspond grossly to the size of the shunt. The other characteristic feature is abnormal septal motion, which is termed "paradoxic" because the interventricular septum moves anteriorly toward the right ventricle in systole.[7, 8] Paradoxic septal motion and right ventricular dilation can occur with most lesions causing right ventricular volume overload and sometimes with lesions causing pressure overload.[9] Also, movement of the pulmonic valve cusps may be affected by the pulmonary hypertension that may develop with large shunts. In normal circumstances, when right ventricular and pulmonary artery pressures are low, right atrial contraction may partially open the pulmonic valve, producing an "a" kick on the pulmonic valve echo. If right atrial contraction does not produce a pressure sufficient to exceed an elevated pulmonary artery pressure, the "a" kick will not be seen.[10] None of these M-mode findings are pathognomonic, and although they may be highly suggestive of atrial septal defect, definitive diag-

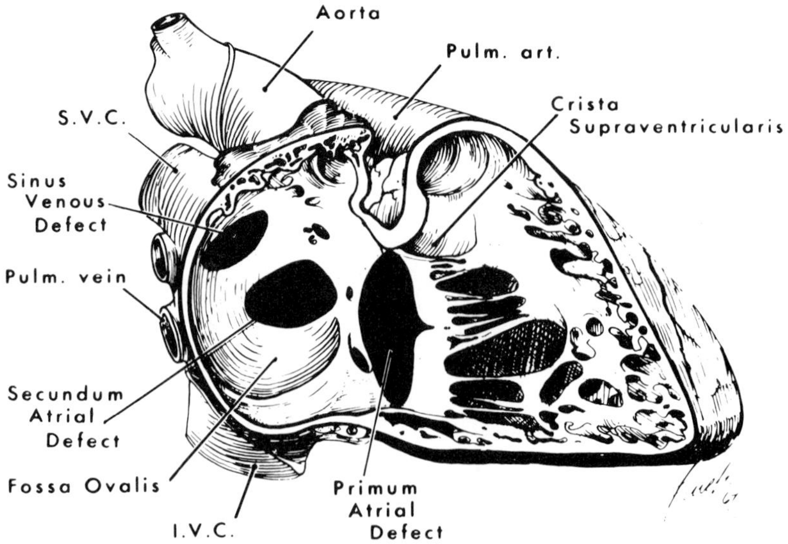

Fig 21–1.—Composite locations of atrial defects. *SVC* = superior vena cava; *IVC* = inferior vena cava. (From Friedman W.R.: Congenital heart disease in infancy and childhood, in Braunwald E. (ed.): *Heart Disease: A Textbook of Cardiovascular Medicine.* Philadelphia, W. B. Saunders, 1980, p. 985. Used by permission.)

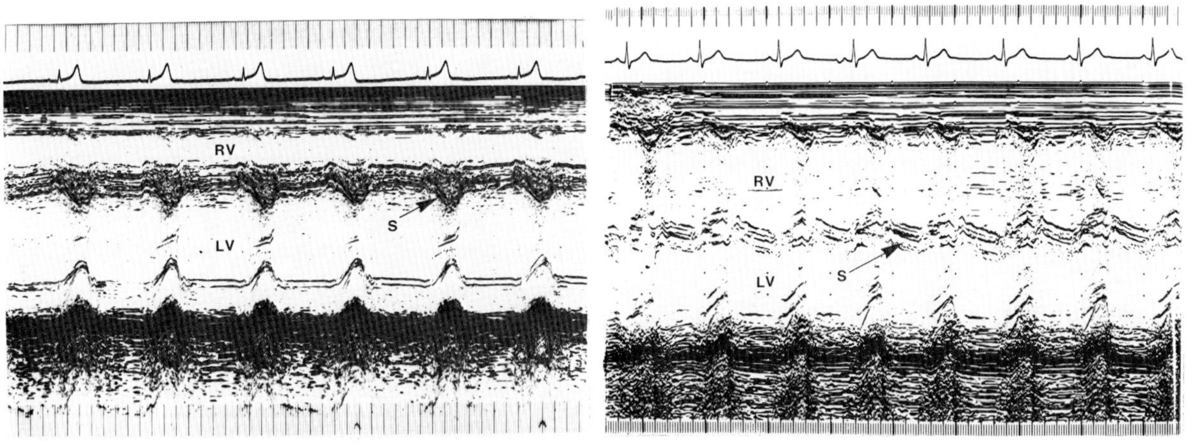

Fig 21–2.—Echograms from a normal subject *(left)* and a patient with an ostium secundum atrial septal defect *(right)*. In the patient, the right ventricle *(RV)* is enlarged and there is paradoxic septal *(S)* motion. *LV* = left ventricle.

nosis is not usually possible with this technique.

With 2DE both right-sided chambers can be more fully delineated. The interatrial septum can be visualized with both the apical four-chamber and short-axis views. Because the interatrial septum lies along the axis of the ultrasound beam in these projections, it is difficult to distinguish between a true defect in the septum and artifactual "dropout" of echoes in the area of the fossa ovalis. In neonates and infants, this problem has been overcome by using a subcostal approach, directing the beam through the liver with the interatrial and interventricular septa lying perpendicularly to the ultrasound beam.[11] The appearances of the various types of atrial septal defects are shown schematically in Figure 21–3. In normal infants the interatrial septum appears as a linear echo with some thinning in the region of the foramen ovale (see *a*, Fig 21–3). A secundum defect appears centrally in the area normally occupied by the

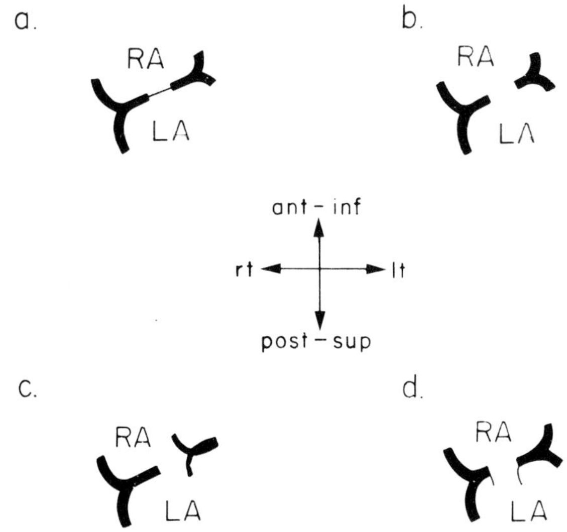

Fig 21–3.—Appearances of the interatrial septum in different types of atrial septal defect as imaged in the subcostal view. *a*, normal; *b*, secundum type of defect; *c;* primum type of defect; *d*, septal defect after balloon septostomy. (Adapted from Bierman F.Z. and Williams R.G.: Subxiphoid two dimensional imaging of the interatrial septum in infants and neonates with congenital heart disease. *Circulation* 60:80, 1979.)

foramen ovale. The intact portion of the septum can be seen at both ends of the defect (see *b,* Fig 21–3). The primum type of defect is located immediately adjacent to the atrioventricular valves and interventricular septum, and no remnant of interatrial septum can be seen between the defect and the interventricular septum (see *c,* Fig 21–3). The defect created by balloon septostomy appears as a secundum defect, often with visualization of the flail remnants of the torn septum (see *d,* Fig 21–3).

Echocardiography after a peripheral vein injection of agitated saline or other echographic contrast solution can easily demonstrate a right-to-left shunt at the atrial level when shunt reversal has occurred.[5, 12] A small right-to-left shunt usually also occurs in uncomplicated atrial septal defects and can be accentuated by respiratory changes in intrathoracic pressure. Contrast echocardiography, especially when performed with the Valsalva maneuver, has demonstrated a right-to-left shunt in most patients who have not developed pulmonary hypertension, including those with so small a right-to-left shunt that it could not be detected by traditional oximetry methods at catheterization.[13] Right-to-left shunting of injected bubbles can be seen to pass directly from right to left atrium on 2DE. On M-mode echocardiography the right and left atria cannot be visualized simultaneously. The presence of an atrial septal defect is inferred from the simultaneous appearance of contrast in the right and left ventricles and can be shown to enter the left ventricle at the level of the mitral valve (Fig 21–4).

Most patients with atrial septal defect do not have complicating pulmonary hypertension, and many reach adulthood without this condition having been detected. The more significant shunt in this case is, of course, from left to right and may sometimes be shown with 2DE by the negative contrast technique. The echo-dense contrast passing through the right atrium is displaced by the jet of contrast-free blood from the left atrium (Fig 21–5). While these negative contrast techniques have been reported to be both highly sensitive and highly specific for detecting shunts at the atrial level, they are less reliable than actually seeing bubbles cross from the right to left side of the heart.[6] Attempts to quantify the size of the shunt by contrast techniques have not proved reliable.

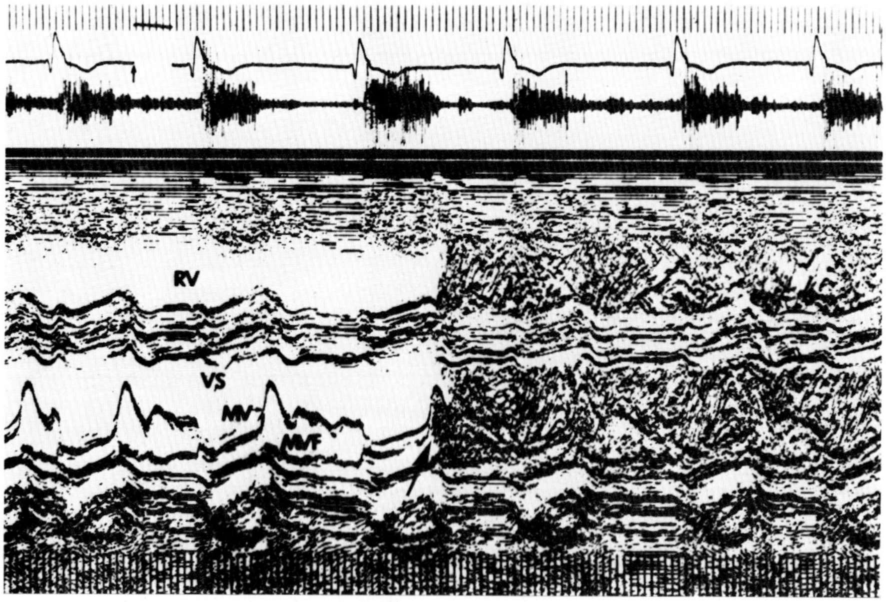

Fig 21–4.—Contrast echocardiogram after venous injection in a patient with right-to-left shunt at the atrial level. Contrast reaches the right and left ventricles simultaneously and enters the left ventricle through the mitral valve funnel *(arrow). RV* = right ventricle; *VS* = ventricular septum; *MV* = anterior mitral valve leaflet; *MVF* = mitral valve funnel. (From Tajik A.J. and Seward J.B.: Contrast echocardiography. *Cardiovasc. Clin. North Am.* 9:2, 1979.)

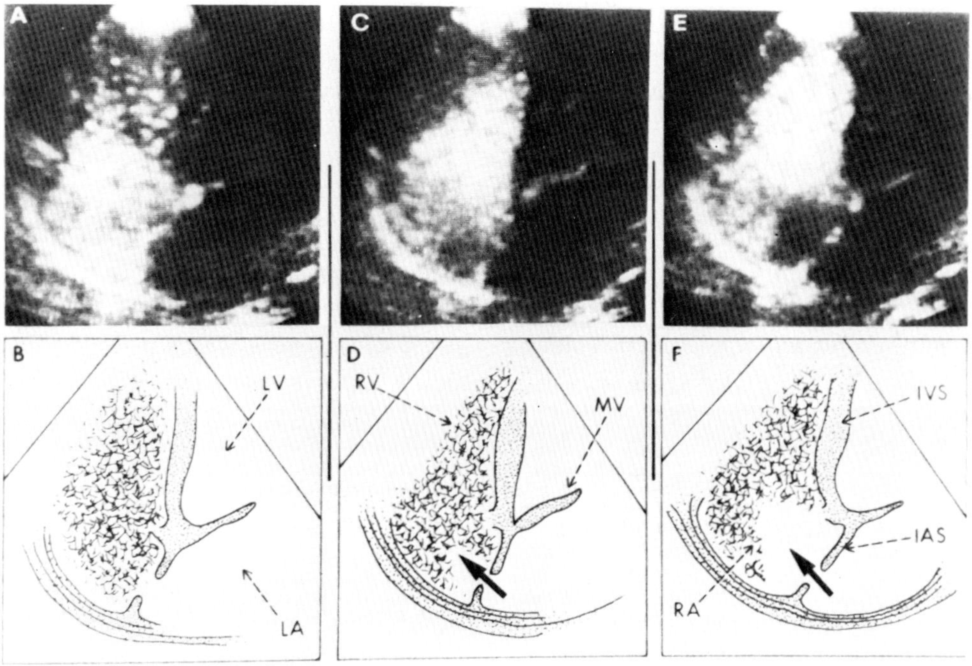

Fig 21–5.—Negative contrast effect. Sequential late diastolic stop-frame videotape images (panels *A, C, E*) in apical four-chamber view with accompanying schematic diagrams (panels *B, D, F*) from a patient with secundum atrial septal defect. Blood without microcavitations (negative contrast) enters the right atrium (panels *C* and *D*) and partially fills it (panels *E* and *F*). *IVS* = interventricular septum; *IAS* = interatrial septum; *LV* = left ventricle; *RV* = right ventricle; *LA* = left atrium; *RA* = right atrium; *MV* = mitral valve. (From Fraker T.D., et al.: Detection and exclusion of interatrial shunts by two-dimensional echocardiography and peripheral venous injection. *Circulation* 59:383, 1979.)

Anomalous Pulmonary Venous Drainage

This lesion most commonly occurs with an atrial septal defect of the sinus venosus type but may occur alone. If a significant left-to-right shunt is created, the appearance will be of a right ventricular volume overload. Most patients have only one or two pulmonary veins draining into the right atrium with an associated atrial septal defect, and the appearance of the echo is indistinguishable from that of a pure atrial septal defect. When all four pulmonary veins enter the right atrium, the confluence of these veins may appear as an extra chamber behind the left atrium (Fig 21–6).[14]

Endocardial Cushion Defects

Endocardial cushion defects comprise a spectrum of malformations involving either singly or in combination the interatrial septum, the interventricular septum, and one or both atrioventricular valves. The most common and least severe form is the ostium primum atrial septal defect described above, and the most severe form is the complete atrioventricular canal. It is unusual for persons to reach adulthood with the more serious malformations undetected. Two-dimensional echocardiography has proved most useful in defining the anatomy of these defects. With primum defects of the partial endocardial cushion type, the features of atrial septal defect are as described above, with localization of the defect immediately adjacent to the atrioventricular valves and interventricular septum, as shown in Figure 21–3, part *c*.[11, 15] Defects in the interventricular septum may also be detected in this view. The mitral valve is the more commonly affected of the atrioventricular valves, and the anterior leaflet is often cleft and displaced toward the interventricular septum. This may present a variety of appearances on the M-mode echogram,[15, 16] depending on the degree

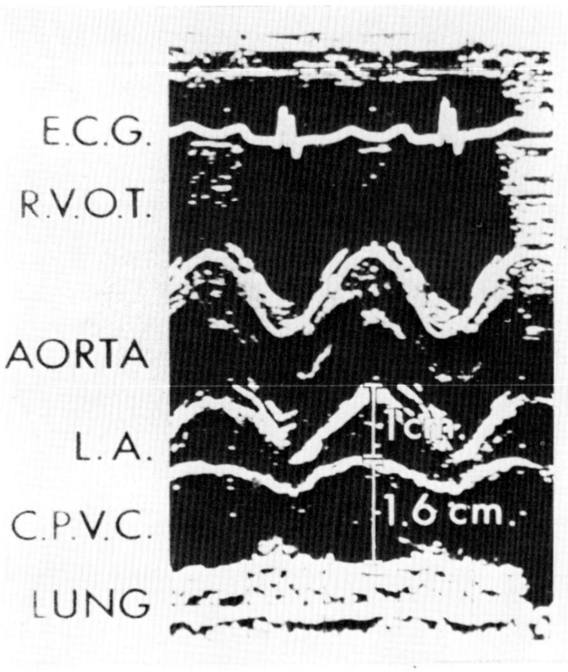

Fig 21–6.—M-mode echocardiogram of a patient with total anomalous pulmonary venous drainage showing a common pulmonary venous chamber *(CPVC)* behind the left atrium. *RVOT* = right ventricular outflow tract; *LA* = left atrium. (From Paquet M. and Gutgesell H.: Echocardiographic features of total anomalous pulmonary venous connection. *Circulation* 51:599, 1975.)

of differentiation of the atrioventricular leaflets. One striking finding in patients with a completely undivided leaflet is the apparent motion of the common valve leaflet traversing the interventricular septum during the cardiac cycle (Fig 21–7). The complete atrioventricular canal can be best appreciated from the apical four-chamber and subcostal views, in which dropout of echoes from both the ventricular and atrial septa in the regions contiguous with the atrioventricular valve can be seen. These views also allow differentiation of divided and undivided, attached and free-floating common atrioventricular valves (Fig 21–8).

Patent Ductus Arteriosus

In patent ductus arteriosus in the absence of pulmonary hypertension, blood passes from the aorta into the pulmonary artery. Shunted blood increases the flow through the left atrium and left ventricle, and these chambers may dilate in response to the increased flow. The principal findings on M-mode echocardiography in patients with a large shunt are a dilated left atrium and a hyperdynamic left ventricle. The ratio of left atrial dimension to aortic root dimension has been used to assess the size of the shunt.[1, 17] The accuracy of this method has been improved using the two-dimensional technique for assessing left atrial size.

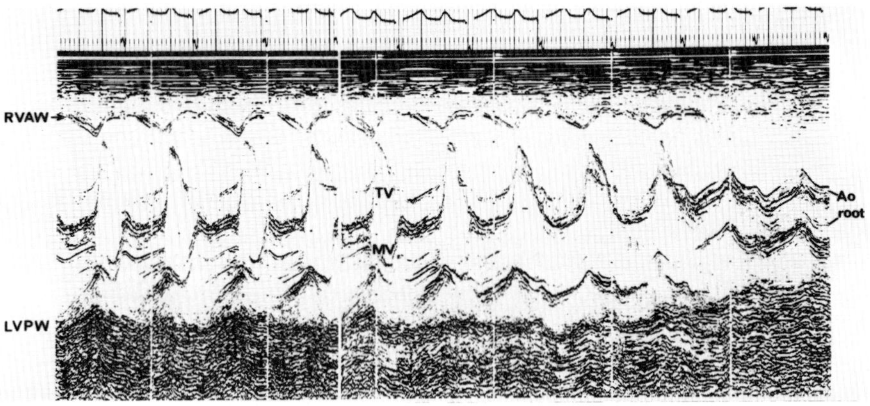

Fig 21–7.—At surgery, this patient had a complete atrioventricular canal with divided mitral and tricuspid portions of the atrioventricular valve. Note that the tricuspid portion *(TV)* of the valve appears within the right ventricle and moves toward the right ventricular anterior wall *(RVAW),* while the mitral portion *(MV)* of the inferior leaflet moves posteriorly into the left ventricle toward the *LVPW.* This is the appearance of the "smiling crocodile," which is strongly suggestive of complete atrioventricular canal but does not differentiate between a single or divided atrioventricular valve. (Courtesy of Dr. Roberta Williams.) (From Parisi A.F. and Tow D.E.: *Noninvasive Approaches to Cardiovascular Diagnosis.* New York, Appleton-Century-Crofts, 1979.)

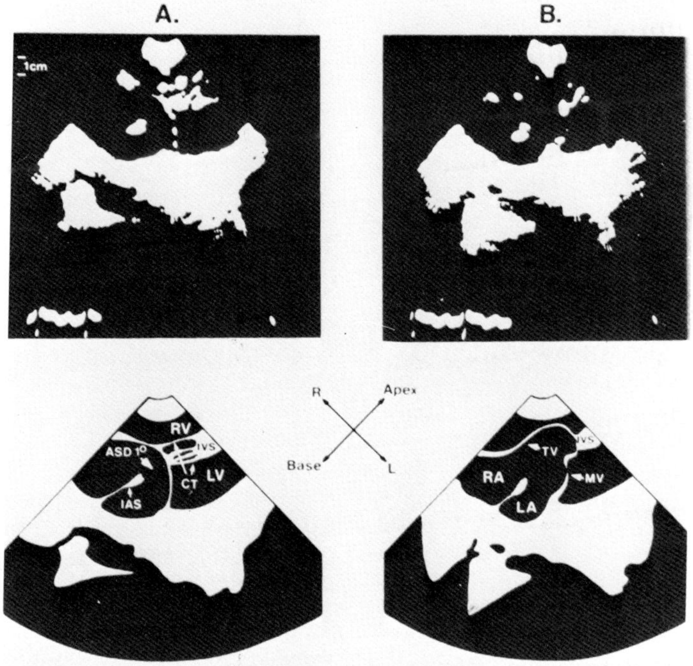

Fig 21–8.—Subcostal view of a two-dimensional echocardiogram in a patient with a complete endocardial cushion defect. A common atrioventricular valve that is septally attached **(A)** and appears to be divided during diastole **(B)** is demonstrated. *RV,* right ventricle; *LV,* left ventricle; *LA,* left atrium; *RA,* right atrium; *MV,* mitral valve portion; *ASD 1°,* primum atrial septal defect; *CT,* chordal structures; *IAS,* interatrial septum; *IVS,* interventricular septum; *TV,* tricuspid valve portion. (From Kotler M.N., et al.: Two-dimensional echocardiography in congenital heart disease. *Am. J. Cardiol.* 46:1237, 1980.)

Neonates with a large shunt may develop left heart failure and a respiratory distress syndrome, and these echocardiographic findings have proved invaluable in making the differential diagnosis between primary lung disease and primary cardiac disease due to a patent ductus arteriosus.[17] Left atrial size may diminish dramatically following surgical closure of the ductus. Similarly, gradual diminution of left atrial size may follow spontaneous closure of the ductus. Echocardiography has proved to be a valuable tool in following the progress of these patients.[1, 17] Direct visualization of the patent ductus with the two-dimensional technique has been described in infants.[18]

In Figure 21–9, a short-axis view through the aorta, the patent ductus appears as an echo-free space between the pulmonary artery and descending aorta. Further studies are needed to confirm the reliability of this technique. Doppler echocardiography has been used to demonstrate flow through a patent ductus. It has been suggested that this method can also determine the presence of pulmonary hypertension. With normal pulmonary artery pressure flow across the ductus is pandiastolic, but in pulmonary hypertension the diastolic flow is cut short.[19]

Contrast echocardiography has also been used to demonstrate abnormal flow in patent ductus arteriosus. Injection of contrast material at the level of the ductus via an umbilical catheter can demonstrate the passage of contrast material from the aorta into the pulmonary artery. This method is facilitated by the indwelling umbilical artery catheter commonly used in such critically ill neonates.[20]

Ventricular Septal Defect

Ventricular septal defect is one of the most prevalent congenital anomalies and may occur as

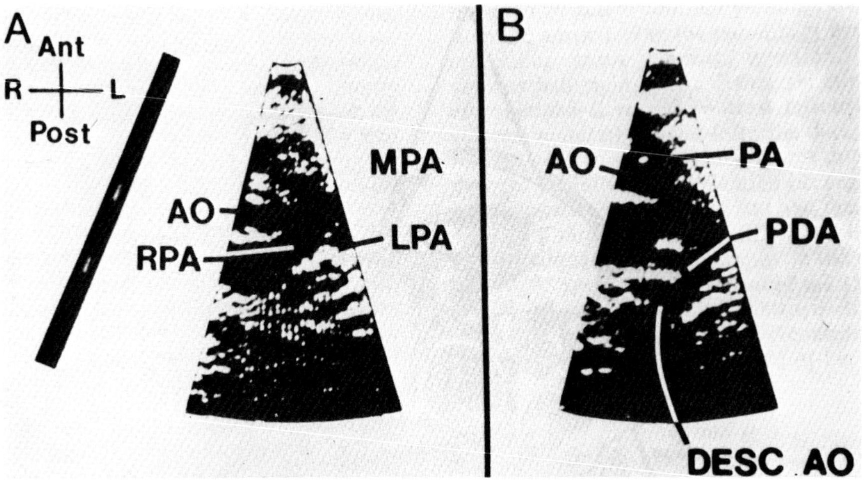

Fig 21–9.—Two still-frame echo images show identification of a patent ductus arteriosus *(PDA)*. From the scan plane of the main pulmonary artery *(MPA)* and its bifurcation **(A),** the scan plane is rotated slightly superiorly to the plane of the ductus arteriosus **(B).** *AO,* aorta; *RPA,* right pulmonary artery; LPA, left pulmonary artery; *DESC AO,* descending aorta. (From Sahn D.J. and Allen H.D.: Real-time cross-sectional echocardiographic imaging and measurement of the patent ductus arteriosus in infants and children. *Circulation* 58:343, 1978.)

an isolated defect or in combination with other malformations. The membranous part of the septum is most commonly affected, but a defect can occur anywhere in the interventricular septum. The degree of functional disturbance depends both on the size of the defect and on the status of the pulmonary vascular bed. A small defect will allow only a small left-to-right shunt, but a large defect will allow a large shunt if there is no associated pulmonary stenosis or increased pulmonary vascular resistance. As in patent ductus arteriosus, the left atrium and left ventricle conduct an increased flow of blood, and the left atrium-aortic root ratio has been suggested as an index of the degree of left-to-right shunting. This ratio has not proved as reliable, however, in ventricular septal defect as in patent ductus.[21] Both ventricles carry an increased volume of blood and septal motion may be exaggerated but is usually normal. With small defects all the cardiac chambers will appear normal.

Direct visualization of the defect may be made with the M-mode technique, but this method is insensitive, and only patients with a large defect consistently show loss of contiguity of septal echoes. False positive results are frequently recorded because of artifactual echo dropout due to such variables as transducer position. Ventricular septal defects have been directly visualized with consid-

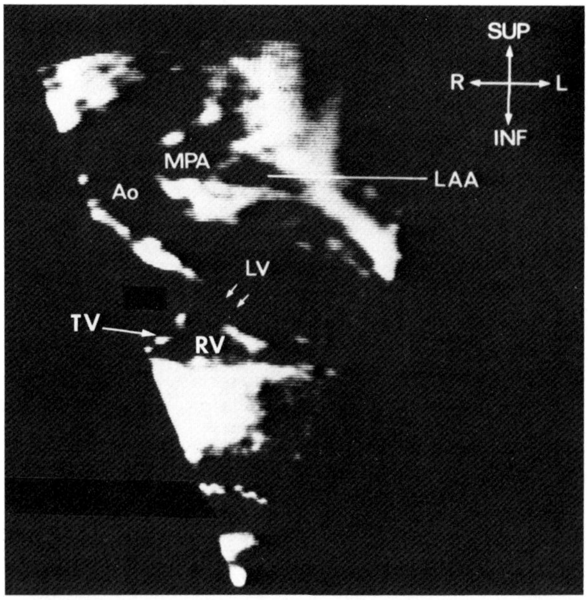

Fig 21–10.—Subcostal two-dimensional echocardiogram in a long-axis view of the left ventricle *(LV)* and aorta *(Ao)*. The right atrium is at bottom left of the picture, adjacent to which are leaflets of the tricuspid valve *(TV)* and right ventricle *(RV)*. A ventricular septal defect is indicated by two arrows. The left atrial appendage *(LAA)* is adjacent to the aorta, and the main pulmonary artery *(MPA)* can be seen as it passes posteriorly before dividing. (Courtesy of Dr. Roberta Williams.)

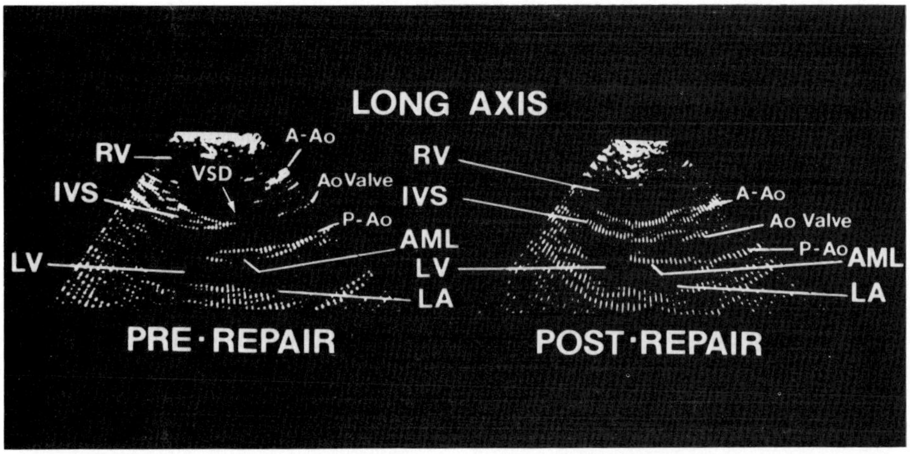

Fig 21–11.—Pre- and postoperative long-axis two-dimensional echocardiograms of a patient with tetralogy of Fallot. The ventricular septal defect *(VSD)* is seen in the preoperative recording. Continuity between the interventricular septum *(IVS)* and anterior wall of the aorta *(A-Ao)* is restored following repair. *RV* = right ventricle; *LV* = left ventricle; *AML* = anterior mitral leaflet; *LA* = left atrium; *P-Ao* = posterior aortic wall. (From Caldwell R.L., et al.: Right ventricular outflow tract assessment by cross-sectional echocardiography in tetralogy of Fallot. *Circulation* 59:395, 1979.)

erably greater success by 2DE.[22] This technique is most reliable when the defect can be visualized in more than one axial plane. Various views may be required to detect defects in different anatomical positions within the interventricular septum. Anterior defects are usually best visualized on the long-axis view and posterior defects on the apical four-chamber view. The parasternal short-axis view, which traverses the heart at the level of the pulmonic and mitral valves, permits visualization of subpulmonic defects. Some workers have found that many defects can be best detected by making serial images of the heart from the subcostal approach, since the interventricular septum lies perpendicular to the ultrasound beam in this plane.[23] Such a defect is shown in Figure 21–10. These techniques allow measurement of the size of the defects, and such estimates have been used to predict the clinical course of patients.[24]

The ventricular septal defect that is secondary to malalignment, such as occurs in tetralogy of Fallot, is the easiest to detect echocardiographically. On M-mode echocardiography the anterior aortic wall is seen to lie anteriorly to the interventricular septum. On the 2DE long-axis view the aorta is seen to override the interventricular septum. Proper continuity between anterior aortic wall and the interventricular septum is restored following surgery (Fig 21–11).[25]

As in atrial septal defect and patent ductus arteriosus, contrast echocardiography can be helpful in detecting the direction of a shunt. A right-to-left shunt may occur with right ventricular outflow tract obstruction or with increased pulmonary vascular resistance, and on 2DE, contrast bubbles may be seen to stream across the defect directly from the right ventricle to the left ventricle. On M-mode echocardiography bubbles appear in the right ventricle and immediately thereafter in the left ventricular outflow tract, in contrast to atrial septal defect, in which bubbles flow through the inflow tract or mitral valve.[25] As with atrial septal defects, a left-to-right shunt may produce a negative contrast effect.

OBSTRUCTIONS TO VENTRICULAR OUTFLOW

Left ventricular outflow tract obstruction can occur at the level of the aortic valve, above it, or below it. Echocardiography, especially two-dimensional echocardiography, has proved to be an accurate method of identifying and localizing the level of obstruction.[26]

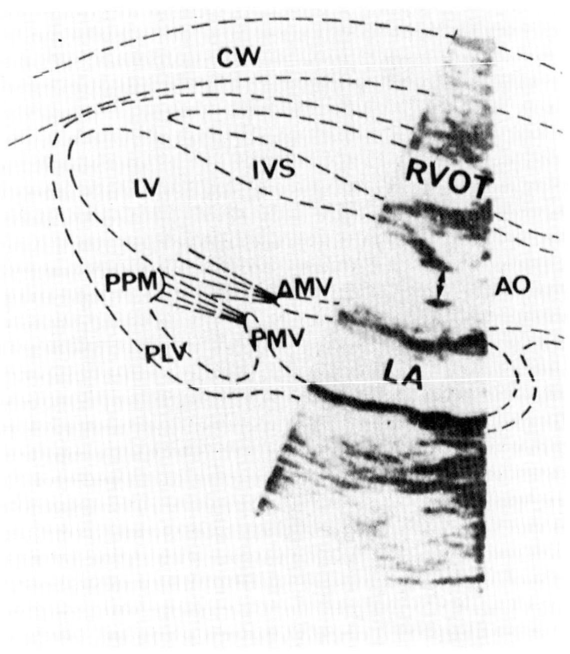

Fig 21–12.—Cross-sectional echocardiogram from a patient with congenital aortic stenosis demonstrating systolic doming of the aortic valve. The thickened anterior and posterior cusp tissue produces relatively strong echoes that arc toward the center of the aorta during systole. The valve orifice is indicated by the arrow. *RVOT,* right ventricular outflow tract; *LA,* left atrium; *AO,* aorta; *IVS,* interventricular septum; *LV,* left ventricle; *AMV,* anterior mitral valve; *PMV,* posterior mitral valve; *PLV,* posterior left ventricular wall; *PPM,* posterior papillary muscle; *CW,* chest wall. (From Weyman A.E., et al.: Localization of left ventricular outflow tract obstruction by cross-sectional echocardiography. *Am. J. Med.* 60:33, 1976.)

Aortic Valve Stenosis

In congenital aortic stenosis features of the echogram usually differ from those of acquired aortic stenosis. In the congenital form, detected in childhood or early adult life, the valve cusps are not as thickened and are not calcified. In contrast to the normal aortic valve, in which the leaflets separate in systole against the aortic walls, the congenitally stenotic valve assumes a domed shape in systole. This can be clearly seen on the two-dimensional echogram in Figure 21–12. Indeed, the demonstration of doming has proved virtually specific for congenital stenosis of both aortic and pulmonary valves (see Fig 21–17) and has greatly enhanced the usefulness of echocardiography in the diagnosis of congenital disease.[27] The M-mode echogram is much less useful and may appear normal even with markedly stenotic valves. If the M-mode echo beam traverses the base of the dome formed by the aortic cusps, the cusps will appear to separate normally, giving the false impression of a normal aortic valve orifice.

Bicuspid Aortic Valve

A bicuspid aortic valve is one of the most common congenital anomalies. Its principal importance is that it may be subject to infective endocarditis, and in later life it may calcify and become significantly stenotic. On the M-mode echogram normal aortic valve leaflets coapt in the midline in diastole, thus creating an echo equidistant from the walls of the aortic root. In the bicuspid valve the cusps are usually not of equal size, and in diastole they meet at an eccentric point in the aortic root. This sign has not, however, proved to be as reliable as visualization of a bicuspid aortic valve by 2DE in the short-axis view (Fig 21–13). Some workers have been able to identify the bicuspid aortic valve in 95% of patients by 2DE, compared to 75% of patients by M-mode echocardiography.[28]

Subvalvular Aortic Stenosis

Discrete subaortic stenosis may be due to a membrane, a fibromuscular ridge or collar, or a fibromuscular tunnel.[26]

One M-mode echocardiographic feature that occurs with all types of subvalvular obstruction, whether discrete or dynamic, is systolic closure of the aortic valve. Because the discrete membrane type of lesion often lies parallel to the ultrasound beam, the M-mode technique has not proved useful in detecting this type of lesion. By scanning from left ventricle to the aorta through the left ventricular outflow tract, fibromuscular narrowing can readily be appreciated (Fig 21–14). Two-dimensional echocardiography in the parasternal long-axis view provides the most accurate means of differentiating the various types of subaortic stenosis.[26] Quantitative assessment of the degree of obstruction by direct measurement has not as yet been successful. The echocardiographic features of idiopathic hypertrophic subaortic stenosis are ab-

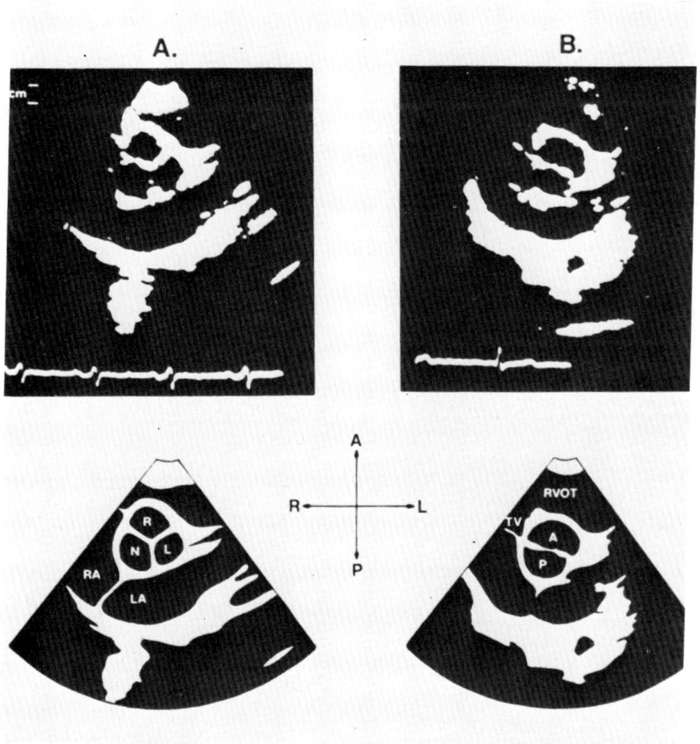

Fig 21–13.—**A,** parasternal short-axis view in a patient showing a normal trileaflet aortic valve. **B,** parasternal short-axis view in a patient with a bicuspid aortic valve. The anterior *(A)* and posterior *(P)* leaflet are separated by a single commisure. *L,* left coronary cusp; *N,* noncoronary cusp, *R,* right coronary cusp; *LA,* left atrium; *RA,* right atrium; *RVOT,* right ventricular outflow tract; *TV,* tricuspid valve. (From Kotler M.D., et al.: Two-dimensional echocardiography in congenital heart disease. *Am. J. Cardiol.* 46:1237, 1980.)

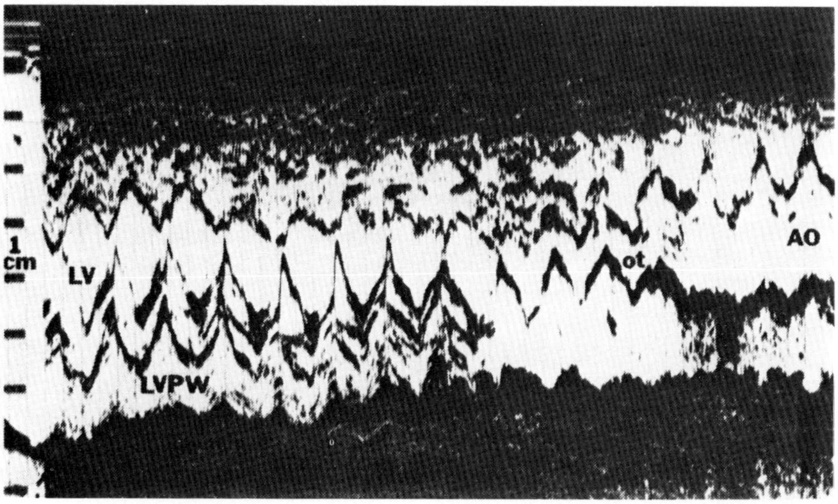

Fig 21–14.—M-mode echocardiogram from a subject with fibromuscular collar around the left ventricular outflow tract. The transducer was swept from the body of the left ventricle *(LV)* on the left to the level of the aorta *(AO).* Note the small size of the outflow tract *(ot)* in comparison with the aorta. (From Popp R.L., et al.: Echocardiographic findings in discrete subvalvular aortic stenosis. *Circulation* 49:226, 1974.)

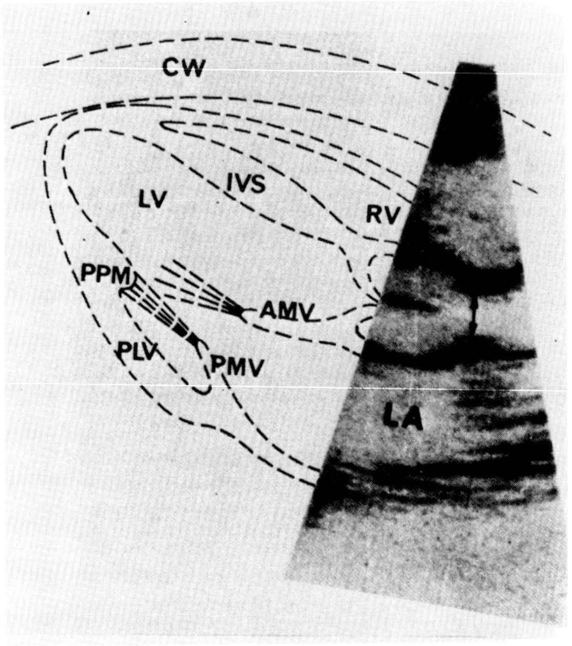

Fig 21–15.—Long-axis echogram from a patient with supravalvular aortic stenosis. The area of obstruction is distal to the aortic valve *(arrow).* Return of the aortic root toward normal can be seen distal to the area of obstruction. The linear echo in the center of the aorta proximal to the area of obstruction is produced by the coapted aortic valve leaflets. Abbreviations same as in Figure 21–12. (From Weyman A.E., et al.: Localization of left ventricular outflow obstruction by cross-sectional echocardiography. *Am. J. Med.* 60:33, 1976.)

normal septal thickness, systolic anterior motion of the mitral valve, and systolic closure of the aortic valve.

Supravalvular Aortic Stenosis

This is an uncommon anomaly and may be associated with other congenital heart defects. Detection of this defect by M-mode echocardiography is difficult, as the ultrasound beam must be scanned along the length of the aorta without deviating from its center or a false impression of narrowing may be created. Two-dimensional echocardiography, by expanding the field of vision and providing spatially orientated information, is more accurate.[26] Figure 21–15 is a two-dimensional echocardiogram from a patient with supravalvular stenosis and shows the narrowed area above the aortic valve.

Coarctation of the Aorta

Visualization of the thoracic aorta is now possible with 2DE when the suprasternal approach is used. Weyman et al. were able to visualize directly the narrowed segment of the descending aorta in 16 of 18 patients studied.[29] The major branches of the aorta and the location of the narrowed segment can be identified. A coarctation characteristically located in the region of the left subclavian artery is shown in Figure 21-16. In addition, prominent systolic pulsation of the aortic arch proximal to the obstructed segment can be seen in real time imaging.

Pulmonic Stenosis

This is a common congenital anomaly and may occur in isolation or in association with other malformations. It is not always possible to visualize the pulmonic valve by M-mode echocardiography. The characteristic finding on M-mode is a prominent "a" wave created by forceful atrial contraction, but this sign is not specific and may occur in patients with bradycardia or a large stroke volume. The pulmonic valve can be more frequently visualized by 2DE[30] and, like the congenitally stenotic aortic valve, has a domed appearance (Fig 21–17).

Subpulmonic Stenosis

Subpulmonic stenosis occurs in tetralogy of Fallot and in other congenital anomalies. Systolic fluttering of the pulmonic valve may be seen on M-mode echocardiography as the jet of blood passes over the valve cusps, but this sign is not specific and may occur in normal individuals.[31]

MALALIGNMENT OF CHAMBERS AND GREAT VESSELS

In the complex congenital malformations, many of which cause cyanosis, no a priori assumptions can be made about the number or spatial relationships of the atria, ventricles, and great arteries. With the ability of 2DE to provide tomographic images in several planes reconstruction of the an-

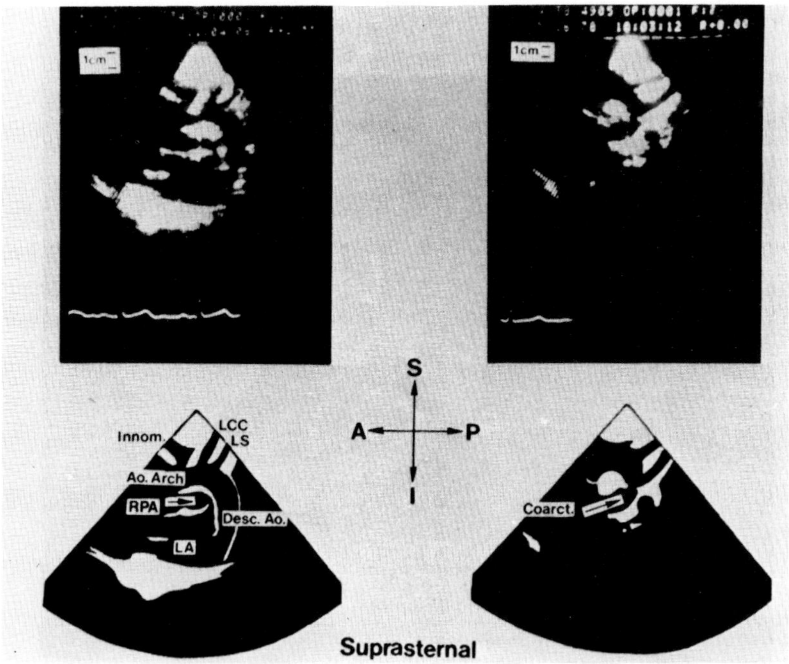

Fig 21–16.—Coarctation of the aorta. Suprasternal views of two-dimensional echocardiogram of aortic arch in a normal subject *(left)* and in a patient with coarctation *(coarct) (right).* In the normal subject the aortic arch and its branches are visible. The narrowed segment *(arrow)* is clearly seen in the right panel. *Desc Ao,* descending aorta; *Innom,* right innominate artery; *LCC,* left common carotid artery; *LS,* left subclavian artery; *RPA,* right pulmonary artery. (From Kotler M.N., et al.: Clinical uses of two-dimensional echocardiography. *Am. J. Cardiol.* 45:1061, 1980.)

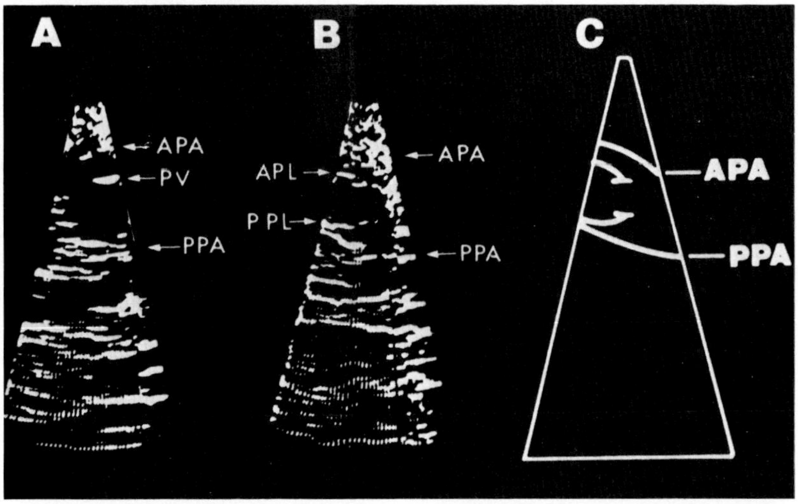

Fig 21–17.—Long-axis echocardiogram of the pulmonary artery and pulmonic valve (PV) from a patient with valvular pulmonic stenosis. *A* was recorded in diastole and depicts the linear echo in the midportion of the pulmonary artery produced by the coapted pulmonary leaflets. *B* illustrates the domed systolic configuration of the pulmonary leaflets. *C* is a line drawing corresponding to the domed systolic appearance of the leaflets in *B. APA,* anterior pulmonary artery; *PPA,* posterior pulmonary artery; *APL,* anterior pulmonic valve leaflet; *PPL,* posterior pulmonic valve leaflet. (From Weymann A.E., et al.: Cross-sectional echocardiographic visualization of the stenotic pulmonary valve. *Circulation* 56:769, 1977.)

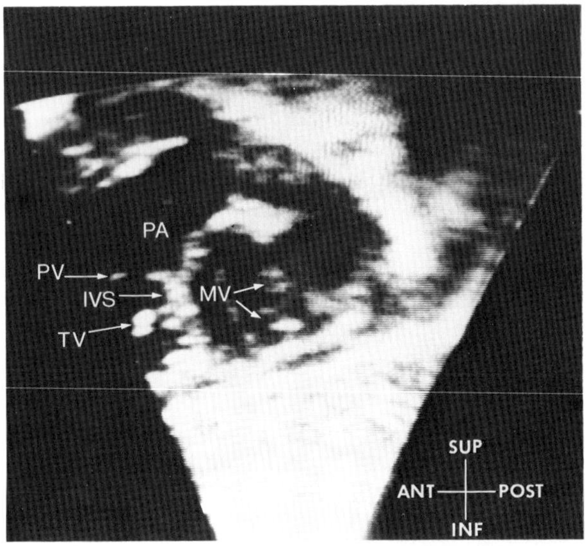

Fig 21–18.—Subcostal two-dimensional echocardiogram of a normal subject in the transverse plane at the level of the right ventricular outflow tract. The left ventricle is identified by the presence of the two papillary muscles of the mitral valve *(MV, arrows)*. The right ventricle lies more anteriorly, and one of the papillary muscles of the tricuspid valve *(TV)* can be seen near the interventricular septum *(IVS)*. The pulmonic valve *(PV)* is seen in this view and communicates with the pulmonary artery *(PA)*, which divides superiorly. (Courtesy of Dr. Roberta Williams.)

atomical relationships of the chambers and major vessels can be made in a manner similar to that used by pathologists at autopsy. Several methods involving different echocardiographic windows and projections have been described. The standard parasternal, apical,[32, 33] suprasternal,[34] and subcostal [11, 24, 35, 36] views all have their advocates. Because of the complexity of many congenital malformations, the pediatric echocardiographer should be familiar with one standard approach that will enable him to study systematically the anatomy of each patient. Because of the wide and easily accessible acoustic window available with the subcostal approach, in which the heart is imaged through the liver, this approach is widely used. The heart is imaged in serial sections in both the short-axis or transverse (sagittal) plane and in the long-axis or coronal plane. This approach enables the echocardiographer to determine atrial situs, ventricular situs, and the relationship of the great arteries to each other and to the ventricles from which they arise. The subcostal approach views the interatrial and interventricular septa at right angles to the echo beam, and this allows the clear est definition of septal defects (see Figs 21–3 and 21–10). With this approach the anatomy of even the most complex malformations can be elucidated. This information, combined with data from other noninvasive studies, often allow a diagnosis to be made without the use of cardiac catheterization.

The remainder of this section outlines the subcostal approach, and anomalies are described in

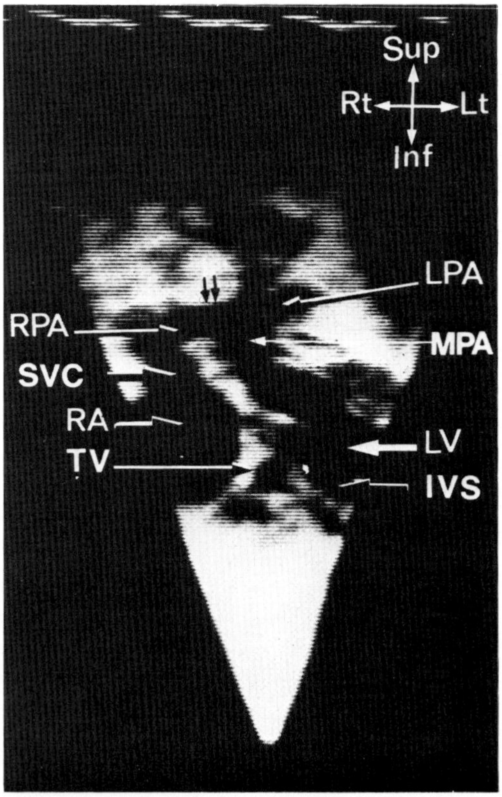

Fig 21–19.—Subcostal two-dimensional echocardiogram from a patient with D-transposition of the great arteries. In this view the left ventricle is seen in long axis. The main pulmonary artery *(MPA)* arises from the left ventricle *(LV)* and divides at right angles into the left and right pulmonary arteries *(LPA, RPA)*. The double arrow indicates the point of division of the main pulmonary artery. *SVC,* superior vena cava; *RA,* right atrium; *TV,* tricuspid valve; *IVS,* interventricular septum. (From Bierman F.Z. and Williams R.G.: Prospective diagnosis of D-transposition of the great arteries in neonates by subxiphoid two-dimensional echocardiography. *Circulation* 60:1496, 1979.)

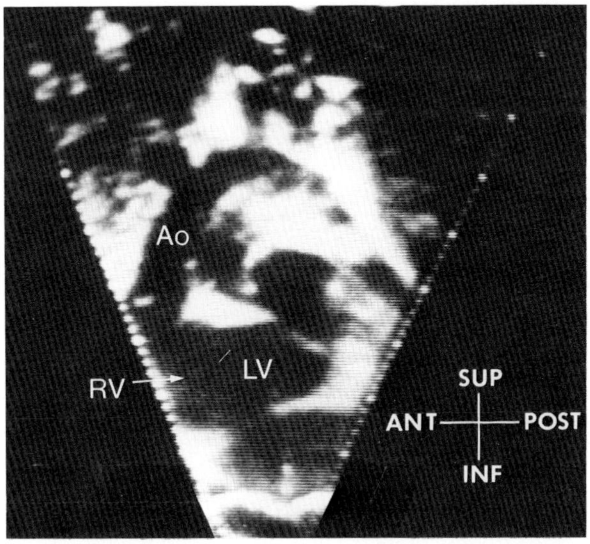

Fig 21–20.—Subcostal two-dimensional echocardiogram of patient in Figure 21–19 with D-transposition of the great arteries. In this transverse plane, the aortic arch *(Ao)* arises from the anterior or right ventricle *(RV)*. Compare this appearance to the example of normal great artery positions in Figure 21–18, where the main pulmonary artery arises from the right ventricle and subsequently divides at right angles. (Courtesy of Dr. Roberta Williams.)

the context of such an approach. This description is a general one but most applicable to pediatric echocardiography. More detailed descriptions are available in the publications of Bierman and Williams[11, 36] and Lange et al.[35]

The first step in the subcostal examination is to identify the inferior vena cava, viewed through the liver in the horizontal plane. It can be distinguished from the aorta by its elliptical shape and by the entry of the hepatic veins. The inferior vena cava is followed superiorly to the right atrium, and in this way atrial situs is defined, since the right atrium is always supplied by the inferior vena cava. As described earlier, the interatrial septum can be examined for defects (see Fig 21–3) and for signs of volume or pressure overload of either atrium, which may cause bulging of the interatrial septum. Once both atria have been identified, a slight rotation of the transducer inferiorly and laterally will reveal all four cardiac chambers; with further cranial angulation, a longitudinal view of the left ventricle, the left ventricular outflow tract, and the posterior great artery can be obtained. This view may demonstrate defects in the interventricular septum (see Fig 21–10). From these views it can be determined whether two ventricles are present or if there is only a single ventricle. The relative sizes of the ventricles and atrioventricular valves can be assessed, and in this way the *hypoplastic left heart syndrome* may be identified. Further cranial angulation of the transducer will identify which great artery is arising from the posterior ventricle. The aorta forms an arch and branches toward the head, while the pulmonary artery bifurcates at right angles into its left and right branches. Ventricular situs can be partly determined from this view, the morphological left ventricle usually lying posteriorly with an atrioventricular valve with two papillary muscles. The right ventricle, the right ventricular infundibulum, and its associated great vessel are best examined in the short-axis or transverse view, which is approximately at right angles to the coronal views described above. These views are similar to the par-

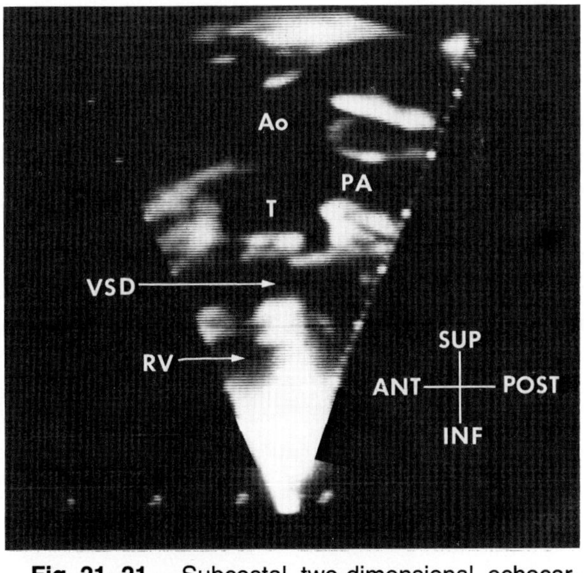

Fig 21–21.—Subcostal two-dimensional echocardiogram of a patient with truncus arteriosus. In this transverse plane, the right ventricle *(RV)* lies anteriorly, and the tricuspid valve has one leaflet attached to the interventricular septum. Overriding the interventricular septum is a large truncus *(T)*, and just below the truncal valves is a ventricular septal defect *(VSD)*. The truncus divides after a short course into the aorta *(Ao)* and pulmonary artery *(PA)*. (Courtesy of Dr. Roberta Williams.)

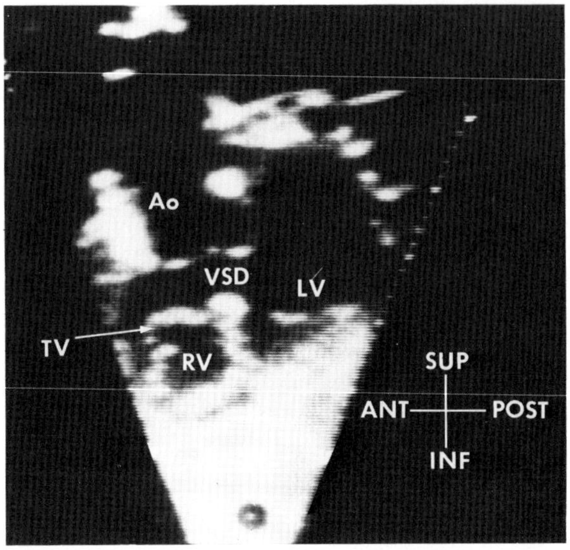

Fig 21–22.—Subcostal two-dimensional echocardiogram of a patient with tetralogy of Fallot. In this transverse view, the aorta *(Ao)* is displaced anteriorly and overrides the interventricular septum, creating a malalignment type of ventricular septal defect *(VSD)*. The tricuspid valve *(TV)* is well seen. The origin of the pulmonary artery is not well seen in this example, but this is also a useful view for assessing the degree of pulmonary stenosis or atresia occurring with tetralogy of Fallot. (Courtesy of Dr. Roberta Williams.) *LV,* left ventricle; *RV,* right ventricle.

asternal short-axis views but give a better view of all right-sided structures. Figure 21–18 is a subcostal two-dimensional echocardiogram showing the left ventricle, right ventricle, and pulmonary artery in such a transverse view. It can be appreciated that ventricular situs is readily determined in this view by identifying the tricuspid and mitral valves and their associated papillary muscles.

A combination of these transverse and longitudinal views can elucidate many of the malformations involving the great vessels. Figure 21–19 is an example of *d-transposition of the great arteries;* in the longitudinal view the pulmonary artery can be identified arising from the posterior and morphological left ventricle. In the transverse view (Fig 21–20) the aorta is seen to be displaced anteriorly and to arise above the right ventricle before giving branch vessels to the head and neck. Similarly, the degree of overriding of a great vessel may be determined. Figure 21–21 shows an example of *truncus arteriosus* in which the truncus can be seen to arise above both right and left ventricles. In *tetralogy of Fallot* the degree of anterior displacement of the aorta in relationship to the interventricular septum can be appreciated (Fig 21–22). Because the right ventricular outflow tract is also well seen in the transverse plane, any de-

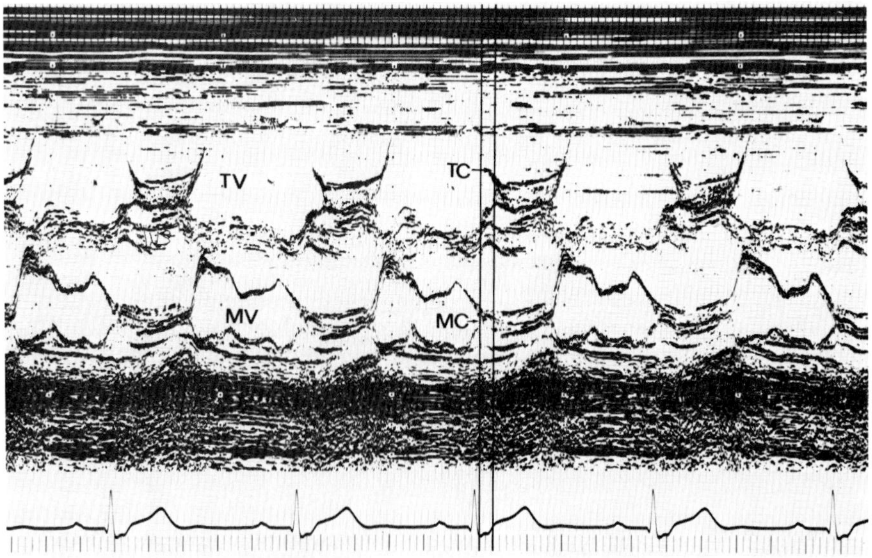

Fig 21–23.—The large sail-like excursion of the tricuspid valve *(TV)* anterior leaflet is seen in this patient with Ebstein's anomaly. The interval between mitral *(MC)* and tricuspid closure *(TC)* is characteristically prolonged in this disorder, as seen in this patient (80 msec). (*MV,* mitral valve). (Courtesy of Dr. Roberta Williams.) (From Parisi A.F. and Tow D.E.: *Noninvasive Approaches to Cardiovascular Diagnosis.* New York, Appleton-Century-Crofts, 1979.)

gree of pulmonary atresia can be determined. This transverse plane is also useful for viewing the interventricular septum, and particularly for identifying ventricular septal defects of the malalignment type such as occur in tetralogy of Fallot.

In transverse plane the morphological left ventricle can be distinguished by the presence of two papillary muscles, neither of which is attached to the interventricular septum (see Fig 21–18). In this way ventricular situs may be determined, which is important for conditions in which ventricular inversion may occur, such as corrected or *L-transposition of the great arteries*. Right ventricular size and the tricuspid valve can be assessed in the transverse plane, and in conjunction with the four-chamber longitudinal view obtained in the coronal plane, an accurate diagnosis of *tricuspid atresia* may be made. Similarly, further assessment of the size of the left ventricle, the mitral valve, and its papillary muscles can be made, which is useful in the assessment of *mitral atresia* and the *hypoplastic left heart syndrome*. By following this systematic approach, other complex malformations such as double outlet right ventricle and double outlet left ventricle can be identified.

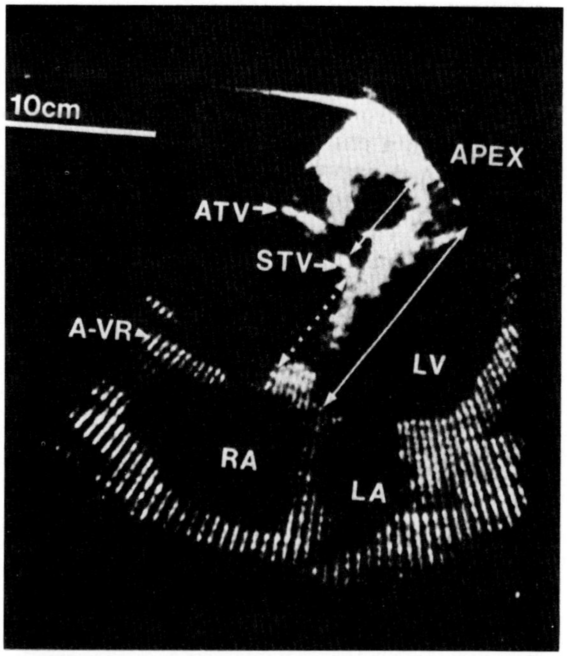

Fig 21–24.—Apical four-chamber view of a patient with Ebstein's anomaly. Note the severe displacement of anterior and septal tricuspid leaflets into the right ventricle, resulting in a large "atrialized" right ventricle. The longer solid arrow indicates the mitral valve-to-apex distance; the shorter solid arrow indicates the tricuspid valve-to-apex distance. The ratio of 2:1 is diagnostic of Ebstein's anomaly. *ATV,* anterior tricuspid valve leaflet; *A-VR,* atrioventricular ring; LA, left atrium; LV, left ventricle; RA, right atrium; STV, septal tricuspid valve leaflet. (From Ports T.A., et al.: Two-dimensional echocardiographic assessment of Ebstein's anomaly. *Circulation* 58:336, 1978.)

OTHER MALFORMATIONS

Ebstein's Anomaly

In Ebstein's anomaly the tricuspid valve is displaced toward the apex of the right ventricle away from the tricuspid valve annulus. The tricuspid and mitral valves can usually be viewed simultaneously in M-mode, with the tricuspid valve displaying a large sail-like excursion. The most consistent finding on M-mode echocardiography is delayed closure of the tricuspid valve.[37] The normal tricuspid valve closes within 30 msec of mitral valve closure, but in this anomaly the delay may be 50 msec or longer (Fig 21–23). With the 2DE apical or subcostal four-chamber view, the displacement of the tricuspid valve into the right ventricle can be seen.[38] Because this view allows simultaneous visualization of the atrioventricular ring and the tricuspid valve, the size of the "atrialized" right ventricle and right atrium can be determined. The severity of tricuspid displacement can also be assessed by comparing the position of the mitral and tricuspid valves relative to the cardiac apex (Fig 21–24).

REFERENCES

1. Goldberg S.J., Allen H.D., Sahn D.J.: *Pediatric and Adolescent Echocardiography*. Chicago, Year Book Medical Publishers, Inc., 1980.
2. Meyer R.A.: *Pediatric Echocardiography*. Philadelphia, Lea & Febiger, 1977.

3. Williams R.G., Tucker C.R.: *Echocardiographic Diagnosis of Congenital Heart Disease*. Boston, Little Brown & Co., 1977.
4. Gramiak R., Shah P.M., Kramer D.H.: Ultrasound cardiography: Contrast studies in anatomy and function. *Radiology* 92:939, 1969.
5. Seward J.B., Tajik A.J., Hagler D.J., et al.: Peripheral venous contrast echocardiography. *Am. J. Cardiol.* 39:202, 1977.
6. Weyman A.E., Wann L.S., Caldwell R.L., et al.: Negative contrast echocardiography: A new method for detecting left-to-right shunts. *Circulation* 59:498, 1979.
7. Radtke W.E., Tajik A.J., Gau G.T., et al.: Atrial septal defect: Echocardiographic observations. Studies in 120 patients. *Ann. Intern. Med.* 84:246, 1976.
8. Hayashida N., Umeda T., Furuta S., et al.: Echocardiographic study on interventricular septal movement in atrial septal defect. *J. Cardiogr.* 6:349, 1976.
9. McCann W.D., Harbold N.B., Giuliani E.R.: The echocardiogram in right ventricular overload. *J.A.M.A.* 221:1243, 1972.
10. Weyman A.E.: Pulmonary valve echo motion in clinical practice. *Am. J. Med.* 62:843, 1977.
11. Bierman F.Z., Williams R.G.: Subxiphoid two-dimensional imaging of the interatrial septum in infants and neonates with congenital heart disease. *Circulation* 60:80, 1979.
12. Fraker T.D., Harris P.J., Behar V.S., et al.: Detection and exclusion of interatrial shunts by two-dimensional echocardiography and peripheral venous injection. *Circulation* 59:379, 1979.
13. Kranik G., Slany J., Moesslacher H.: Contrast M-mode echocardiography in diagnosis of atrial septal defect in acyanotic patients. *Circulation* 59:372, 1979.
14. Paquet M., Gutgesell H.: Echocardiographic features of total anomalous pulmonary venous drainage. *Circulation* 51:599, 1975.
15. Bass J.L., Bessinger F.B., Lawrence C.: Echocardiographic differentiation of partial and complete atrioventricular canal. *Circulation* 57:1144, 1978.
16. Williams R.G., Rudd M.: Echocardiographic features of endocardial cushion defects. *Circulation* 49:418, 1974.
17. Sahn D.J., Vaucher Y., Williams W.E., et al.: Echocardiographic detection of large left-to-right shunts and cardiomyopathies in infants and children. *Am. J. Cardiol.* 38:73, 1976.
18. Sahn D.J., Allen H.D.: Real-time cross-sectional echocardiographic imaging and measurement of the patent ductus arteriosus in infants and children. *Circulation* 58:343, 1978.
19. Stevenson J.G., Kanabon I., Guntheroth W.G.: Noninvasive detection of pulmonary hypertension in patent ductus arteriosus by pulsed Doppler echocardiography. *Circulation* 60:355, 1979.
20. Allen H.D., Sahn D.J., Goldberg S.J.: A new serial contrast technique for assessment of left-to-right shunting patent ductus arteriosus in the neonate. *Am. J. Cardiol.* 41:288, 1978.
21. Lester L.A., Vitullo D., Soot P., et al.: An evaluation of the left atrial/aortic root ratio in children with ventricular septal defect. *Circulation* 60:364, 1979.
22. Seward J.B., Tajik A.J., Hagler D.J., et al.: Visualization of isolated ventricular septal defect with wide-angled two-dimensional sector echocardiography, abstracted. *Circulation* 58(suppl. II):202, 1978.
23. Bierman F.Z. Williams R.G.: Prospective diagnosis of ventricular septal defects in infants by subxiphoid two-dimensional echocardiography, abstracted. *Circulation* 60(suppl. II):112, 1979.
24. Williams R.G., Bierman F.Z., Sanders S.P.: Echocardiographic ventricular septal defect measurement as an indicator of clinical course, abstracted. *Circulation* 64(suppl. IV):166, 1981.
25. Caldwell R.L., Weyman A.E., Hurwitz R.A., et al.: Right ventricular outflow tract assessment by cross-sectional echocardiography in tetralogy of Fallot. *Circulation* 59:395, 1978.
26. Weyman A.E., Feigenbaum H., Hurwitz R.A., et al.: Localization of left ventricular outflow obstruction by cross-sectional echocardiography. *Am. J. Med.* 60:33, 1976.
27. Weyman A.E., Feigenbaum H., Hurwitz R.A., et al.: Cross-sectional echocardiographic assessment of the severity of aortic stenosis in children. *Circulation* 55:773, 1977.
28. Fowles R.E., Martin R.P., Abrams J.M., et al.: Two-dimensional echocardiographic features of bicuspid aortic valve. *Chest* 75:434, 1979.
29. Weyman A.E., Caldwell R.L., Hurwitz R.A., et al.: Cross-sectional echocardiographic detection of aortic obstruction: II. Coarctation of the aorta. *Circulation* 57:498, 1978.
30. Weyman A.E., Dillon J.C., Feigenbaum H., et al.: Echocardiographic patterns of pulmonic valve motion in pulmonic stenosis. *Am. J. Cardiol.* 34:644, 1974.
31. Weyman A.E., Dillon J.C., Feigenbaum H., et al.: Echocardiographic differentiation of infundibular from valvular pulmonary stenosis. *Am. J. Cardiol.* 36:21, 1975.
32. Henry W.L., Maron B.J., Griffin J.M.: Cross-sectional echocardiography in the diagnosis of congenital heart disease: Identification of the relation of the ventricles and great arteries. *Circulation* 56:267, 1977.
33. Henry W.L.: Evaluation of older children and adults with congenital heart disease by M-mode and cross-sectional echocardiography, in Roberts W.L. (ed.): *Congenital Heart Disease in Adults*. Philadelphia, F.A. Davis Co., 1979.
34. Snider R.A., Silverman N.H.: Suprasternal notch echocardiography. A two-dimensional technique for

evaluating congenital heart disease. *Circulation* 63:165, 1981.
35. Lange L.W., Sahn D.J., Allen H.D., et al.: Subxyphoid cross-sectional echocardiography in infants and children with congenital heart disease. *Circulation* 59:513, 1979.
36. Bierman F.Z., Williams R.G.: Prospective diagnosis of d-transposition of the great arteries in neonates by subxyphoid, two-dimensional echocardiography. *Circulation* 60:1496, 1979.
37. Farooki Z.Q., Henry J.G., Green E.W.: Echocardiographic spectrum of Ebstein's anomaly of the tricuspid valve. *Circulation* 53:63, 1976.
38. Ports T.A., Silverman N.H., Schiller N.B.: Two-dimensional echocardiographic assessment of Ebstein's anomaly. *Circulation* 58:336, 1978.

RADIONUCLIDE IMAGING

Charles A. Boucher and Richard R. Liberthson

THE ROLE OF RADIONUCLIDE IMAGING in the evaluation of patients with congenital heart disease is still evolving, and its ultimate status relative to ultrasound and cardiac catheterization in delineating the anatomy and physiology of these patients has not yet been determined. While echocardiography is preferable for some purposes because of superior resolution and the absence of a radiation burden, for other purposes, radionuclide imaging is superior. As with cardiac catheterization, clinical input from the managing physician is essential to the optimal use of this technique.

Among our present uses for radionuclide imaging for patients with congenital heart disease are (1) detection and quantification of left-to-right shunting, (2) assessment of the direction of blood flow through the great veins, cardiac chambers, and great arteries, (3) detection of right-to-left cardiac shunting, (4) delineation of ventricular size and morphology, (5) evaluation of ventricular function both at rest and with exercise, and (6) assessment of myocardial perfusion. This chapter analyzes the technical considerations of radionuclide imaging measurements and reviews their clinical role in the evaluation and management of patients with specific congenital heart lesions.

TECHNICAL CONSIDERATIONS

Left-to-Right Shunts

Radionuclide techniques permit accurate noninvasive detection and quantitation of left-to-right shunting.[1–4] The increased flow of blood through the lungs is monitored externally by recording the first-pass transit of an intravenous bolus of technetium 99m. A region of interest is located over the lung, and a time-activity curve of the passage of the tracer through the pulmonary circulation is generated. In normal subjects there is an uninterrupted monoexponential washout of tracer from peak pulmonary activity on the first pass (Fig 22–1). In patients with a left-to-right shunt, however, this monoexponential washout is interrupted by early reappearance of activity in the pulmonary artery and lungs.

The most widely used method of left-to-right shunt analysis was developed by Treves.[3] A gamma-variate computer fit is applied to the initial and recirculation curves, allowing a mathematical separation of lung activity washing out from that recirculating. The area under the derived time-activity curve representing the entire early recirculation relative to the area under the derived curve representing the entire initial circulation is the shunt fraction (the fraction of the pulmonary blood flow shunted left to right). The pulmonary-to-systemic flow ratio (Qp/Qs) is then derived as a 1(1 − shunt fraction). This quantitative analysis utilizes indicator-dilution principles and therefore requires a bolus injection of tracer into or close to the superior vena cava, usually via an external jugular or central venous catheter. The adequacy of the bolus should be confirmed by determining the width of the time-activity curve of the passage

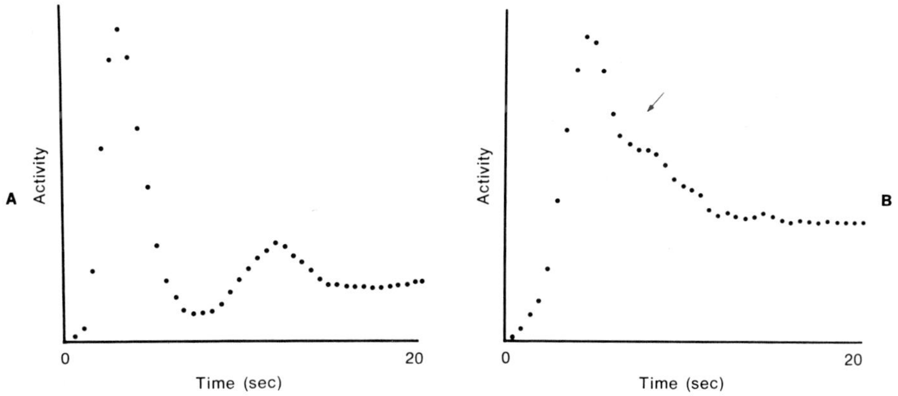

Fig 22–1.—Pulmonary time-activity curves in a normal patient **(A)** and in a patient with a large left-to-right shunt **(B).** Normally, there is a single spike with rapid washout, representing passage of tracer through the lung. The second peak represents recirculation. With a left-to-right shunt, the initial washout is interrupted by early recirculation *(arrow),* representing left-to-right shunt flow. The area between the recirculation curve and a mathematical extrapolation of the initial washout is proportional to shunt size.[38] (Reproduced with permission of the C.V. Mosby Co.)

of the tracer through the superior vena cava. The bolus width should be no more than 2.5 seconds in the superior vena cava to produce reliable data for shunt analysis. This method is not reliable in patients in whom there is bolus dispersion due to low cardiac output, severe heart failure, valvular regurgitation, right-to-left shunting, or extensive bronchial collaterals. In addition, it may not be sensitive enough to detect small left-to-right shunts (Qp/Qs $<$ 1.2). These radionuclide shunt measurements have a high potential for error, and considerable experience is needed for their proper implementation.

A more direct method of assessing left-to-right shunting involves the use of carbon dioxide labeled with oxygen 15, a two-minute half-life, positron-emitting radionuclide.[5, 6] After inhalation, $C^{15}O_2$ is immediately converted by the action of the enzyme, carbonic anhydrase, to $^{15}O_2$-labeled water, which enters as a bolus into the pulmonary veins and left heart. Washout of $^{15}O_2$-labeled water from the lung is monoexponential, similar to

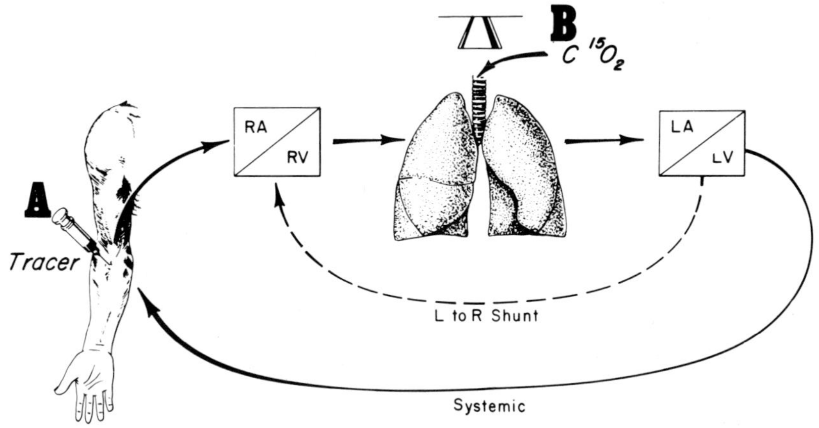

Fig 22–2.—Comparison of the intravenous **(A)** and inhalation **(B)** methods of left-to-right shunt analysis. Because intravenous tracers pass through the right heart before entering the left heart, there may be bolus dispersion, which limits the accuracy of the intravenous approach for shunt detection. Inhalation of $^{15}O_2$-labeled carbon dioxide provides a direct infusion of tracer into the left heart, avoiding such bolus dispersion.

that of the intravenous tracer, and it is interrupted by early recirculation in a left-to-right shunt. The size of the second peak is also proportional to the shunt fraction and may be readily calculated. The differences in these two techniques for the left-to-right shunt measurement are shown in Figure 22–2. These techniques do not require cardiac imaging, and reliable time-activity curves may be derived using a nonimaging probe placed over the lung. We have found the inhalation approach particularly helpful in younger patients, who generally are more cooperative with this method because the tracer can be administered without the need for a "needle."

A recent report has suggested that an atrial shunt may also be evaluated by measuring the severity of the volume overload on the right ventricle (the ratio of right ventricular to left ventricular stroke counts).[7] This technique has the advantage of permitting shunt quantitation from a gated equilibrium study. Patients with large left-to-right shunts usually have ratios above 3. Normal patients have ratios near unity. However, although the elevated ratio is a result of the left-to-right shunt, the ratio does not closely correlate with the pulmonary-to-systemic flow ratio.[3] Furthermore, postoperatively the ratio may remain elevated despite successful closure of the atrial defect, most likely due to technical limitations in the analysis of relative right and left ventricular stroke volumes, such as inclusion of right atrial activity within the right ventricular region of interest (see Chap. 16). The value obtained does not give as accurate information as more direct left-to-right shunt measurements, and therefore its clinical role appears limited.

Direction and Course of Blood Flow

First-pass nuclear imaging can provide information on the direction and course of blood flow through the heart in ways similar to early contrast angiography techniques using venous dye injections. Sequential half-second images usually provide adequate temporal and spatial resolution to identify the course of cardiac blood flow. We presently use a single-plane first-pass injection in the projection which best separates the right from the left ventricle, usually a left anterior oblique view (Fig 22–3), except in patients with cardiac malpositions or ventricular inversion.

One limitation of first-pass studies is the long half-life of the ^{99m}Tc (six hours) relative to the brief duration (15–30 seconds) of the first-pass imaging study itself. Due both to accumulation of background activity and to patient dosimetry using ^{99m}Tc, there is a practical limit of three first-pass studies in one setting. A shorter-lived tracer with comparable imaging properties would be particularly useful. Recently, Treves et al. have reported the successful use of a new tracer, iridium 191, in first-pass evaluations.[8] Its short, 5-second half-life permits multiple injections at a higher dose with minimal background accumulation. Therefore, it

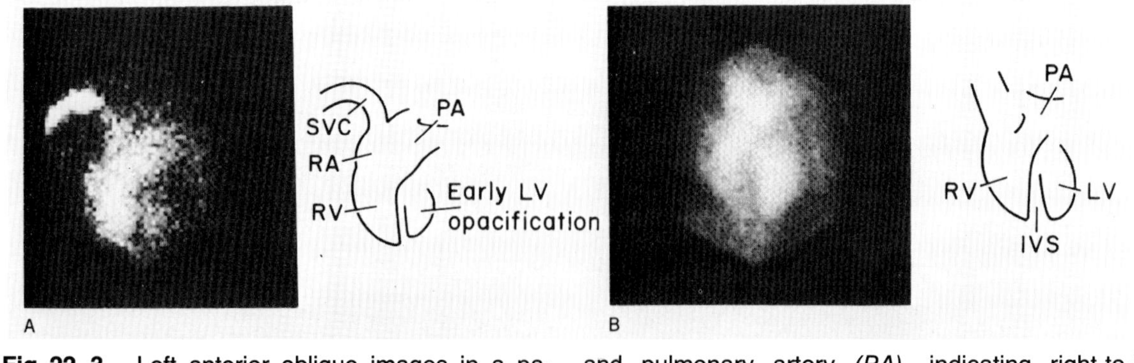

Fig 22–3.—Left anterior oblique images in a patient with a right-to-left shunt at the ventricular level due to Eisenmenger's syndrome. **A,** the first-pass study shows sequential filling of the superior vena cava *(SVC),* right atrium *(RA)* and right ventricle *(RV).* There is simultaneous opacification of the left ventricle *(LV)* and pulmonary artery *(PA),* indicating right-to-left shunting at the ventricular level. **B,** the equilibrium views demonstrate the size and orientation of the two ventricles. The interventricular septum *(IVS)* is well seen, thus ruling out a common or single ventricle.[13] (Reproduced with permission of Little, Brown & Co.)

has considerable potential value for patients with complex lesions as well as for younger patients, in whom minimization of the radiation burden is particularly important.

Right-to-Left Shunts

In delineating the presence and location of right-to-left (pulmonary-to-systemic) shunting, a tracer attached to 10μ or larger particles (such as ^{99m}Tc-labeled macroaggregated albumin) is injected intravenously.[1–3] Normally, 97% or more of the injected dose is trapped in the lung and less than 3% reaches the systemic circulation.[3] Right-to-left shunting results in systemic uptake of the tracer. Imaging of an organ which has a high systemic blood flow, such as the brain or kidney, demonstrates abnormal activity (Fig 22–4). This method is sensitive for even small right-to-left shunts, and the risk of ischemic damage to a systemic organ is small because of the relatively small number of particles used. Because this is the same approach as is used for conventional lung scanning, a right-to-left shunt may be fortuitously detected by observing myocardial activity on a lung scan.[9] In addition, the shunt flow may be quantified as the ratio of pulmonary counts to whole body counts, pulmonary-to-systemic flow ratio.

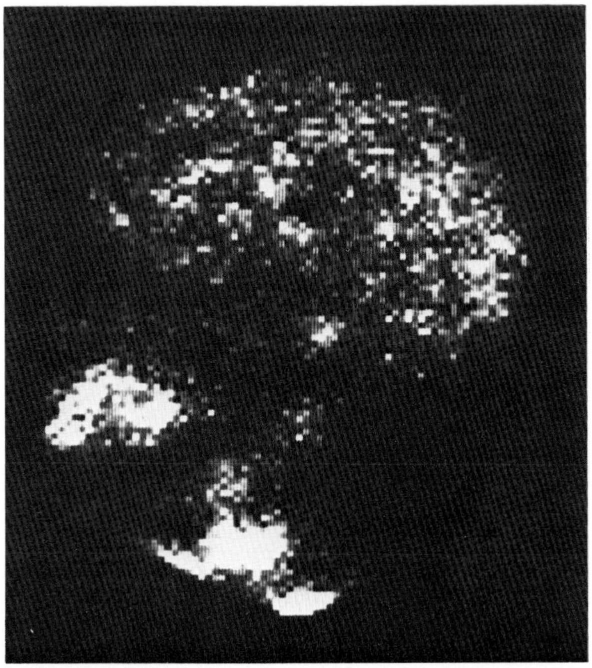

Fig 22–4.—Lateral view static image of the head after injection of ^{99m}Tc-labeled macroaggregated albumin in a patient with Eisenmenger's syndrome. Prominent systemic uptake in the head confirms a right-to-left intracardiac shunt. The bright regions below are the apices of the lung fields.

An alternative to static imaging of the systemic organs is direct visualization of the flow of tracer within the circulation during first-pass imaging. Normally, the left heart opacifies shortly after appearances of activity in the right heart and lungs. With right-to-left shunting, there is early appearance of activity in the left heart prior to transit of the tracer through the lungs. Direct visualization also indicates the level of the shunt—whether atrial, ventricular, or in the great artery.

It is important to be aware of potential complications of an intravenous injection in a patient with a right-to-left shunt, especially systemic embolization of air or particles injected into the venous circulation. Therefore, meticulous care is essential when using indwelling catheters or with intravenous injections.

Chamber Size and Anatomy

Radionuclide blood pool imaging is ideally suited to measuring relative chamber size and position and to assessing the presence of ventricular septation and the status of the great arteries and veins. In addition, as with angiographic studies, radionuclide studies are useful in assessing specific ventricular anatomy and differentiating between the anatomical right and left ventricle.

Thallium 201 imaging has also been used to assess right ventricular hypertrophy. Normally, there is minimal uptake of ^{201}Tl by the right heart.[10] In patients with right ventricular hypertrophy, however, there is prominent right ventricular uptake.[11]

Ventricular Function

Because ventricular function is an important determinant of clinical course and prognosis in patients with congenital heart disease, radionuclide blood pool imaging has particular value in measuring both right and left ventricular global and regional function. Details of the general use of radionuclides to assess ventricular function are provided in Chapter 4.

Congenital Abnormalities of Coronary Circulation

Radionuclide techniques, particularly myocardial perfusion imaging using ^{201}Tl, have been valuable in assessing patients with suspected congenital coronary artery abnormalities. Thallium 201, usually injected at peak exercise stress, is distributed in the myocardium in relation to coronary flow. Subsequent serial imaging is used to demonstrate myocardial viability in regions with reduced flow. In patients in whom blood pool imaging demonstrates a severe regional wall motion abnormality, the thallium uptake in that wall suggests the extent to which the asynergy is due to infarction or to potentially reversible ischemia.

CLINICAL APPLICATIONS

The clinical use of radionuclide techniques in the evaluation of patients with congenital heart disease requires detailed knowledge of the cardiac anatomy and physiology of the individual entities.[12, 13] In this section, we review the major disorders in which we have found nuclear imaging to be helpful clinically. The role of radionuclide studies in postoperative patients will also be considered.[14, 15]

Left-to-Right Shunt Assessment

Regardless of the level of the shunt, whether atrial, ventricular, or in the great artery (such as a patent ductus arteriosus), the presence and magnitude of left-to-right shunting can be readily determined by intravenous or inhalation imaging techniques.[1–6] Differentiation of the specific level and type of shunt can usually be made by clinical means and rarely requires imaging. However, the different left-to-right shunts have a different effect on the individual cardiac chambers and great arteries which receive the increased volume of shunted blood, and this is readily apparent on the nuclear studies. An uncomplicated atrial shunt causes right atrial, right ventricular, and pulmonary artery enlargement with a normal-sized left heart and aorta. An uncomplicated ventricular septal defect causes biventricular, left atrial, and pulmonary arterial enlargement with a normal-sized right atrium and aorta. In contrast, an uncomplicated patent ductus arteriosus causes left atrial, left ventricular, aortic, and pulmonary arterial enlargement with a normal-sized right heart.

Atrial Septal Defect

Cardiac catheterization is still the optimal method of preoperative evaluation in patients with an atrial septal defect. Therefore, radionuclide imaging is usually not necessary, particularly in the uncomplicated young patient. However, some investigators favor a nuclear and ultrasound assessment and do not catheterize such patients prior to surgery. Radionuclide studies are particularly useful in differentiating atrial septal defect from lesions which closely mimic it on clinical examination. These include the straight back syndrome, pectus excavatum, kyphoscoliosis, mild pulmonic stenosis, and, occasionally, mitral valve stenosis.[16]

Another use of the scans is to evaluate ventricular function. In the older patient with complicated atrial septal defect, right ventricular dysfunction may develop and affect the postoperative course. Therefore we often use scan as well as catheterization data in these patients. As illustrated in Figure 22–5, when preoperative right ventricular contraction is normal, the postoperative clinical course is usually excellent and right ventricular size and contraction generally return to normal. In contrast, when preoperative right ventricular contraction is diminished significantly, there is some postoperative improvement, but residual symptoms and a right ventricular contraction abnormality often persist.[17] Patients with atrial septal defect have also been reported to have depression of left ventricular function on rest and exercise, although the clinical significance of these observations is unclear.[14, 15, 17–19] These changes have been attributed to left ventricular distortion secondary to chronic right ventricular overload and they appear to be reversible after atrial septal defect closure.

Ventricular Septal Defect

Patients with small, uncomplicated, and asymptomatic ventricular septal defects do not require

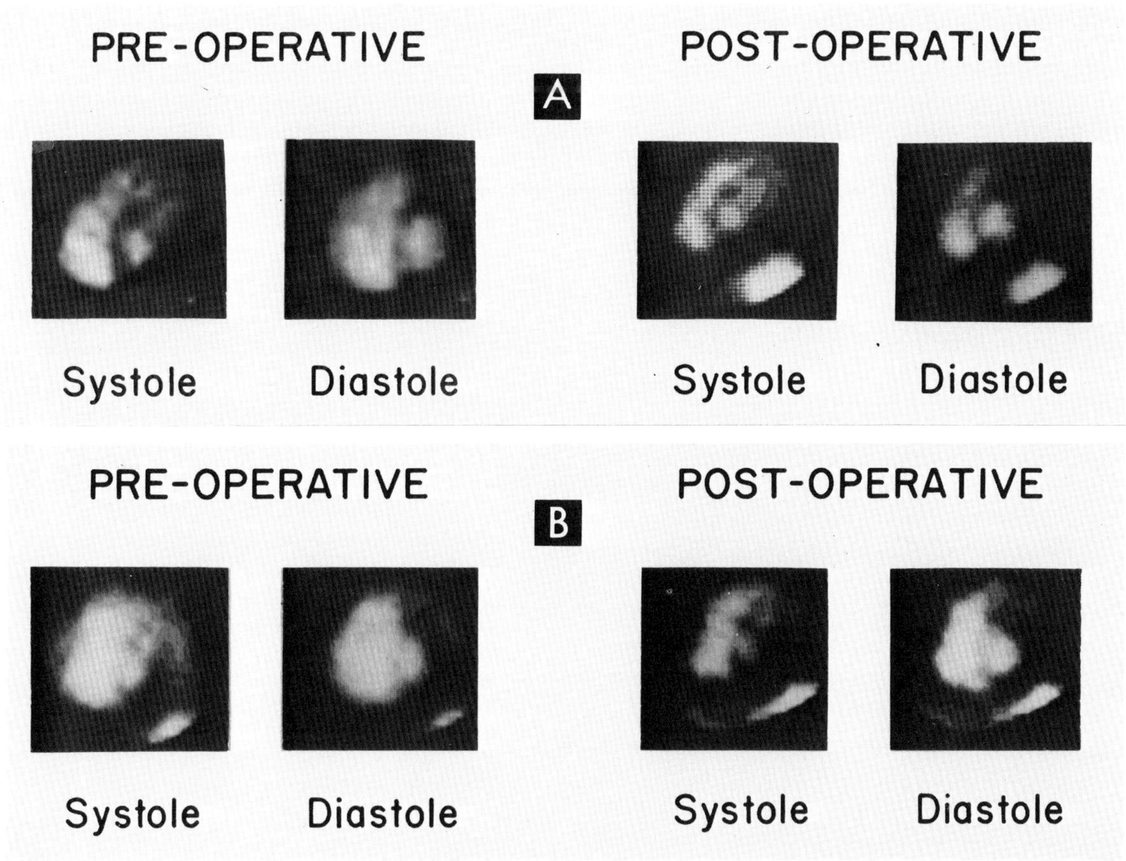

Fig 22–5.—Left anterior oblique images before and after atrial septal defect closure. **A,** scans of a 25-year-old asymptomatic patient. Preoperatively, the right ventricle is dilated but has normal wall motion. Postoperatively, there is decreased right ventricular size and normal wall motion. **B,** scans of a 58-year-old patient with moderate pulmonary hypertension and heart failure. Preoperatively, the right ventricle is markedly dilated and severely hypokinetic. Postoperatively, there is a decrease in right ventricular size but persistent right ventricular hypokinesis.[17] (Reproduced with permission of the *American Journal of Cardiology*.)

radionuclide angiography or catheterization. Those with large shunts require catheterization, and therefore nuclear imaging adds little and is not needed. However, if the ventricular septal defect is of uncertain size, a radionuclide assessment of shunt size may help identify patients with large left-to-right shunts who should then have catheterization. Echocardiography is a useful adjunct to the nuclear study in more precisely delineating the anatomy of the defect and the presence of associated valvular lesions. In selected patients, serial shunt flow measurements may help in their clinical management, since some defects spontaneously decrease in size over time. In others, progressive pulmonary hypertension or secondary right ventricular infundibular stenosis may also decrease left-to-right shunt flow.[13] For postoperative patients who are suspected of having residual left-to-right shunting, radionuclide imaging may also be helpful.

The gated blood pool scan is useful in defining ventricular anatomy prior to catheterization in selected patients with complicated ventricular septal defects including patients who have had prior pulmonary artery banding or who have associated lesions such as pulmonary stenosis or atresia. In such patients, radionuclide imaging can be an adjunct to the contrast angiographic studies. The presence of two distinct ventricular chambers and an interventricular septum distinguishes patients with a large ventricular septal defect from those with a single or common ventricle.

Older patients with long-standing ventricular septal defect may develop both right and left ventricular contraction abnormalities, which can be assessed by radionuclide imaging and which may have clinical consequences postoperatively. Those with abnormal right or left ventricular contraction often have a less satisfactory postoperative course and do not regain normal ventricular function postoperatively, although their condition may improve.

Patent Ductus Arteriosus

Children and adults with uncomplicated patent ductus arteriosus are usually readily diagnosed clinically. Because they usually undergo preoperative catheterization, they rarely require nuclear imaging. However, in the neonate with lung disease, assessment of the presence and size of the left-to-right shunt may be useful in determining the relative component of pulmonary versus cardiac right-to-left shunting.[2, 3] In older symptomatic adults with a long-standing large patent ductus arteriosus, preoperative left ventricular contraction abnormalities can be identified by radionuclide imaging and often predict a less than complete postoperative improvement, in contrast to those with normal preoperative left ventricular function.

Eisenmenger's Physiology

Eisenmenger's physiology (right-to-left shunting through a large cardiac or great vessel defect as a result of a severe elevation in pulmonary vascular resistance) may be a complication of any large left-to-right shunt.[20, 21] In these patients, the level of the shunt may no longer be evident clinically because of the altered hemodynamics. Because cardiac catheterization has a well-recognized high risk in these patients, nuclear imaging is particularly appropriate in their evaluation. The first-pass and gated equilibrium study can delineate the level of these shunt defects (see Fig 22–3). The clinical importance of this differentiation is that the different lesions may have a different natural course; patent ductus arteriosus is often associated with greater longevity than Eisenmenger's syndrome, due to the placement of intracardiac shunts.[13] In addition, although patients with Eisenmenger's syndrome are no longer surgically approachable, they may be difficult to distinguish from patients with other forms of surgically correctable cyanotic congenital heart disease, and in this regard the scan may also be helpful.[22]

Differentiation between congenital heart disease and pulmonary disorders such as multiple pulmonary emboli, primary pulmonary hypertension, and severe cor pulmonale can be difficult clinically and is helped by nuclear imaging. A right-to-left shunt study is particularly useful in these patients to rule out a primary cardiac defect. Patients with systemic embolization in whom a "paradoxical embolus" which has crossed from the right to the left heart is suspected may also be studied with this technique. It is important to recognize, however, that patients with advanced pulmonary hypertension and right heart failure may develop late patency of their foramen ovale and right-to-left shunting at this level that are not due to intrinsic congenital heart disease.

Pulmonic Stenosis, Aortic Stenosis, and Coarctation of the Aorta

Most patients with pulmonic stenosis do not warrant nuclear imaging study. In patients with moderate pulmonic stenosis, the demonstration of impairment of right ventricular function on exercise might help in determining the timing of surgery, but this is not yet established. Occasional patients with severe postoperative pulmonary regurgitation secondary to a large outflow tract patch develop late right ventricular dysfunction.[14] Assessment of right ventricular function on rest and exercise in these patients may be useful but has not been systematically studied. Recent studies have also suggested that thallium imaging may be used to follow the regression of right ventricular hypertrophy after correction of pulmonic stenosis. We have not used thallium imaging in this context because such information is usually evident clinically without a radiation burden.

Radionuclide studies are seldom needed in patients with aortic stenosis. The resolution is inadequate to define the level or severity of the stenosis, and the radionuclide assessment of left ventricular function does not correlate with the severity of the obstruction, timing of surgery, or prognosis.[23, 24] In a rare patient, the scan may be useful in identifying hypertrophic cardiomyopathy associated with either valvular or discrete subvalvular stenosis.[25, 26] The scan may also be useful in evaluating a patient with postoperative or postendocarditic aortic regurgitation (see Chap. 16) or potential ischemic damage to the myocardium during surgery.

In coarctation of the aorta, the present level of resolution of radionuclide angiography does not permit this study to be substituted for a contrast angiographic study of the arch, of the coarctation anatomy, or of the collateral circulation.[27] Therefore, it does not add to the requisite preoperative angiographic assessment. In the rare patient with atypical clinical findings for a congenital coarctation, precatheterization gated imaging of the aorta may distinguish aortic obstruction secondary to aortitis (Takayasus' obstruction), dissection, or mediastinal tumor that are not necessarily localized from congenital coarctation, which is usually localized to the juxtaductal region.

Tetralogy of Fallot

Nuclear studies are rarely indicated in typical uncomplicated tetralogy of Fallot, since preoperative cardiac catheterization and angiography are essential. In older patients with unusual findings, however, blood pool imaging may be useful as a screening method along with ultrasound study. Differentiation between tetralogy of Fallot and single ventricle with pulmonic stenosis can be difficult clinically yet is readily achieved by the demonstration of two ventricles and an interventricular septum on the scans. Furthermore, a radionuclide study provides an assessment of right ventricular size and function, especially in older patients and in patients with associated pulmonary atresia, who are more likely to develop right ventricular contraction abnormalities (Fig 22–6).

Nuclear imaging is particularly useful for evaluating patients after surgery for tetralogy of Fallot.[14, 15, 28, 29] Residual left-to-right shunting can be readily detected and quantified. Right and left ventricular rest and exercise function may be readily assessed. Postoperative right ventricular aneurysms and severe dysfunction secondary to iatrogenic damage to an anomalous left anterior descending or left coronary artery crossing the resected right ventricular outflow tract, an aneurysmal pulmonary artery outflow tract patch, severe pulmonary regurgitation, or a large residual ventricular septal defect all may be identified by gated blood pool or thallium imaging or both, and these studies may help in evaluating the postoperative clinical course.[15, 29]

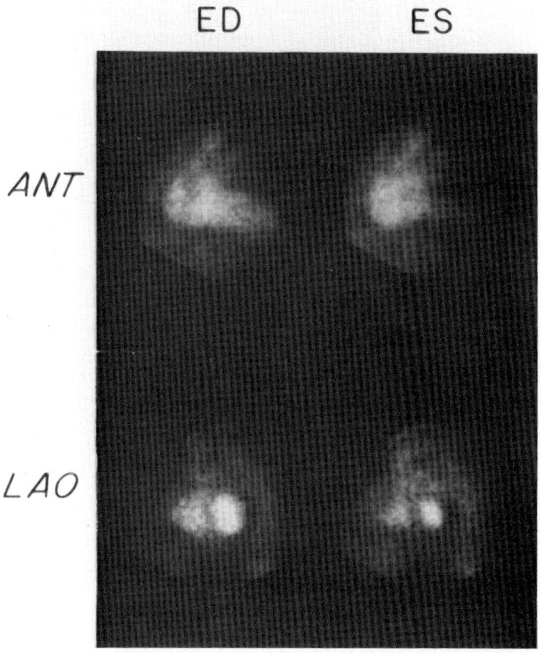

Fig 22–6.—Anterior *(ANT)* and left anterior oblique *(LAO)* equilibrium of a patient with tetralogy of Fallot. Two ventricles and an interventricular septum are well seen, and both ventricles contract normally. *ED,* end-diastole; *ES,* end-systole.

Ebstein's Anomaly

In Ebstein's anomaly, there is variable displacement downward of the attachments of the tricuspid valve (particularly the septal and inferior leaflets) away from the tricuspid annulus, with variable compromise in the resulting size and function of the remaining right ventricle.[13] Radionuclide angiography is useful in demonstrating the size and function of the actual right ventricle in these patients as well as the presence of associated right-to-left shunting through the interatrial communication (Fig 22-7). These findings are im-

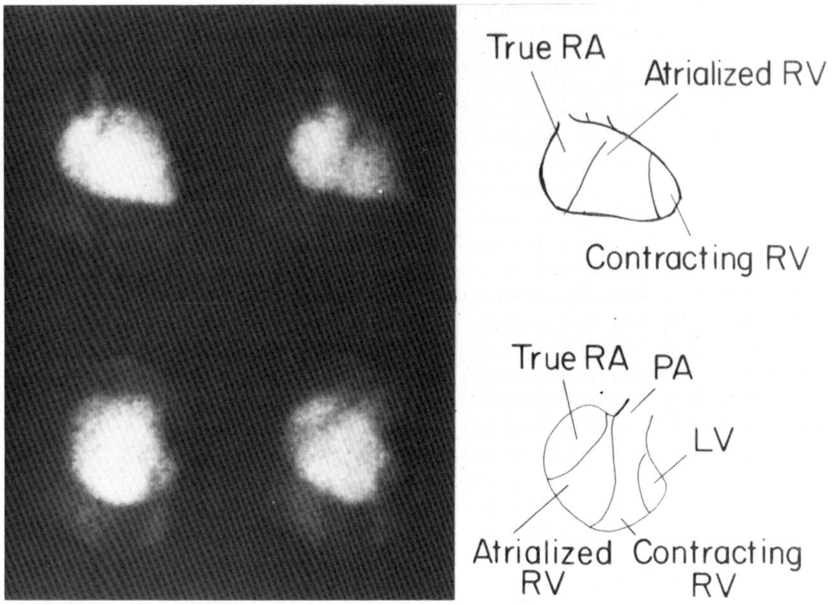

Fig 22–7.—Anterior *(top)* and left anterior oblique *(bottom)* equilibrium blood pool images in a patient with Ebstein's anomaly. A large right atrium *(RA)* and atrialized right ventricle *(RV)* are seen. The contracting right ventricle is small.

portant with regards to operability, because optimal surgical results require an adequately sized and functioning right ventricle. In some but not all patients, the gated blood pool scan can thus be a useful precatheterization screening device along with ultrasound in selecting patients for cardiac catheterization. Because catheterization does have a significant risk, it should not be undertaken without careful noninvasive assessment.

Tricuspid Atresia

Patients with tricuspid atresia are readily identified by first-pass imaging because blood enters the right atrium and shunts right to left to fill the left atrium and left ventricle before entering the great arteries. Right ventricular filling from the right atrium is conspicuously absent (Fig 22–8). Blood pool scan assessment of size and function of

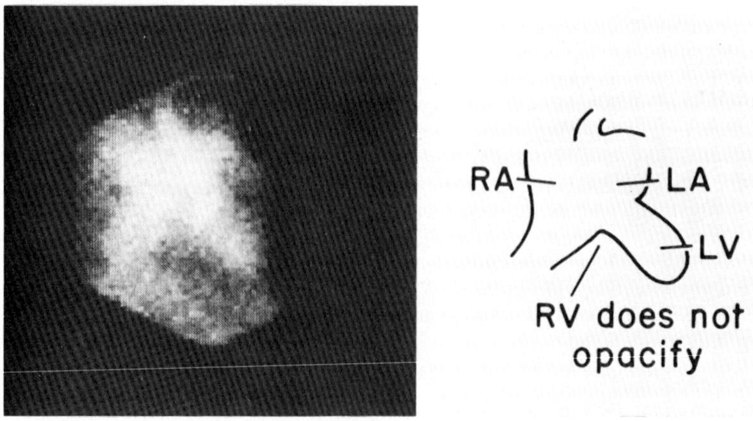

Fig 22–8.—Anterior view gated blood pool scan in patient with tricuspid atresia. The right atrium *(RA)*, left atrium *(LA)*, and left ventricle *(LV)* are seen, but the right ventricle *(RV)* is unopacified.[13] (Reproduced with permission of Little, Brown & Co.)

the left ventricle and, when present, the right ventricle (via a ventricular septal defect) is possible, and in selected, but not all, patients it may be a useful adjunct to ultrasound imaging and contrast angiography prior to surgical intervention.

Congenitally Corrected (L-Type) Transposition (Ventricular Inversion)

First-pass flow and gated equilibrium imaging can be useful in the noninvasive delineation of a congenitally corrected transposition. In the young asymptomatic patient, it adds only minimally to the ultrasound assessment. Both noninvasive techniques can identify the ventricular inversion as well as the presence of two adequately sized ventricles, thus differentiating these patients from patients with a single ventricle and an inverted small outlet chamber, who have a similar clinical presentation (Fig 22–9).[13] In the older symptomatic patient and in those with associated lesions, these studies are superior to ultrasound and even to contrast angiography in assessing rest and exercise ventricular function, which is of prime importance in these patients because the anatomical right ventricle supplies the aorta.

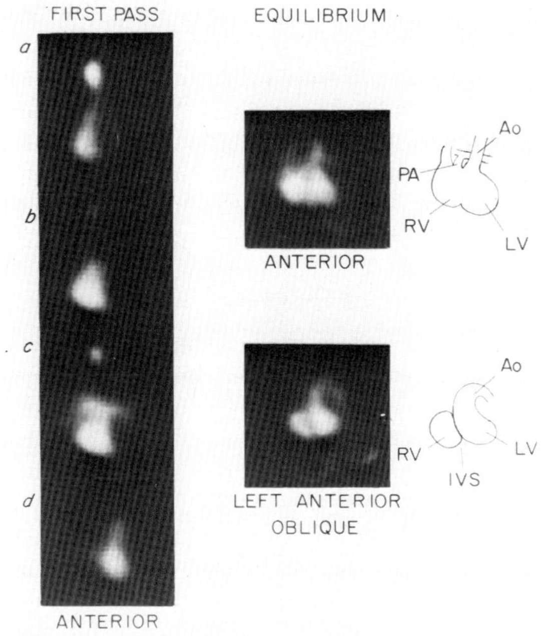

Fig 22–9.—First-pass *(left)* and equilibrium *(right)* radionuclide angiograms in a 51-year-old woman with ventricular inversion. The venous return enters a morphological left ventricle *(RV)* *(a, b)* and empties into a right-sided pulmonary artery *(PA)* without an infundibulum *(c)*. The system ventricle *(LV)* then empties into a left-sided anterior aorta *(AO)*, which is side-by-side with the pulmonary artery *(d)*.

Transposition of the Great Arteries

Transpositions are among the more difficult congenital abnormalities to evaluate because anatomy and blood flow are abnormal and there are usually multiple associated cardiac abnormalities. The great arteries arise abnormally—the aorta from the right ventricle and the pulmonary artery from the left ventricle.[30, 31] In addition, the transposed great arteries differ from their normal counterparts in that the aorta is anterior and to the right of the pulmonary artery.

The clinical value of radionuclide imaging in the evaluation of the patient with transposition of the great arteries is limited by the fact that all patients require detailed preoperative cardiac catheterization and angiography. However, in selected patients with transposition of the great arteries, particularly in those who have survived by virtue of having earlier palliative procedures or fortuitous associated defects or who have developed pulmonary vascular disease, both first-pass flow studies and equilibrium imaging may be useful in the preliminary screening evaluation. The course of blood flow from the great veins to the great arteries, the presence of right-to-left or left-to-right shunting, and the position of the cardiac chambers and interventricular septum can be readily determined. In addition, these studies are well suited to the evaluation of the efficacy and function of the interatrial baffling in the postoperative patient. The flow studies show whether blood flow has been appropriately corrected in the "physiologic" sense. Patients with clinical evidence of systemic venous obstruction secondary to baffle obstruction caused by inadequate repair may be identified (Fig 22–10).[14, 15]

There have been several recent reports of the use of radionuclide imaging for measuring ventricular function on rest and exercise in patients with transposition of great arteries following interatrial

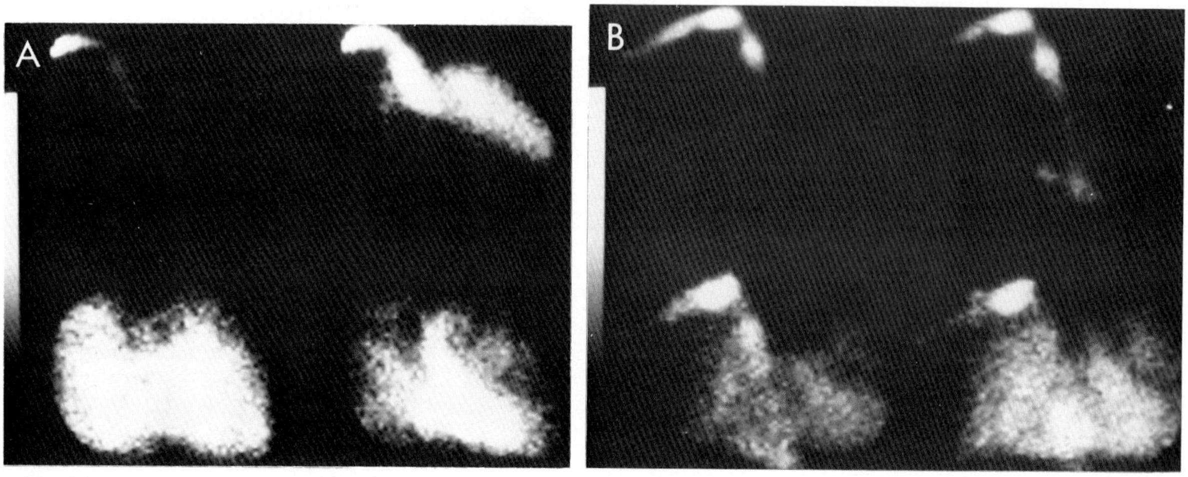

Fig 22–10.—Sequential first-pass anterior view images in two patients following a Mustard procedure for transposition of the great arteries. **A,** a good postoperative result demonstrating normal flow of the tracer. **B,** a patient with near-total superior vena caval obstruction. Even in the last frame there is considerable activity remaining above the obstruction.

baffling.[14, 15] These methods have obvious importance because the anatomical right ventricle must bear the lifetime burden of the systemic circulation. Inadequacy of ventricular function may contribute to the frequent problem of late postoperative arrhythmias in these patients.

Malpositions

Radionuclide techniques are often useful for the noninvasive assessment of congenital heart lesions associated with body situs abnormalities in which venous drainage, cardiac chamber situs, and great artery connections may be highly variable. In malpositions, the cardiac chambers often lose their normal right-left and anteroposterior orientation, and careful selection of the optimal plane for imaging is important. Study of patients with right-sided hearts (dextrocardia) requires detailed knowledge of expected variations.[13] There are three forms of dextrocardia: mirror-image dextrocardia, isolated dextrocardia (dextroversion), and mixed dextrocardia.[13] Patients with mirror-image dextrocardia (situs inversus and right-sided heart) should have imaging in the right anterior oblique projection to optimally view the course of blood flow, to separate the right and left ventricles, and to visualize the interventricular septum. In contrast, in patients with isolated dextrocardia or mixed dextrocardia (normal situs and right-sided heart), optimal imaging for blood flow and chamber morphology should be made in the anteroposterior view, since the chambers lie side by side. First-pass flow studies readily differentiate these entities, and this information has clinical importance because each form of dextrocardia has different associated intracardiac lesions and therefore different prognostic and management implications (Figs 22–11 and 22–12).

Abnormalities of the Coronary Circulation

Clinically important abnormalities of the coronary circulation include anomalous origin of the left coronary artery from the pulmonary artery, aberrant origin of the left coronary artery from the anterior sinus of Valsalva of the aorta, and coronary arteriovenous fistula.[32–34]

Patients with anomalous origin of the left coronary artery from the pulmonary artery may develop ischemia and infarction of the anterolateral wall of the left ventricle. Although most of these patients die during infancy, a small number survive by evolving collateral circulation from the normally arising right coronary artery to the territory normally perfused by the left coronary artery. In these patients, the myocardium perfused by this artery may be normal, but more often it is ischemic or infarcted, depending on the adequacy of the collateral myocardial blood flow. Serial ^{201}Tl

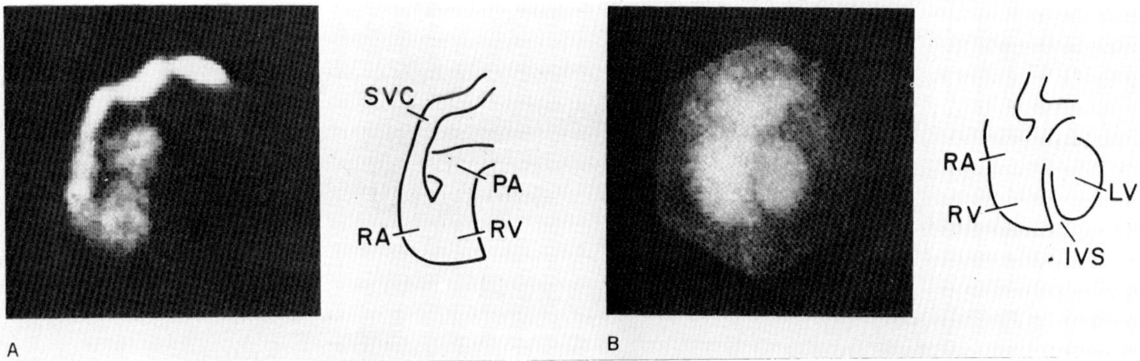

Fig 22–11.—Radionuclide study in a 29-year-old patient with dextroversion. **A,** the first-pass study demonstrates sequential flow from the right-sided superior vena cava *(SVC)* to the right atrium *(RA),* right ventricle *(RV),* and then pulmonary artery *(PA).* **B,** the gated equilibrium study is taken in the anterior view. The RV and LV are side-by-side with the "on end" interventricular septum *(IVS)* in this projection, which is typical for dextroversion.[13] (Reproduced with permission of Little, Brown & Co.)

imaging can be useful in assessing myocardial perfusion in this abnormality and in characterizing the state of myocardium (Fig 22–13).[35–37] Blood pool imaging permits visualization of the extent of the anterolateral wall motion abnormality. Some patients develop anterolateral aneurysms and mitral regurgitation. In some patients, left ventricular dilation and dysfunction are due to large collateral vessels between the right coronary artery and the anomalous left coronary artery, which cause a coronary steal of blood shunted from the right coronary artery to the pulmonary artery. Left ventricular function in these patients may be markedly abnormal and is readily seen by radionuclide angiography. Although the actual left-to-right shunting is often relatively small, it may be detected by a left-to-right shunt nuclear study. Hot spot (pyrophosphate) imaging may be useful in documenting the acute myocardial infarction that may occur in these patients. Postoperative radionuclide studies can be helpful in assessing the extent of improvement in perfusion and contraction.[35]

Patients with aberrant origin of the left coronary artery from the anterior sinus of Valsalva of the aorta may develop left ventricular ischemia, ventricular arrhythmias, and sudden death secondary to acute hypoperfusion of the left ventricle. This has been attributed to proximal kinking of the aberrantly arising left coronary artery. Exercise ^{201}Tl imaging can identify left ventricular

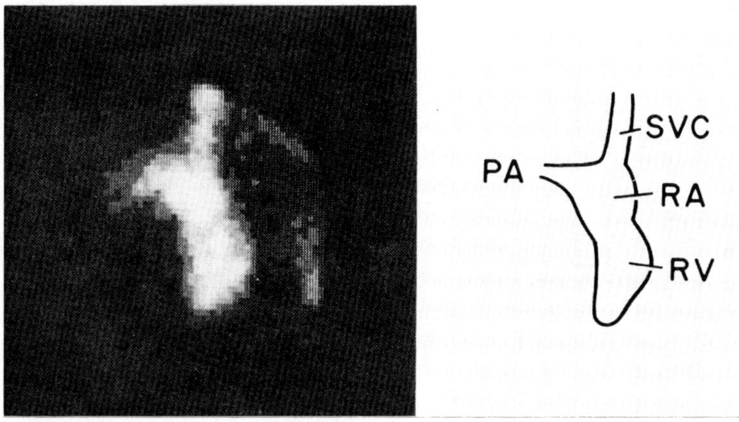

Fig 22–12.—First-pass study in a 42-year-old patient with mirror-image dextrocardia. There is a left-sided superior vena cava *(SVC),* "right atrium" *(RA),* and "right ventricle" *(RV)* which lead to the pulmonary artery *(PA).*[13] (Reproduced with permission of Little, Brown & Co.)

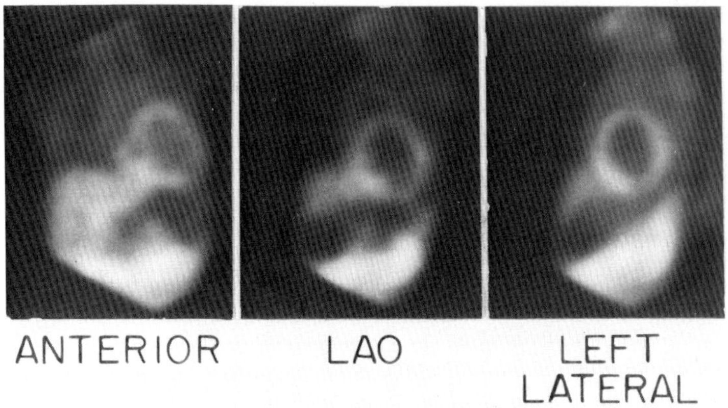

Fig 22–13.—Thallium images in a 14-month-old infant with severe heart failure due to an anomalous origin of the left coronary artery from the pulmonary artery. The heart is markedly dilated and occupies over half of the thorax. The apex is thinned.

perfusion abnormalities in these patients (Fig 22–14), which may be instrumental in determining whether coronary bypass grafting to the left anterior descending and left circumflex coronary arteries is appropriate. When this diagnosis is suspected, stress thallium imaging may be useful as a screening test.

In selected patients with congenital coronary arteriovenous fistula, radionuclide studies may also add valuable information to the clinical assessment. Fistulous connections most often go between the right coronary or circumflex artery and the right atrium, coronary sinus, or right ventricle, and less often to the pulmonary artery or the left heart. Shunt size in these patients is usually small and therefore a radionuclide left-to-right shunt is often normal, although it is still appropriate. This entity rarely causes symptoms or complications in young patients; however, after many years of even small shunting, ventricular function may deteriorate.[34] Thus in older patients with coronary arteriovenous fistula, rest and exercise radionuclide angiographic assessment of ventricular size and function can be helpful. In these patients, when function is impaired, the decision to perform surgical ligation of the fistula may be strengthened. In addition, some patients with coronary arteriovenous fistula develop angina due to a coronary artery steal phenomenon through the fistula, which diverts myocardial perfusion from the normal distal coronary artery.[34] Ischemia can be detected by thallium imaging, which may also be used to support the decision for surgical intervention and to evaluate the patients postoperatively.

In summary, the radionuclide approaches are clearly useful in the physiologic assessment of patients with congenital heart disease. We have reviewed some of the potential clinical roles of these studies. However, these studies are not necessary

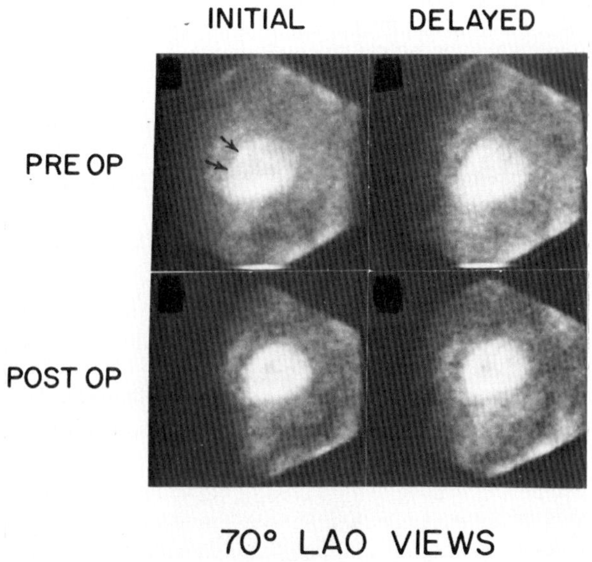

Fig 22–14.—Preoperative and postoperative serial exercise thallium 201 images in a patient with an aberrant origin of the left anterior descending coronary artery from the right coronary artery. Preoperatively, there is a transient defect *(arrows).* After coronary bypass surgery, the images are normal.

or indicated in all patients with these entities, because similar and more complete data are often obtained from other diagnostic tests, particularly cardiac catheterization, which may be necessary for other reasons. Therefore, presence of a lesion is not in itself an indication for imaging, and the decision to perform these tests should be carefully designed to answer specific questions. Optimal clinical use and technical performance of radionuclide imaging require close involvement of the clinician managing these patients. Finally, because the clinical utility of radionuclide imaging relative to both ultrasound and cardiac catheterization is continually evolving, it should not be isolated from these other diagnostic modalities for its optimal application.

REFERENCES

1. Greenfield L.D., Bennett L.R.: Detection of intracardiac shunts with radionuclide imaging. *Semin. Nucl. Med.* 3:139–152, 1973.
2. Parker J.A., Treves S.: Radionuclide detection, localization and quantitation of intracardiac shunts and shunts between the great arteries. *Prog. Cardiovasc. Dis.* 20:121–150, 1977.
3. Treves S.: Detection and quantitation of cardiovascular shunts with commonly available radionuclides. *Semin. Nucl. Med.*10:16–26, 1980.
4. McIlveen B.M., Murray I.P.C., Giles R.W., et al.: Clinical application of radionuclide quantitation of left-to-right cardiac shunts in children. *Am. J. Cardiol.* 47:1273–1278, 1981.
5. Boucher C.A., Ahluwalia B., Block P.C., et al.: Inhalation imaging with oxygen-15 labeled carbon dioxide for detection and quantitation of left-to-right shunts. *Circulation* 56:632–640, 1977.
6. Watson D.D.: Shunt detection with the short-lived radioactive gases. *Semin. Nucl. Med.* 10:27–38, 1980.
7. Bough E.W., Gandsman E.J., Benham I.S., et al.: Detection and quantitation of atrial shunts by gated radionuclide angiography, abstracted. *Am. J. Cardiol.* 45:409, 1980.
8. Treves S., Cheng C., Samuel A., et al.: Iridium-191 angiocardiography for the detection and quantitation of left-to-right shunting. *J. Nucl. Med.* 21:1151–1157, 1980.
9. Weissmann H.S., Steingart R.M., Kiely T.M., et al.: Myocardial visualization on a perfusion lung scan. *J. Nucl. Med.* 21:745–746, 1980.
10. Cook D.J., Bailey I., Strauss H.W., et al.: Thallium-201 for myocardial imaging: Appearance of the normal heart. *J. Nucl. Med.* 17:583–589, 1976.
11. Ohsuzu F., Handa S., Kondo M., et al.: Thallium-201 myocardial imaging to evaluate right ventricular overloading. *Circulation* 61:620–625, 1980.
12. Rudolph A.M.: *Congenital Diseases of the Heart.* Chicago, Year Book Medical Publishers, 1974.
13. Liberthson R.R.: Congenital heart disease in the child, adolescent and adult patient. in Johnson R.A., Haber E., Austen W.G. (eds.): *The Practice of Cardiology.* Boston, Little, Brown & Co., 1980, pp. 755–893.
14. Morriss J.H., McNamara D.G.: Residuae, sequelae, and complications of surgery for congenital heart disease. *Prog. Cardiovasc. Dis.* 18:1–25, 1975.
15. Graham T.P. Jr.: Myocardial performance after anatomic or physiologic corrective surgery. *Prog. Cardiovasc. Dis.* 18:439–449, 1975.
16. Burchell H.B.: Possibly unrecognized forms of heart disease. *Circulation* 28:1153–1164, 1963.
17. Liberthson R.R., Boucher C.A., Strauss H.W., et al.: Right ventricular function in adult atrial septal defect: Preoperative and postoperative assessment and clinical implications *Am. J. Cardiol.* 47:56–60, 1980.
18. Hung J., Uren R.F., Richmond D.R., et al.: The mechanism of abnormal septal motion in atrial septal defect: Pre- and postoperative study by radionuclide ventriculography in adults. *Circulation* 63:142–148, 1981.
19. Bonow R.O., Borer J.S., Rosing D.R., et al.: Left ventricular functional reserve in adult patients with atrial septal defect: Pre- and postoperative studies. *Circulation* 63:1315–1322, 1981.
20. Young D., Mark H.: Fate of the patient with the Eisenmenger syndrome. *Am. J. Cardiol.* 28:679, 1971.
21. Brammell H.L., Vogel J.H.K., Pryor R., et al.: The Eisenmenger syndrome. *Am. J. Cardiol.* 48:679, 1981.
22. Konstam M.A., Levine B.W., Strauss H.W., et al.: Left superior vena cava to left atrial communication diagnosed with radionuclide angiography and with differential right to left shunting. *Am. J. Cardiol.* 43:149–153, 1979.
23. Gunther S., Grossman W.: Determinants of ventricular function in pressure-overload hypertrophy in man. *Circulation* 59:679–688, 1979.
24. Boucher C.A., Okada R.D., Pohost G.M.: Current status of radionuclide imaging in valvular heart disease. *Am. J. Cardiol.* 46:1153–1163, 1980.
25. Block P.C., Powel W.J., Dinsmore R.E., et al.: Coexistent fixed congenital and idiopathic hypertrophic subaortic stenosis. *Am. J. Cardiol.* 31:523, 1973.
26. Pohost G.M., Vignola P.A., McKusick K.A., et al.: Hypertrophic cardiomyopathy: Evaluation by gated cardiac blood pool scanning. *Circulation* 55:92–96, 1977.
27. Liberthson R.R., Pennington D.G., Jacobs M.L., et al.: Coarctation of the aorta: Review of 234 patients and clarification of management problems. *Am. J. Cardiol.* 43:835–840, 1979.
28. Garson A.Jr., Nihill M.R., McNamara D.G., et al.:

Status of the adult and adolescent after repair of tetralogy of Fallot. *Circulation* 59:1232–1240, 1979.
29. Reduto L.A., Berger H.J., Johnstone D.E., et al.: Radionuclide assessment of right and left ventricular exercise reserve after total correction of tetralogy of Fallot. *Am. J. Cardiol.* 45:1013–1018, 1980.
30. Shaher R.M.: *Complete Transposition of the Great Arteries*. New York, Academic Press, 1973.
31. Attie F., Cuaron A., Marquez M., et al.: Qualitative radionuclide angiocardiography in the diagnoses of corrected transposition. *Am. Heart J.* 97:141–146, 1979.
32. Ogden J.A.: Congenital anomalies of the coronary arteries. *Am. J. Cardiol.* 25:474–479, 1970.
33. Liberthson R.R., Dinsmore R.E., Fallon J.T.: Aberrant coronary artery origin from the aorta: Report of 18 patients, review of literature and delineation of natural history and management. *Circulation* 59:748–754, 1979.
34. Liberthson R.R., Sagar K., Berkoben J., et al.: Congenital coronary arteriovenous fistula: Report of 13 patients, review of the literature and delineation of management. *Circulation* 59:849–854, 1979.
35. Verani M.S., Marcus M.L., Ehrhardt J.C., et al.: Demonstration of improved myocardial perfusion following aortic implantation of anomalous left coronary artery. *J. Nucl. Med.* 19:1032–1035, 1978.
36. Moodie D.S., Cook S.A., Gill C.G., et al.: Thallium-201 myocardial imaging in young adults with anomalous left coronary artery arising from the pulmonary artery. *J. Nucl. Med.* 21:1076–1079, 1980.
37. Gutgesel H.P., Pinsky W.W., DePuey G.E.: Thallium-201 myocardial perfusion imaging in infants and children: Value in distinguishing anomalous left coronary artery from congestive cardiomyopathy. *Circulation* 61:596–599, 1980.
38. Treves S., Parker J.A.: Detection and quantitation of intracardiac shunts. in Strauss H.W., Pitt B., (eds.): *Cardiovascular Nuclear Medicine*, ed. 2. St. Louis, C.V. Mosby Co., 1979, p. 151.

PART XII

Pericardial Disease

ECHOCARDIOGRAPHY

Satish C. Sharma and Alfred F. Parisi

THE ORIGINAL DESCRIPTION, in the 1960s, of echocardiographic findings in pericardial effusion by Feigenbaum and co-workers[1, 2] was a major impetus to the development of echocardiography as a diagnostic method in cardiology. In the ensuing years, important additional experience has been acquired with pericardial disease. In fact, echocardiography has now become the method of choice for diagnosis of pericardial effusion, completely replacing such invasive techniques as contrast angiography and diagnostic pericardiocentesis. Echocardiography may also be helpful in the diagnosis of cardiac tamponade, pericardial thickening or constriction, and pericardial masses and cysts.

NORMAL ANATOMY OF PERICARDIUM

Two layers of pericardium normally surround the heart. The inner layer is a serous membrane known as the *visceral pericardium* or *epicardium*. The visceral pericardium is continuous with the outer fibrous layer (parietal pericardium) so that there is a potential space between the two layers, which normally contains 10–20 ml of pericardial fluid. It is in this space that a pericardial effusion may accumulate. Behind the left atrium, the pericardium reflects from the pulmonary veins in a manner which tends to obliterate the pericardial space. As a result, pericardial fluid usually does not accumulate behind the left atrium. However, in the presence of large pericardial effusions, fluid may accumulate in the oblique sinus of the pericardium, which is located in the area of pericardial reflections between the pulmonary veins.

On a normal echocardiogram, the anterior wall of the right ventricle is in direct contact with the stationary echoes of the chest wall, whereas the posterior left ventricular wall (epicardium) is in direct contact with the posterior pericardium and pleura. When pericardial effusion develops, fluid separates the two layers of pericardium; this is visualized as a relatively echo-free space between posterior epicardium and parietal pericardium. With large pericardial effusions, a relatively echo-free space may be present both anteriorly as well as posteriorly with respect to the heart. The presence of a relatively echo-free space anteriorly without a posterior space is not sufficient for diagnosis of pericardial effusion.

ECHOCARDIOGRAPHIC TECHNIQUE FOR EVALUATING THE PERICARDIUM

The pericardium is a strong reflector of ultrasound and is imaged as the most echo-dense structure related to the posterior left ventricular wall. In a standard echocardiographic examination, the heart is scanned from base to the apex, with the gain and reject controls continually ad-

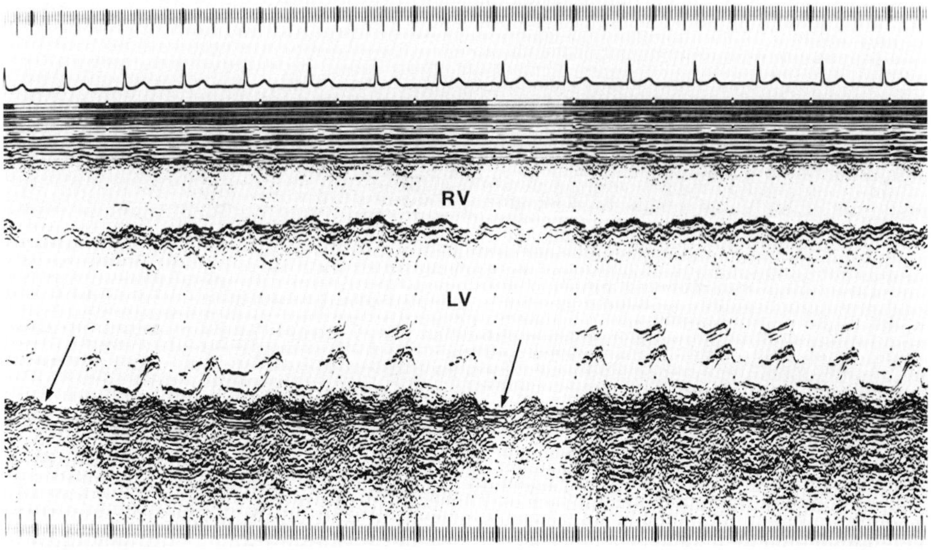

Fig 23–1.—M-mode echocardiogram from a normal subject demonstrating normal pericardium with damping *(arrows)*. There is no space between the posterior epicardium and pericardium. *RV*, right ventricle; *LV*, left ventricle.

justed. The posterior pericardium is defined by damping the energy of the ultrasonic beam so that echoes are reflected from the highly reflective posterior pericardium only. When the ultrasonic beam is directed just below the level of the mitral valve, the beam traverses the anterior chest wall, the anterior right ventricular wall, the right ventricular cavity, the interventricular septum, the left ventricular cavity, the posterior left ventricular wall. and the posterior pericardium. Figure 23–1 shows the normal echocardiographic appearance of the pericardium in the absence of pericardial effusion. The arrows indicate areas of increased damping so that the only structure imaged is the posterior pericardium. There is no space between posterior epicardium and pericardium and hence there is no effusion.

PERICARDIAL EFFUSION

As fluid accumulates in the pericardium, the two pericardial layers become separated by a space that appears relatively echo free. The distribution of pericardial fluid depends on its volume and the patient's posture. When the subject is recumbent, fluid initially collects directly behind the heart; with increasing volume, it tends to distribute laterally and around the apex.[3] Figure 23–2 shows the echocardiogram from a patient with a moderately large pericardial effusion. A relatively echo-free space can be seen between the epicardium and parietal pericardium behind the left ventricle, as well as anterior to the right ventricle. Figure 23–3 demonstrates the disappearance of the relatively echo-free space (pericardial effusion) behind the left atrium.

At high gain settings, pericardial fluid does produce echoes (Fig 23–4); therefore it is important that the term "relatively echo-free" be used when describing pericardial fluid.[4]

Another echocardiographic hallmark of pericardial effusion is poor or absent motion of the posterior parietal pericardium. This results from the buffering action of the pericardial fluid between the posterior wall of the left ventricle and the pericardium. However, in the presence of small effusions, the motion of the posterior parietal pericardium may be preserved (Fig 23–5).

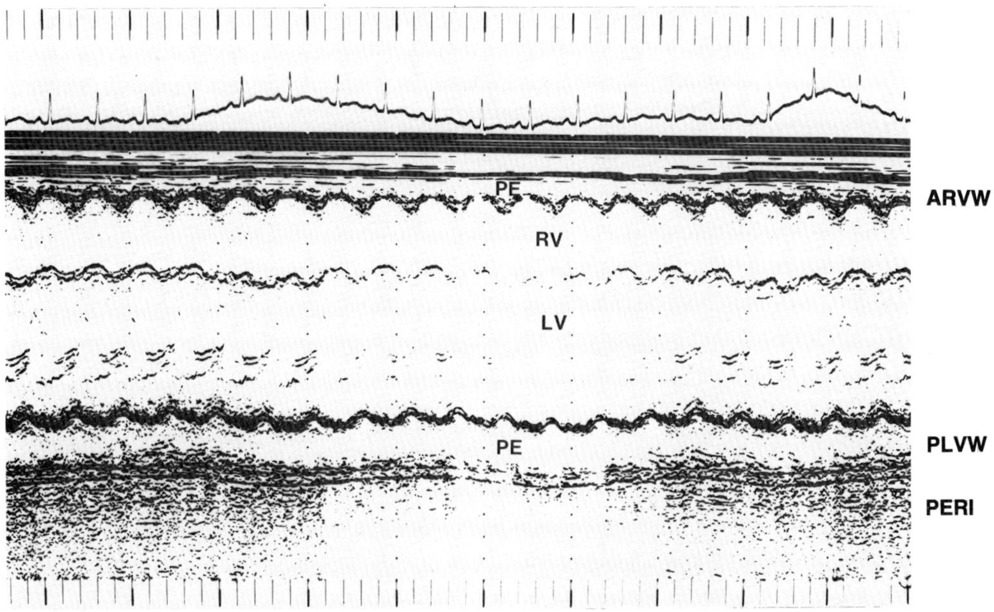

Fig 23–2.—M-mode echocardiogram of a patient with moderate amount of pericardial effusion *(PE)*. A relatively echo-free space can be seen anterior to the anterior right ventricular wall *(ARVW)* and posterior to the posterior left ventricular wall *(PLVW)*. Note that the posterior pericardium *(PERI)* is flat without motion. *RV*, right ventricle; *LV*, left ventricle.

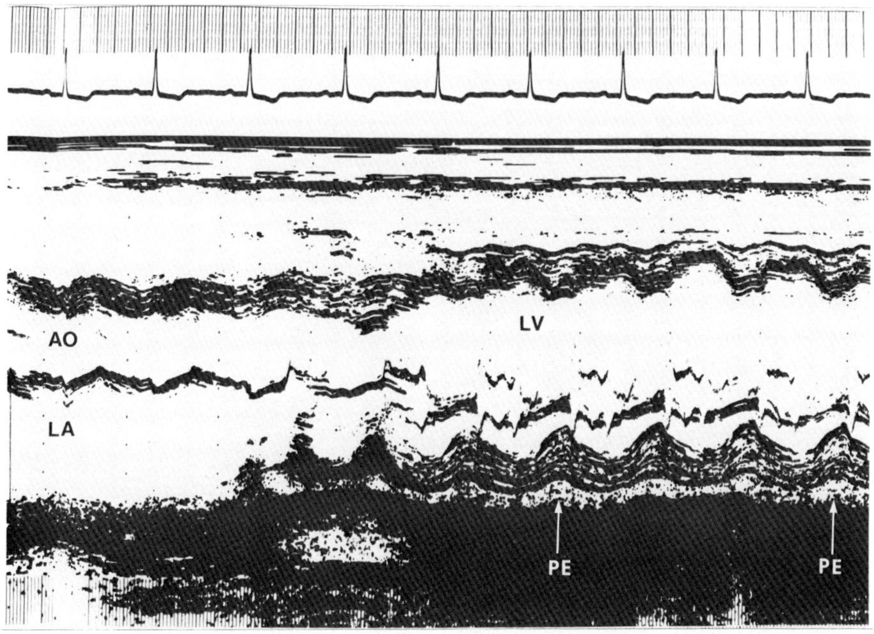

Fig 23–3.—M-mode echocardiogram of a patient with a pericardial effusion. A relatively echo-free space is seen behind the left ventricle but it disappears as the ultrasonic beam is directed toward the left atrium. *PE*, pericardial effusion; *LV*, left ventricle; *LA*, left atrium; *AO*, aortic root.

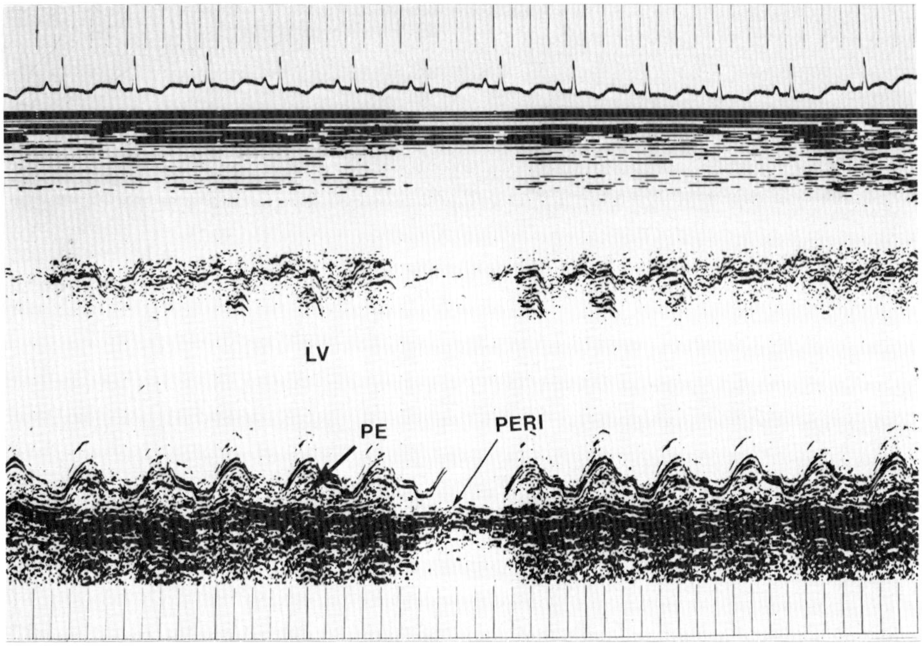

Fig 23–4.—M-mode echocardiogram showing echoes produced by pericardial fluid if gain is too high. *PE,* pericardial effusion; *PERI,* pericardium; *LV,* left ventricle.

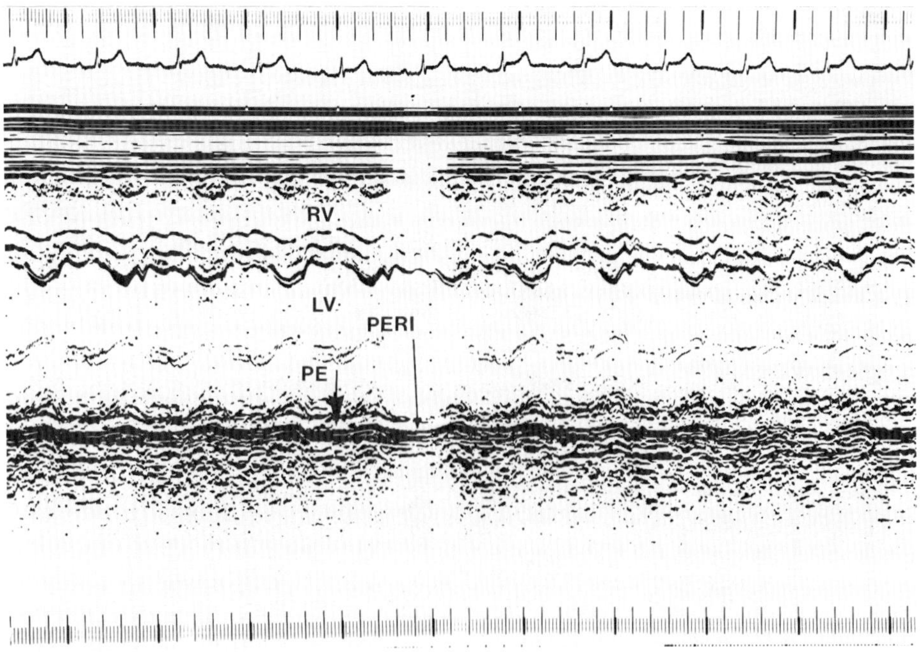

Fig 23–5.—M-mode echocardiogram of a patient demonstrating a small posterior pericardial effusion *(PE)* with intact pericardial motion. *PERI,* pericardium; *RV,* right ventricle; *LV,* left ventricle.

With large pericardial effusions, the heart tends to exhibit increased motion within the pericardial sac. When effusion is massive, cardiac mobility is further increased and may exhibit the rocking or swinging motion considered to be pathognomonic of a large pericardial effusion.[5] At its extreme, swinging may distort the normal motion patterns of septum, mitral valve, and posterior wall (Fig 23–6).[6] The mitral valve has been shown to exhibit a pattern of pseudoprolapse as a result of swinging cardiac motion.[7–9] Figure 23–7 shows the echocardiogram of a patient with large pericardial effusion with distortion of wall motion and pseudoprolapse of the mitral valve.[10]

Swinging cardiac motion can result in the ECG phenomenon of electric alternans (see Fig 23–7). The principle underlying this phenomenon is that the heart depolarizes in relatively anterior and posterior positions on alternate beats, resulting in larger and smaller QRS forces on every other complex of the ECG.

QUANTIFICATION OF PERICARDIAL FLUID

The degree of separation of the posterior pericardium from the posterior heart wall has been found to correlate roughly with the amount of pericardial fluid present. Several studies have attempted to correlate the amount of pericardial fluid with the distance between the posterior epicardium and parietal pericardium.

Horowitz et al.[11] correlated the amount of pericardial fluid recovered in patients undergoing cardiac surgery with the findings of M-mode echocardiograms obtained preoperatively. They found that as little as 16 ml of fluid could produce slight separation of the two pericardial layers, thus demonstrating the very high sensitivity of this technique. They emphasized, however, that such small amounts of pericardial fluid are not clinically important and that to diagnose an abnormal accumulation of pericardial fluid, complete separation between the posterior epicardium and pericardium should be demonstrated throughout the cardiac cycle. They also proposed a formula for predicting the volume of pericardial effusion. In this

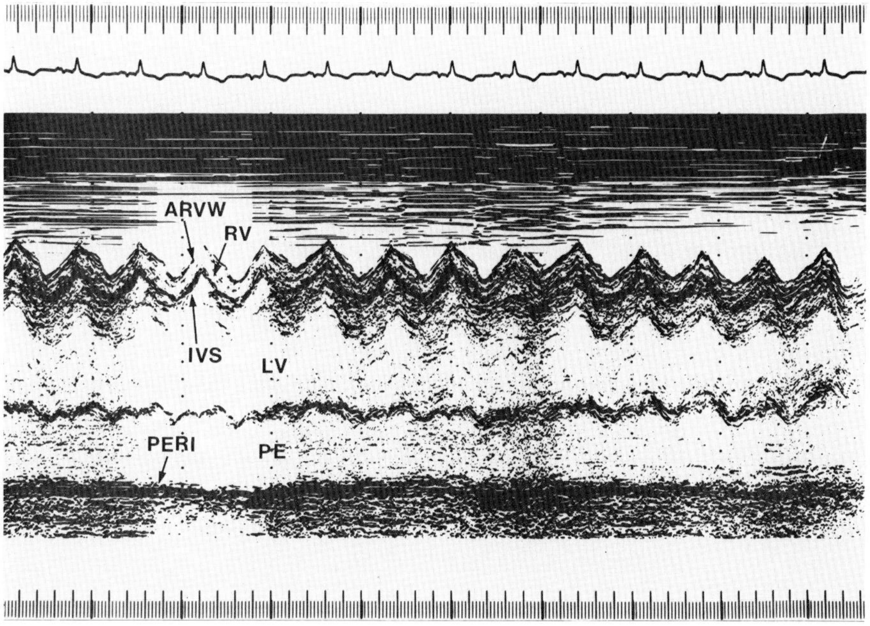

Fig 23–6.—M-mode echocardiogram of a patient with massive pericardial effusion demonstrating swinging of the heart within the fluid-filled pericardial space. *PERI,* pericardium; *PE,* pericardial effusion; *LV,* left ventricle; *IVS,* interventricular septum; *RV,* right ventricular cavity; *ARVW,* anterior right ventricular wall.

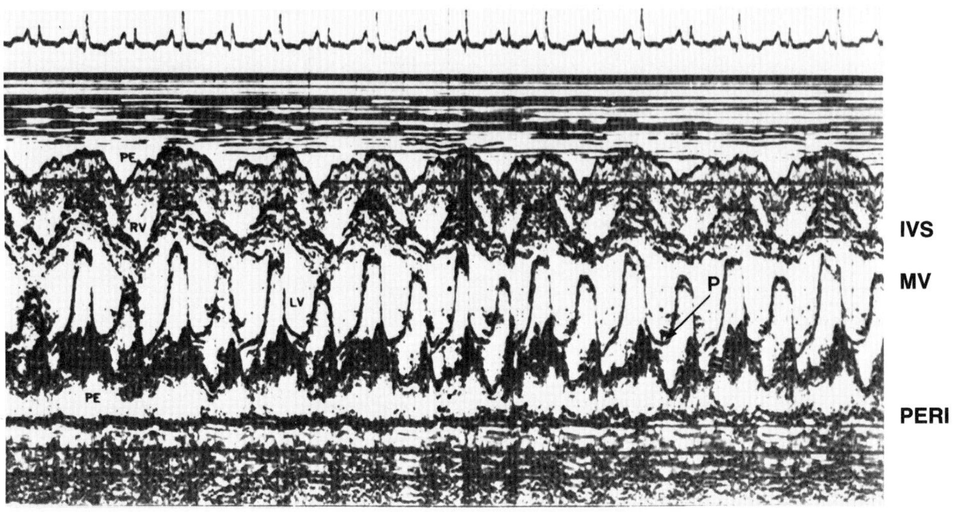

Fig 23–7.—M-mode echocardiogram of a patient with chronic renal failure and massive pericardial effusion. Note that cardiac oscillation occurs with every other cardiac cycle, causing electrical alterans. Systolic posterior motion with every other cycle simulates mitral valve prolapse *(P)*. *PE,* pericardial effusion; *RV,* right ventricle; *IVS,* interventricular septum; *MV (arrow),* anterior mitral leaflet; *LV,* left ventricle; *PERI,* pericardium. (From Jacobs W.R., et al.: *Arch. Intern. Med.* 138:622, 1978; copyright 1978, American Medical Association. Reproduced by permission.)

method cubed diameters from the anterior to posterior pericardium and from the anterior to posterior epicardium are calculated at end-diastole, and the difference between the two gives the volume of pericardial fluid.

Most investigators have concluded that one can only grossly estimate the quantity of pericardial fluid by echocardiography.[2, 12, 13] We believe that the echocardiographic quantification of pericardial fluid has been overemphasized in the literature. It is far more important to ascertain whether a given amount of pericardial fluid is producing undesirable hemodynamic effects. These effects do not necessarily correlate with the size of the pericardial effusion. With penetrating chest wall injuries, for example, a small to moderate amount of hemorrhage into the pericardium can cause acute tamponade, even though the cardiac silhouette may not even appear enlarged on a chest x-ray film. On the other hand, with slowly developing effusions, huge quantities of the pericardial fluid may be able to accumulate without causing hemodynamic compromise.

It is important, however, for the physician to determine whether a pericardial effusion detected by echocardiography is disproportionate to the severity of underlying cardiac disease in a particular patient. Small amounts of echocardiographically demonstrable pericardial fluid are found in patients with advanced heart disease and should not lead to an unnecessary workup to determine the etiology of the effusion. On the other hand, if effusion is present without associated valvular or myocardial disease or if it is out of proportion to the severity of cardiac disease in a given patient, further evaluation is warranted.

DIFFERENTIATION OF PERICARDIAL FROM PLEURAL EFFUSION AND RETROCARDIAC STRUCTURES

In the presence of large left-sided pleural effusions, a large relatively echo-free space may be seen behind the left ventricle, giving rise to confusion in interpretation. Usually, however, a pleural effusion can be differentiated from a pericardial effusion by echocardiography. A pleural effusion

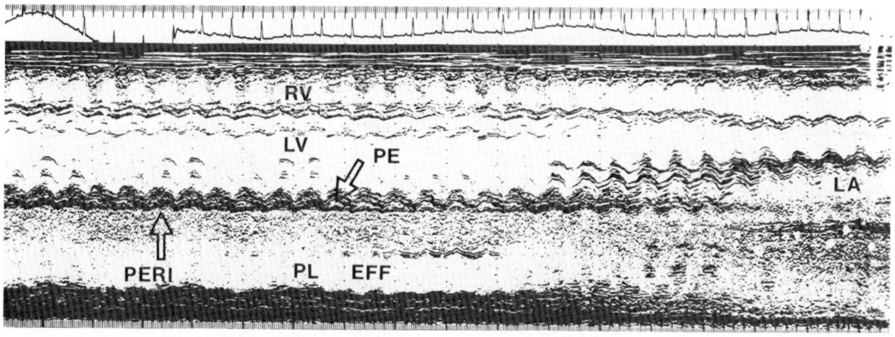

Fig 23–8.—M-mode echocardiogram of a patient with a small pericardial effusion *(PE)* demonstrated by the systolic separation of posterior pericardium *(PERI)* from the epicardium. The large relatively echo-free space posterior to the heart is due to a large pleural effusion which persists behind the left atrium *(LA)*. *RV,* right ventricle; *LV,* left ventricle; *PL EFF,* pleural effusion.

commonly produces a large, relatively echo-free space posterior to the heart without an anterior echo-free space (Fig 23–8).

The posterior relatively echo-free space occasionally varies with respiration in the presence of pleural but not pericardial effusion. If pleural and pericardial effusions coexist, the parietal pericardium may occasionally be seen separating two relatively echo-free spaces (see Fig 23–8).

Rarely, it may be extremely difficult to differentiate between pleural and pericardial effusion, particularly if the pleural effusion is small and unaccompanied by pericardial fluid. Two-dimensional echocardiography (2DE) may be helpful under such circumstances.[14]

LIMITATIONS OF M-MODE ECHOCARDIOGRAPHY

The accuracy of M-mode echocardiography exceeds 90% in the diagnosis of pericardial effusion. It does have some pitfalls, however, because of a small "anatomic window" available to the sonographer. Normal retrocardiac structures such as the thoracic aorta, lower pulmonary veins, and coronary sinus may occasionally cause a relatively echo-free space behind the heart. Other causes of false positive echocardiographic results include too much medial angulation of transducer, posterior diaphragmatic hernia,[13] giant left atrium,[15] mitral anulus calcification,[16] and tumor encapsulating the entire heart.[17, 18] Mediastinal tumors[19] and pericardial cysts[20] have been reported to separate the heart from the anterior chest wall. False negative findings have been reported with loculated fluid[2, 21] and in patients with chest wall deformities.

TWO-DIMENSIONAL ECHOCARDIOGRAPHY

With the advent of two-dimensional, wide-angle echocardiography, the scope of ultrasonography in diagnosis of pericardial diseases has increased further. In most instances, M-mode echocardiography is sufficient for diagnosis of pericardial effusion and 2DE is probably superfluous. However, the narrow field of M-mode echocardiography has led to errors in the diagnosis of pericardial effusion in certain circumstances (see above). In these instances, 2DE appears to have a significant advantage over M-mode echocardiography, for it permits simultaneous visualization of the entire heart and surrounding pericardium in multiple, tomographic planes (Fig 23–9). It has been found to be particularly useful in diagnosing loculated pericardial effusion (Fig 23–10).[22]

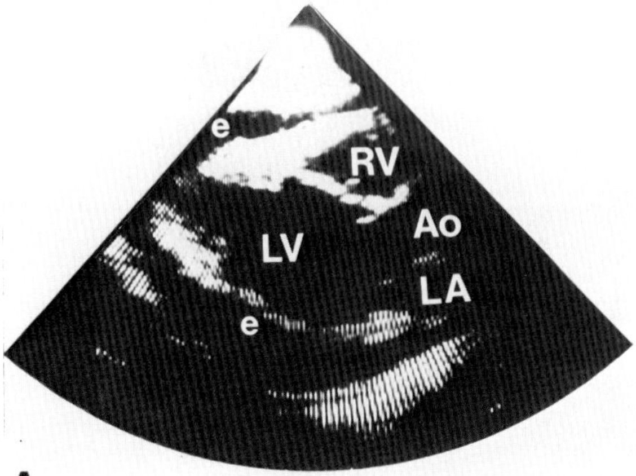

A.

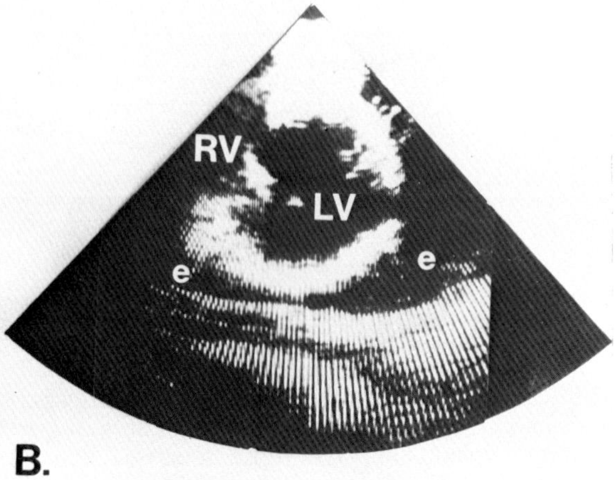

B.

Fig 23–9.—Pericardial effusion demonstrated by two-dimensional echocardiography in long- and short-axis views. **A,** long-axis view of the heart in a patient with moderate pericardial effusion. Effusion *(e)* can be seen anterior to the right ventricle *(RV)* as well as posterior to the left ventricle *(LV)* and also toward the apical region. *LA,* left atrium; *AO,* aorta. **B,** short-axis view in the same patient demonstrating pericardial effusion *(e)* posteriorly as well as laterally. (From Parisi A.F., et al.: *J. Cardiovasc. Med.* 5:39, 1980. Reproduced by permission.)

The real-time format is invaluable in studying the various patterns of cardiac motion and in differentiating a pericardial effusion from pleural effusion and retrocardiac structures. Two-dimensional echocardiography also offers advantages over M-mode echocardiography in the diagnosis of pericardial effusion in the presence of abnormal chest wall anatomy. A patient with severe pectus excavatum, recently studied in our laboratory, presented with massive enlargement of cardiac silhouette over a three-week period. No effusion could be detected on standard M-mode echocardiography. Two-dimensional echocardiography documented that the effusion was distributed laterally on either side of the heart but was not directly posterior to the left ventricle (Fig 23–11).

Schiller has recently described a technique for quantification of pericardial effusion by 2DE.[14] In this method, a light pen computational system is used to outline freeze-frame video images of the epicardium and pericardium from an apical four-chamber view of the heart. Volumes of each outline are computed by the area-length single-plane method. The difference between the volumes of pericardial outline and epicardial outline is the volume of the pericardial fluid.

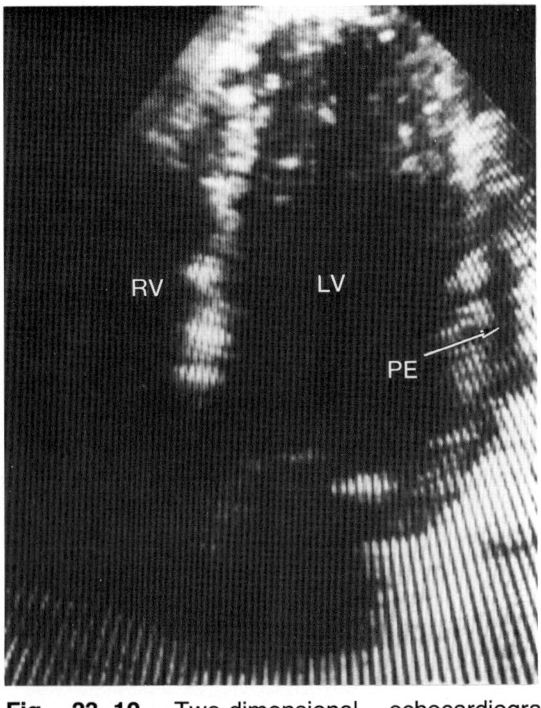

Fig 23–10.—Two-dimensional echocardiogram *(apical view)* demonstrating loculated pericardial effusion *(PE, arrow)*. *LV,* left ventricle; *RV,* right ventricle.

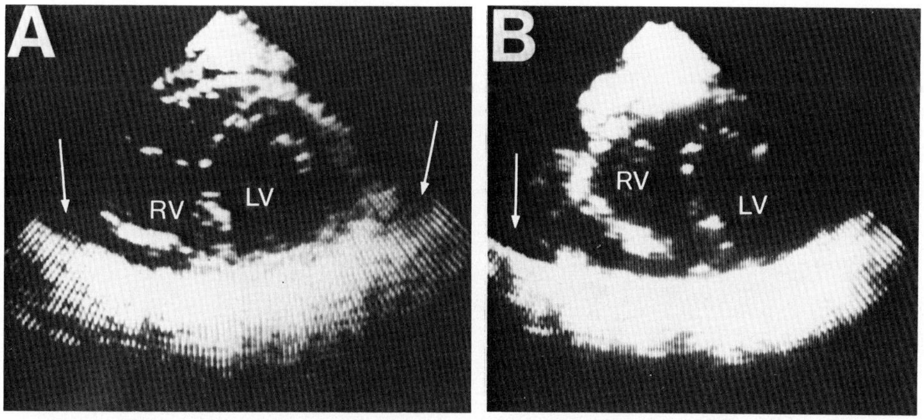

Fig 23–11.—Two-dimensional echocardiograms recorded from the subcostal view in a patient with severe pectus excavatum. Note that effusion *(Panel A)* can be seen laterally *(arrows)* but not directly posterior to the heart. In *Panel B,* the transducer beam has been directed to define more of the right ventricular free wall. *RV,* right ventricle; *LV,* left ventricle.

SELECTED DISORDERS

Cardiac Tamponade

Cardiac tamponade is a medical emergency characterized clinically by systemic hypotension, elevated venous pressure, and pulsus paradoxus. It occurs when pericardial effusion increases the intrapericardial pressures so greatly that left ventricular filling is severely compromised. Echocardiography can be helpful in this setting, for cardiac tamponade is very unlikely in the absence of echocardiographically demonstrable pericardial effusion. Furthermore, several other echocardiographic features have been reported in tamponade (Table 23–1).

The sensitivity and specificity of many of these echocardiographic clues to cardiac tamponade have been debated.[29] In the series of Schiller and Botvinick,[23] almost all patients with cardiac tamponade had an end-expiratory right ventricular end-diastolic dimension (RVID*d*) of less than 7 mm. It was considered to be the most specific finding for diagnosis of cardiac tamponade. However, Settle et al.[25] studied 14 patients with proved tamponade and found that the mean end-expiratory RVID*d* was 1.8 cm. A possible explanation for the differences in the right ventricular dimensions in the two series is the difference in the position of patients (left oblique vs. supine)[23, 25] used by these investigators for imaging the right ventricular internal dimension. In any event, further studies are required to elaborate on these findings.

It cannot be overemphasized that, while echocardiography can provide important clues to the presence of cardiac tamponade, this primarily remains a clinical, bedside diagnosis.

Figure 23–12,A shows an echocardiogram of a

TABLE 23–1.—ECHOCARDIOGRAPHIC FEATURES OF CARDIAC TAMPONADE

FINDING	STUDY
Right ventricular compression at end-expiration (RVIDd < 7 mm)	Schiller and Botvinick[23]
Diminished EF slope (< 50 mm/sec)	Vignola et al.,[24] Settle et al.[25]
Inspiratory increase in RV internal dimension with reciprocal decrease in LV internal dimension	Settle et al.,[25] D'Cruz et al.[26]
Notched right ventricular epicardial echo in early systole	Vignola et al.[24]
Beat-to-beat variation in RV and LV internal dimensions with beat-to-beat variation in mitral valve diastolic excursion	Zoneraich et al.[27]
Significant decrease in the size of all chambers	Schiller[14]
Immediate reversibility of above findings with pericardiocentesis	Schiller[14]
Diastolic collapse of the RV outflow tract	Armstrong et al.[28]

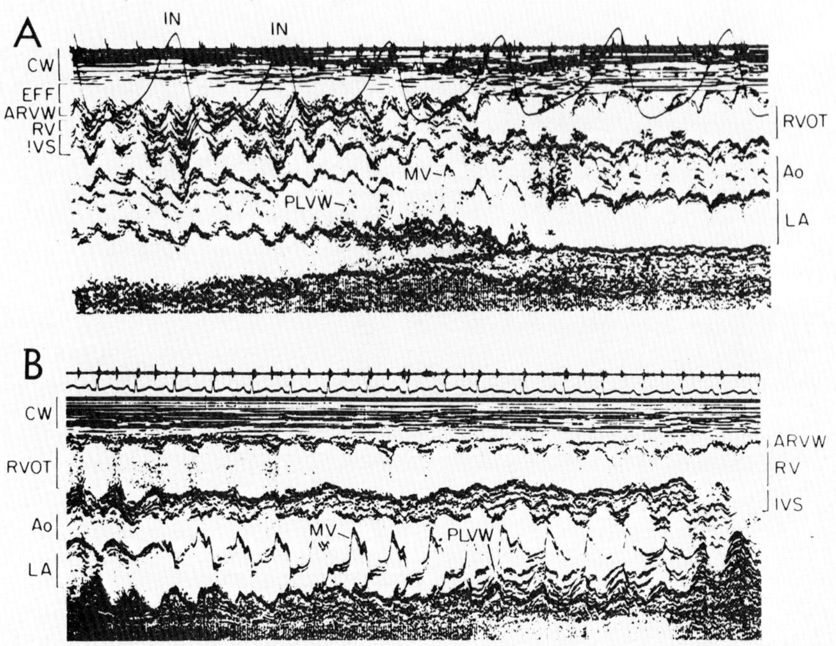

Fig 23–12.—A, continuous echocardiographic scan from the left ventricle to the aortic root *(Ao)* in a patient with cardiac tamponade. Right ventricular *(RV)* cavity is compressed with minimal expansion during inspiration *(IN).* **B,** M-mode scan from the same patient after pericardiocentesis showing the expansion of the RV cavity. Effusion is now difficult to identify. *CW,* chest wall; *EFF,* effusion; *ARVW,* anterior right ventricular wall; *IVS,* interventricular septum; *MV,* mitral valve; *RVOT,* right ventricular outflow tract; *PLVW,* posterior left ventricular wall; *LA,* left atrium. (From Schiller N.B., Botvinick E.H.: *Circulation* 56:774, 1977. Reproduced by permission of the American Heart Association, Inc.)

patient with large pericardial effusion and clinical findings of cardiac tamponade. Note that there is slight right ventricular expansion during inspiration but the right ventricular cavity is markedly compressed during expiration. Figure 23–12,B demonstrates immediate reversal of these abnormalities following pericardiocentesis. Similar changes in right and left ventricular dimensions with respiration can be demonstrated with 2DE.

Echocardiography may be falsely negative in cardiac tamponade caused by acute hemopericardium. There is experimental evidence that the presence of clots in the pericardium may mask an otherwise relatively echo-free space.[30]

Constrictive Pericarditis

Diagnosis of constrictive pericarditis can be extremely difficult to establish by noninvasive means. Echocardiography can provide important clues to this condition. Several workers[4, 31, 32] have reported a "flattening" of the left ventricular posterior wall motion during diastole due to an abrupt cessation of the rapid filling phase in constrictive pericarditis. In a recent study reported from our laboratory,[33] it was demonstrated that this flattening comprised less than 1 mm of the posterior diastolic motion of the left ventricular posterior wall as measured from the crystal artifact (Fig 23–13).

Gibson et al.[34] reported an abnormal interventricular septal motion in eight of ten patients with constrictive pericarditis. In another study,[35] an early diastolic septal notch was found to be present in chronic constrictive pericarditis. However, several authors have reported a septal notch in conditions other than constrictive pericarditis, including amyloidosis[14] and endomyocardial fibrosis.[36]

In chronic constrictive pericarditis, the pericardium may be thickened, but there is considerable overlap with the thickness of pericardium seen in

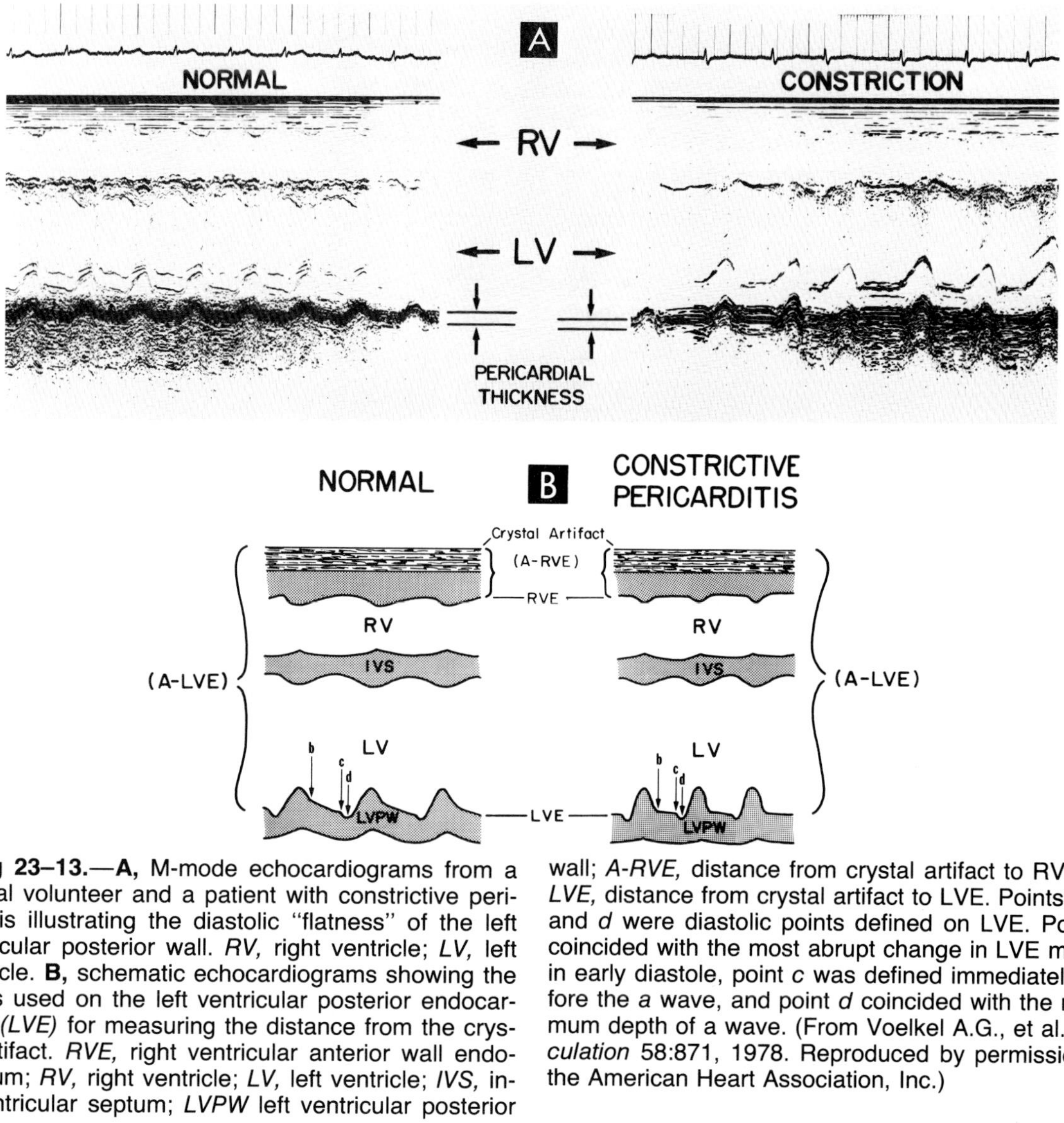

Fig 23–13.—**A,** M-mode echocardiograms from a normal volunteer and a patient with constrictive pericarditis illustrating the diastolic "flatness" of the left ventricular posterior wall. *RV,* right ventricle; *LV,* left ventricle. **B,** schematic echocardiograms showing the points used on the left ventricular posterior endocardium *(LVE)* for measuring the distance from the crystal artifact. *RVE,* right ventricular anterior wall endocardium; *RV,* right ventricle; *LV,* left ventricle; *IVS,* interventricular septum; *LVPW* left ventricular posterior wall; *A-RVE,* distance from crystal artifact to RVE; *A-LVE,* distance from crystal artifact to LVE. Points *b, c,* and *d* were diastolic points defined on LVE. Point *b* coincided with the most abrupt change in LVE motion in early diastole, point *c* was defined immediately before the *a* wave, and point *d* coincided with the maximum depth of a wave. (From Voelkel A.G., et al.: *Circulation* 58:871, 1978. Reproduced by permission of the American Heart Association, Inc.)

normal patients. Voelkel et al.[33] were not able to differentiate between normal volunteers and patients with constrictive pericarditis on the basis of pericardial thickness by echocardiography (see Fig 23–13,A). Unusually thickened pericardium (> 1 cm) is rare in the idiopathic variety of constrictive pericarditis and should arouse suspicion of tumor in the pericardium as the etiology for constriction (Fig 23–14).[37]

With 2DE, we have observed a phenomenon of "freezing" of the late diastolic motion of both ventricles in constrictive pericarditis. Normally, in an apical four-chamber view, the ventricles continue to expand gradually after the rapid filling phase of early diastole. In constrictive pericarditis, there is sudden cessation of expansion (freezing) after the rapid filling phase of diastole.

Mimics of Pericardial Constriction and Tamponade

There have been several reports in the literature of right ventricular infarction mimicking pericardial constriction or tamponade.[38, 39] He-

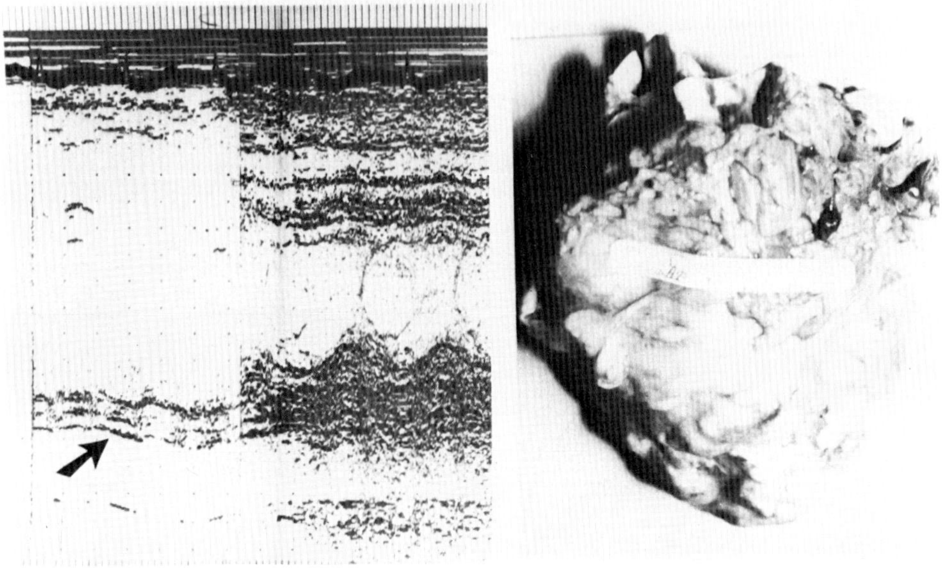

Fig 23–14.—M-mode echocardiogram from a patient with pericardial tumor and constrictive pericarditis. *Left,* unusually thickened posterior pericardium *(arrow). Right,* pathologic specimen with pericardial tumor nodules as the cause of constriction. (From Parisi A.F., Tow D.E. [eds.]: *Noninvasive Approaches to Cardiovascular Diagnosis.* New York, Appleton-Century-Crofts, 1979, p. 176. Reprinted by permission.)

modynamically significant right ventricular infarction usually occurs in the setting of acute inferior or posteroinferior myocardial infarction. It can present with systemic hypotension and shock along with increased jugular venous pressure. Noninvasive methods, including echocardiography and gated blood pool scintigraphy, are extremely helpful in differentiating this entity from cardiac tamponade by demonstrating the absence of pericardial effusion and the presence of a dilated and noncontractile right ventricle.[40] Table 23–2 summarizes some features of cardiac tamponade, constrictive pericarditis, and right ventricular infarction.

Congenital or Acquired Absence of the Pericardium

Partial or complete absence of the pericardium is a rare congenital anomaly which may be manifested in several ways—by the complete absence of the left hemipericardium, by the partial absence of the left hemipericardium, by the partial absence of the right hemipericardium, and by the total absence of the pericardium.[41–43] The most common manifestation is the complete absence of the left hemipericardium. In this condition, there is an exaggerated motion of the left ventricular posterior wall, which in turn displaces the interventricular septum anteriorly during systole so that it appears to move paradoxically. In addition, the heart is displaced leftward due to the absent left pericardium, thus making more of the right ventricle visible on M-mode echocardiography from the standard parasternal position. As a result, the right ventricle appears dilated. Similar findings have been reported after surgical removal of the pericardium (acquired absence of the pericardium) (Fig 23–15). Thus, the echocardiographic findings with congenital or acquired absence of the pericardium include exaggerated motion of the left ventricular posterior wall, paradoxic septal motion, and right ventricular dilation. These findings resemble those of right ventricular volume overload,[44] and it may be impossible to distinguish the two conditions by M-mode echocardiography. Two-dimensional echocardiographic differentiation of these conditions has not yet been reported.

Pericardial Tumors

There is little information available in the literature on the echocardiographic findings in pa-

TABLE 23–2.—Features of Cardiac Tamponade, Constrictive Pericarditis, and Right Ventricular Infarction

Feature	Cardiac Tamponade	Constrictive Pericarditis	Right Ventricular Infarction
Etiology	Rapidly accumulating pericardial effusions due to any cause; hemopericardium due to penetrating chest injuries, acute myocardial infarction, after cardiac surgery, during invasive procedures such as cardiac catheterization and insertion of pacemakers	Usually idiopathic; other causes include tuberculosis, tumor, viral pericarditis	Usually occurs in the setting of acute inferior or posteroinferior myocardial infarction
Clinical features	Systemic hypotension (shock), increased venous pressure, pulsus paradoxus	Increased venous pressure, positive Kussmaul's sign, pericardial knock, ascites, peripheral edema	Sinus bradycardia, occasional complete heart block, systemic hypotension (shock), increased venous pressure, pulsus paradoxus (occasionally), Kussmaul's sign (occasionally)
Echocardiographic features	Evidence of pericardial effusion both anterior as well as posterior to the heart; end-expiratory compression of right ventricle; inspiratory increase in RV internal dimension with reciprocal decrease in LV internal dimension	Flattening of diastolic motion of left ventricular posterior wall; thickening of pericardium	Dilated RV, increased RV/LV minor axis ratio, paradoxic septal motion
Gated blood pool scintigraphy	Evidence of fluid in the pericardium; small vigorously contracting cardiac chambers	Small, vigorously contracting cardiac chambers	Dilated, akinetic RV, decreased RV ejection fraction
Hemodynamic features	Diastolic pressure equilibration in all cardiac chambers; right atrial pressure tracing shows prominent X′ descent; Y descent usually obliterated	Diastolic pressure equilibration in all cardiac chambers; right atrial pressure tracing shows prominent a and v waves with a prominent y descent (M pattern); RV pressure tracing shows characteristic early dip and plateau configuration (square root sign)	Diastolic pressure equilibration in right heart chambers; right heart filling pressures may be higher than left heart filling pressure; RV pressure tracing may show an early dip and plateau configuration; right atrial cineangiogram demonstrates dilated, noncontractile right ventricle
Therapy	Pericardiocentesis; volume expansion while preparing for pericardiocentesis	Pericardiectomy; diuretic therapy for selected cases	Volume expansion, pressors, temporary pacemakers if complete heart block occurs, afterload reduction in selected cases with concomitant LV infarction

tients with pericardial tumors. Pericardial effusion is common, and therefore its presence in a patient with systemic malignancy such as lymphoma, leukemia, carcinoma of lung or breast, or malignant melanoma should raise the suspicion of pericardial metastases. A recently published study demonstrated the usefulness of cross-sectional echocardiography in detection of pericardial metastases.[45] Seven of nine patients with pericardial metastases and effusion were found to have irregular cauliflower-like masses protruding from the pericardium (Fig 23–16). These masses demonstrated a to-and-fro motion within the pericardial space with contraction of the heart.

Pericardial Cysts

Pericardial cysts are outpouchings of pericardium which may occur as a congenital anomaly or as a result of chronic pericardial inflammation.

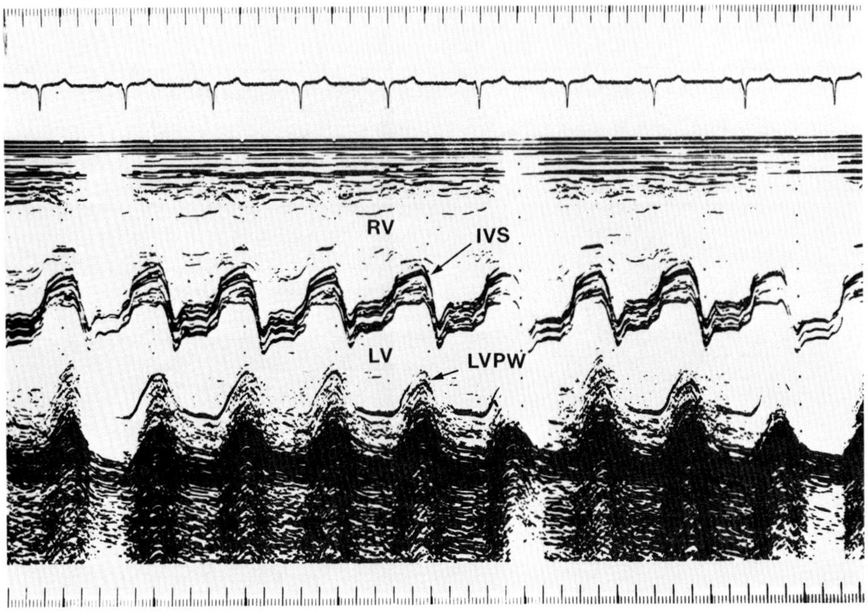

Fig 23–15.—M-mode echocardiogram from a patient after pericardiectomy (acquired absence of pericardium). Note exaggerated left ventricular posterior wall *(LVPW)* and septal excursion and paradoxic motion of the interventricular septum *(IVS)*. Right ventricular dilation is also present. *RV*, right ventricle; *LV*, left ventricle.

These cysts are usually benign, cause no symptoms, and are discovered on routine chest roentgenograms. Occasionally, however, symptoms of chest pressure or pain, or signs of obstruction of venous return to the right heart have been reported. The diagnosis is made by chest roentgenography, which shows the cyst to be a sharply outlined semicircular or oval structure protruding from the cardiac silhouette, usually from its lower right border, occasionally from its left side. Lung markings can often be seen through the density.

On ultrasonic examination, a relatively echo-free space is usually present between the chest wall and the anterior right ventricular wall with no such

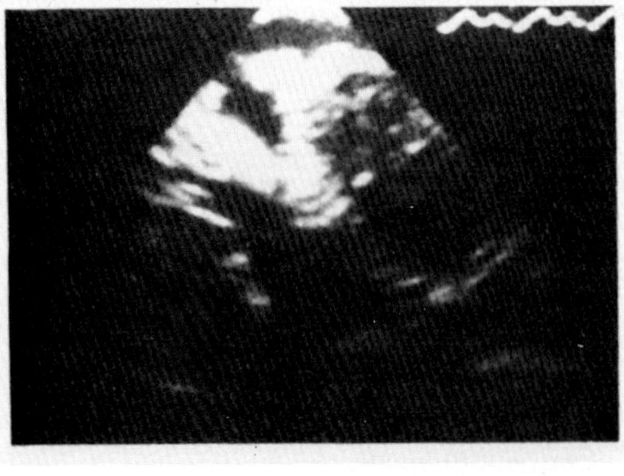

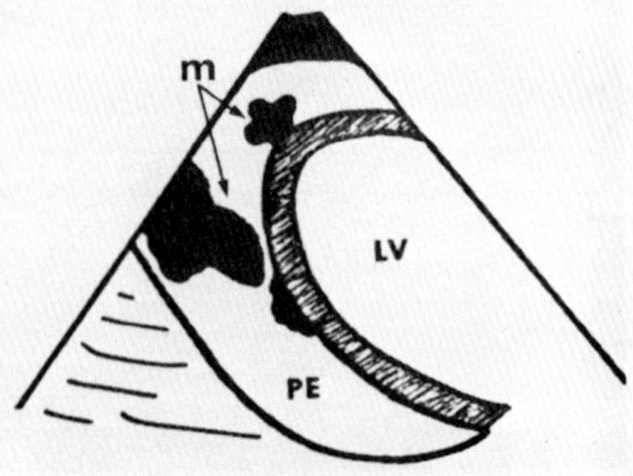

Fig 23–16.—Long-axis view of a two-dimensional echocardiogram illustrating pericardial effusion *(PE)* with irregular masses *(m)*, most likely pericardial metastases, protruding into the pericardial sac. *LV*, left ventricle. (From Chandraratna P.A.N., Aronow W.S.: *Circulation* 63:197, 1981. Reproduced by permission of the American Heart Association, Inc.)

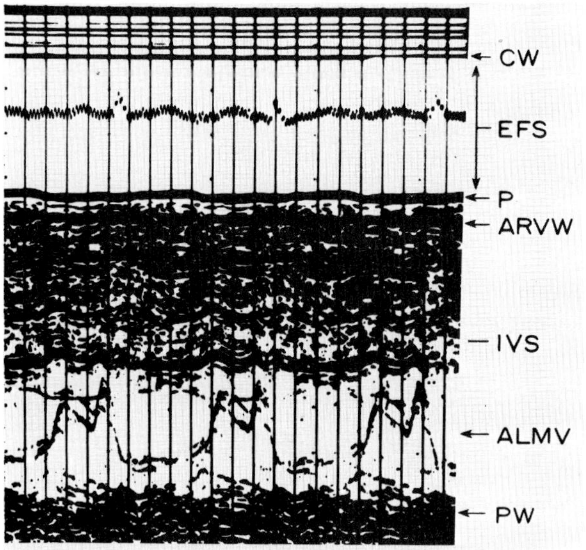

Fig 23–17.—M-mode echocardiograms showing a large, relatively echo-free space anteriorly but not posteriorly. A large pericardial cyst was found at surgery. The space disappeared postoperatively. *CW,* chest wall, *EFS,* echo-free space; *P,* echo comprising the interface between the lesion and the pericardium; *ARVW,* anterior right ventricular wall; *IVS,* interventricular septum; *ALMV,* anterior mitral valve leaflet; *PW,* posterior wall. (From Felner J.M., et al.: *Chest* 68:386, 1975. Reproduced by permission.)

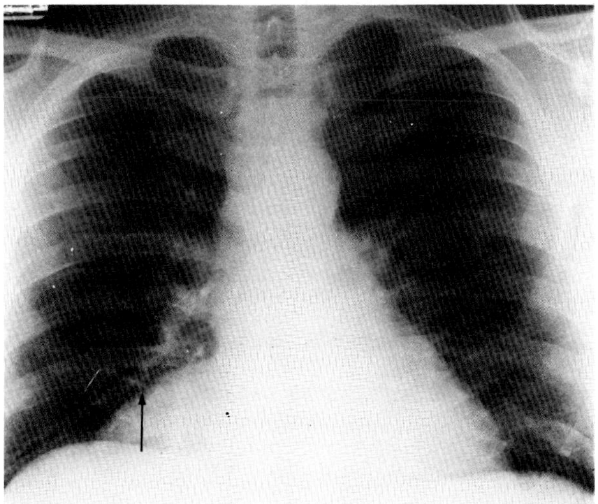

Fig 23–18.—Chest roentgenogram taken in an asymptomatic patient demonstrates the rounded density, along the lower right border of the cardiac silhouette, that most likely represents a pericardial cyst.

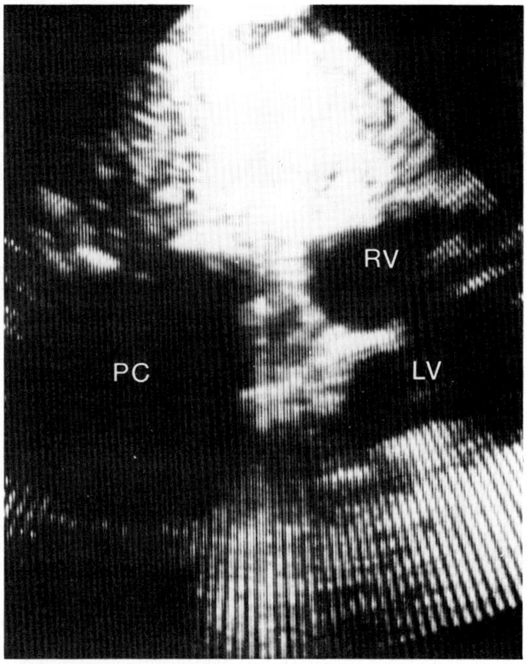

Fig 23–19.—Two-dimensional echocardiogram (subcostal view) demonstrating a large, circular, echo-free space consistent with a pericardial cyst. *PC,* pericardial cyst; *RV,* right ventricle; *LV,* left ventricle.

space posterior to the heart. Figure 23–17 shows the M-mode echocardiogram of a patient who presented with precordial pain and an enlarging mediastinal mass on the chest x-ray film.[46] A relatively echo-free space could be seen anteriorly but not posteriorly. At surgery, a large pericardial cyst containing clear fluid was found anterior to the heart. Postoperatively, the relatively echo-free space was no longer present. Figure 23–18 shows the routine chest roentgenogram of an asymptomatic patient. An M-mode echocardiogram was essentially unremarkable. Two-dimensional echocardiography from the subcostal approach (Fig 23–19) revealed a large, relatively echo-free space consistent with a pericardial cyst posteriorly and to the right of the ventricular chambers. This example points out the advantages of 2DE when one is dealing with localized pericardial disease.

REFERENCES

1. Feigenbaum H., Waldhausen J.A., Hyde L.P.: Ultrasound diagnosis of pericardial effusion. *J.A.M.A.* 191:711, 1965.

2. Feigenbaum H., Zaky A., Waldhausen J.A.: Use of reflected ultrasound in detecting pericardial effusion. *Am. J. Cardiol.* 19:84-90, 1967.
3. Martin R.P., French J.W., Pittman M.M., et al.: Identification and localization of pericardial effusion by real-time two-dimensional echocardiography. *Ultrasound Med.* 3A:211, 1976.
4. Feigenbaum H.: *Echocardiography,* ed. 2. Philadelphia, Lea & Febiger, 1976.
5. Feigenbaum H.: Echocardiographic diagnosis of pericardial effusion. *Am. J. Cardiol.* 26:475, 1970.
6. Warren B.H., Lynn R.R., Allen F.H.: Echocardiographic observation of ventricular volume changes and swinging septal motion in massive pericardial effusion. *J. Clin. Ultrasound* 3:383-386, 1975.
7. Nanda N.C., Gramiak R., Gross C.J.: Altered motion of the cardiac valves in pericardial effusion. *Circulation* 52(suppl. II):528, 1975.
8. Levisman J., Abbasi A.: Abnormal motion of the mitral valve with pericardial effusion: Pseudoprolapse of the mitral valve. *Am. Heart J.* 91:18–20, 1976.
9. Owens J.S., Kotler M.N., Segal B.L., et al.: Pseudoprolapse of the mitral valve in a patient with pericardial effusion. *Chest* 69:214, 1976.
10. Jacobs W.R., Talano J.V., Loeb H.S.: Echocardiographic interpretation of pericardial effusion. *Arch. Intern. Med.* 138:622, 1978.
11. Horowitz M.S., Schultz C.S., Stinson E.B., et al.: Sensitivity and specificity of echocardiographic diagnosis of pericardial effusion. *Circulation* 50:239–246, 1974.
12. Gramiak R., Shah P.M.: Cardiac ultrasonography. *Rad. Clin. North Am.* 9:446, 1971.
13. Popp R.L., Harrison D.C.: Echocardiography, in Weissler A.M. (ed): *Noninvasive Cardiology.* New York, Grune & Stratton, 1974.
14. Schiller N.B.: Echocardiography in pericardial disease. *Med. Clin. North Am.* 64:253–282, 1980.
15. Ratshin R.A., Smith M.K., Hood W.P. Jr.: Possible false-positive diagnosis of pericardial effusion by echocardiography in the presence of large left atrium. *Chest* 65:112, 1974.
16. Walinsky P.: Pitfalls in the diagnosis of pericardial effusion. *Cardiovasc. Clin.* 9:111–122, 1978.
17. Millman A., Meller J., Motro M., et al.: Pericardial tumor or fibrosis mimicking pericardial effusion by echocardiography. *Ann. Intern. Med.* 86:434, 1977.
18. Foote W.C., Jefferson C.M., Price H.L.: False-positive echocardiographic diagnosis of pericardial effusions: Result of tumor encasement of the heart simulating constrictive pericarditis. *Chest* 71:546-549, 1977.
19. Child J.S., Abbasi A.S., Pearce M.L.: Echocardiographic differentiation of mediastinal tumors from primary cardiac disease. *Chest* 67:108, 1975.
20. Felner J.N.: Fleming W.H., Franch R.H.: Echocardiographic identification of a pericardial cyst. *Chest* 68:386, 1975.
21. Casarella W.J., Schneider B.O.: Pitfalls in the ultrasonic diagnosis of pericardial effusion. *Am. J. Roentgenol.* 110:760, 1970.
22. Friedman M.J., Sahn D.J., Haber K.: Two-dimensional echocardiography and B-mode ultrasonography for the diagnosis of loculated pericardial effusion. *Circulation* 60:1644, 1979.
23. Schiller N.B., Botvinick E.H.: Right ventricular compression as a sign of cardiac tamponade. *Circulation* 56:774, 1977.
24. Vignola P.A.; Pohost G.M., Curfman G.D., et al.: Correlation of echocardiographic findings and clinical findings in patients with pericardial effusion. *Am. J. Cardiol.* 37:701, 1976.
25. Settle H.P., Adolph R.J., Fowler N.O., et al.: Echocardiographic study of cardiac tamponade. *Circulation* 56:951, 1977.
26. D'Cruz I.A., Cohen H.C., Prabhu R., et al.: Diagnosis of cardiac tamponade by echocardiography: Changes in mitral valve motion and ventricular dimensions, with special reference to paradoxical pulse. *Circulation* 52:460, 1975.
27. Zoneraich S., Zoneraich O., Rhee J.J.: New, poorly recognized echocardiographic findings. *J.A.M.A.* 236:1954, 1976.
28. Armstrong W.F., Schilt B.F., Helper D.J., et al.: Diastolic collapse of the right ventricle with cardiac tamponade: An echocardiographic study. *Circulation* 65:1491, 1982.
29. Child J.S., Kaufman J.: Echocardiogram in cardiac tamponade, letter. *Am. J. Cardiol.* 39:761, 1977.
30. Kerber R.E., Payvandi M.N.: Echocardiography in acute hemopericardium: Production of false negative echocardiograms by pericardial clots, abstracted. *Circulation* 56(suppl. III):24, 1977.
31. Popp R.L.: Echocardiographic assessment of cardiac disease. *Circulation* 54:538, 1976.
32. Horowitz M.S., Rossen R.M., Harrison D.C., et al.: Ultrasonic evaluation of constrictive pericardial disease, abstracted. *Circulation* 50(suppl. III):III–87, 1974.
33. Voelkel A.G., Pietro D.A., Folland E.D., et al.: Echocardiographic features of constrictive pericarditis. *Circulation* 58:871–875, 1978.
34. Gibson C., Grossman W., McLaurin L.P., et al.: An echocardiographic study of the interventricular septum in constrictive pericarditis. *Br. Heart J.* 38:738, 1976.
35. Candell-Riera J., Garcia Del Castillo H., Permanger-Miralda G., et al.: Echocardiographic features of the interventicular septum in chronic constrictive pericarditis. *Circulation* 57:1154, 1978.
36. Acquatella H., Puigbo J.J., Suarez C., et al.: Sudden early diastolic anterior movement of the septum in endomyocardial fibrosis, letter. *Circulation* 59:847, 1979.
37. Kurzel R.B., Parisi A.F., Harrington J.J., et al.: Echocardiographic detection of tumor invasion of

the heart resulting in constrictive pericarditis. *J.A.M.A.* 236:2601, 1977.

38. Lorell B., Leinbach R.C., Pohost G.M., et al.: Right ventricular infarction: Clinical diagnosis and differentiation from cardiac tamponade and pericardial constriction. *Am. J. Cardiol.* 43:465, 1979.
39. Cohn J.N., Guiha N.H., Broder M.I., et al.: Right ventricular infarction: Clinical and hemodynamic features. *Am. J. Cardiol.* 33:209, 1974.
40. Sharpe D.N., Botvinick E.H., Shames D.M., et al.: The noninvasive diagnosis of right ventricular infarction. *Circulation* 57:483, 1978.
41. Teichholz L.E.: Echocardiographic evaluation of pericardial diseases. *Prog. Cardiovasc. Dis.* 21:133–140, 1978.
42. Glover L.B., Barcia A., Reeves T.J.: Congenital absence of the pericardium: A review of the literature with demonstration of a previously unreported fluoroscopic finding. *Am. J. Roentgenol.* 106:542–549, 1969.
43. Heinz H., Raizner A.E., Chahine R.A., et al.: Congenital absence of the left pericardium: An unusual palpation finding and echocardiographic demonstration of the defect. *South. Med. J.* 69:1222, 1976.
44. Payvandi M.N., Kerber R.E.: Echocardiography in congenital and acquired absence of the pericardium. *Circulation* 53:86, 1976.
45. Chandraratna P.A.N., Aronow W.S.: Detection of pericardial metastases by cross-sectional echocardiography. *Circulation* 63:197, 1981.
46. Felner J.M., Fleming W.H., Franch R.H.: Echocardiographic identification of a pericardial cyst. *Chest* 68:386, 1975.

COMMENT: PERICARDIAL DISEASE

Alfred F. Parisi

HISTORICALLY, the ability to provide objective confirmation of pericardial effusion was a major advance in the differential diagnosis of cardiomegaly. Prior to radionuclide imaging and echocardiography, the diagnosis of pericardial effusion could only be confirmed by invasive procedures. These usually involved right atrial angiography using carbon dioxide injections or contrast medium. In many centers diagnostic pericardial centesis was used as a pragmatic, albeit hazardous, approach to this problem.

Early in the 1960s radionuclide angiography became popular as a way to confirm that the striking cardiomegaly caused by large pericardial effusions was indeed due to fluid accumulation around the heart. The diagnosis was usually based on the disproportion between the size of the intracardiac blood pool and the cardiac silhouette on chest x-ray or on the obvious separation by a prominent pericardial halo of the cardiac blood pool from the intravascular pool in the liver and lungs. The success of this approach requires a large amount of pericardial fluid to be present in order to be detected and was soon eclipsed by M-mode echocardiography.

Because of the exquisite sensitivity and portable instrumentation of M-mode echocardiography, the diagnosis of pericardial effusion was made feasible in even the sickest of patients. Throughout the world today, M-mode echocardiography is the single most valuable noninvasive technique for the differential diagnosis of cardiomegaly, since it can readily distinguish the presence of important amounts of pericardial fluid from a large cardiac silhouette due to dilation and /or hypertrophy of the ventricles; furthermore, echocardiography allows a judgment to be made as to the specific contributions of the left atrium, right ventricle, and left ventricle to the overall degree of heart enlargement. In some regards echocardiography is too sensitive for assessing fluid around the heart, inasmuch as small degrees of pericardial effusion may be seen about 15% of the time in patients with a variety of cardiac disorders and are probably more likely as heart disease progresses. Thus, it remains a matter of clinical judgment whether the detection of a small amount of pericardial fluid by echocardiography is consistent with a patient's ongoing cardiac disease process or represents a hemodynamically or etiologically important contribution to the present illness.

Two-dimensional echocardiography extends the sensitivity of the ultrasonic technique to detection of pericardial fluid. Overall spatial orientation is much more readily appreciated. It is possible to approach the heart from multiple windows, with a clear delineation of anatomy. This allows detection of fluid when a parasternal window does not suffice, as well as detection of loculated fluid that is not directly posterior to the heart. Echocardiography can also be used as a guide to pericardiocentesis, improving the safety of this procedure. With the increasing availability of portable two-dimensional instruments, echocardiographic guidance of pericardiocenteses is likely to receive increased attention.

Radionuclide imaging of pericardial fluid is not a practical method for detecting pericardial effusion in the average patient. In special circumstances, however, the technique has some value. Its use is usually restricted to patients with cardiomegaly in whom technically adequate echocardiograms cannot be obtained or when there is atypical location of substantial amounts of fluid which are not directly posterior to the heart yet separate cardiac from pericardial structures.

The value of echocardiography in pericardial disease transcends its ability to detect pericardial fluid. While most sensitive in this role, it can provide important clues to other pericardial diseases such as constriction, tumor nodules, cysts, and even absence of the pericardium. No echocardiographic examination should be considered complete unless the pericardium is identified and its anatomical and functional relationship to the walls of the heart clearly ascertained.

PART XIII

Future Directions in Noninvasive Cardiac Imaging

OTHER METHODS

Gerald M. Pohost and Samuel Z. Goldhaber

THE PREVIOUS CHAPTERS have dealt primarily with echocardiography and gamma camera radionuclide imaging, which are presently the most important and most widely available noninvasive imaging methods for evaluating the heart. Other newer methods promise to have important impact on noninvasive evaluation of the heart. These include digital subtraction angiography (DSA),[1–20] x-ray computed (transmission) tomography,[21–34] positron or gamma photon (emission) tomography,[35–43] and nuclear magnetic resonance (NMR) approaches (imaging or in vivo spectroscopy). These modalities are compared in Table 24–1. This chapter reviews the two newest approaches, DSA and NMR. Readers interested in the techniques of transmission and emission tomography as they apply to the heart are referred to several excellent publications.[21–43]

DIGITAL SUBTRACTION ANGIOGRAPHY

Angiographic visualization of cardiovascular structures has usually depended on administration of adequate amounts of radiopaque contrast medium directly into the vessel or cardiac chamber under investigation. Photographic film has been used to record the contrast injection for future evaluation. Intravenous injections have been used to visualize the heart chambers, but this approach has led to suboptimal definition of cardiovascular structures.[1] During the past decade investigators have used modern computer and television technology to improve the visibility of cardiovascular structures so that the small concentrations of contrast material delivered by the safer intravenous rather than arterial injections can be visualized. This approach, called digital subtraction angiography, subtracts a computer-acquired preinjection image (the mask) from later images of contrast-filled cardiovascular structures. The remaining image, displayed on a television monitor, is that of the contrast medium in the cardiovascular structure free of background. Digital contrast enhancement methods are applied to the image to further improve its appearance. As Mistretta described it, functionally, this approach defines the needle in the haystack by subtracting the haystack.

Radiographic (analog) subtraction techniques have been used for several decades. The analog method uses two films, one taken before and one after contrast injection. A negative of one of the images is added to the other, and the subtraction image shows the contrast medium alone. The use of a digital computerized approach has added enormous flexibility. It allows easy readjustment of image density after acquisition and application of computer approaches for data storage and contrast enhancement. Accordingly, the contrast medium dose can be reduced with the maintenance of images of diagnostic quality.

Intravenous angiocardiography was first described in 1937 by Robb and Steinberg.[2] Large amounts of contrast medium (100 ml) were injected into both antecubital veins with 12-gauge intravenous cannulas, and images of the heart and

TABLE 24–1.—COMPARISON OF NEW, NONINVASIVE IMAGING MODALITIES

METHOD	POTENTIAL BIOLOGIC HAZARD	PARAMETERS EVALUATED	CARDIOLOGY APPLICATIONS
Digital subtraction angiography (DSA)	Ionizing radiation, radiopaque contrast medium	Distribution and concentration of radiopaque contrast medium	Angiographic anatomy using an intravenous injection of contrast medium Ventricular function ?Coronary angiography
Transmission computed tomography	Ionizing radiation, radiopaque contrast medium	Distribution of differently attenuated x-rays	Tomographic distribution of contrast medium
Emission computed tomography	Ionizing radiation	Distribution and concentration of radionuclides	Metabolism of labeled substrate; blood flow distribution
Nuclear magnetic resonance imaging (zeumatography) In vivo spectroscopy	Unknown, probably none	Distribution and concentration of H-1, and relaxation parameters T_1 and T_2 Concentration of sensitive nuclei (e.g., C-13, F-19, Na-23, and P-31) and frequency shift due to differences in chemical form	Three-dimensional evaluation of structure, flow, ? tissue integrity, wall motion Evaluation of metabolism and tissue integrity in one region of interest

great vessels were obtained. These images were frequently of poor quality. The contrast agents were relatively toxic, and there were no devices for rapid changing of films. Digital subtraction angiography makes it possible to obtain more consistent, reasonable-quality images of cardiovascular structures with substantially lower doses of contrast medium.

A clinically useful digital angiographic system requires a high-quality cesium iodine intensifier and a video camera with a high dynamic range. The video signal from the camera is logarithmically amplified prior to digitization. The amplified video signal is then digitized and stored in one of the two digital memories. Digital subtraction images can be stored on digital or analog disks or on magnetic tape.[1] Conspicuity—the degree to which a target stands out from the background—is enhanced by the subtraction process to produce a clearly defined, time-dependent signal. This two-dimensional pattern of iodine contrast material is represented in computer memory by a pixel value that can be described as the "attenuation thickness." Digital subtraction angiography has a contrast material sensitivity superior to that of the conventional film screen subtraction techniques, enabling visualization of small levels of iodine not previously identifiable with a peripheral venous injection.[3]

Power injections of contrast medium were initially administered through a short catheter into the antecubital vein. However, contrast medium occasionally extravasated and often refluxed into neck veins. More recently, a 55-cm 5 F catheter with an end hole and four side holes has been used. The catheter is placed percutaneously into an antecubital vein and positioned in the superior vena cava. A total of 40–60 ml of contrast is injected at the rate of 12–14 ml/second.

For a successful DSA study, the subject must remain essentially motionless during the contrast injection.[4] Patients are instructed to avoid the

TABLE 24–2.—PROMISING APPLICATIONS OF DSA IN CARDIAC DIAGNOSIS

Quantitative left ventricular wall motion assessment
Quantitative right ventricular wall motion assessment
Evaluation of aortic configuration to detect distention
Evaluation of aorta and femoral arteries prior to insertion of intra-aortic balloon pump
Pulmonary artery patency to detect pulmonary embolism
Coronary artery bypass graft patency
Cerebrovascular disease, especially carotid arteries
Renovascular disease, especially renal arteries
? Coronary artery stenosis—? after contrast injection into aortic root—? after intravenous injection

Valsalva maneuver to prevent slowing of cardiac filling and trapping of contrast material in neck veins.[5] The iodine content on the arterial side must be at least 2 mg/ml, which accounts for the rather large bolus of contrast needed. Cardiac disease with large chambers and reduced ejection fraction or valvular incompetence will dilute the contrast material centrally, resulting in lower-quality DSA images.[5] Furthermore, the x-ray system must be capable of delivering a dose of 0.5–1.0 mrad to the intensifier face to provide sufficient flux for detection and characterization of these low-contrast arterial images.[4] In general, the projections used are the same as those for routine angiography.[6]

Even in this relatively early phase of development, considerable commercial and industrial interest in DSA techniques has been expressed. At least 13 companies are either manufacturing such systems or have announced their intention of becoming involved with DSA.[7] Although the exact role of DSA remains to be determined, it is estimated that more than 3,000 patients have been evaluated with digital angiocardiography and arteriographic techniques at the universities of Wisconsin and Arizona, the Cleveland Clinic, and the Kinderklinik in Kiel.[7]

Promising applications in cardiac diagnosis (Table 24–2) include analysis of ventricular wall motion,[8] calculation of cardiac ejection fraction,[8–12] and evaluation of coronary artery bypass graft patency.[7] Figure 24–1 illustrates a digital subtraction angiogram after intravenous injection of radiopaque contrast medium into the superior vena cava. It may soon be possible to assess the left ventricle quantitatively using densitometric measurements without the need to make assumptions regarding left ventricular configuration that are necessary with conventional angiography.[7] Digital processing of video angiograms can also be applied to studies of regional arterial blood flow.[13] To date, however, the most dramatic and easily accomplished studies have been of the carotid,[14–16] renal,[17–19] and peripheral arterial[20] systems.

Because the coronary arteries are small, continuously moving vessels, and because they directly overlie the large left ventricular blood pool, the ability to clearly define the coronary arteries using DSA after an intravenous or intra-aortic injection of contrast medium is unlikely with present technology. However, improvements in data recording, storage and retrieval methods, display approaches, and data transfer rates may make this exciting noninvasive technique applicable to coronary artery imaging in the future. Initial application of DSA to evaluating the coronary arteries will include development of densitometric methods to quantitate severity of stenosis. Assessment of myocardial perfusion is also feasible. Vogel et al. have developed an innovative method for evaluating the phase of myocardial perfusion after an intracoronary injection of contrast medium.[10] This method involves taking the end-diastolic frame from several cardiac cycles after intracoronary contrast injection. Color coding distinguishes between the arterial phase, the capillary phase, and the venous phase on a single functional image.[10] By the same token, global myocardial perfusion pattern might be assessed using intra-aortic contrast administration.

NUCLEAR MAGNETIC RESONANCE

Nuclear magnetic resonance spectroscopy is a technique used since the 1940s principally by chemists for determining the structure of molecules. Only recently has the methodology been applied to the study of biochemistry of intact organ systems and to imaging various parts of the body, including the heart and brain. Application of much of the technology made available through the development of computerized x-ray tomography has allowed reconstruction of tomographic images using NMR. Nuclear magnetic resonance studies of intact living muscle and red blood cells has elicited certain metabolic information unavailable through any other technique. The possibility of extracting important clinical information from spectra and from images, information which cannot be derived from presently available approaches, is prompting the rapid evolution of this

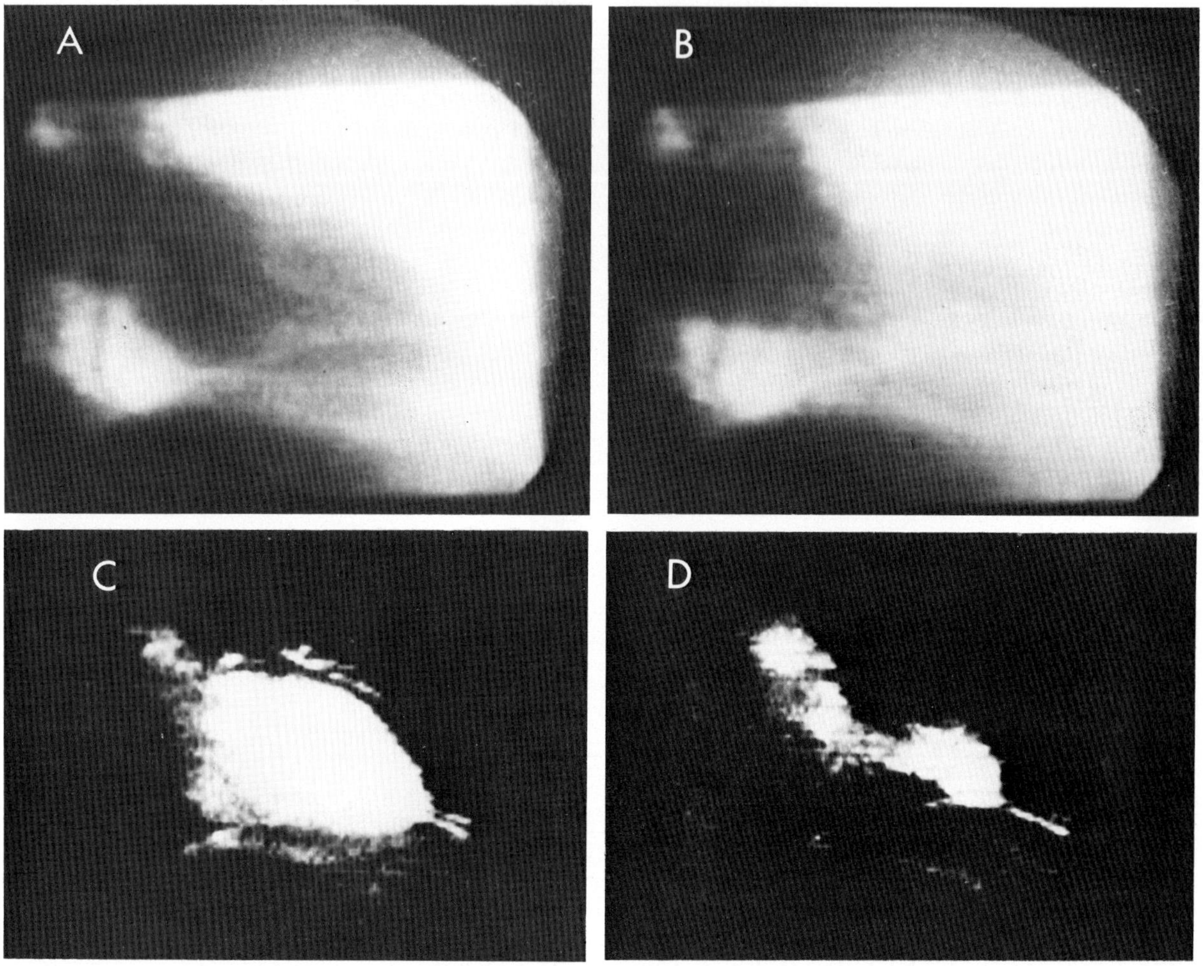

Fig 24–1.—Digital angiogram acquired after injection of 30 cc of radiopaque contrast medium into the superior vena cava. A computer is employed to store a mask of the bones and soft tissues prior to contrast injection and to subtract this mask from 128 × 128 pixel frames acquired at 30 per second. The end-diastolic (**A** and **C**) and end-systolic (**B** and **D**) frames are shown, before (**A** and **B**) and after (**C** and **D**) mask correction.

technology. The physical principles of NMR are introduced below. The reader is referred to several excellent references for a more comprehensive description.[44-46]

Nuclear Magnetic Resonance Spectroscopy

Nuclear magnetic resonance spectroscopy relies on the spinning of the charged nuclei of certain isotopes with unpaired nucleons (protons or neutrons), such as hydrogen ions, carbon 13, and phosphorus 31. Because a moving charge produces a magnetic field, these nuclei behave as though they were tiny magnets. Such nuclei become aligned when placed within an external magnetic field. If a short burst of radiofrequency radiation (radiowaves) is applied, the nuclei are "tilted" from their aligned position and begin to precess, just as a child's gyroscope precesses within the earth's gravitational field when tipped from its vertical position. As they realign themselves with the external magnetic field, the precessing nuclei gradually lose energy to the environment by emitting radiofrequency radiation that can be detected by an antenna coil. Fourier transformation is applied to the decaying emitted signal to generate frequency spectra. A frequency spectrum will show multiple peaks, each reflecting a different chemical species of a given nuclear species. Nuclear magnetic resonance is a powerful tool for analytic chemists because both molecular structure and concentration can be analyzed.

Other potentially useful data that can be derived from NMR spectroscopy are relaxation times. Relaxation times (known as T_1 and T_2) represent exponential decay constants that describe how quickly the excited nuclei return to equilibrium. Relaxation times of hydrogen ions change with evolving abnormalities in cell viability, such as those associated with ischemia.[47]

Because natural NMR signals are weak and various factors, including thermal motion, may reduce the signal-to-noise ratio, it is necessary to pulse samples with radiofrequency radiation numerous times and to average the resulting spectra to obtain useful information. Thus, the longer the sample remains within the spectrometer, the more highly resolved the resultant spectrum. Examples of nuclei which are NMR-sensitive and have biologic relevance include hydrogen 1 (proton), carbon 13, flourine 19, sodium 23, and phosphorus 31.

Protons are highly sensitive and the most abundant nuclei in biology. They are located in water, fats, proteins, and other biologic forms. Accordingly, protons are the nuclei most easily imaged. Carbon 13 and ^{19}F might be useful as NMR "tracers" when attached to appropriate metabolic substrates or other biochemicals. Sodium 23 may provide a means of evaluating the cardiac blood pool. Finally, ^{31}P is located in the high-energy phosphates adenosine triphosphate (ATP) and creatine phosphate. These phosphates in specific cell compartments are involved in the energy-dependent processes of myocardial contraction and ion transport and, accordingly, in cell viability. Fossel et al.[48] have studied phosphate metabolism in isolated beating rat hearts using NMR spectroscopy. At the onset of ischemia, the creatine phosphate concentration begins to decrease within seconds, while the ATP concentration decreases more slowly. There is a concomitant increase in the concentration of inorganic phosphate since its rate of incorporation into the high-energy phosphates decreases. If ischemia is reversed and the cells remain viable, the concentrations of high-energy phosphates return toward normal. However, if cell death occurs, the high-energy phosphates are not resynthesized, and the inorganic phosphate gradually leaks out through the disrupted cell membrane. Fossel et al. also demonstrated the changes that occur in high-energy phosphates during the cardiac cycle, using ECG gating to acquire data in selected aspects of the cardiac cycle.[49] In addition, Hollis et al.[50] have used shifts in the position of the inorganic ^{31}P NMR peak to monitor changes in intracellular pH.

Nuclear Magnetic Resonance Imaging

In the early 1970s Lauterbur[51] recognized that images could be derived by using the emitted NMR signal. In contrast to the homogeneous field used in NMR spectroscopy, the magnetic field for imaging is made nonhomogeneous, and the resultant emitted radiofrequency contains spatial information. Using a computer, images can be constructed.

Several methods for producing NMR images have been reported. These methods differ in the way that the nonhomogeneous magnetic field is produced.[45] Since NMR signal information is intrinsically three-dimensional, it is possible to produce three-dimensional images.

One approach, the "sensitive point" technique pioneered by Hinshaw,[52] utilizes rapidly alternately orthogonal "perpendicular" magnetic field gradients superimposed on the static field. By adjusting the gradients appropriately, a single point or line can be defined in the object to be imaged where the alternating gradients are zero. These alternating field gradients are analogous to a child's seesaw. A time exposure photograph of the seesaw when it is moving will show only the fulcrum clearly, while the remainder of the seesaw will be blurred. The fulcrum is analogous to the sensitive point, while a line of fulcrums of many aligned seesaws is analogous to the sensitive line. It is from this point or line that the NMR signal is gathered and stored in a computer; signals from all other locations are eliminated. The sensitive locus can then be moved electronically through the sample by adjusting the field gradients, and the completed image is displayed as a tomogram.

Another means of imaging is known as "selective irradiation." In this technique, rapidly changing magnetic field gradients are combined with programming of a radiofrequency phase profile to allow selective excitation of sensitive nuclei in a single plane.[53] Ordidge and colleagues have utilized an approach called "echo planar" imaging to allow extremely fast data collection times.[54] Of the reported imaging approaches, the echo planar approach has the most exciting potential for imaging of the heart. By this approach, images can be generated from a time period as short as 30 msec, which would allow heart motion to be "frozen." But even without high-speed imaging, it is possible to obtain reasonable-quality NMR images of the heart by acquiring the NMR signal at various phases of the cardiac cycle using physiologic gating.

Proton Imaging

Protons are the only nuclei that have been used in intact animals and in man to generate NMR images. The reason for this is twofold. First, water has two protons in each molecule, and there is plenty of water in biologic tissue. Second, protons provide the most sensitive nucleus for NMR detection. In addition to water protons, the mobile protons of lipids and other biochemicals also contribute to the NMR image. Accordingly, protons are the most feasible species for NMR imaging.

In addition to differences in water content, the relaxation times T_1 and T_2 may also differ with the type of tissue and in the presence of disease. Although changes in relaxation times reflect differences in water content, they have been shown to be affected by other factors, including the biochemical environment, ionic strength, and some less well defined factors. Since ischemia may lead to changes in tissue water content and thence to alterations in relaxation times, proton NMR imaging may provide a means for evaluating ischemia. Specifically, this approach might allow differentiation between ischemic tissue which is irreversibly damaged and tissue which is not. Initial work by Buonanno et al.[47, 55] from the laboratory at Massachusetts General Hospital demonstrated that experimental ischemic stroke in the cat can be detected as early as two hours after middle cerebral artery ligation. Clinical data from Young and co-workers demonstrated that proton NMR imaging, in contrast to x-ray CT, depicts the degenerative brain damage consequent to multiple sclerosis with great sensitivity.[56]

The application of the radiofrequency (RF) pulse or pulses can be varied to emphasize one or more of the NMR imaging parameters (proton density, T_1 and T_2). A saturation-recovery pulse sequence occurs when the appropriate RF is applied for a long enough time to displace the magnetized protons by 90 degrees from their position aligned with the external magnetic field. Then the RF emitted by the protons during their realignment (relaxation) in the external magnetic field is collected. These signals are converted into images which are primarily related to both proton density and T_1. If 90-degree RF pulses are applied frequently enough to keep the protons in the excited state, that is, each pulse applied before the completion of relaxation initiated by the previous pulse, then the pulse sequence is known as steady-state-free-precession (SSFP). Such a pulse sequence produces images which are related to all three NMR parameters. Other pulse sequences include inversion-recovery, which highlights T_1, and spin-echo approaches, which highlight T_2.[45]

Paramagnetic substances such as manganese alter the NMR signal and provide a means of tracing the distribution of blood flow. Studies using radioactive isotopes of manganese (Mn-52m) have demonstrated that after intravenous administration, the distribution of ionic Mn^{++} is closely related to blood flow. Lauterbur et al.[57] have suggested the potential utility of this agent in evaluating the damage from myocardial infarction. We used a prototype imaging system with a cylindric superconducting magnet with a 3-in. bore and imaging was performed using selective irradiation and an SSFP pulse sequence to study circumflex coronary artery occlusion in a canine model.[58] The myocardial radiotracer thallium 201 and a manganese ion ($MnCl_2$) were given intravenously 90 minutes after coronary ligation and the animal was sacrificed. The heart was removed from the animal and NMR tomograms were obtained (Fig 24–2). Then the heart was sliced to produce samples that matched the levels of the tomographic im-

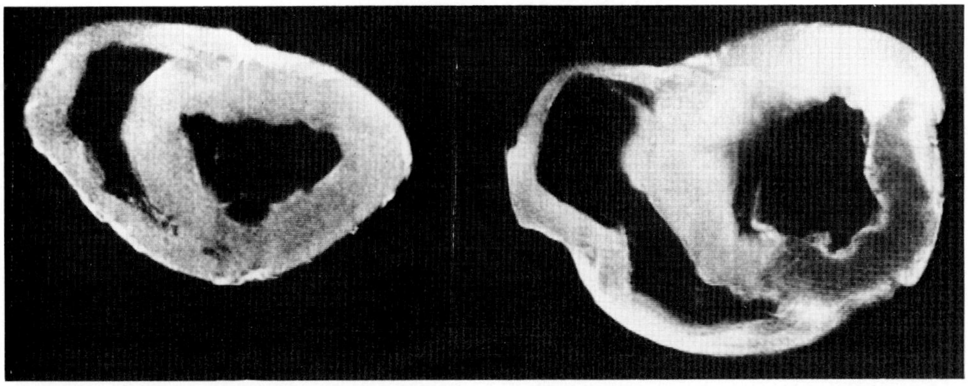

Fig 24–2.—Proton NMR tomograph at the midventricular level obtained on excised dog hearts using the steady-state free precession approach. Both hearts were obtained from dogs with 90 minutes of left circumflex coronary occlusion. *Left,* study shows no distinct delineation of the zone of reduced perfusion; *right,* study shows excellent delineation of the nontransmural distribution of perfusion deficit. The perfusion delineation was accomplished with the intravenous injection of $MnCl_2$.

ages. Gamma camera images of the slices were obtained, and the slices were stained with a dye to identify the viable tissue. The NMR images showed the anatomy of the heart in detail. More importantly, the heart muscle supplied by the occluded coronary demonstrated reduced NMR signal intensity. The region of reduced signal correlated well with the region of myocardial infarction as demonstrated by lack of staining with the supravital dye, triphenyl tetrazolium chloride.

The mechanism by which manganese alters image contrast is related to its paramagnetic behavior. Paramagnetic substances diminish the T_1 relaxation time. Since manganese concentration is proportional to blood flow after intravenous injection, relaxation times of the water in poorly perfused myocardium are different from relaxation times in the normally perfused myocardium. Using NMR imaging methods, however, it may be possible to detect and quantify myocardial infarction without paramagnetic contrast administration. It is likely that approaches that depict T_1 or T_2 relaxation times will be successful, since these parameters change during ischemic insult.

Application of NMR to Nuclei Other Than Protons

The use of ^{31}P NMR to study myocardial ischemia and infarction is an exciting potential application. Nuclear magnetic resonance offers a means of noninvasively determining the concentration of high-energy phosphates, such as ATP and creatine phosphate, and of inorganic phosphate. Changes in the concentration of these phosphates are related to the state of health of the cell and ultimately to cell viability. Evaluation of the presence of the phosphates and their concentration may permit definition of the extent of ischemic damage and its reversibility. However, in contrast to protons, ^{31}P NMR imaging will be extremely difficult, owing both to the relative insensitivity of ^{31}P NMR detection (it is only about 7% as sensitive as protons) and to its relatively low concentration in biologic tissue. Whereas protons are approximately 70M in tissue, phosphorus is present in millimolar quantities. Thus a 10^4-fold decrease in sensitivity of phosphorus compared to proton would be anticipated. But by using higher magnetic fields and accepting lower spatial resolution, it may be possible to obtain images of high-energy phosphate distribution.

Topical Magnetic Resonance

An approach which does not generate images but rather produces a spectrum of ^{31}P or other NMR-sensitive nuclei is called "topical magnetic resonance," or TMR. This approach involves the use of a relatively high-magnetic field and the isolation of a sensitive volume within the object to be studied from which a spectrum is derived. Thus far studies have been performed of the ^{31}P and proton concentrations in human limbs at rest and with exercise, and of animal models. Ross et al.[59] demonstrated absence of the normal reduction in the intracellular pH of the exercising forearm in patients with McArdle's syndrome by using TMR evaluations of chemical shifts of the inorganic phosphorus peak. It is likely that this approach will be applied to the clinical evaluation of the heart in the future. Carbon 13, an NMR-sensitive nucleus, is only 1% naturally abundant, and therefore provides a potential label and tracer for metabolic substrates.

Sodium 23 is also sensitive to NMR detection but, like ^{31}P, has a sensitivity lower than that of protons. Sodium is relatively abundant in extracellular fluid, comprising nearly 1% by weight. Because of the substantially higher sodium concentration in blood compared to concentrations within cells, it may be possible to use ^{23}Na as a blood pool imaging agent. DeLayre and co-workers recently published gated blood pool images of the isolated perfused beating rat heart.[60] It is possible that as ischemia develops and progresses, the active sodium-potassium pump located in the cell membrane breaks down and the leakage of sodium into the cell may be detectable by NMR methods. At present, work needs to be done to establish the role of NMR methods in medical practice. It is clear even from the few reported studies that NMR methods have enormous potential for application to medical practice.

Safety

There is no known biologic hazard associated with NMR imaging. Persons exposed to high-level magnetic fields such as those associated with particle accelerators have had no ill effects. The radiofrequency energy loss in the tissues has been calculated to be far below the recommended safe maximal long-term exposure limit. Patients with cardiac pacemakers may be adversely affected, since pacemakers may switch to a fixed rate mode or may reprogram in the midst of an intense magnetic field. But images of human beings without pacemakers have been obtained thousands of times without incident. There are literally thousands of patient-hours of NMR imaging time with no reported untoward effects. Nuclear magnetic resonance imaging does not use an ionizing type of radiation such as that associated with x-ray or radionuclide techniques. As with ultrasound, the only potentially deleterious effect of magnetic and radiofrequency fields is heating of tissue. However, no evidence of significant heating has been reported, even with the higher fields employed in topical magnetic resonance studies.

Organ Motion

Motion of an organ such as the heart during NMR imaging may present problems not found in imaging more stationary organs such as the brain. Sensitivity to motion is related to the imaging method employed. Images obtained by Hutchison and co-workers appeared less sensitive to motion than other techniques.[61] Their images of the chest demonstrated a tomographic cross-section through the heart. The right and left ventricular cavities, myocardium, and interventricular septum were seen; these structures displayed an apparent end-diastolic configuration. By using ECG or pressure signals to synchronize the energy bursts from the NMR radiofrequency transmitter with the cardiac cycle, it is possible to obtain NMR images in a fashion analogous to that used with the gated radionuclide blood pool imaging (Fig 24–3). The technique described by Ordidge et al. may allow tomographic imaging data to be acquired in a matter of tens of milliseconds and to accomplish near real-time imaging.[53]

In summary, promising new approaches for the future of cardiac diagnosis are digital subtraction angiography and NMR. Digital angiography permits evaluation of regional and global ventricular function and of arterial patency using an intravenous dose of radiopaque contrast medium. In addition, DSA permits computer quantitative approaches to be applied to both intravenous and direct catheter-injected approaches. NMR imaging is in its infancy, and its medical potential appears enormous.[62] The ability to derive biochemical and metabolic information noninvasively without the intravenous injection of tracers would allow assessment of tissue health without the confounding impact of tracer perfusion. Further, high-resolution tomographic or three-dimensional imaging of the heart with possible tissue characterization using proton NMR has exciting poten-

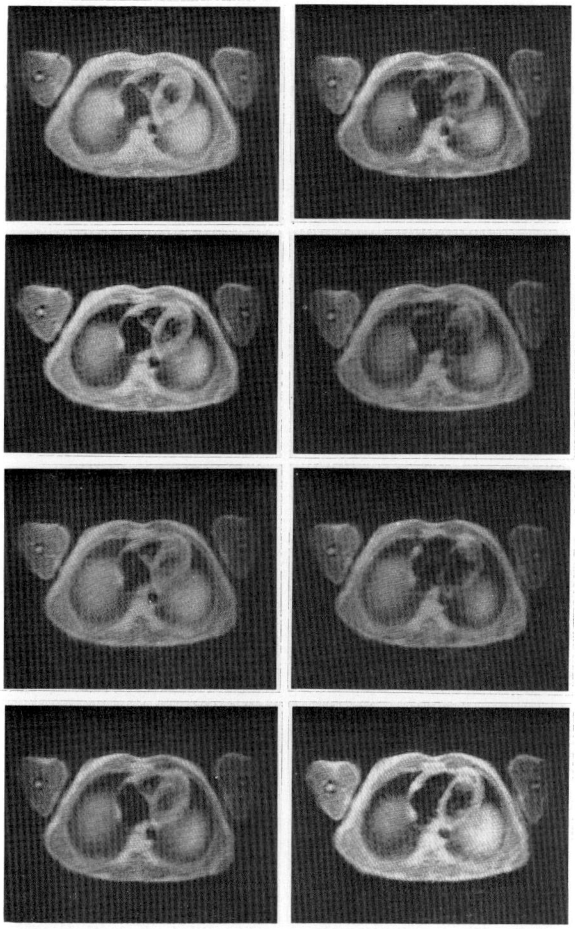

Fig 24–3.—Gated proton NMR tomographic study through the lower thorax demonstrating excellent delineation of the heart. The patient's arms are seen adjacent to the thorax. The domes of the diaphragms are seen in each hemithorax. Anterior is facing upward; posterior is facing downward. The *upper left* image shows early systole. The right and left ventricles are clearly observed. In the left ventricle the two papillary muscles are well defined. The descending aorta is seen just posterior to the heart. The tricuspid valve plane and right atrium are visualized posteromedially to the right ventricle. The *lower right* image shows end-diastole. (Images courtesy of Technicare, Solan, Ohio.)

tial. Thus the differentiation among normal tissues, ischemic but viable tissues, and irreversibly damaged tissues might be accomplished using biochemical rather than indirect structural or flow-dependent markers. This is not possible using other techniques.

REFERENCES

1. Mistretta C.A., Crummy A.B., Strother C.M.: Digital angiography: A perspective. *Radiology* 139:273–276, 1981.
2. Robb G.P., Steinberg I.: Visualization of the chambers of the heart, the pulmonary circulation, and the great blood vessels in man. *A.J.R.* 41:1–17, 1939.
3. MacIntyre W.J., Pavlicek W., Gallagher J.H., et al.: Imaging capability of an experimental digital subtraction angiography unit. *Radiology* 139:307–313, 1981.
4. Ovitt T.W., Christenson P.C., Fisher H.D. III, et al.: Intravenous angiography using digital video subtraction: X-ray imaging system. *A.J.R.* 135:1141–1144, 1980.
5. Meaney T.F., Weinstein M.A., Buonocore E., et al.: Digital subtraction angiography of the human cardiovascular system. *A.J.R.* 135:1153–1160, 1980.
6. Crummy A.B., Strother C.M., Sackett J.F., et al.: Computerized fluoroscopy: Digital subtraction for intravenous angiocardiography and arteriography. *A.J.R.* 135:1131–1140, 1980.
7. Mistretta C.A., Crummy A.B.: Diagnosis of cardiovascular disease by digital subtraction angiography. *Science* 214:761–765, 1981.
8. Gerber K., Bhargava V., Slutsky R., et al.: Quantitation of regional and global left ventricular (LV) function by digital intravenous ventriculography (DIV) with functional image analysis. *Circulation* 64(suppl. IV):219, 1981.
9. Kronenberg M.W., Price R.R., Domanski M.J., et al.: Digital subtraction angiography for measuring left ventricular performance: Early results in man. *Circulation* 64(suppl. IV):219, 1981.
10. Vogel R., LeFree M., Foster R., et al.: Integral signed ECG-synchronized difference (ISED): A new technique for performing digital ventriculography. *Circulation* 64(suppl. IV):220, 1981.
11. Lipton M.J., Gould R.G.: Digital subtraction fluoroscopy: A dual video system. *Circulation* 64(suppl. IV):220, 1981.
12. Bogren H.G., Bursch J.H., Brennecke R., et al.: Intravenous angiocardiography using digital image processing: Experience with axial projections in normal pigs. *Circulation* 64(suppl. IV):220, 1981.
13. Bursch J.H., Hahne J.H., Brennecke R., et al.: Assessment of arterial blood flow measurements by digital angiography. *Radiology* 141:39–47, 1981.
14. Christenson P.C., Ovitt T.W., Fisher H.D. III, et al.: Intravenous angiography cervicocerebrovascular angiography. *A.J.R.* 135:1145–1152, 1980.
15. Chilcote W.A., Modic M.T., Pavlicek W.A., et al.: Digital subtraction angiography of the carotid arteries: A comparative study in 100 patients. *Radiology* 139:287–295, 1981.
16. Brody W.R., Enzmann D.R., Deutsch L.-S., et al.:

Intravenous carotid arteriography using line-scanned digital radiography. *Radiology* 139:297–300, 1981.

17. Hillman B.J., Ovitt T.W., Nudelman S., et al.: Digital video subtraction angiography of renal vascular abnormalities. *Radiology* 139:277–280, 1981.
18. Buonocore E., Meaney T.F., Borkowski G.P., et al.: Digital subtraction angiography of the abdominal aorta and renal arteries: Comparison with conventional aortography. *Radiology* 139:281–286, 1981.
19. Hillman B.D., Ovitt T.W., Capp M.P., et al.: The potential impact of digital video subtraction angiography on screening for renovascular hypertension. *Radiology* 142:577–579, 1982.
20. Crummy A.B., Strother C.M., Lieberman R.P., et al.: Digital video subtraction angiography for evaluation of peripheral vascular disease. *Radiology* 141:33–37, 1981.
21. Ter-Pogossian M.M., Weise E.S., Coleman R.E.: Computed tomography of the heart. *A.J.R.* 127:79, 1976.
22. Powell W.R., Jr., Wittenbert J., Maturi R.A., et al.: Detection of edema associated with myocardial ischemia by computerized tomography in isolated, arrested canine hearts. *Circulation* 55:99, 1977.
23. Wood E.H.: New vistas for the study of structural and functional dynamics of the heart, lungs, and circulation by noninvasive numerical tomographic vivisection. *Circulation* 56:506–520, 1977.
24. Huang H.K., Mazziotta J.C.: Heart imaging from computerized tomography. *Comput. Tomogr.* 2:37–44, 1978.
25. Hessel S.J., Adams D.F., Judy P.F., et al.: Detection of myocardial ischemia in vitro by computed tomography. *Radiology* 127:413, 1978.
26. Gray W.R., Buja L.M., Hagler H.K., et al.: Computed tomography for localization and sizing of experimental acute myocardial infarcts. *Circulation* 58:497, 1978.
27. Guthaner D.F., Wexler L., Harell G.: CT demonstration of cardiac structures. *A.J.R.* 133:75–81, 1979.
28. Cormack A.M.: Early two-dimensional reconstruction and recent topics stemming from it. *Science* 209:1482–1486, 1980.
29. Hounsfield G.N.: Computed medical imaging. *Science* 210:22–28, 1980.
30. Schelbert H., Phelps M., Hoffman E.J., et al.: Regional myocardial perfusion assessed with N-13 ammonia and positron computer tomography. *Am. J. Cardiol.* 43:209–218, 1979.
31. Moncada R., Salinas M., Churchill R., et al.: Patency of saphenous aortocoronary bypass grafts demonstrated by computed tomography. *N. Engl. J. Med.* 303:503–505, 1980.
32. Tomoda H., Hoshiai M., Furuya H., et al.: Evaluation of left ventricular thrombus with computed tomography. *Am. J. Cardiol.* 48:573–577, 1981.
33. Kahl F., Wolfman N.T., Watts L.E.: Evaluation of aortocoronary bypass graft status by computed tomography. *Am. J. Cardiol.* 48:304–310, 1981.
34. Doherty P.W., Lipton M.J., Berninger W.H., et al.: Detection and quantitation of myocardial infarction in vivo using transmission computed tomography. *Circulation* 63:597–606, 1981.
35. Phelps M.E.: Emission computed tomography. *Sem. Nucl. Med.* 7:337–365, 1977.
36. Sobel B.E., Weiss E.S., Welch M.J., et al.: Detection of remote myocardial infarction in patients with positron emission transaxial tomography and intravenous C-11-palmitate. *Circulation* 55:853–857, 1977.
37. Weiss E.S., Siegel B.A., Sobel B.E., et al.: Evaluation of myocardial metabolism and perfusion with positron-emitting radionuclides. *Prog. Cardiovasc. Dis.* 20:191–206, 1977.
38. Keyes J.W., Leonard P.F., Brody S.L., et al.: Myocardial infarct quantitation in the dog by single photon emission computed tomography. *Circulation* 58:227–232, 1978.
39. Keyes J.W., Lenard P.F., Svetkoff D.J., et al.: Myocardial imaging using emission computed tomography. *Radiology* 127:809–812, 1978.
40. Phelps M.E., Hoffman E.J., Huang S.C., et al.: ECAT: A new computerized tomographic imaging system for positron-emitting radiopharmaceuticals. *J. Nucl. Med.* 19:635–647, 1978.
41. Vogel R.A., Kirch D., LeFree M., et al.: A new method of multiplanar emission tomography using a seven pinhole collimator and an Anger scintillation camera. *J. Nucl. Med.* 19:648–654, 1978.
42. Harrison D.C.: Research related to noninvasive instrumentation. *Circulation* 60:1569–1574, 1979.
43. Holman B.L., Hill T.C., Wynne J., et al.: Single-photon transaxial emission computed tomography of the heart in normal subjects and in patients with infarction. *J. Nucl. Med.* 20:736–740, 1979.
44. Crooks L., Kaufman L., Margules A.: *Nuclear Magnetic Resonance Imaging in Medicine*. New York, Igaku-Shoin Medical Publishers, 1981.
45. Pykett I., Newhouse J., Buonanno F.S., et al.: Principles of NMR imaging. *Radiology* 143:157–168, 1982.
46. Goldman M.R., Pohost G.M., Ingwall J.S., et al.: NMR imaging: Potential clinical applications. *Am. J. Cardiol.* 46:1278–1283, 1980.
47. Buonanno F.S., Pykett I.L., Brady T.J., et al.: Proton NMR imaging in experimental ischemic infarction. *Stroke*, to be published.
1030, 1980.
48. Fossel E.T., Kramer M.F., Taegtmeyer H., et al.: P-31 nuclear magnetic resonance of perfused rat hearts. Studies during anoxia and recovery, abstracted. *Circulation* 56(suppl. II):227, 1977.
49. Fossel E.T., Morgan H.E., Ingwall J.S.: Measurement of changes in high-energy phosphates in the cardiac cycle using gated P-31 nuclear magnetic resonance. *Proc. Natl. Acad. Sci.* 77:5471–5475, 1980.

50. Hollis D.P., Nunnally R.L., Taylor G.J., et al.: P-31 NMR studies of heart physiology. *J. Magnet. Reson.* 29:319–330, 1978.
51. Lauterbur P.C.: Image formation by induced local interactions: Examples employing nuclear magnetic resonance. *Nature* 242:190–191, 1973.
52. Hinshaw W.S.: Image formation by NMR: The sensitive point method. *J. Appl. Physiol.* 47:3709, 1976.
53. Edelstein W.A., Hutchinson J.M.S., Johnson G., et al.: T-spin warp NMR imaging and applications to human whole-body imaging. *Phys. Med. Biol.* 25:751–756, 1980.
54. Ordidge R.J., Mansfield P., Doyle M., et al.: Real time moving images by NMR, in *NMR Imaging: Proceedings of an International Symposium on Nuclear Magnetic Resonance Imaging*. Bowman Gray School of Medicine, Winston-Salem, North Carolina, 1982.
55. Buonanno F.S., Pykett I.L., Kistler J.P., et al.: Cranial anatomy and detection of ischemic stroke in cats by nuclear magnetic resonance imaging. *Radiology,* 143:187–196, 1982.
56. Young I.R., Hall A.S., Pallis C.A., et al.: Nuclear magnetic resonance imaging of the brain in multiple sclerosis. *Lancet* 2:1063–1066, 1981.
57. Lauterbur P.C., Dias M.H.M., Rudin A.M.: Augmentation of tissue water proton spin-lattice relaxation rates by in vivo addition of paramagnetic ions, in *Frontiers of Biological Energetics*. New York, Academic Press, 1978, vol. 1, pp. 752–759.
58. Brady T.J., Goldman M.R., Pykett I.L., et al.: Proton nuclear magnetic resonance imaging of regional ischemic canine hearts: Effect of paramagnetic proton signal enhancement. *Radiology,* to be published.
59. Ross B.D., Radda G.K., Gadian D.G., et al.: Examination of a case of suspected McArdle's syndrome by ^{31}P nuclear magnetic resonance. *N. Engl. J. Med.* 304:1339–1342, 1981.
60. DeLayre J.L., Ingwall J.S., Malloy C., et al.: Measurement of ejection fraction in isolated perfused working rat hearts using gated Na-23 nuclear magnetic resonance imaging. *Science* 212:935–936, 1981.
61. Hutchison J., Edelstein W., Johnson G.: A whole-body NMR imaging machine. *J. Phys.* [*E.*] 13:903–1030, 1980.
62. Pohost G.M.: NMR: Diagnostic wave of the future. *West. J. Med.*, to be published.

INDEX

R